Neurosurgical Operative Atlas

Second Edition

Neuro-Oncology

American Association of Neurological Surgeons

and the American Association of Neurosurgeons

American Association of Neurosurgeons • Rolling Meadows, Illinois

Thieme

Neurosurgical Operative Atlas

Second Edition

Neuro-Oncology

Behnam Badie, M.D., F.A.C.S.
Director
Department of Neurosurgery
Director
Brain Tumor Program
City of Hope Medical Center
Duarte, California

Thieme
New York • Stuttgart

American Association of Neurosurgeons
Rolling Meadows, Illinois

Thieme Medical Publishers, Inc.
333 Seventh Ave.
New York, NY 10001

American Association of Neurosurgeons (AANS)*
5550 Meadowbrook Drive
Rolling Meadows, Illinois, 60008-3852

* *The acronym AANS refers to both the American Association of Neurological Surgeons and the American Association of Neurosurgeons.*

Associate Editor: Birgitta Brandenburg
Assistant Editor: Ivy Ip
Vice President, Production and Electronic Publishing: Anne T. Vinnicombe
Production Editor: Print Matters, Inc.
Sales Director: Ross Lumpkin
Associate Marketing Director: Verena Diem
Chief Financial Officer: Peter van Woerden
President: Brian D. Scanlan
Compositor: Thomson Digital

Library of Congress Cataloging-in-Publication Data

Neurosurgical operative atlas. Neuro-oncology / [edited by] Behnam Badie. – 2nd ed.
p. ; cm.
Includes bibliographical references and index.
ISBN 1-58890-340-0 (US : hc.) – ISBN 3-13-141951-2 (GTV : hc.)
1. Nervous system–Surgery–Atlases. I. Badie, Behnam. II. Title: Neuro-oncology.
[DNLM: 1. Nervous System Neoplasms–surgery–Atlases. WL 17 N4943 2006]
RD593.N43 2006
617.4'800223–dc22
2006044644

Important note: Medical knowledge is ever-changing. As new research and clinical experience broaden our knowledge, changes in treatment and drug therapy may be required. The authors and editors of the material herein have consulted sources believed to be reliable in their efforts to provide information that is complete and in accord with the standards accepted at the time of publication. However, in view of the possibility of human error by the authors, editors, or publisher of the work herein or changes in medical knowledge, neither the authors, editors, or publisher, nor any other party who has been involved in the preparation of this work, warrants that the information contained herein is in every respect accurate or complete, and they are not responsible for any errors or omissions or for the results obtained from use of such information. Readers are encouraged to confirm the information contained herein with other sources. For example, readers are advised to check the product information sheet included in the package of each drug they plan to administer to be certain that the information contained in this publication is accurate and that changes have not been made in the recommended dose or in the contraindications for administration. This recommendation is of particular importance in connection with new or infrequently used drugs.

Some of the product names, patents, and registered designs referred to in this book are in fact registered trademarks or proprietary names even though specific reference to this fact is not always made in the text. Therefore, the appearance of a name without designation as proprietary is not to be construed as a representation by the publisher that it is in the public domain.

The material presented in this publication by the AANS is for educational purposes only. The material is not intended to represent the only, nor necessarily the best, method or procedure appropriate for the medical or socioeconomic situations discussed, but rather it is intended to present an approach, view, statement, or opinion of the faculty, which may be helpful to others who face similar situations.

Neither the content, the use of a specific product in conjunction therewith, nor the exhibition of any materials by any parties coincident with this publication, should be construed as indicating endorsement or approval of the views presented, the products used, or the materials exhibited by the AANS, or its Committees, Commissions, or Affiliates.

5 4 3 2

TMP ISBN 1-58890-340-0
978-1-58890-340-2
GTV ISBN 3-13-141951-2
978-3-13-141951-4

This book is dedicated to my father, Mehdi Badie, whose wisdom, devotion, and love for life and humanity will continue to illuminate my path.

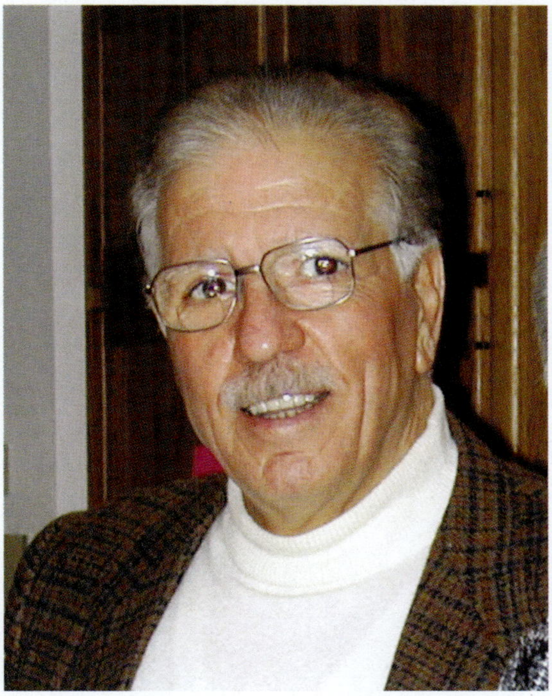

Contents

Continuing Medical Education Credit Information and Objectives

◆ Objectives

After reading this book, the reader should:

1. Recognize current management of brain tumors.
2. Discuss modern surgical techniques for approaching most common brain tumors.
3. Describe the indications, preoperative evaluation, and complication avoidance for surgical treatment of brain tumors.

◆ Accreditation

This activity has been planned and implemented in accordance with the Essentials and Standards of the Accreditation Council for Continuing Medical Education through the American Association of Neurological Surgeons (AANS*). The AANS is accredited by the Accreditation Council for Continuing Medical Education to provide continuing medical education for physicians.

◆ Credit

The AANS designates this educational activity for a maximum of 15 AMA PRA Category 1 credits.™ Physicians should only claim those hours of credit commensurate with the extent of their participation in the activity.

The Home Study Examination is online on the AANS Web site at: http://www.aans.org/education/books/atlas1.asp

Estimated time to complete this activity varies by learner, and activity equaled is up to 15 Category 1 credits of CME.

**The acronym AANS refers to both the American Association of Neurological Surgeons and the American Association of Neurosurgeons.*

◆ Release/Termination Dates

Original Release Date: November 15, 2006

The CME termination date is: November 15, 2009

Disclosure Information

The AANS controls the content and production of this CME activity and attempt to ensure the presentation of balanced, objective information. In accordance with the Standards for Commercial Support established by the Accreditation Council for Continuing Medical Education, speakers, paper presenters/authors and staff (and the significant others of those mentioned) are asked to disclose any relationship they or their co-authors have with commercial companies which may be related to the content of their lecture.

Speakers, paper presenters/authors and staff (and the significant others of those mentioned) who have disclosed a relationship* with commercial companies whose products may have a relevance to their presentation are listed below.

Author Name	Disclosure	Type of Relationship
Behnam Badie	Scanlon International MN	Royalties, Other Support
Marvin Bergsneider	Siemens	Grant Support
Jeffrey N. Bruce	NIH	Grant
Iman Feiz-Erfan	Zimmer Spine	Grant for Clin. Fellowship
Amin B. Kassam	Stryker, STORZ, Baxter, Radionics	Consultant Fee
Linda M. Liau	Siemens Medical Systems	Research Grant
Robert Maciunas	Medtronic, BrainLAB AG	Industry Grant
Daniel R. Pieper	Michigan Head and Spine Institute	Stock and Shareholder
Daniel K. Resnick	Medtronic	Consultant Fee
Timothy Ryken	Medtronics, Nirthwest Biotherapeutics	Industry Grant
	Ivax, Xenova, MGI Pharma, Abbot Spine	Industry Grant
	Abbot Spine	Consultant Fee
	MGI Pharma, Schering	Speakers Bureau
Andrew E. Sloan	Brain Lab	Consultant Fee
Mark M. Souweidane	Aesculap	Honorarium
Robert E. Wallace	North American Scientific-Isotopes	Consultant Fee (Ongoing)
	Aptium Oncology -Rad Onc Svcs at Cedars-Sinai Med Ctr	Salary
John S. Yu	NIH	University Grants
	Guilford	Speaker's Bureau

*Relationship refers to receipt of royalties, consultantship, funding by research grant, receiving honoraria for educational services elsewhere, or any other relationship to a commercial company that provides sufficient reason for disclosure.

Speakers, their paper presenters/authors and staff (and the significant others of those mentioned) who have reported they do not have any relationships with commercial companies:

Author Name:

Ossama Al-Mefty
Joachim M. Baehring
Asis Kumar Bhattacharya
Stephen P. Beals
Vallo Benjamin
Nathaniel Brooks
Michael Chicoine
William T. Couldwell
John Diaz Day
Franco DeMonte
Aaron S. Dumont
Kurt Eichholz
Mark B. Eisenberg
James J. Evans
Abhijit Guha
Patrick J. Gullane
Behrooz Hakimian
Wayne Hamm
Greg Karl Hartig
Bermans J. Iskandar
Jay Jagannathan
John A. Jane Jr.
John A. Jane Sr.
Edward F. Joganic
Sarah C. Jost
Paulo A. S. Kadri
Ajit Krishnaney
Ali F. Krisht
Jeong-Taik Kwon
Frederick F. Lang
Samir B. Lapsiwala
Joung H. Lee
Salvatore C. Lettieri
James K. Liu
Anne Luptrawan
Michael W. McDermott
Joshua Medow
L. Madison Michael II
Roham Moftakhar
Peter C. Neligan
Christine B. Novak
Eylem Ocal
Michael J. Odell
Alfred T. Ogden
Andrew T. Parsa
Joseph Piepmeier
Randall W. Porter
Mark Pyle
Sharad Rajpal
Jon H. Robertson
Stephen M. Russell
Madjid Samii
William Sharp
Robert F. Spetzler
Michael P. Steinmetz
Stephen B. Tatter
Gregory Trost
Joseph Wiley
Kevin C. Yao

Series Foreword

The Publications Committee of the American Association of Neurological Surgeons began publishing the first edition of the *Neurosurgical Operative Atlas* in 1991. To allow for timely publication, coverage of six operations was published at bimonthly intervals in looseleaf format in the order finished manuscripts were received. The completed series had nine volumes and covered the entire spectrum of neurosurgery.

The goal was to publish a comprehensive reference that included well-established neurosurgical procedures as practiced in the United States and Canada by authors who are respected in the field.

Working together, the AANS Publications Committee and Thieme New York have organized the second edition of this atlas series. The atlas's main purpose remains the same, to be a ready reference for well-established neurosurgical procedures for trainees and practitioners of neurosurgery worldwide. The new edition contains five volumes, covering neuro-oncology, spine and peripheral nerves, functional, pediatric, and vascular neurosurgery. For each volume, one or more lead editors with known expertise in the subject area were selected. Each volume editor had complete freedom to add, revise, or delete chapters. The number of chapters per volume is approximately the same as the number of chapters in that particular subject area found in the first edition.

Each chapter is designed to teach a specific surgical technique or approach. The illustrations of the techniques are a vital part of the work, and the authors commissioned most of the drawings in color. The text in each chapter covers the case selection, the operative indications and contraindications, special points in the anesthetic technique, a step-by-step detailed description of the operation, and postoperative complications. Detailed discussion of diagnostic techniques, pathology, mechanisms of disease, histology, and medical management are not included since they are logically outside the scope of a surgical atlas. Detailed tables, reference lists, and statistical analysis of results are also not included because they are readily available in standard texts.

We hope you find this reference of value in your practice of neurosurgery.

Robert Maciunas, M.D.
Chair, AANS Publications Committee
Professor of Neurosurgery
University Hospitals of Cleveland
Cleveland, Ohio

Foreword

Few subspecialties in surgery can boast as many and as varied technical procedures as neurosurgery. Without question, neurosurgery is a technically driven subspecialty that has advanced significantly in the past 25 years, arguably more so than any other surgical subspecialty. This is perhaps nowhere more apparent than in the technical procedures that are used to treat patients with brain or spinal column tumors.

In this second edition of the *Neurosurgical Operative Atlas* on the topic of *Neuro-Oncology*, Behnam Badie and colleagues have provided us with a unique opportunity to view firsthand how neurosurgery has changed since the first edition was published. Once again, tumors that occur in all the main compartments of the brain and skull base are comprehensively covered. However, in the current atlas, we are provided with a window into the future of neurosurgery with chapters devoted exclusively to minimally invasive neurosurgery for sellar, skull base, and intraventricular tumors. Of course, refinements in approaches to complex tumors of the skull base have also taken place and are well described in the chapters on the preauricular transzygomatic subtemporal and infratemporal approach, the transmaxillary approach to the clivus, and the transmandibular approach to the skull base. What has become more apparent in the present edition of the *Neurosurgical Operative Atlas* is the awareness by all authors of the importance of preserving critical neural structures at all costs. At the end of a long case, and at the end of the day, neurosurgeons performing these complex procedures as described here are most interested in patient outcome and quality of life.

This edition of the *Operative Atlas* also teaches us that the neurosurgeon must also be a neurosurgical oncologist ready to deliver brachytherapy via balloon catheters and radiosurgery for selected benign and malignant lesions as needed. Other adjuncts to safe neurosurgical resections for patients with brain tumors described in the text include the use of intraoperative magnetic resonance imaging and the continued use of stereotaxy at the outset and throughout many neurosurgical oncology procedures.

Even though several novel treatment strategies are outlined within the pages of this atlas, there continues to be no substitute for standard microneurosurgical approaches to a variety of the more common types of tumors, including meningiomas of the clinoid, tentorium, and petroclival regions. For both technically difficult and straightforward brain and skull base tumors, the *Atlas* is very accessible to the reader, with familiar subheadings of Patient Selection, Preoperative Preparation, Operative Procedure, and Postoperative Management within all chapters.

It is hard to believe the speed with which the practice of neurosurgery for brain and skull base tumors has advanced this past decade. From a functional standpoint, neurosurgical patients are doing better immediately following their brain tumor resections than ever before. This is in no small part due to the artistry and wizardry that the authors of the chapters within the *Atlas* have used to take care of their patients with brain tumors, and that these same authors have written about so cogently and clearly herein. The second edition of the *Neurosurgical Operative Atlas: Neuro-Oncology* by Dr. Badie and colleagues will serve as a lasting contribution to the field of neurosurgery.

James T. Rutka, M.D., Ph.D., F.R.C.S.C., F.A.C.S., F.A.A.P.
Professor and Chairman
Department of Neurosurgery
The University of Toronto
Division of Neurosurgery
The Hospital for Sick Children
Toronto, Canada

Preface

This second edition of the *Neurosurgical Operative Atlas* is a collection of current manuscripts on neurosurgical management of central and peripheral nervous system neoplasms. The text is organized by sections on tumor anatomical locations, tumor types, and surgical approaches. Specific sections are dedicated to spine and peripheral nerve tumors, meningiomas, and skull base approaches. Most chapters are accompanied by high-quality illustrations that help readers better understand the technical aspects of surgical approaches. This book is not meant to be a comprehensive neurosurgical atlas, but for beginning neurosurgeons or those with less experience in surgical neuro-oncology it should provide adequate guidance to grasp and utilize basic surgical concepts.

The art of neurosurgery will undoubtedly continue to evolve as new technology and techniques are introduced. Experience in skull base surgery, for example, has provided us with anatomical lessons that have paved the road for the development of less invasive neurosurgical methods. Similarly, advances in stereotactic radiation therapy and neuroimaging have had a tremendous impact on neurosurgery. Refinement and availability of these modalities have led to earlier diagnosis of brain tumors (often before they become symptomatic) and have improved our ability to address and manage these tumors. These new tools have also transformed our thinking and have changed our approach to these tumors.

Future neurosurgeons, however, should not be content with the status quo. Although books such as this remind us of our technical skills, we continue to have major obstacles in dealing with the most common, and unfortunately most fatal, brain tumors. It is not our hands but our minds that will ultimately lead us to prevail in the battle against malignant gliomas. Future surgical neuro-oncologists need to devise ways to merge technology and science to deliver specific, targeted therapies for gliomas in a noninvasive fashion. Until these discoveries are made, let books such as this continue to guide our hands.

Acknowledgments

I would like to thank the AANS publications committee for giving me the opportunity to oversee this project. Special gratitude is expressed to the colleagues and friends who have contributed to this book.

Ms. Birgitta Brandenburg and her team at Thieme Medical Publishers deserve special recognition for their skill, hard work, and persistence in helping me publish this book in a timely fashion.

Contributors

Ossama Al-Mefty, M.D.
Chairman
Department of Neurosurgery
University of Arkansas Medical Center
Little Rock, Arkansas

Behnam Badie, M.D., F.A.C.S.
Director
Department of Neurosurgery
Director
Brain Tumor Program
City of Hope Medical Center
Duarte, California

Joachim M. Baehring, M.D.
Assistant Professor of Neurology and Neurosurgery
Department of Neurosurgery
Yale University School of Medicine
New Haven, Connectictut

Stephen P. Beals, M.D.
Southwest Craniofacial Center
Phoenix, Arizona

Vallo Benjamin, M.D.
Professor of Neurosurgery
New York University School of Medicine
New York, New York

Marvin Bergsneider, M.D.
Associate Professor
Division of Neurosurgery
University of California–Los Angeles
Los Angeles, California

Asis Kumar Bhattacharyya, M.S., M.Ch.
Clinical Fellow
Division of Neurosurgery
Toronto Western Hospital
University Health Network
Toronto, Canada

Nathaniel Brooks, M.D.
Department of Neurosurgery
University of Wisconsin Hospital and Clinics
Madison, Wisconsin

Jeffrey N. Bruce, M.D.
The Neurological Institute
Department of Neurological Surgery
Columbia University
New York, New York

Ricardo L. Carrau, M.D.
Professor
Departments of Neurosurgery and Otolaryngology
University of Pittsburgh Medical Center
Pittsburgh, Pennsylvania

Michael Chicoine, M.D.
Department of Neurological Surgery
Washington University School of Medicine
St. Louis, Missouri

William T. Couldwell, M.D.
Department of Neurosurgery
University of Utah
Salt Lake City, Utah

John Diaz Day, M.D.
Colorado Neurologic Institute
Rocky Mountain Neurosurgical Alliance, P.C.
Englewood, Colorado

Franco DeMonte, M.D.
Professor
Deputy Chairman
Medical Director
Brain and Spine Center
Department of Neurosurgery
The University of Texas
M. D. Anderson Cancer Center
Houston, Texas

Aaron S. Dumont, M.D.
Department of Neurological Surgery
University of Virginia School of Medicine
Charlottesville, Virginia

Kurt Eichholz, M.D.
Department of Neurosurgery
University of Iowa Hospitals and Clinics
Iowa City, Iowa

Mark B. Eisenberg, M.D.
Great Neck, New York

James J. Evans, M.D.
The Cleveland Clinic Foundation
Cleveland, Ohio

Iman Feiz-Erfan, M.D.
Resident
Barrow Neurological Institute
St. Joseph's Hospital and Medical Center
Phoenix, Arizona

Paul A. Gardner, M.D.
Resident
Department of Neurosurgery
University of Pittsburgh Medical Center
Pittsburgh, Pennsylvania

Abhijit Guha, M.D., M.Sc., F.R.S.C.
Professor for Neurosurgery
Toronto Western Hospital
University Health Network
Toronto, Canada

Patrick J. Gullane, M.B., F.R.C.S.C., F.A.C.S.
Department of Otolaryngology—Head and Neck Surgery
Toronto General Hospital
University Health Network
Toronto, Canada

Behrooz Hakimian, M.D.
Department of Radiation Oncology
Cedars-Sinai Medical Center
Los Angeles, California

Wayne Hamm, C.R.N.A.
Department of Neurosurgery
The University of Tennessee at Memphis
Memphis, Tennessee

Gregory Karl Hartig, M.D.
Associate Professor
Division of Otolaryngology
University of Wisconsin Hospital and Clinics
Madison, Wisconsin

Bermans J. Iskandar, M.D.
Department of Neurosurgery
University of Wisconsin Hospital and Clinics
Madison, Wisconsin

Jay Jagannathan, M.D.
Department of Neurological Surgery
University of Virginia School of Medicine
Charlottesville, Virginia

John A. Jane Jr., M.D.
Assistant Professor of Neurological Surgery
Department of Neurological Surgery
University of Virginia Health System
Charlottesville, Virginia

John A. Jane Sr., M.D.
Chairman
David W. Weaver Professor of Neurosurgery
Department of Neurological Surgery
University of Virginia Health System
Charlottesville, Virginia

Edward F. Joganic, M.D.
Southwest Craniofacial Center
Phoenix, Arizona

Sarah C. Jost, M.D.
Resident
Department of Neurological Surgery
Washington University School of Medicine
St. Louis, Missouri

Paulo A. S. Kadri, M.D.
Department of Neurosurgery
University of Arkansas Medical Center
Little Rock, Arkansas

Amin B. Kassam, M.D.
Associate Professor
Departments of Neurosurgery and Otolaryngology
University of Pittsburgh Medical Center
Pittburgh, Pennsylvania

Ajit Krishnaney, M.D.
Brain Tumor Institute and Department of Neurosurgery
The Cleveland Clinic Foundation
Cleveland, Ohio

Ali F. Krisht, M.D.
Department of Neurosurgery
University of Arkansas Medical Center
Little Rock, Arkansas

Jeong-Taik Kwon, M.D., Ph.D.
The Cleveland Clinic Foundation
Cleveland, Ohio

Frederick F. Lang, M,D.
Department of Neurosurgery
MD Anderson Cancer Center
Houston, Texas

Samir B. Lapsiwala, M.D.
Department of Neurosurgery
University of Wisconsin Hospital and Clinics
Madison, Wisconsin

Joung H. Lee, M.D.
Cleveland Clinic Foundation
Cleveland, Ohio

Salvatore C. Lettieri, M.D.
Chief
Division of Plastic Surgery
Department of Surgery
Mayo Clinic College of Medicine
Rochester, Minnesota

Linda M. Liau, M.D., Ph.D.
Associate Professor
Co-Director
Comprehensive Brain Tumor Program
Division of Neurosurgery
David Geffen School of Medicine
University of California–Los Angeles
Los Angeles, California

James K. Liu, M.D.
Department of Neurosurgery
University of Utah School of Medicine
Salt Lake City, Utah

Anne Luptrawan, M.S.N., F.N.P.
Neurosurgical Institute
Cedars-Sinai Medical Center
Los Angeles, California

Joseph C. Maroon, M.D.
Professor
Department of Neurosurgery
University of Pittsburgh Medical Center
Pittsburgh, Pennsylvania

Michael W. McDermott, M.D., F.R.C.S.C.
Professor
Vice Chair
Director of Patient Care Services
Robert and Ruth Halperin Chair in Meningioma Research
Department of Neurological Surgery
University of California, San Francisco
San Francisco Medical Center
San Francisco, California

Joshua Medow, M.D.
Department of Neurosurgery
University of Wisconsin Hospital and Clinics
Madison, Wisconsin

L. Madison Michael II, M.D.
Semmes-Murphy Neurologic and Spine Institute
Memphis, Tennessee

Arlan H. Mintz, M.Sc., M.D.
Assistant Professor
Department of Neurosurgery
University of Pittsburgh Medical Center
Pittsburgh, Pennsylvania

Roham Moftakhar, M.D.
Department of Neurosurgery
University of Wisconsin Hospital and Clinics
Madison, Wisconsin

Peter C. Neligan, M.B., F.R.C.S.(I.), F.R.C.S.(C.), F.A.C.S.
Professor and Chair
Division of Plastic Surgery
University Health Network
Toronto, Canada

Christine B. Novak, P.T., M.S.
Research Associate
Wharton Head and Neck Centre
University Health Network
Toronto, Canada

Eylem Ocal, M.D.
Yale–New Haven Hospital
New Haven, Connecticut

Michael J. Odell, B.Sc., M.D., F.R.C.S.(C.)
Head and Neck Fellow
Department of Otolaryngology—Head and Neck Surgery
University Health Network
Toronto, Canada

Alfred T. Ogden, M.D.
The Neurological Institute
Department of Neurological Surgery
Columbia University
New York, New York

Andrew T. Parsa, M.D., Ph.D.
Assistant Professor
Department of Neurological Surgery
University of California, San Francisco
San Francisco, California

Daniel R. Pieper, M.D.
Director of Cerebrovascular and Skull Base Surgery
Michigan Head and Spine Institute
Southfield, Michigan

Joseph Piepmeier, M.D.
Department of Neurosurgery
Yale University School of Medicine
New Haven, Connectictut

Randall W. Porter, M.D.
Chief
Intradisciplinary Skull Base Section
Barrow Neurological Institute
St. Joseph's Hospital and Medical Center
Phoenix, Arizona

Nader Pouratian, M.D., Ph.D.
Department of Neurological Surgery
University of Virginia School of Medicine
Charlottesville, Virginia

Mark Pyle, M.D.
Division of Otolaryngology
University of Wisconsin Hospital and Clinics
Madison, Wisconsin

Sharad Rajpal, M.D.
Department of Neurosurgery
University of Wisconsin Hospital and Clinics
Madison Wisconsin

Daniel K. Resnick, M.D.
Department of Neurosurgery
University of Wisconsin Hospital and Clinics
Madison, Wisconsin

Jon H. Robertson, M.D.
Department of Neurosurgery
The University of Tennessee at Memphis
Semmes-Murphy Neurologic and Spine Institute
Memphis, Tennessee

Stephen M. Russell, M.D.
Chief Resident
Department of Neurosurgery
Belleview Hospital
New York, New York

Timothy Ryken, M.D.
Associate Professor
Department of Neurosurgery
University of Iowa College of Medicine
Iowa City, Iowa

Madjid Samii, M.D.
Neurosurgery Clinic
Nordstadt Hospital
Hannover, Germany

William Sharp, M.D.
Division of Vascular Surgery
Department of Surgery
University of Iowa Hospitals and Clinics
Iowa City, Iowa

Andrew E. Sloan, M.D., F.A.C.S.
Director of Radiosurgery
Associate Professor of Neurosurgery and Radiation Oncology
H. Lee Moffitt Cancer Center and Research Institute
Tampa, Florida

Carl H. Snyderman, M.D.
Departments of Neurosurgery and Otolaryngology
Director of Center for Cranial Base Surgery
Department of Neurosurgery
University of Pittsburgh Medical Center
Pittsburgh, Pennsylvania

Mark M. Souweidane, M.D.
Associate Professor and Vice Chairman
Department of Neurological Surgery
Weill Medical College of Cornell University
New York, New York

Robert F. Spetzler, M.D.
J. N. Harber Chairman of Neurological Surgery
Director
Neurovascular Research and Pediatric Neurosurgical Research Laboratory
Barrow Neurological Institute
St. Joseph's Hospital and Medical Center
Phoenix, Arizona

Michael P. Steinmetz, M.D.
The Cleveland Clinic Foundation
Cleveland, Ohio

Stephen B. Tatter, M.D.
School of Medicine
Wake Forest University
Winston-Salem, North Carolina

Ajith Thomas M.D.
Department of Neurosurgery
University of Pittsburgh Medical Center
Pittsburgh, Pennsylvania

Gregory Trost, M.D.
Department of Neurosurgery
University of Wisconsin Hospital and Clinics
Madison, Wisconsin

Ugur Türe, M.D.
Department of Neurosurgery
Marmara University School of Medicine
Istanbul, Turkey

Robert E. Wallace
Department of Radiation Oncology
Cedars-Sinai Medical Center
Los Angeles, California

Joseph Wiley, M.D.
Graduate Student
Arthur and Sonia Labotts Brain Tumor Center
The Hospital for Sick Children
Toronto Western Hospital
Toronto, Canada

Kevin C. Yao, M.D.
Assistant Professor
Department of Neurosurgery
Tufts–New England Medical Center
Boston, Massachusetts

John S. Yu, M.D.
Neurosurgical Institute
Cedars-Sinai Medical Center
Los Angeles, California

Section I

Sellar and Parasellar Tumors

1

Transsphenoidal Approaches to the Sella and Suprasellar Region

Nathaniel Brooks and Behnam Badie

◆ Patient Selection

Since its introduction nearly a century ago, the transsphenoidal approach to the sella has undergone significant transformation. Scloffer first reported the initial successful removal of a pituitary tumor through a transethmoidal-transsphenoidal approach in 1907. To improve cosmetic results, the procedure was further modified by surgeons such as Kochler, Kanavel, Mixter, Quakenboss, Halstead, and Hirsch and finally evolved into the sublabial-transseptal approach. From 1910 to 1925 Cushing reported employing this approach in 231 patients with an operative mortality of 5.6%. Despite this relatively good outcome, he abandoned the transsphenoidal approach for craniotomy because of the better optic nerve decompression achieved with the latter approach. Although many neurosurgeons in North America followed suit, with the development and implementation of the operating microscope, the transnasal-transsphenoidal pituitary surgery once again became popular in the 1960s. This approach, as modified by Hardy, is presently used by many neurosurgeons to reach pituitary tumors.

As described later, the classic transsphenoidal approaches to the sella involve mucosal incisions and submucosal dissection of the anterior nasal septum. Perhaps this submucosal dissection of the septum was incorporated into the procedure to reduce the risk of postoperative meningitis seen during the early introduction of this technique. The extensive mucosal dissection and soft tissue trauma, however, are drawbacks to the procedure, being responsible for most of the postoperative pain and discomfort and the sinonasal complications such as septal perforation. In 1987, Griffith and Veerapen described the direct endonasal approach, which involves an anterior sphenoidotomy without mucosal dissection. Although others used this approach thereafter, it was not until the introduction of endoscopy that the endonasal approach became even more popular. Early reports by our group and others have demonstrated the efficacy and safety of the endonasal approach to be comparable to the classic approaches. The endonasal approach to the sella has become the procedure of choice for surgical treatment of most pituitary and intrasellar tumors.

This chapter discusses the most popular transsphenoidal approaches to the sella; namely, the direct endonasal (EN), the sublabial (SL), and the endonasal transseptal (TS). The EN procedure will be described first because this approach provides adequate exposure for resection of most pituitary tumors. Surgeons' familiarity with the SL and TS approaches, however, is still necessary for their implementation in larger pituitary and superior clival tumors. The traditional SL approach, although more invasive, provides a wider view of the sella and the parasellar region and may be employed for removal of tumors with parasellar extension or in pediatric patients with small nasal passages.

◆ Preoperative Preparation

Preoperative assessment of patients undergoing pituitary surgery is of critical importance no matter what surgical approach is employed. A full history and physical exam, detailed endocrine screening, and neuro-ophthalmologic evaluation should be completed prior to the planned operation. Routine endocrine tests include basal measurements of prolactin, growth hormone, insulin-like growth factor (IGF)-1, thyroxine, triiodothyronine, thyroid-stimulating hormone (TSH), cortisol, adrenocorticotropic hormone (ACTH), follicle-stimulating hormone (FSH), luteinizing hormone (LH), and testosterone (in men).

Review of the preoperative magnetic resonance imaging (MRI) studies is also crucial prior to every surgery. A dedicated pituitary MRI that consists of coronal and sagittal T1- and T2-weighted images before and after infusion of paramagnetic contrast, consisting of gadolinium and pentetic acid (Gd-DTPA), is obtained in every patient. For patients with small microadenomas, a "dynamic" study, where sellar imaging is performed every 10 seconds during contrast infusion, may better delineate the tumor. Besides tumor characteristics, several other factors are inspected on preoperative images. Sphenoid sinus anatomy such as ossification and its septal anatomy should be closely evaluated. Furthermore, the location and the course of the carotid arteries should be carefully observed. Ectatic carotid arteries that course too medially may minimize surgical exposure and even preclude the transsphenoidal approach. It is also important to recognize the location of the residual pituitary gland in macroadenomas because this structure appears as a thin rim of enhancement on coronal and sagittal images **(Fig. 1–1)**.

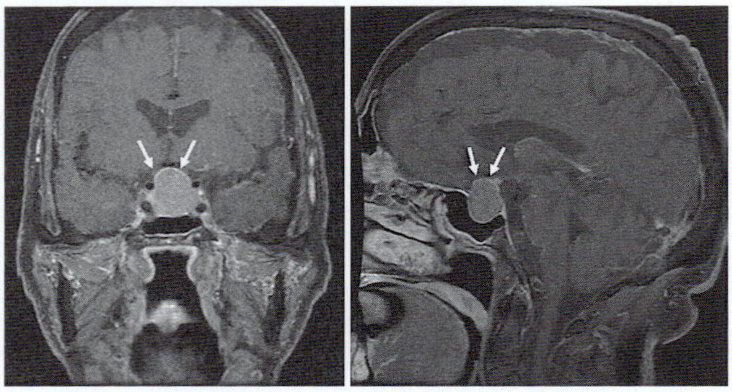

Figure 1–1 T1-weighted coronal (left) and sagittal magnetic resonance imaging after administration of contrast demonstrating a macroadenoma with suprasellar extension. Note the location of the residual pituitary gland (arrows), which appears as a rim of enhancing tissue superior and posterior to the tumor.

◆ Operative Procedure

Direct Endonasal Approach

Positioning

Patient positioning and operating room setup are identical for all of the transsphenoidal approaches discussed in this chapter **(Fig. 1–2)**. The patient is placed supine with the right shoulder at the right-hand corner of the table. The endotracheal tube, nasogastric tube, and temperature probe are brought to the left side of the mouth. The head, slightly elevated to improve venous drainage, is placed in a Mayfield three-point clamp to incorporate frameless stereotaxy. The head is slightly tilted to the patient's left (10 to 15 degrees), rotated to the right (10 to 20 degrees), and slightly extended. In our experience the use of frameless stereotaxy for guidance to the sella turcica is superior to the traditional fluoroscopy because it provides guidance in both vertical and lateral directions. Furthermore, frameless stereotaxy can be very valuable at teaching institutions where neurosurgical residents first become familiar with endonasal anatomy.

Antiseptic solution (e.g., Povidone-iodine) is applied to the nose and the left lower abdominal quadrant where adipose tissue may be harvested for repair of cerebrospinal fluid (CSF) leakage. For EN surgeries, mucosal prepping is unnecessary. For the SL and TS approaches, however, lidocaine with 1:100,000 epinephrine is injected submucosally along the septum (only on the side of entry), the floor of each nostril, and the upper buccal mucosa (for SL only). Finally, the oropharynx is packed with 2 in. gauze to avoid aspiration of blood during surgery.

Instrumentation

The EN approach used at our institution only requires a few additional tools besides the standard transsphenoidal instruments. These include: 0, 30, and 45 degree endoscopes,

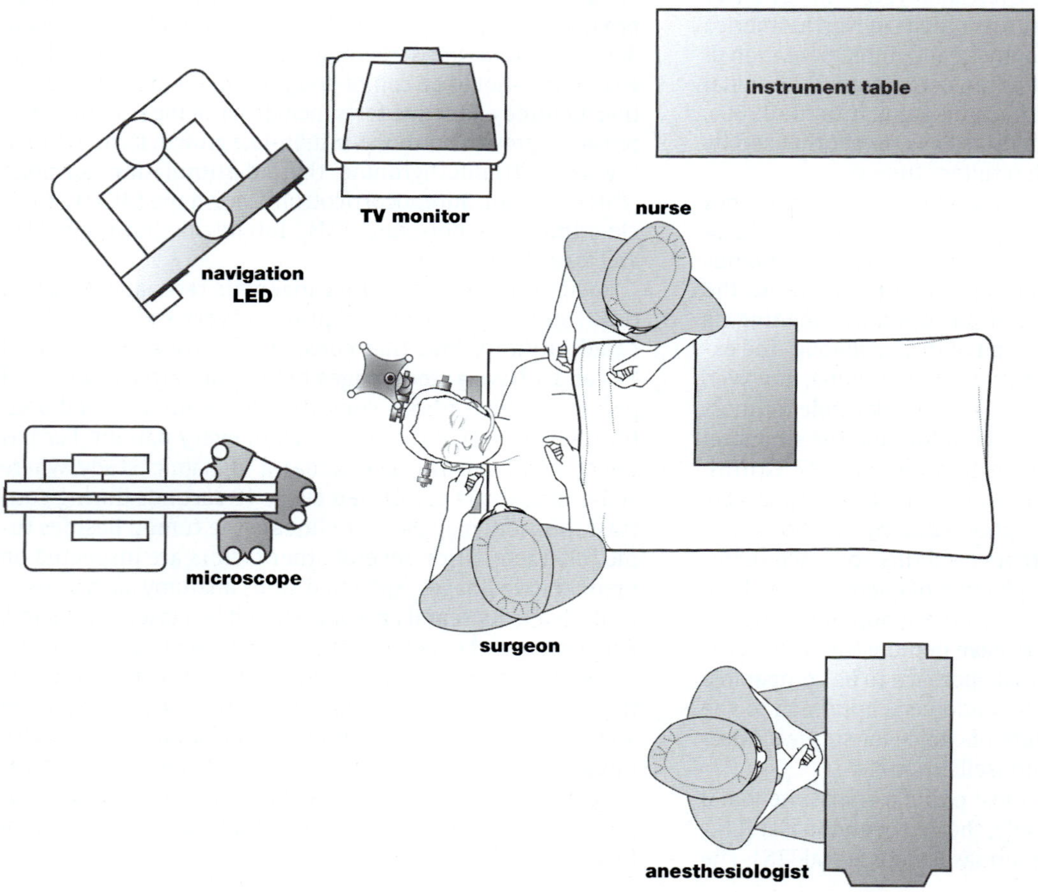

Figure 1–2 Operating room and patient positioning for transsphenoidal surgery LED, light-emitting diode.

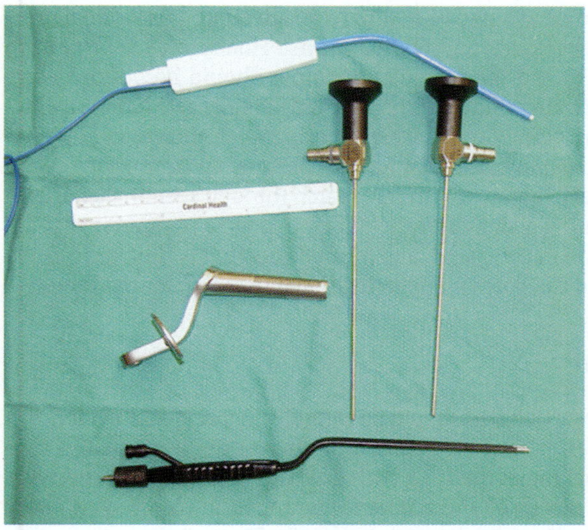

Figure 1–3 Additional transsphenoidal instruments used for endonasal pituitary surgery include: 0, 30, and 45 degree endoscopes, modified narrow nasal speculum, suction-monopolar-coagulator, and the Badie Suction Bipolar Forceps.

modified narrow nasal speculum, suction-monopolar-coagulator, and the Badie Suction Bipolar Forceps (Scanlan International, St. Paul, MN) **(Fig. 1–3).**

Operative Technique

Our endoscopically guided pituitary operations are performed through only one nostril, usually the one opposite the side of the tumor. For midline tumors, the wider nasal cavity is selected. The endoscope is initially inserted into the nostril and the anatomy of the turbinates is explored **(Fig. 1–4).** For a wide nasal passage, the endoscope is then passed between the septum medially and the middle turbinate laterally. The middle turbinate is gently pushed laterally as the endoscope is passed deeper into the nasal cavity. For narrower corridors, we use the larger space between the inferior turbinate and the nasal septum to visualize the choana, and as the scope is angulated in a cephalad direction, the shaft of the endoscope is used to displace the middle turbinate. The posterior attachment of the middle turbinate is used as a landmark to localize the sphenoid sinus.

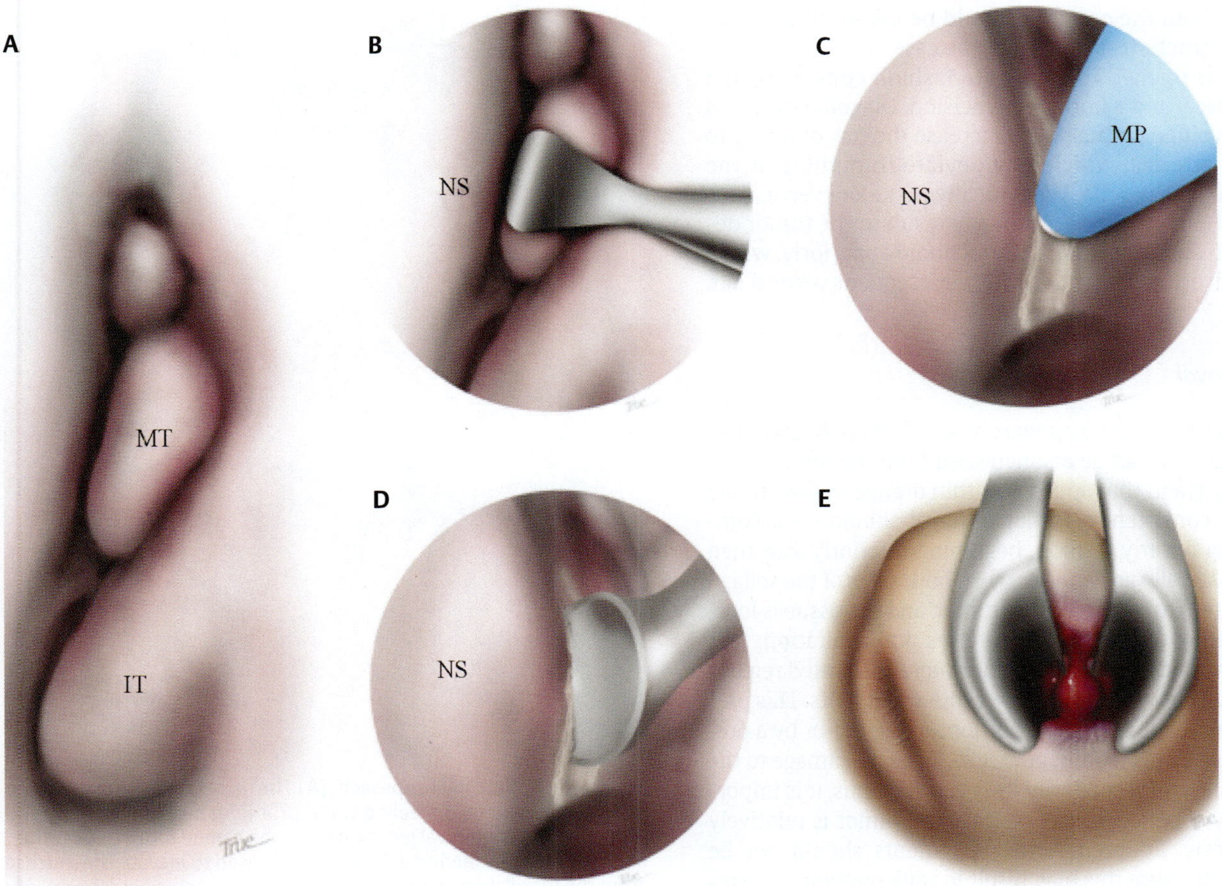

Figure 1–4 Endonasal anatomy as seen through an endoscope. **(A)** The endoscope is passed through the patient's left nares and slowly advanced between the septum medially and the middle turbinate laterally. **(B)** As the endoscope is advanced, the flat end of a Penfield Dissector no. 1 can be used to push the middle turbinate laterally. **(C)** The mucosa over the sphenoid sinus is coagulated using a suction-monopolar and **(D)** the posterior aspect of the nasal septum is fractured from the vomer using the sharp end of a Penfield-one. **(E)** A narrow speculum is then advanced under endoscopic guidance to the sphenoid face and gently opened. IT, inferior turbinate; MP, suction monopolar; MT, middle turbinate; NS, nasal septum.

After the location of the entry into the sphenoid sinus is confirmed with the navigation system, mucosa over the sphenoid sinus is cut using a suction-monopolar-coagulator, and the posterior aspect of the nasal septum is fractured from the vomer. A narrow speculum is then advanced under endoscopic guidance to the sphenoid face. An anterior sphenoidotomy is then performed.

Although the endoscope is still used to optimize the extent of anterior sphenoidotomy and exposure of the sella, the actual tumor removal is performed using a microscope. By freeing the surgeon's hands and providing stereoscopic visualization, the microscope can reduce the operative time and allow easier control of bleeding.

Once inside the sphenoid sinus, the endoscope is used to inspect the septal anatomy and localize the sella. The optic and carotid prominences can also be easily visualized through the endoscope. The sphenoid mucosa is preserved and is only partially coagulated to reveal the anterior wall of the sella turcica. Frameless stereotactic guidance is also useful to target the floor of the sella turcica, which generally reveals itself as a smooth bulge in the superior midline region of the sinus.

The sella can then be opened with a small dissector, curette, drill, or osteotome. The opening should not extend to the chiasmatic sulcus or tuberculum sellae because this can increase the likelihood of a postoperative CSF leak. The opening can be extended using a micro Kerrison punch. All bone taken from the opening should be saved for the final sellar reconstruction at the end of the case.

The dura is opened in a cruciate fashion consisting of a midline vertical and a horizontal incision. Diagonal incisions should be avoided because they increase the risk of injury to the carotid arteries, which may deviate to midline at the upper aspect of the sella. We typically make the vertical incision first. A horizontal incision may result in the tumor decompression and descent of the arachnoid superiorly, which may be inadvertently opened with a subsequent vertical cut.

Tumor Removal

A typical macroadenoma appears as a soft grayish, granular-textured mass and can be distinguished from the remnants of the pituitary gland that appears as thin orange-yellow tissue with firmer consistency. Tumor removal should be accomplished in an orderly fashion, beginning inferiorly and then proceeding laterally and superiorly on both sides of the sella. A ringed curette is used to enter the tumor, and the tissue is loosened and removed with blunt curettes and aspiration. It is helpful to proceed first with the more laterally situated regions of the tumor followed by the more central segments. This prevents entrapment of the lateral portions of the tumor by a prematurely descending diaphragma sella. To avoid damage to the pituitary stalk, and secondarily the hypothalamus, it is important to delay superior dissection until the tumor is relatively freed inferiorly. Adherent tumor fragments should not be pulled down because this may result in stalk traction and irreversible diabetes insipidus. Often, with removal and decompression of the intrasellar portion of the tumor, the suprasellar tumor will prolapse into view. If this does not occur, a Valsalva maneuver by the anesthesiologist will facilitate herniation of residual tumor. Thus early arachnoid tears and CSF leaks should be avoided to maintain an adequate intracranial pressure necessary for this maneuver. Finally, visual inspection with 30 and 45 degree endoscopes should be performed to look for any residual tumor located laterally and superiorly. Hemostasis can often be achieved using soft Gelfoam packing.

Microadenomas that are not present on the surface of the pituitary require a systemic search through seemingly normal-appearing gland. After the dura is opened a transverse incision is made in the gland, and blunt dissection is then performed around the normal-appearing tissue to search for the tumor.

Closure

The resection bed should be carefully inspected for evidence of CSF leak or arachnoid tears. If no obvious CSF leak is noted, simple packing of the sella with Gelfoam is sufficient. Otherwise, small pieces of abdominal fat wrapped in oxidized cellulose (Surgicel) can be placed intradurally. The anterior sellar wall is

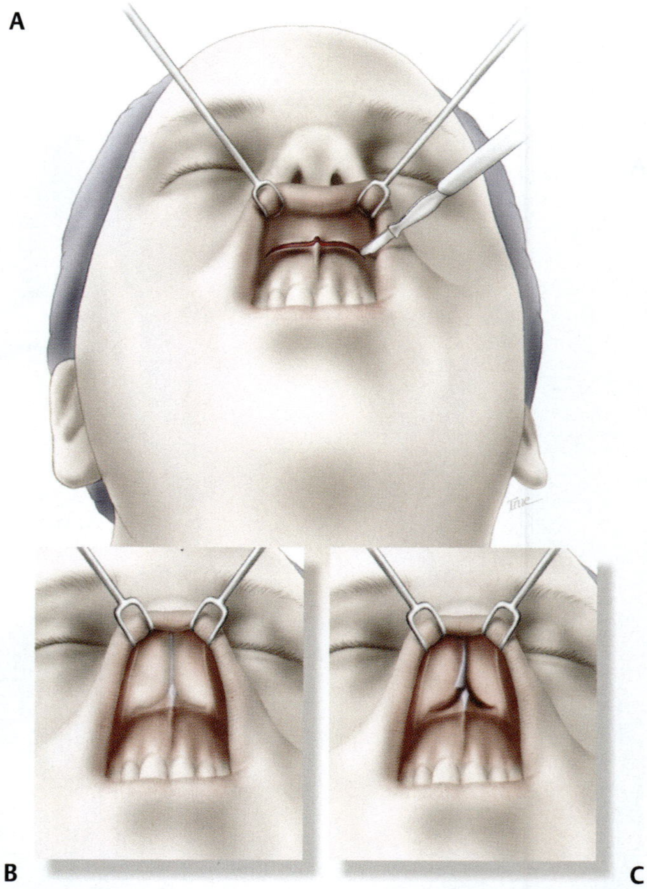

Figure 1–5 Sublabial approach. **(A)** The upper lip is retracted using handheld retractors revealing the septum. An incision is performed along the buccogingival junction from one canine tooth to the other, ~3.5 to 4 cm. Subperiosteal dissection is used to elevate the mucosa from the maxillary ridge along the anterior nasal spine until the inferior border of the piriform aperture is reached (left inset). A submucosal plane is then developed along the left side of the septum and floor of each nostril (right inset). **(B)** A submucoperichondrial flap is developed along one side of the nasal septum. **(C)** The cartilaginous nasal septum is dislocated from the vomer and reflected to the opposite side using firm blunt dissection. A nasal speculum is inserted.

then reconstructed by intradural placement of a small, flat piece of bone removed at the initial exposure. To avoid injury to the arachnoid membrane situated superiorly, the bone should be placed in a horizontal orientation and locked into place against dural or bone edges. If indicated the reconstruction will be reinforced with fibrin glue. The sphenoid sinus itself is not packed with fat. If the dural leak is large, which can often be signified by pooling of CSF in the sphenoid sinus, a lumbar drain should be placed at the end of the case.

After the nasal speculum is removed, the middle turbinate and the nasal septum are realigned into normal anatomical orientation. Insertion of a lubricated fifth digit into the contralateral nares is often sufficient to check for septal alignment. Postoperative nasal packing is not used.

Since our first reported experience with the endoscopically guided direct EN route to the sella 4 years ago, we have used this approach in nearly 200 patients with pituitary tumors. We have not experienced any cosmetic complications or nasal perforations using this technique. Most patients are discharged to home within 48 hours.

Sublabial and Transseptal Approaches

SL and TS approaches provide a larger surgical corridor and are more suitable for tumors with parasellar extension. The SL approach, however, has fallen out of favor for resection of most pituitary tumors because it requires extensive submucosal dissection that tends to increase postoperative patient discomfort and recovery time.

The SL approach begins along the buccogingival margin and extends submucosally to the sphenoid face. Patient positioning remains identical to the EN approach already described. For the SL approach, the upper lip is retracted and an incision is performed along the buccogingival junction from one canine tooth to the other, ~3.5 to 4 cm **(Fig. 1–5A).** The mucosa from the maxillary ridge along the anterior nasal spine is elevated until the inferior border to the piriform aperture is reached. A submucoperichondrial flap is then developed along one side of the nasal septum, and submucosal dissection is extended into the nasal floor on both sides. Using a curved dissector the mucosa inferior to either nares is dissected away from the surface of the hard palate superiorly back to the perpendicular plate of the ethmoid. The cartilaginous nasal septum is then dislocated and reflected to the opposite side using firm blunt dissection **(Fig. 1–5B).** The transsphenoidal retractor can then be introduced and gently opened **(Fig. 1–5B).** With the retractor in place the keel of the vomer should be well visualized **(Fig. 1–5C).** The mucosa on the rostrum of the sphenoid is elevated laterally on both sides until the sphenoid ostia are visualized. A standard anterior sphenoidotomy is then performed under the microscope. The tips of the nasal speculum should never be placed into the sphenoid sinus after the completion of the anterior sphenoidotomy. Overexpansion of the nasal speculum in such instances can fracture the sphenoid bone and the optic canals and thus result in catastrophic optic nerve injury.

For the TS approach an intranasal incision just behind the mucosal–cutaneous junction is made **(Fig. 1–6).** A submucoperichondrial plane is then developed and the submucosal

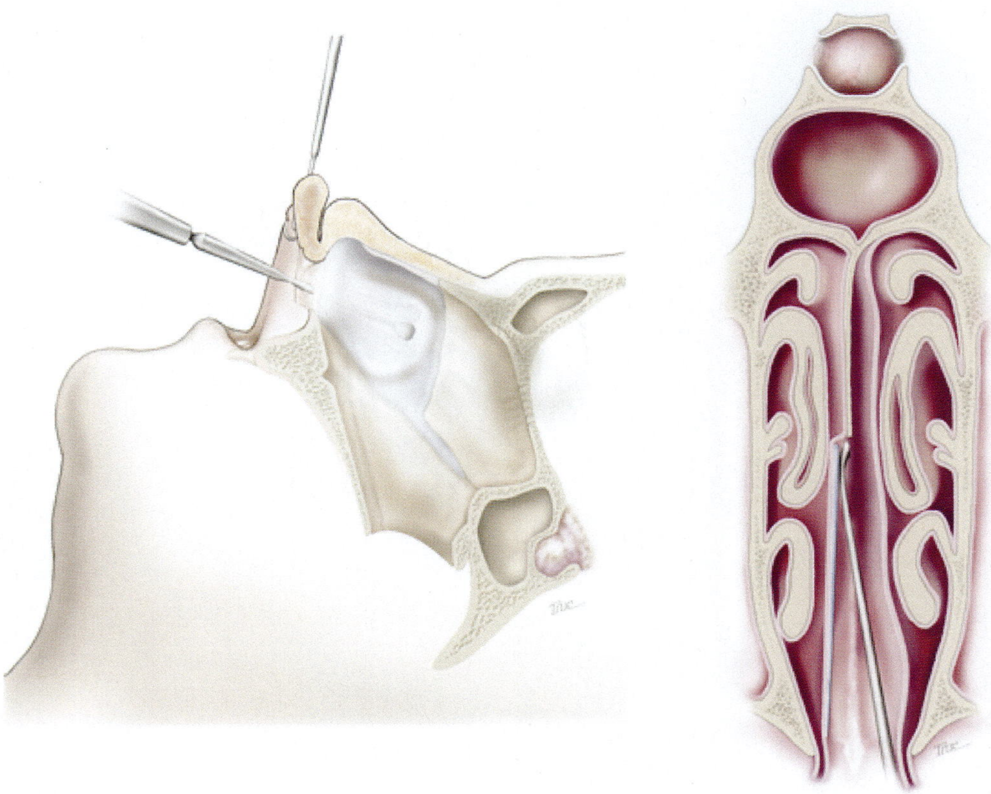

A B

Figure 1–6 Transseptal approach. **(A)** An intranasal incision just behind the mucosal–cutaneous junction is made and a **(B)** submucoperichondrial plane is developed along the nasal septum.

dissection is extended onto the nasal floor on one side. The nasal septum can then be fractured to the other side or partially excised to reach the vomer. The rest of the operation is similar to the EN and SL approaches.

At the completion of the surgery, the nasal septum is reapproximated in the midline and the mucosal and buccogingival incisions closed with 4.0 catgut or Vicryl sutures. For the SL approach, postoperative nasal packing can be used for 1 to 2 days to prevent septal hematoma or bleeding. For the TS approach, we do not routinely use nasal packing postoperatively unless there is difficulty with hemostasis.

◆ Postoperative Management

The patient should be observed for further CSF leakage, which may require lumbar drainage or reexploration. Also, the patient's fluid balance should be strictly monitored. Postoperative diuresis is not uncommon in any surgical patient but urine outputs greater than 300 mL/h for 2 consecutive hours often trigger serum sodium and urine specific gravity measures. In our patient population diabetes insipidus is uncommon, but if seen, it is only transient. We do not treat the patient with vasopressin right away but rather liberalize the patient's fluid intake to keep up with output. If the diabetes insipidus persists beyond 24 hours, or if the patient is unable to match the input and output, then vasopressin is administered intranasally. Serum sodium levels are then monitored daily to avoid hyponatremia.

Exogenous steroid treatment is tapered fairly rapidly postoperatively. If there is concern for decreased pituitary–adrenal axis function then maintenance doses of steroids are administered until appropriate endocrine follow-up can be obtained.

Our patients also receive prophylactic antibiotics postoperatively. Augmentin (750 mg/d orally for 14 days) has been effective in reducing postoperative sinusitis.

◆ Conclusion

In our experience transsphenoidal operations can be efficiently, effectively, and safely performed through an EN approach. The combination of the endoscope, operating microscope, and frameless stereotaxy has been instrumental in improving this approach. The translabial approach is used less frequently but can be helpful in the approach to larger tumors with parasellar extension. The key to a successful transsphenoidal operation remains strict adherence to the midline, preservation of normal tissue, and careful postoperative care.

2

Surgical Approaches to Craniopharyngiomas

Ali F. Krisht and Ugur Türe

Craniopharyngiomas are benign tumors that arise from squamous cell rests that lie along the pituitary stalk. These tumors are usually very adherent to the stalk and are capable of infiltrating the region of the tuber cinereum and insinuating themselves into the hypothalamic tissue, inducing severe reactive astrogliosis. Hypopituitarism from compression of the pituitary gland and diabetes insipidus from compression of the pituitary stalk may ensue. Craniopharyngiomas often compress the optic chiasm and fill the entire third ventricular region when very large, blocking the foramina of Monro and inducing secondary hydrocephalus.

Despite their benign nature, the location of craniopharyngiomas and their close proximity to important suprasellar and parasellar structures render their surgical excision hazardous. Recent refinements in microsurgical techniques and advances in endocrinology have significantly impacted the management of craniopharyngiomas. Total surgical excision has become possible in up to 70% of cases, and the postoperative morbidity rate has been significantly improved with adequate hormone replacement therapy.

◆ Preoperative Preparation

Diagnostic Evaluation

In addition to obtaining a detailed history of the current illness, complete neurological, neuro-ophthalmologic, and endocrinologic evaluations are performed on all patients. Basic hormonal studies that evaluate the anterior pituitary function are routinely obtained. In our practice, these include a.m. serum cortisol, 17-hydroxycorticosteroid, growth hormone, prolactin, T4, luteinizing hormone, follicle-stimulating hormone, testosterone in men and estradiol in women, and urinary free cortisol. In addition, determination of serum and urine osmolalities prior to and after 12 hours of water deprivation is indicated when diabetes insipidus is suspected.

Modern imaging techniques, including computed tomography and magnetic resonance imaging (MRI), play an important role in the preoperative evaluation by providing information about the tumor's consistency and its relationship to the surrounding structures, which helps in determining the appropriate surgical approach. Sagittal and coronal MRI helps in discerning whether the suprasellar portion of the tumor has infiltrated the substance of the third ventricle or is merely causing compression. This is important because many tumors that appear to be within the third ventricular substance are, in fact, only in the suprasellar region and can be removed totally by extra-axial approaches.

◆ Choice of Surgical Approach

Craniopharyngiomas have different growth patterns, which are probably related to the exact location from which they arise along the pituitary stalk. Tumors arising from the distal portion of the pituitary stalk may grow either in the intrasellar compartment **(Fig. 2–1A)** or extend superiorly into the suprasellar region. Those arising from the middle portion of the stalk may fill either the suprasellar compartment **(Fig. 2–1B,C)** or extend superiorly into the third ventricular compartment **(Fig. 2–1D)**. Tumors arising from the proximal portion of the pituitary stalk may be restricted to the third ventricular region **(Fig. 2–1E)** or may grow in a manner similar to that of the tumors arising from the middle portion of the stalk, impinging on the structures in the suprasellar region and extending into the ventricle **(Fig. 2–1D)**. Their consistency can be mixed, with solid and cystic components. The tumors can enlarge to a giant size. Their growth and relationship to the optic apparatus vary depending on the size of the tumor and the location of the optic chiasm. They occasionally grow in the suprasellar region between the optic nerves, pushing them laterally **(Fig. 2–1B)**. If the chiasm is in a prefixed position, the entire suprasellar portion of the optic apparatus may be pushed anteriorly and superiorly, with flattening of the chiasm region **(Fig. 2–1C)**.

The decision regarding the surgical approach varies with each case and is generally based on the location and size of the tumor. **Table 2–1** shows our decision-making algorithm based on these criteria. Tumors growing in the intrasellar compartment with no suprasellar component **(Fig. 2–1A)** are approached through the transnasal-transsphenoidal route (this approach is not discussed in this chapter). Large intrasellar tumors with suprasellar extensions **(Fig. 2–1B,C)** and small suprasellar tumors are approached through the pterional-transsylvian route. Tumors located in the suprasellar compartment that are large and have significant extension into the third ventricular compartment **(Fig. 2–1D)** are operated on through a combined pterional- and transcallosal-transventricular approach, as described by Yasargil. Tumors

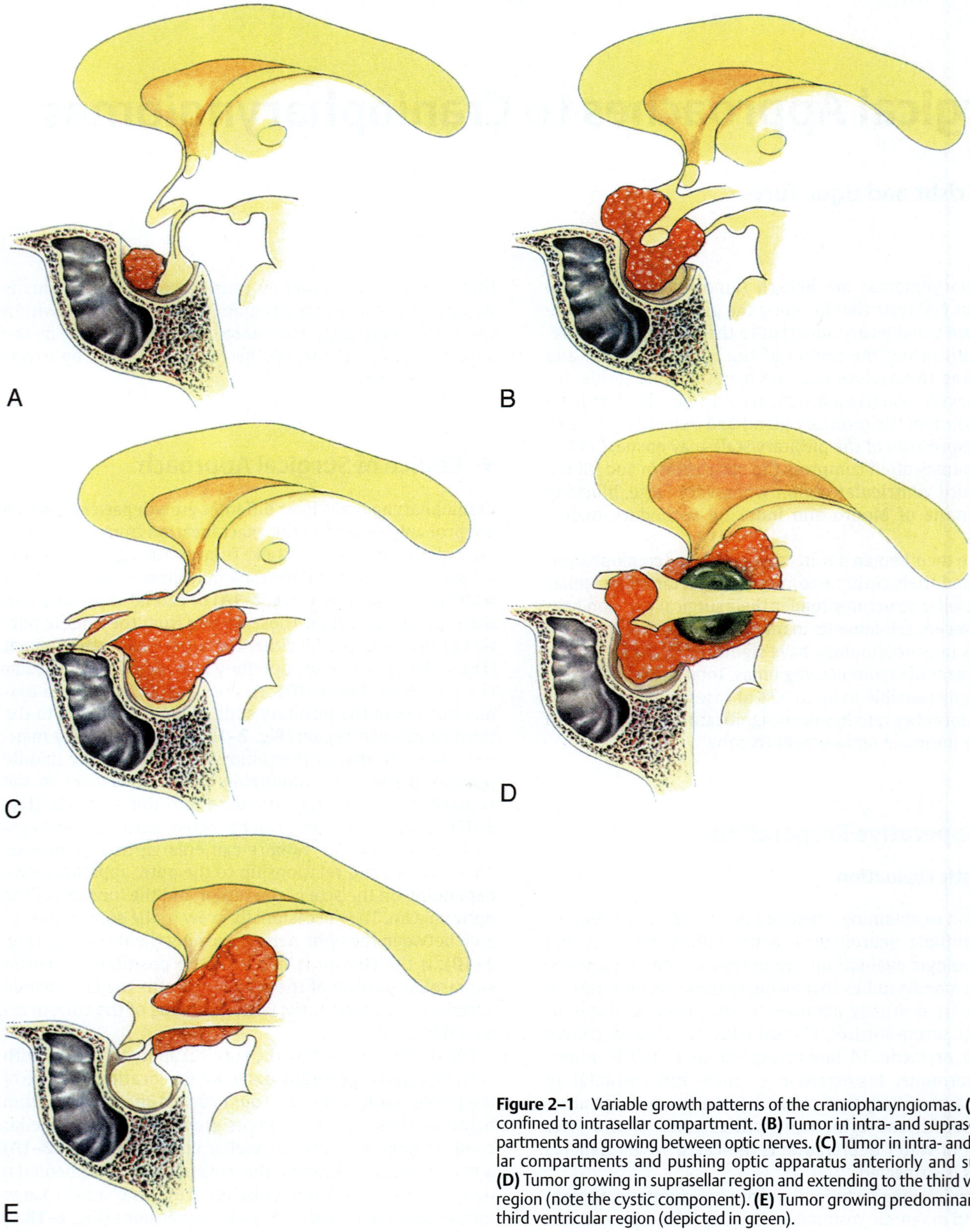

Figure 2–1 Variable growth patterns of the craniopharyngiomas. **(A)** Tumor confined to intrasellar compartment. **(B)** Tumor in intra- and suprasellar compartments and growing between optic nerves. **(C)** Tumor in intra- and suprasellar compartments and pushing optic apparatus anteriorly and superiorly. **(D)** Tumor growing in suprasellar region and extending to the third ventricular region (note the cystic component). **(E)** Tumor growing predominantly in the third ventricular region (depicted in green).

Table 2–1 Surgical Approach Based on Tumor Location and Size

Tumor Location	Size	Approach
Intrasellar	Small	Transsphenoidal
	Large	Pterional-transsylvian
Suprasellar	Small	Pterional-transsylvian
	Large	Pterional-transsylvian or combined*
Intraventricular		
Suprasellar		Combined*
Intraventricular		Transcallosal-transventricular

*Combined pterional-transsylvian and transcallosal-transventricular.

that are purely intraventricular **(Fig. 2–1E)** are usually approached via the transcallosal-transventricular route, but in many cases we prepare for the combined approach if complete tumor removal is not possible through the pterional approach.

◆ Operative Procedure

Anesthesia

Patients are routinely treated with appropriate doses of parenteral hydrocortisone in the immediate preoperative period to enable them to withstand the stress of a major procedure. Hydrocortisone can be substituted with dexamethasone in the postoperative period to reduce brain swelling. In the perioperative period, patients are also given prophylactic antibiotics and anticonvulsants.

Anesthesia is induced with thiopental and a muscle relaxant. For the major part of the procedure, a combination of a muscle relaxant, a narcotic, and nitrous oxide is used. Inhalational anesthetics are usually avoided, especially when increased intracranial pressure is suspected. The patient is given 20 to 40 mg of Lasix (furosemide) after induction of anesthesia to achieve a negative fluid balance. A total of no more than 500 mL of intravenous fluids is allowed for the entire procedure. Hypotension is avoided, with normotension being the goal.

Patient Positioning

Patients are positioned in the supine position with the head slightly tilted (10 to 20 degrees) to the side opposite from the side of incision and slightly elevated. The neck is hyperextended to allow the frontal lobes to fall backward with gravity. The head is then fixed with the Mayfield three-point headholder **(Fig. 2–2A)**.

Surgical Technique

Pterional-Transsylvian Approach

The standard pterional approach, described by Yasargil, is used to remove large intrasellar and small suprasellar craniopharyngiomas. The skin incision begins 1 cm anterior to the tragus and extends in a curvilinear fashion behind the hairline to the midsagittal plane. We prefer a right-sided craniotomy for midline tumors. After reflection of the skin flap, an interfascial dissection of the superficial temporalis fascia behind the zygoma is performed to identify and preserve the frontalis branch of the seventh cranial nerve. In most cases, we preserve and reflect the pericranium for possible use as a dural graft later **(Fig. 2–2B)**. We then cut the temporalis muscle and reflect it anteriorly.

For tumors located in the suprasellar region, we have modified our pterional craniotomy to extend medially and inferiorly just above the superior orbital ridge **(Fig. 2–2C)**. This allows a more subfrontal approach to tumors extending between the optic nerves. In this case, the skin incision is extended further in the bicoronal plane for exposure of the larger bone flap.

The bone flap is elevated, and dural tack-up stitches are applied to establish epidural hemostasis. Next, the sphenoid ridge is drilled along its medial extension as far as the lateral aspect of the superior orbital fissure **(Fig. 2–2D)**. This entails coagulating and cutting the meningo-orbital artery. The dura is then opened in a U-shaped fashion above the sylvian fissure, and the opening is extended along the frontal lobe to allow a subfrontal approach to the suprasellar region **(Fig. 2–2E)**. The dura is then reflected. Any further dissection from this point onward is performed using the surgical microscope **(Fig. 2–2F)**.

Our first step is to expose the region of the chiasmatic cistern, open both the chiasmatic and carotid cisterns, and allow the spinal fluid to drain for brain relaxation. After this step is concluded, attention is directed to the distal part of the sylvian fissure, where microdissection of the arachnoid is begun. This transsylvian microdissection is initiated by opening the arachnoid on the frontal side of the superficial middle cerebral veins. Dissection is continued into the depth of the fissure and along the M_1 segment of the middle cerebral artery toward the carotid artery bifurcation. This procedure allows visualization of the A_1 segment and its relationship to the tumor **(Fig. 2–2G)**.

Tumor resection is facilitated by draining any cystic component of the tumor. This step shrinks the tumor and relaxes the stretched optic apparatus. Occasionally, if the tumor is completely solid, we begin by drilling the right optic canal

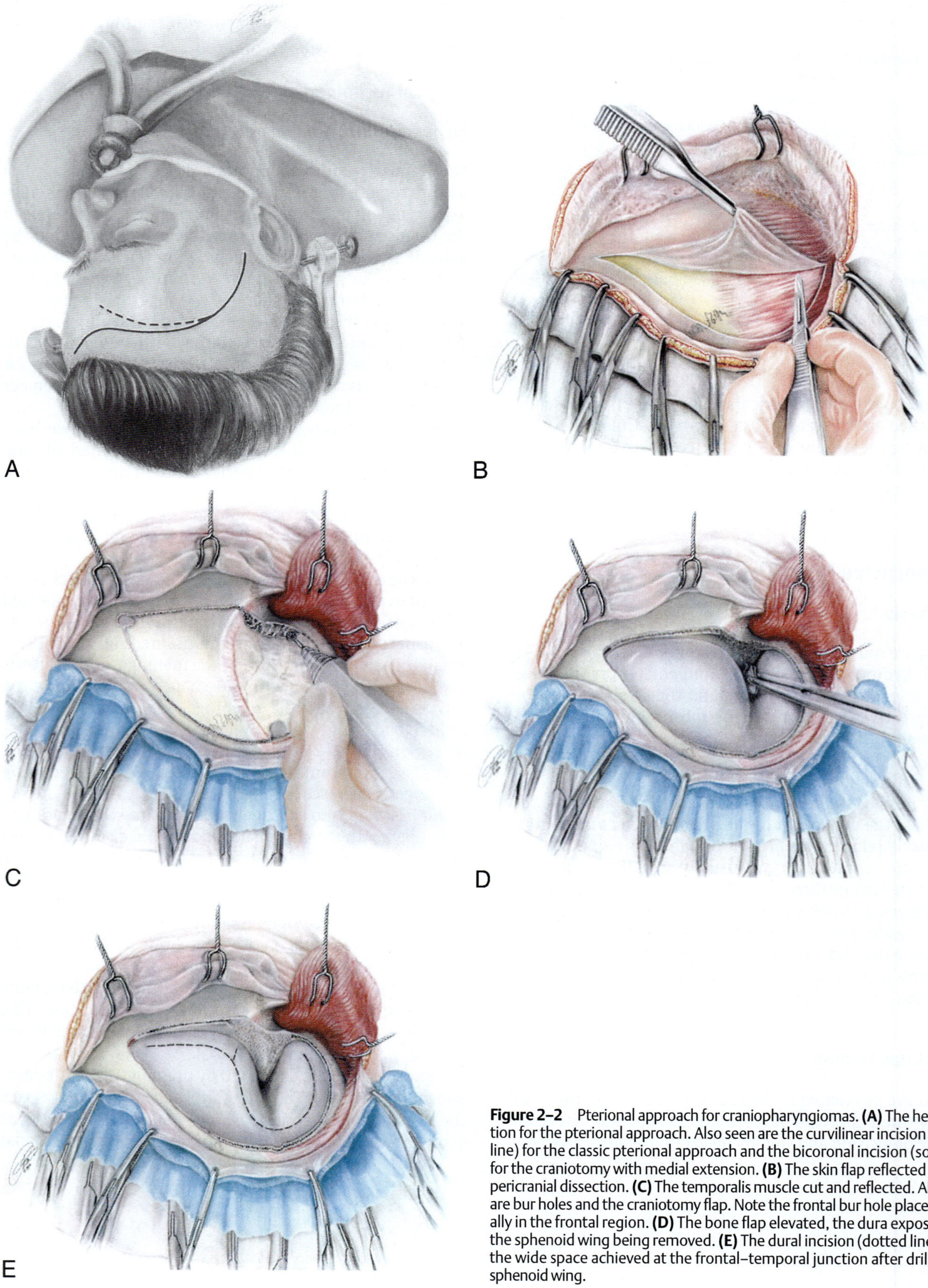

Figure 2–2 Pterional approach for craniopharyngiomas. **(A)** The head position for the pterional approach. Also seen are the curvilinear incision (dotted line) for the classic pterional approach and the bicoronal incision (solid line) for the craniotomy with medial extension. **(B)** The skin flap reflected and the pericranial dissection. **(C)** The temporalis muscle cut and reflected. Also seen are bur holes and the craniotomy flap. Note the frontal bur hole placed medially in the frontal region. **(D)** The bone flap elevated, the dura exposed, and the sphenoid wing being removed. **(E)** The dural incision (dotted line). Note the wide space achieved at the frontal–temporal junction after drilling the sphenoid wing.

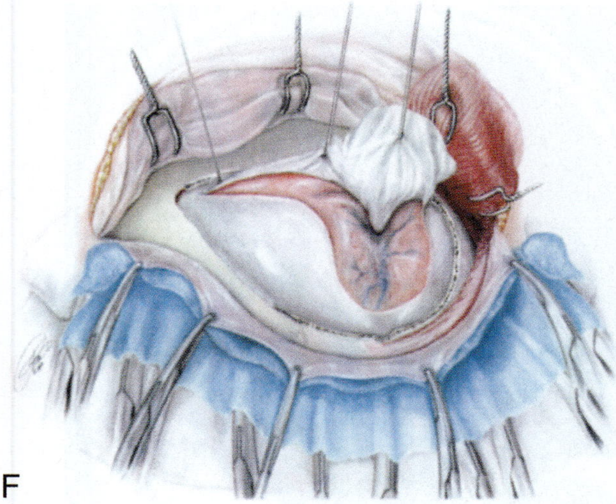

F

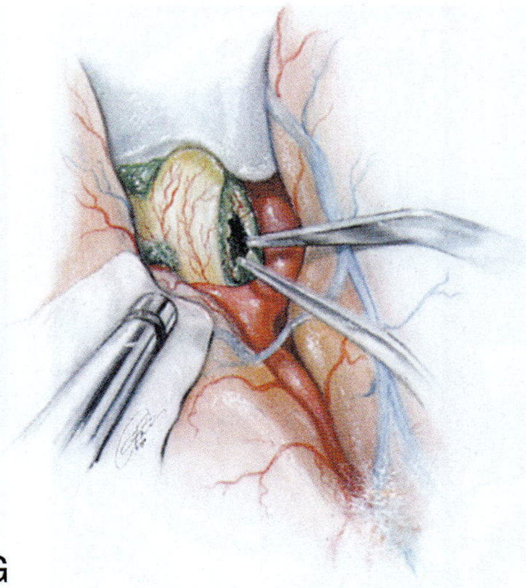

G

(Continued) **(F)** The dura opened and reflected over the sylvian fissure. **(G)** The transsylvian approach to the craniopharyngioma through the opticocarotid space. Note the visualization of the carotid bifurcation that is achieved after splitting the sylvian fissure. (Modified from Yasargil MG. Microneurosurgery, Vol 4B, with permission.)

and then cut the dural fibrous band, the falciform ligament overlying the optic nerve. This maneuver decompresses and relaxes the nerve, allowing it to be more tolerant to manipulation until the bulk of the tumor is removed. The tumor can then be approached through several windows, one of which is the space between the optic nerves. It is attacked by coagulating the overlying arachnoid distal to the chiasm to avoid injury to the blood supply of the chiasm. Tumor debulking is performed using suction and the pituitary rongeur, with gentle traction on the tumor. Occasionally, the ultrasonic aspirator is used. Sometimes, the tumor is calcified and more difficult to remove. In these cases, we attempt to break the large calcific pieces into smaller fragments that become easier to remove from within the tumor bed.

Another window through which the tumor is approached is the opticocarotid space. The arachnoid is dissected through this space, with attention being paid to several small branches that arise from the medial wall of the carotid artery, which is usually stretched around the tumor. A window between these small branches is established, and the tumor is approached. These branches provide the blood supply to the chiasm, the pituitary stalk, and the optic nerve, the preservation of which is essential to prevent postoperative ischemic visual deficits.

The third window that can be used is the lamina terminalis. When stretched and enlarged by the tumor, it can be opened safely and used for removing the tumor. Extra caution is exercised in dissecting the tumor capsule and its attachment to the surrounding gliotic brain in the hypothalamic region. If the tumor has significant suprasellar and intraventricular extensions, there is no need for heroic attempts that risk injury to the hypothalamus. The residual tumor can be safely removed through a combined transcallosal-transventricular approach, and in the same sitting. With small suprasellar tumors, it is possible to identify the pituitary stalk and, in some cases, even save it **(Fig. 2–3)**. This task becomes more difficult with large tumors and has no advantage if it risks leaving residual tumor behind.

The modified pterional craniotomy already described here provides options for several routes to easily access the suprasellar region. In addition, the surgical microscope can be moved from the lateral pterional-transsylvian position to the medial subfrontal position with no difficulty. This approach also allows access to the basal cisterns and drainage of spinal fluid for maximal brain relaxation, which minimizes use of brain retraction that is potentially injurious to the brain **(Fig. 2–4)**.

Transcallosal–Transventricular Approach

The transcallosal-transventricular approach is used for tumors located purely in the third ventricular compartment **(Fig. 2–1E)**. When the combined approach is considered, either a bicoronal or a curvilinear incision extending beyond the midline is used. For the transcallosal part, a triangular craniotomy is established with two bur holes along the midline, as shown in **Fig. 2–5A.** The posterior midline bur hole is made 1 cm behind the coronal suture, and the anterior midline bur hole is made 3 to 5 cm anterior to the coronal suture. The dura is opened and reflected medially. Microdissection of the interhemispheric fissure is performed until the pericallosal arteries and the corpus callosum are identified **(Fig. 2–5B)**. The corpus callosum is divided longitudinally at the level of the coronal suture, and the lateral ventricular cavity is entered. The tumor is then dissected through the foramen of Monro, which is usually enlarged. The septum pellucidum is also opened to approach the tumor from the opposite foramen of Monro and around both fornices. Care is taken to gently retract the forniceal system to avoid its injury. After the

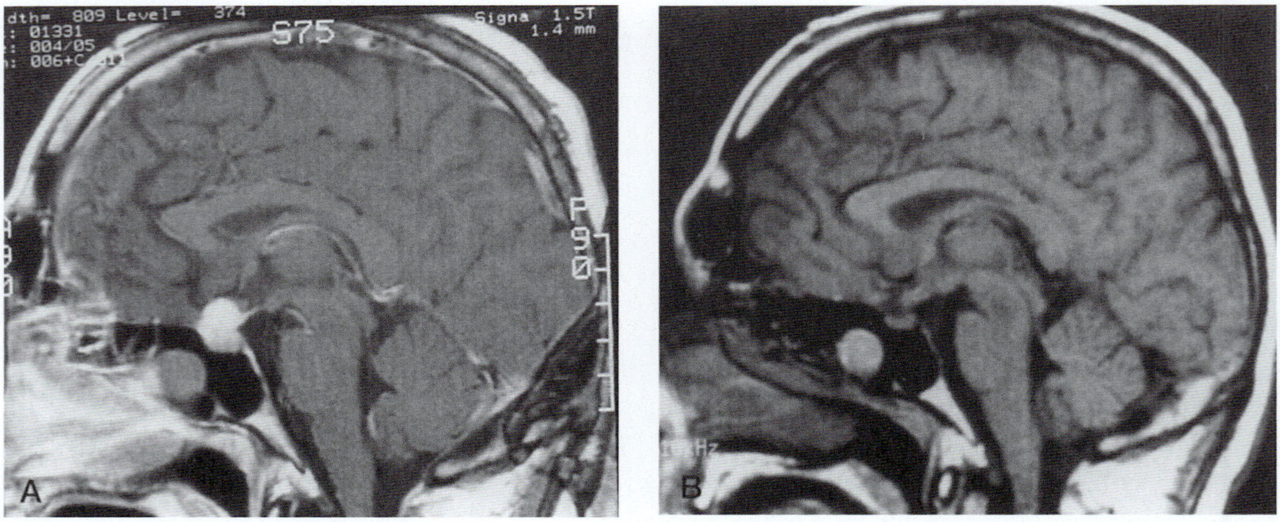

Figure 2–3 **(A)** Preoperative sagittal gadolinium-enhanced T1-weighted magnetic resonance imaging of an intra- or suprasellar craniopharyngioma. **(B)** Postoperative sagittal image showing gross total removal of the tumor with preservation of the pituitary gland and stalk.

septal and thalamostriate veins are identified, the tumor is debulked beginning at its central portion and moving outward **(Fig. 2–5C).** This procedure allows the surrounding tumor capsule to be dissected easily from the surrounding adherent gliotic brain layer. The tumor and its surrounding capsule should be manipulated in a central direction toward the midline to avoid lateral diversion of the dissection, which carries the risk of injuring the hypothalamus and the lateral third ventricular wall. Tumor removal may lead to the interpeduncular fossa; if so, visualization of the basilar artery and its branches becomes important to avoid their injury.

The transcallosal-transventricular approach to craniopharyngiomas is recommended following an attempt at tumor removal through the pterional approach. Starting with the pterional approach has the advantage of achieving good brain relaxation in addition to mobilizing the inferior portion of the tumor and dissecting it from the optic apparatus and the anterior cerebral artery complex and its branches. After the transcallosal part of the tumor resection has been completed, the tumor bed is reinspected through the pterional approach to allow removal of any residual tumor in the retrochiasmatic region or in the interpeduncular fossa. Once total resection is achieved, hemostasis is established, and the wound is closed.

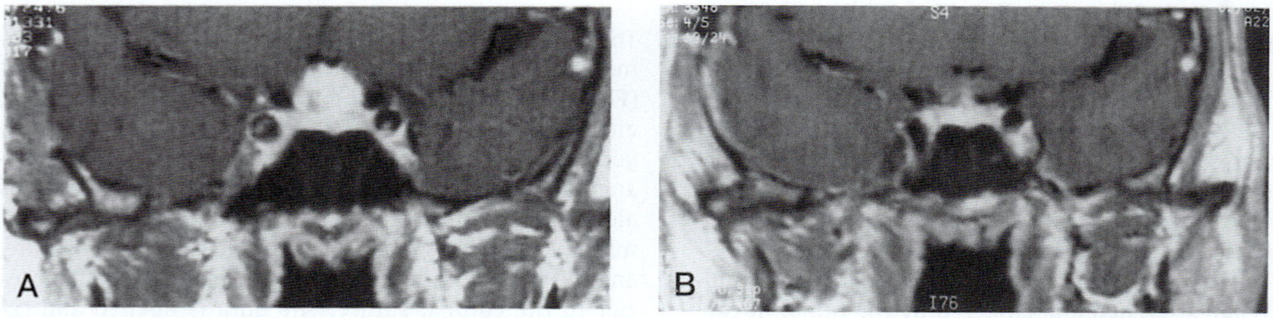

Figure 2–4 **(A)** Preoperative coronal gadolinium-enhanced T1-weighted magnetic resonance imaging of a suprasellar craniopharyngioma. **(B)** Postoperative coronal image showing decompression of the optic apparatus and enhancement along the pituitary stalk. Gross total removal of the tumor was achieved using the pterional-transsylvian approach.

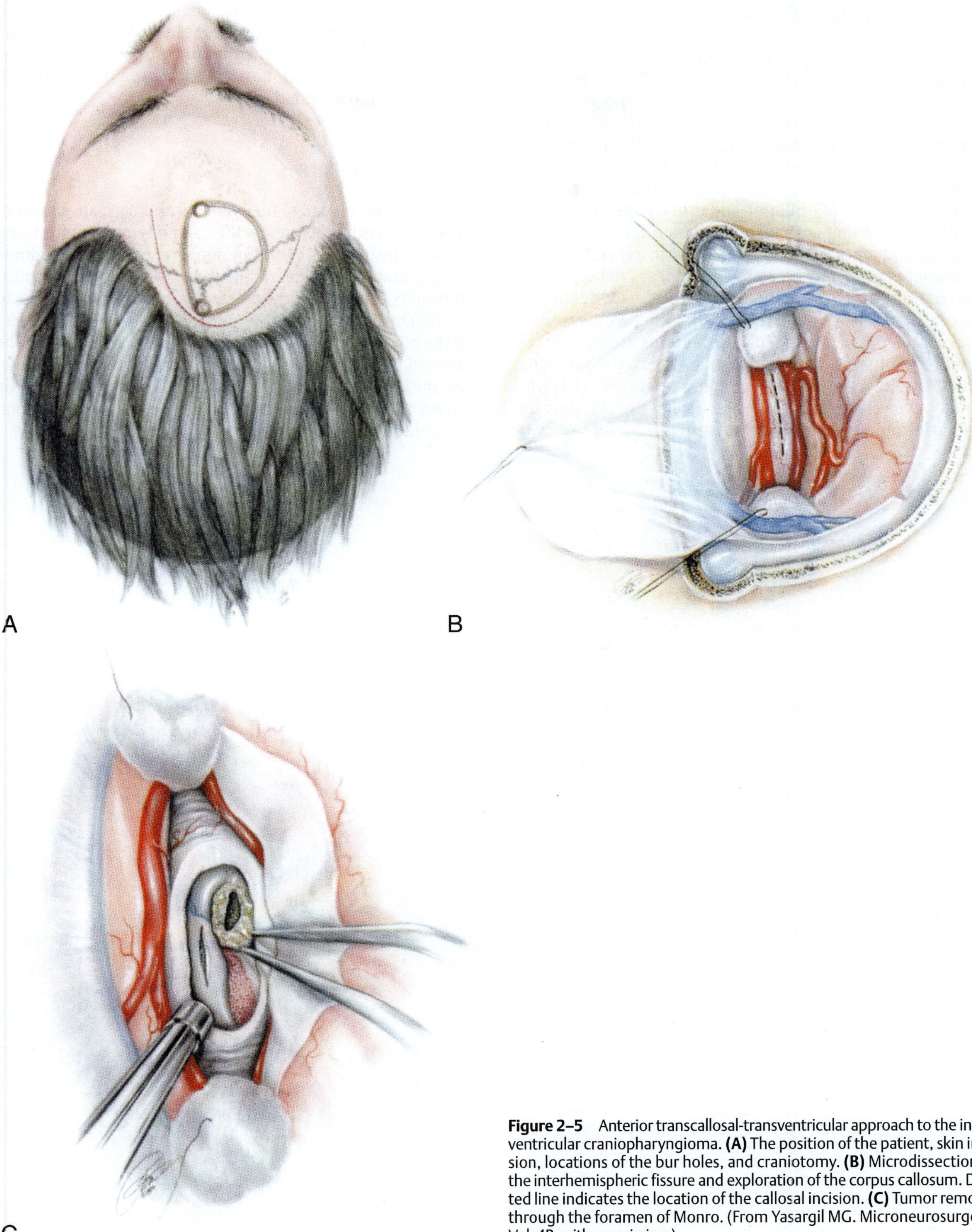

A B C

Figure 2–5 Anterior transcallosal-transventricular approach to the intraventricular craniopharyngioma. **(A)** The position of the patient, skin incision, locations of the bur holes, and craniotomy. **(B)** Microdissection of the interhemispheric fissure and exploration of the corpus callosum. Dotted line indicates the location of the callosal incision. **(C)** Tumor removal through the foramen of Monro. (From Yasargil MG. Microneurosurgery, Vol. 4B, with permission.)

◆ Postoperative Care

Patients usually remain in the intensive care unit for 1 or 2 nights after surgery. They are kept on fluid restriction ($<$500 mL/24 hours) even after resuming food intake by mouth and are carefully monitored for signs of diabetes insipidus. If the urine output is more than 250 mL/h for 2 hours or more than a total of 500 mL for 2 hours, a stat serum sodium is obtained with a urine specific gravity. If the serum sodium is $>$142 mEq/dL and urinary specific gravity is $<$10.10, then 5 units of aqueous Pitressin are given subcutaneously and repeated every 6 hours on an as needed basis.

If diabetes insipidus persists and appears to be permanent, patients are started on desmopressin [1-deamino-8-D-arginine vasopressin (DDAVP)], which is given as a nasal spray once a day at bedtime. Steroids are usually tapered to the maintenance dose of 20 mg in the morning and 10 mg in the evening. An a.m. cortisol level is obtained 1 week after discharge and a day after skipping an a.m. dose to determine if further cortisol replacement is needed. A serum T4 level is obtained before discharge and again 1 week after discharge to evaluate the need for thyroid hormone replacement therapy. An evaluation of the other anterior pituitary hormones is made during the 30-day postoperative period.

◆ Complications

Complications related to the pterional approach are similar to those seen with other neurosurgical intracranial procedures. Diabetes insipidus is very common after craniopharyngioma surgery and is usually permanent due to damage of the pituitary stalk. Hypopituitarism may also result from damage to the pituitary stalk. Visual loss is most commonly due to injury of the blood supply of the optic apparatus. This can best be avoided by the surgeon having a detailed understanding of the microsurgical and microvascular anatomy of the optic nerves and chiasm. Rarely, coma and autonomic dysfunction occur due to hypothalamic injury.

3

Eyebrow Orbitotomy Approach to Parasellar Tumors

Behnam Badie

The eyebrow orbitotomy, also called the orbital roof craniotomy, is a modification of the subfrontal craniotomy through a limited eyebrow incision. This keyhole approach can provide a small corridor into the frontal skull base and suprasellar region while minimizing frontal lobe retraction.

◆ Patient Selection

Eyebrow orbitotomy is ideal for anterior skull base meningiomas such as clinoidal, olfactory groove, tuberculum sellar, and planum sphenoidale meningiomas. It can also be used to access most sellar and parasellar tumors with suprasellar extension. We have used this approach as a less invasive alternative to the frontotemporal approach to resect anterior skull base meningiomas or parasellar tumors such as pituitary adenomas or craniopharyngiomas **(Fig. 3–1)**. An even smaller version of this approach can also be used to repair frontal fossa defects such as meningoceles.

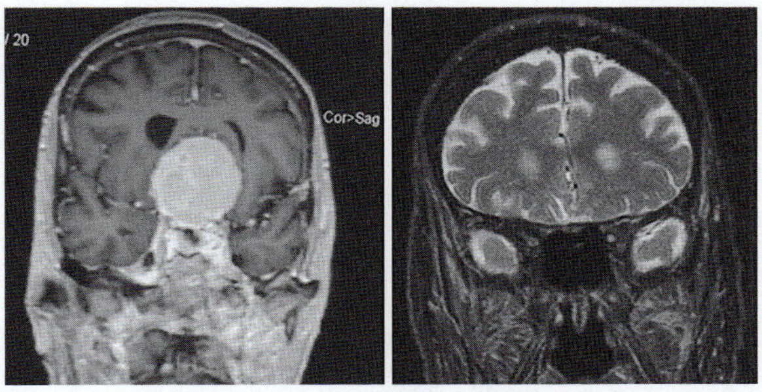

A B

Figure 3–1 **(A)** Preoperative coronal T1 and **(B)** 6-month postoperative coronal T2 images of an 81-year-old female with a planum sphenoidale meningioma completely removed through an eyebrow orbitotomy. Note absence of frontal lobe retraction injury in the postoperative image.

Small subchiasmatic tumors, however, may be difficult to approach through this route if the optic nerves and chiasm are displaced anteriorly (prefixed chiasm).

◆ Preoperative Preparation and Operative Procedure

The patient's head is immobilized in a three-pin holder and, depending on the location of the tumor, rotated 10 to 30 degrees. Ophthalmic antibiotic ointment is applied to the eye, which is kept closed with Tagaderm (3M Health, St. Paul, MN). After prepping and draping, a 4 to 5 cm incision is made through the eyebrow **(Fig. 3–2)**. The

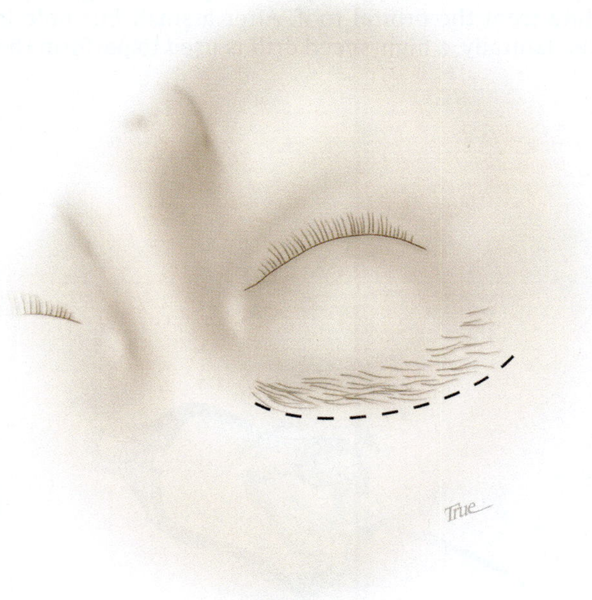

Figure 3–2 The procedure is begun with a 4 to 5 cm incision a few mm above or through the eyebrow.

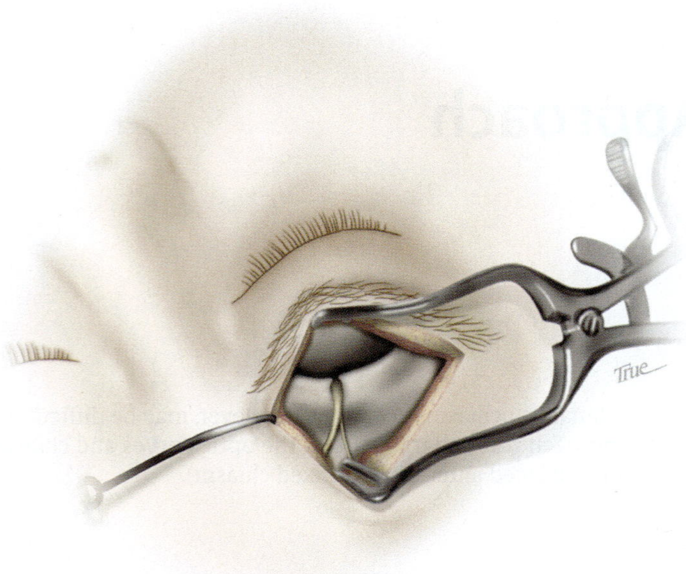

Figure 3–3 The frontalis muscle is divided and the supraorbital nerve is dissected using sharp scissors.

frontalis muscle is divided and the supraorbital nerve is dissected using sharp scissors **(Fig. 3–3)**. Although this nerve can be preserved for small tumors, it is cut in most cases to obtain a larger corridor **(Fig. 3–4)**. The periosteum is then freed from the orbital ridge and frontal bone. This plane is then extended by carefully dissecting the periorbita from the orbital roof. After a small bur hole is placed laterally, a high-speed drill is used to perform the most superior aspect of the craniotomy **(Fig. 3–5)**. While protecting the dura through the bur hole, a limited orbitotomy, which may extend into the frontal sinus medially, is performed using an oscillating saw **(Fig. 3–6)**. A small osteotome is then used to fracture the roof of the orbit, and finally a single bone flap consisting of the orbital ridge and the orbital roof can be removed **(Fig. 3–7)**. The mucosa of the frontal sinus is removed completely and

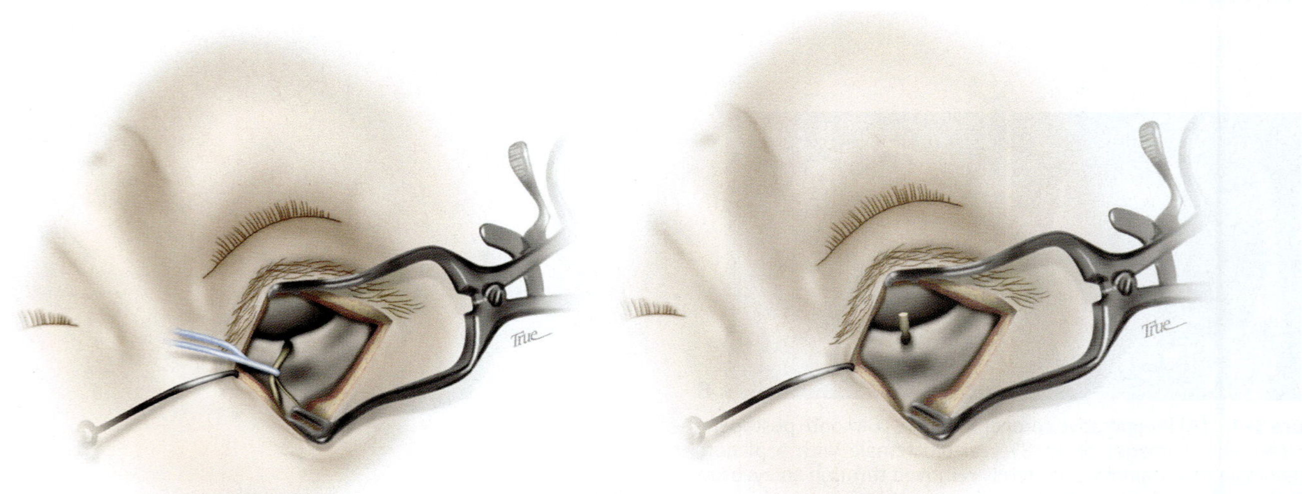

A B

Figure 3–4 **(A)** The supraorbital nerve can be saved and retracted with a vessel loop. **(B)** For larger tumors, however, this nerve is divided to obtain a larger exposure.

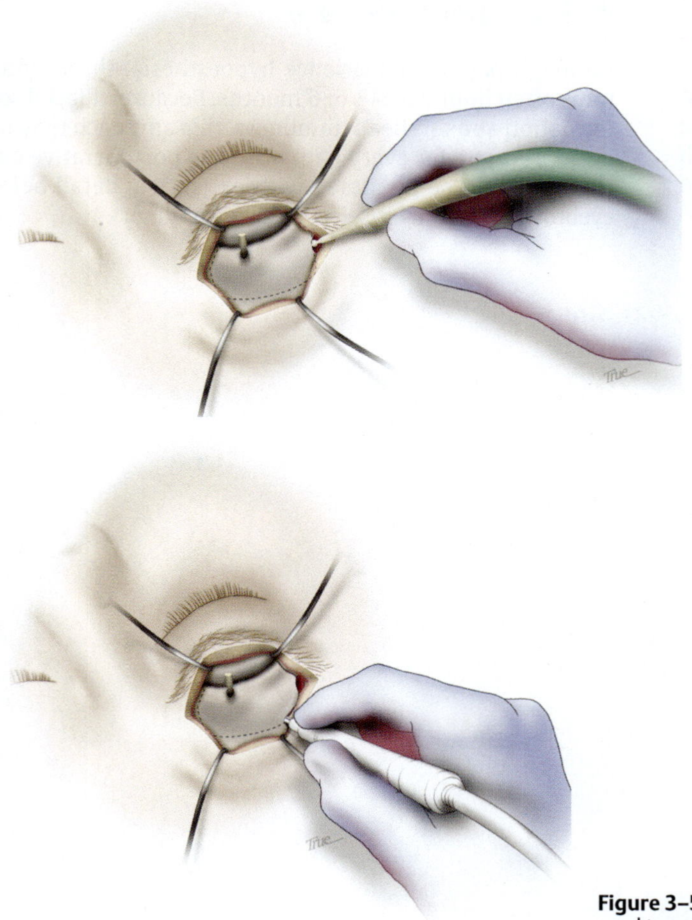

A

B

Figure 3–5 **(A)** A small bur hole is placed laterally and **(B)** a high-speed drill is used to perform the most superior aspect of the craniotomy.

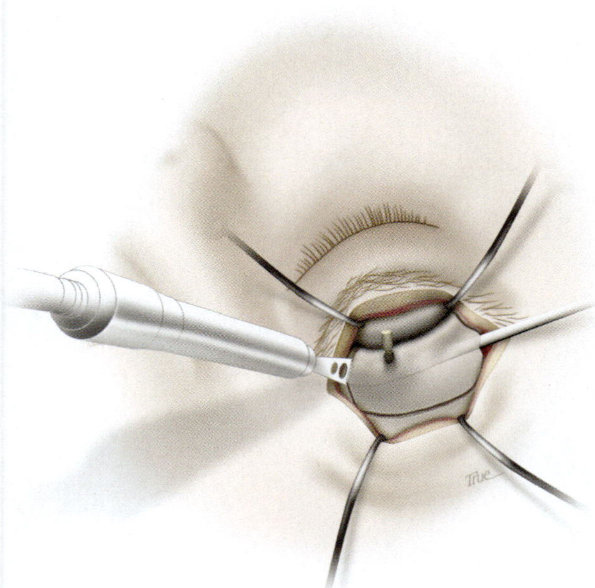

Figure 3–6 An oscillating saw is used to cut the orbital rim laterally and medially. The dura is protected by passing a small dissector through the bur hole.

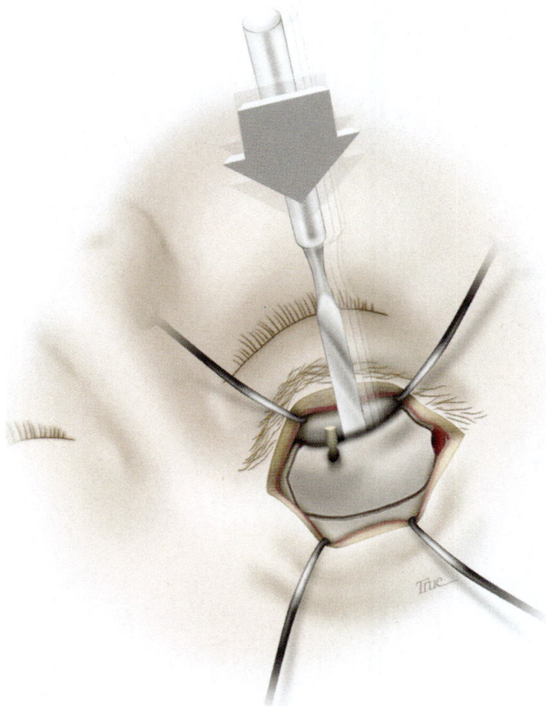

Figure 3–7 A small osteotome is used to fracture the roof of the orbit. A single bone flap consisting of the orbital ridge and the orbital roof can then be removed.

the sinus is packed with pieces of Gelfoam, bone wax, and sometimes abdominal fat. The dura is opened in a curvilinear fashion.

The dura is closed with 4–0 nonabsorbable sutures and the bone flap is fixed with small titanium plates. The frontalis muscle is approximated and the skin closed with 6–0 nylon sutures. The sutures are removed in 5 days to minimize scar formation.

◆ Postoperative Care

Although patients experience hypoesthesia, these symptoms often improve in 3 to 6 months. Because of facial scar formation and forehead numbness, this approach may not be appropriate for every patient. These postoperative outcomes should be discussed with patients in detail before eyebrow orbitotomy is selected for such tumors.

4

Expanded Endonasal Approach to the Sella and Anterior Skull Base

Amin B. Kassam, Arlan H. Mintz, Carl H. Snyderman, Paul A. Gardner, Ricardo L. Carrau, and Joseph C. Maroon

This chapter outlines the technical nuances of a fully endoscopic, completely transnasal approach to the ventral skull base along a midline sagittal plane from the sella through the anterior skull base and crista galli rostrally. The development of endoscopic approaches to the pituitary fossa represents the foundation for this work. We have subsequently expanded from this platform to develop the expanded endonasal approach (EEA). We present a series of modular approaches along the rostral–caudal axis of the ventral skull base facilitating the management of a wide variety of both intradural and extradural pathologies.

In this chapter we describe the technical nuances, key anatomical principles, and specialized equipment required for these approaches. We begin by describing the general approach to the sphenoid sinus and then describe techniques for intrasellar/intradural resection. We then provide the segmental modular EEAs extending to the crista galli. These modules can be used individually or in combination based on the location of the lesion.

◆ Patient Selection

The EEA has been used to treat a variety of nonneoplastic and neoplastic conditions of the ventral skull base. The most common nonneoplastic diagnosis (other than inflammatory sinus disease) is a cerebral spinal fluid leak (traumatic, iatrogenic, and spontaneous). The most common benign neoplasms are pituitary adenomas, meningiomas, and craniopharyngiomas. In terms of malignant lesions, sinonasal cancers with cranial base involvement are the most frequent malignant neoplasms treated. Other neoplasms such as chordomas and olfactory neuroblastomas are being increasingly treated, given their ideal midline position. Although endoscopic techniques have become well established for the treatment of benign extradural and skull base pathology, there are limited data regarding their use for both benign and malignant intradural tumors. Long-term outcome data will be needed to address this question. An ideal application for EEA is to obtain tissue diagnosis. Currently, endoscopic techniques allow a preoperative biopsy with minimal morbidity, often in an outpatient setting.

There are few contraindications to the EEA for pathological conditions of the ventral skull base. In principle there are two factors that need to be considered: patient/tumor characteristics and surgical experience of the operating team.

Patient and Tumor Characteristics

The patient must be a suitable medical candidate for surgery and anesthesia. In our experience, tumor extent has not been a limiting factor and the EEA can achieve the same resection margins as traditional open approaches for ventral skull base lesions, providing the orientation of the neurovascular structures is suitable. This is predicated on the surgeon's experience that is best gained in clearly defined increments (as will be described). If an orbital exenteration or resection of external tissues is necessary, then the EEA does not offer any advantages over an open approach. Dural involvement and brain invasion represent the same degree of contraindications as they would for any open approach. These factors have not been limitations for EEA; specifically, we have been able to achieve a comparable degree of resection in appropriately selected patients as we would with an open approach. Similarly, we have not found tumor type or vascularity to represent an additional limitation when considering an EEA versus an open approach.

The most important tumor characteristic in selecting an open approach versus EEA is the exact relationship of the tumor to critical neurovascular structures. Simply put, if the neurovascular structures are ventral to the tumor they will be encountered prior to the tumor and will need to be retracted and manipulated when approaching from the ventrally oriented EEAs. In this circumstance it is preferable to use an alternative approach. The EEA is an ideal approach for lesions where the critical neurovascular structures are on the perimeter of the tumor, thus allowing for direct access to the tumor with minimal manipulation of normal neurovascular structures. Currently, the EEA is also contraindicated when resection or reconstruction of a major vessel is needed.

In summary, the degree of resection in our experience has been determined based on a combination of several key predetermined factors that define the goals of surgery: patient age; premorbid conditions; symptoms, and natural history of the lesion. These are the same factors that determine the goals of surgery whether an EEA or open approach is being considered.

Surgical Experience of the Team

When selecting this approach, the experience of the surgical team is as important as the aforementioned patient and tumor characteristics. There may be institutional barriers to selecting the EEA, such as availability of equipment or personnel to create the necessary team. The primary contraindication to EEA is the lack of progressive experience that is gained from each module and pathology type before progressing to the next.

◆ Preoperative Preparation

We use intraoperative frameless stereotactic image guidance in all patients. Image-guided surgery (IGS) is of value in identifying critical structures and allows for targeted resection. In the case of pituitary adenomas magnetic resonance imaging (MRI) is preferable because soft-tissue visualization is of paramount importance. For other EEAs, we prefer fine-cut computed tomographic (CT) angiography that allows for the simultaneous visualization of osseous, vascular, and soft tissue anatomy critical in creating a targeted approach.

Following endotracheal intubation the patient is positioned supine with the head in neutral position held by Mayfield pins. Rigid immobilization of the patient's head is preferred because it prevents the potential risk of movement during detailed drilling and dissection. Somatosensory evoked potentials, brain stem evoked responses, and cranial nerve electromyograms (EMGs) are monitored as appropriate. Nasal decongestion is achieved by packing the nasal cavities with pledgets soaked in oxymetazoline 0.05% while the IGS registration is completed. The skin of the external nose and nasal vestibule as well as the abdomen (fat graft donor site) is prepped with a povidone antiseptic solution. The patient is given a fourth-generation cephalosporin for perioperative prophylaxis. The endoscopist and dissecting surgeon stand on the patient's right. The LCD monitors are arranged in an array 270 degrees around the patient's head. To optimize comfort each surgeon uses a different monitor for viewing. The image guidance is placed at the patient's head **(Fig. 4–1A).**

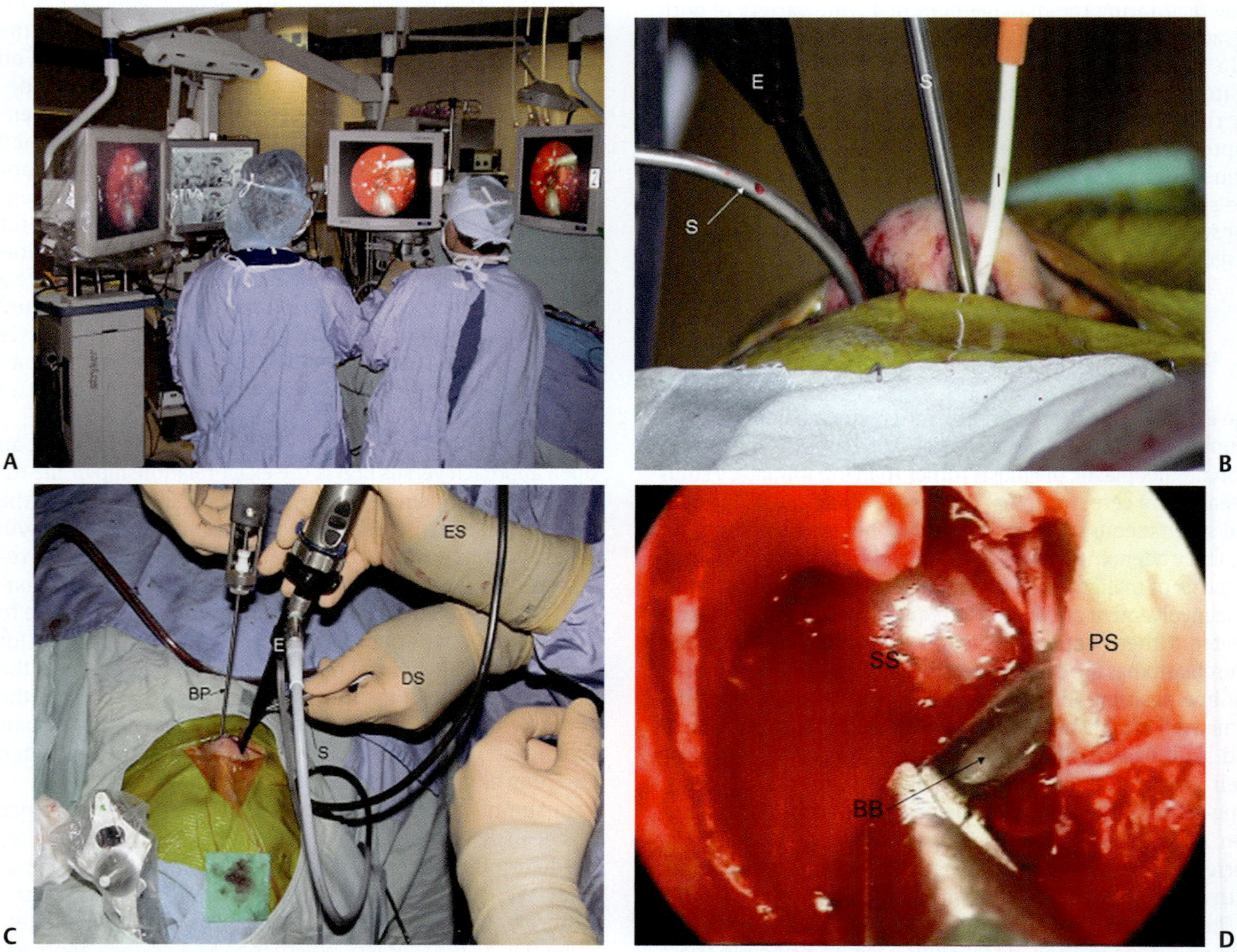

Figure 4–1 **(A)** Patient positioning. **(B,C)** Instrument positioning. E, endoscope; S, suction; I, irrigation; DS, dissecting surgeon; ES, endoscopic surgeon; BP, endoscopic bipolar. **(D)** Resection of the posterior nasal septum. PS, posterior septum; SS, sphenoid sinus; BB, back bitter.

◆ Operative Procedure

General Exposure

Bilateral access to the sphenoid sinus represents the foundation for the initial exposure utilized in all anatomical modules of the EEA. The exposure commences through the right nares using a 0 degree endoscope. The middle turbinate is resected and the ipsilateral sphenoid ostium is identified and opened to fashion a wide sphenoidotomy. The endoscope is then entered into the contralateral nares to mobilize, but not resect, the contralateral middle turbinate. A large, wide, bilateral sphenoidotomy is fashioned extending to the level of the medial pterygoid plates to maximize light delivery. The removal of all intrasphenoidal septae creates a single rectangular cavity. The endoscopist generally completes the initial exposure. As the dissecting surgeon enters the field, to facilitate exposure, the endoscope is positioned superiorly at "12 o'clock" and held by the endoscopist. The dissecting surgeon places the suction at the 6 o'clock position in the right nares. The left nares is used to introduce dissecting instruments **(Figs. 4–1B,C).** To facilitate a bilateral approach, the posterior septum is detached and a 1 to 2 cm portion is resected. Removal of the posterior septum prevents deflection of the septum into the endoscope while using bilateral instrumentation **(Fig. 4–1D).** This bimanual dissection is mandatory for EEA.

Intradural Endoneurosurgical Dissection Techniques

The basic principles of standard microneurosurgical techniques for tumor removal are strictly adhered to in EEA. They consist of internal debulking, capsular mobilization, extracapsular dissection of neurovascular structures, capsular coagulation, and capsule removal.

Tumor debulking techniques are dependent on the tumor consistency. Softer tumors can be resected utilizing the "two-suction technique." When using this technique, the lumen of one suction is used for debulking and the tip and shaft of the other suction are used for blunt dissection and to provide countertraction. Malleable or bent suctions can be used to improve endoscopic visualization. Tumors with firmer consistency can be crushed and removed using pistol grip through-cutting forceps or removed with a modified EEA ultrasonic aspirator. In some cases, use of a drill may be necessary to thin calcified tumors, which can then be resected piecemeal by circumferential dissection.

As the tumor is debulked, the capsule can be mobilized freely with gentle countertraction applied with a fine suction such as a 6 French. To prevent the disastrous complication of tearing extracapsular vessels, countertraction should be done with a suction and not a grasping instrument. Extracapsular dissection is best done sharply or with blunt endoscopic dissectors and a number 4 French suction in the dominant hand to provide countertraction. The capsule is coagulated using an endoscopic bipolar cautery, with care taken to prevent thermal injury to important neurovascular structures. Critical neurovascular structures can be identified during the extracapsular dissection.

Hemostatic Techniques

Hemostatic techniques can be subdivided into venous and arterial, with specific courses of action employed in each. A bipolar cautery with a pistol-grip design (EEA bipolars, Storz Endoscopy, Culver City, CA) is an essential part of the EEA armamentarium. Standard bayonet designs will close prematurely due to the narrow passage of the nares and are often too short. The prevention of bleeding has been the best defense in the control of bleeding, and a sound knowledge of the skull base anatomy allows avoidance of catastrophic bleeding.

Venous Hemostasis

Mucosal and bone bleeding represent diffuse venous bleeding. This type of bleeding responds very well to warm saline irrigation (40°C) delivered extradurally via a red-rubber catheter and intradurally via an external ventricular drain. Focal venous bleeding, such as that encountered with the cavernous sinus or within the tumor bed, is managed with the focal application of INSTAT Collagen Abserbable Hemostat (Johnson & Johnson, New Brunswick, NJ) on a dry cottonoid pledget. This "sandwich" of Instat is applied directly to the bleeding point and may need to be repeated, with multiple exchanges, until bleeding is controlled.

Arterial Hemostasis

Arterial bleeding can be classified as either high flow or low flow, which corresponds to the diameter of the ruptured vessel. With high-flow bleeding, to address the specific site of arterial rupture, it is critical to segmentalize the bleeding to a relatively specific portion of the artery. Isolation of the bleeding portion is generally done with suction, with the goal of having the extravasating blood running directly up the suction. Once the portion of the artery that is bleeding has been identified, the direct application of bipolar coagulation along the sidewall of the vessel is often possible. Because blood has a tremendous capacity for heat dispersion, diffuse coagulation to the vessel will not be as effective as direct application over the vessel tear with the bleeding controlled. Further removal of bone may be necessary to isolate the site of rupture.

The technique is similar for low-flow arterial bleeding. One must be cautious in avoiding thermal injury to small perforating vessels with heat dispersion from the bipolar cautery. Isolated segmental packing with a variety of hemostatic materials can also be used. The packing must be applied focally. There is a significant danger of the vessel retracting or for the bleeding to continue in a retrograde fashion into the adjacent brain, with the subsequent complication of parenchymal hemorrhage with devastating consequences. We therefore rarely use packing as a technique to control arterial bleeding. It is imperative to remember that if an arterial vessel of significant caliber has been sealed with either technique the risk of delayed development of pseudoaneurysm must be considered and appropriately investigated.

Pituitary and Sellar Approaches

Exposure

Exposure of the sella for resection of sellar lesions follows the general exposure already reported. The sellar exposure is widened by extending the bilateral sphenoidotomy through the lateral recess of the sphenoid laterally to the level of the parasellar carotid protuberance. To achieve the rostral margin, the ethmoidal septae are reduced to the level of anterior cranial base. This provides direct visualization of the planum–tuberculum junction. The complete reduction of the sphenoid floor to the level of the clival recess, using a high speed drill, completes the caudal margin. To achieve the required rostral angle, the caudal exposure is critical for macroadenomas with suprasellar extension.

To visualize the critical bony landmarks of the sphenoid sinus, we favor the removal of mucosa of the sphenoid sinus. The critical bony landmarks include the medial opticocarotid recess (mOCR), the carotid protuberance within the parasellar space (ICA), the sellar face, the clival recess, and the strut of bone over the superior intercavernous sinus (SIS) **(Fig. 4–2A).**

The mOCR is the ventral side of the region of the optic canal and tuberculum sella and represents the key anatomical landmark of the sphenoid floor. Simultaneous access to the carotid canal, optic canal, sella, and medial cavernous sinus can be achieved through the mOCR during an EEA. This is analogous to the "key hole" described during a conventional pterional craniotomy. The mOCR does not usually contain tumor unless there is significant suprasellar and lateral extension toward the opticocarotid cistern. For lesions that extend into the anterior cranial fossa, it is mandatory that the strut of bone overlying the superior intercavernous sinus is resected. Our final exposure represents a large rectangle extending rostrally from the SIS to the inferior cavernous sinus caudally and medially from one mOCR to the other **(Fig. 4–2B).**

Intrasellar Dissection

An important distinction from traditional microseptal transsphenoidal tumor dissection is the use of the two-suction technique and the reliance on the principles of microsurgical technique, rather than the use of curettes. The endoscope provides the necessary visualization to utilize these techniques, even within confined spaces such as the sella. Although we appreciate that extracapsular dissection for pituitary tumors is often not possible, we advocate debulking using two suctions or an EEA aspirator for firmer tumors. This method, in our opinion, results in less trauma to the pituitary gland and infundibulum during tumor separation and provides greater control of the cavernous sinus and its contents.

Systematic intrasellar dissection is a key principle to optimize visualization and preserve the normal gland tissue. One must try to prevent premature descent of the diaphragma, and subsequent descent, which will obstruct visualization. Using a sickle knife, the dura is opened in the center of the sella and extended caudally and obliquely toward the 8 o'clock and 5 o'clock positions, creating the inferior flap **(Fig. 4–3A).** To hold the anterior face of the tumor overlying the diaphragma, the superior dural flap is left intact. Macroadenomas will herniate through the inferior opening of the dura, allowing this portion of the tumor to be removed in a posterior trajectory toward the clival–dorsum junction. The inferior portion of the tumor is resected widely between each cavernous sinus laterally and posteriorly to the dorsum using the two-suction technique **(Fig. 4–3B).** Because macroadenomas can thin the dorsum, caution should be exercised during this portion to avoid entering the basilar cistern. At this point, the exposed dura can be coagulated and the lateral dissection along the cavernous–carotid recess can be initiated. The dural opening is now extended superiorly to increase the exposure, and dissection can be completed along the lateral recesses from a caudal to rostral direction.

There are two common sites that should be carefully assessed for retained tumor. The first is the region of the mOCR

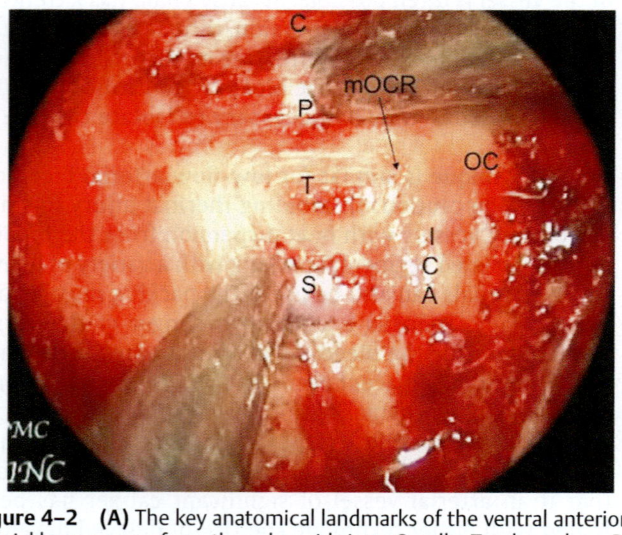

A

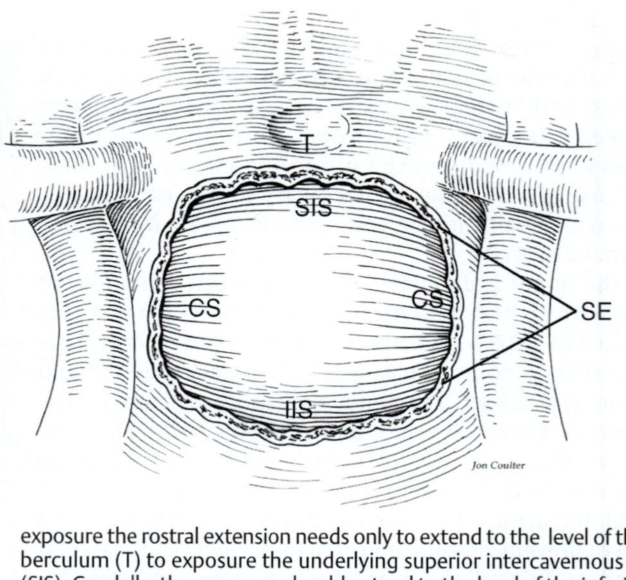

B

Figure 4–2 **(A)** The key anatomical landmarks of the ventral anterior cranial base as seen from the sphenoid sinus. S, sella; T, tuberculum; P, planum; C, crista gali; ICA, internal carotid artery; OC, optic canal; mOCR, medial opticocarotid recess. **(B)** Schematic drawing of the completed sellar exposure (SE) required for a routine pituitary macroadenoma. For this exposure the rostral extension needs only to extend to the level of the tuberculum (T) to exposure the underlying superior intercavernous sinus (SIS). Caudally, the exposure should extend to the level of the inferior intercavernous sinus (IIS). Laterally, the bony removal should exposure the medial portion of the cavernous sinus (CS).

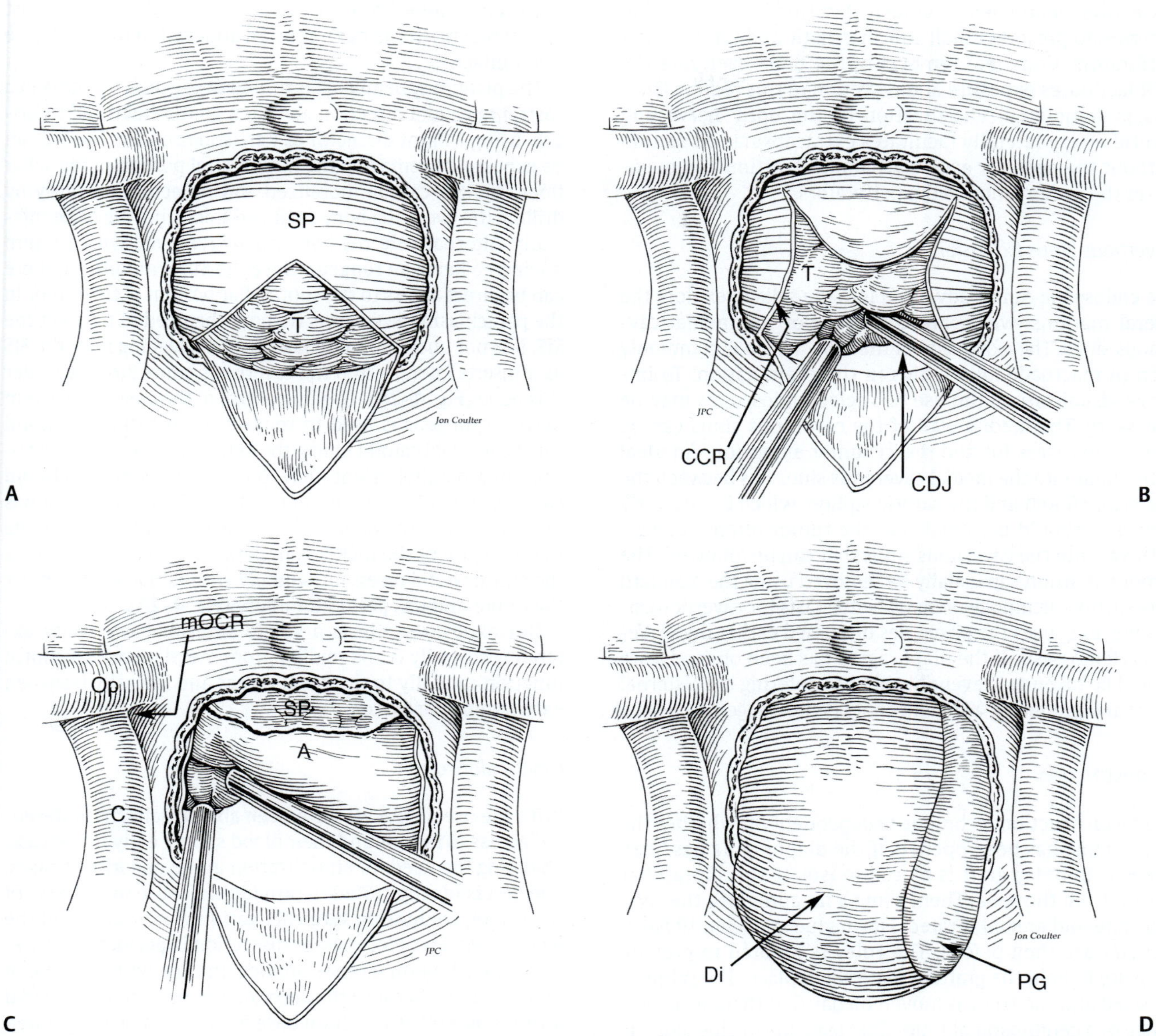

Figure 4–3 Schematic drawing outlining the opening of the sella dura amd the sequence of intrasellar tumor dissection. **(A)** Opening of the inferior leaves of the dura leaving the superior portion (SP) intact to prevent tumor (T) herniation and consequent visual obstruction. **(B)** Tumor (T) removal is initiated inferiorly in a posterior direction to the level of the clival dorsum junction. Then tumor resection continues in an inferior lateral direction along both carotid cavernous recesses (CCR). **(C)** Release of the superior portion (SP) of the dura is followed by superior lateral dissection intradurally along both medial optico (Op) -carotid (C) recesses (mOCR). Tumor along the anterior superior portion of the dura (A) under the SIS will subsequently be removed. **(D)** Final view showing concentric descent of the diaphragma (Di) often having a thin rim of residual pituitary gland (PG) pasted on its surface.

and the opticocarotid angle from inside the sella superolaterally. The other common site is under the anterior lip of dura at the level of the SIS directly beneath the sellar–tuberculum junction **(Fig. 4–3C)**. Removal of tumor along the anterior face overlying the diaphragma optimizes visualization of this segment and this will also allow for the diaphragma to descend resulting in an opening of the superior angle. To optimize visualization, the remaining dura can be coagulated shrinking it back to the SIS and the overlying sellar bone can be removed.

The final inspection of the sella occurs in a systematic way and usually in a clockwise fashion, staring inferiorly at 6 o'clock. Visualization is improved with the use of an angled endoscope if required. During this final inspection, the diaphragma should have descended concentrically. In our experience, the residual gland is most commonly observed to appear as an apron plastered to the undersurface of the diaphragma **(Fig. 4–3D)**. Failure of the diaphragma to descend concentrically usually indicates retained tumor in the suprasellar space. Further dissection to attempt to remove this portion depends on the goals of surgery. In a planned staged surgery, that portion may be left. In the case of optic decompression as the primary goal, tumor removal should continue until pulsations are visible in the diaphragma. If the surgical goal is complete resection and diaphragma descent is not concentric, then the diaphragma is electively opened and tumor in the suprasellar cistern can be removed until the optic nerves are directly visualized. During this portion, we strongly advocate the use of endosurgical dissection techniques previously described, as opposed to curettes, to preserve small subchiasmatic and infundibular perforators. Complete removal of the bone overlying the OCR facilitates exposure and resection in this region. Once this is completed, visualization of the optic nerve and carotid artery laterally facilitates extracapsular dissection without the need for excessive countertraction and maximizes the preservation of the perforators.

Cavernous Sinus Extension

The endoscope can be advanced into the sella to explore the lateral margins, which are composed of the medial cavernous sinus. The expansion of the sella, which is commonly seen in macroadenomas, aids in the examination. To improve visualization, the use of angled endoscopes may be necessary. The medial wall of the cavernous sinus can be opened to assess for and resect tumor extension. An ideal entry point into the medial cavernous sinus lies between the posterior clinoid and the carotid siphon, which is anteriorly placed. It should be noted that the tumor often creates a pathway into the cavernous sinus that can be followed. The tumor extension can usually be removed using the standard two-suction technique. Venous hemostasis for cavernous sinus bleeding uses the principles discussed earlier under Venous Hemostasis. If the diaphragma has been opened, care should be taken to prevent blood from entering the cisternal space and producing a subarachnoid hemorrhage.

Reconstruction

The reconstruction technique is dependent on whether the diaphragma has been opened. If the diaphragma has been opened, an onlay graft is placed to isolate the suprasellar cistern from the sella. Then, using a fat autograft, the sella and sphenoid are obliterated. Fibrin glue and a no. 10 Foley catheter are then placed. The Foley is inflated to provide pressure to hold the grafting material in place. The saline is released and the Foley removed on day 5. If there is no evidence of a cerebrospinal fluid (CSF) leak, fibrin glue alone is placed within the sella.

Transtuberculum/Transplanum Approach

Building on the experience with the sellar and parasellar approaches we have developed a series of modular expanded approaches to address lesions of the skull base, including the transtuberculm/transplanum and transcribriform approaches to the anterior skull base.

Extradural Exposure

This module is initiated by utilizing the general bilateral approach to the sphenoid. The rostral extension is then initiated by completing wide bilateral anterior and posterior ethmoidectomies. Using a high-speed drill the ethmoid septations are drilled flush to the anterior cranial base and laterally to the level of the lamina papyracea.

In the transplanum approach, to avoid compromising olfaction, the exposure should not extend rostral to the level of the posterior ethmoidal arteries and canals, and the most rostral margin of the nasal septum attached to the skull base is left intact.

The planum sphenoidale is drilled to eggshell thinness in a rostral to caudal direction and then gently fractured inferiorly using a blunt dissector or Kerrison rongeur. The SIS can be exposed by removing the most rostral portion of the sellar floor. The SIS can be mobilized and reflected inferiorly by drilling the overlying bony strut and fracturing the bone inferiorly. Alternatively, the bone can be removed with a 1-mm 45 degree Kerrison rongeur. Once the SIS is mobilized, there can be direct access to the suprasellar portion of the tumor in the parachiasmatic cisterns without the need to transect the SIS. It is not uncommon to have venous bleeding from the SIS as it inserts laterally into the cavernous sinus directly under this bone **(Fig. 4–2A).** To gain control of the bleeding a 1-mm Kerrison rongeur is used to remove the paraclinoid carotid canals. To avoid carotid injury, the Kerrison is positioned vertically in a parallel orientation to the underlying subclinoid carotid, and only one third of the distal tip of the Kerrison is used to remove the bone. Drilling the remainder of the bone in the region of the mOCR is imperative to be able to access the opticocarotid recess intradurally without having to retract the tumor and risk perforator injury **(Fig. 4–2A).**

Our exposure reflects a single anterior base cavity extending rostrally in the midline from the planum–cribriform junction caudally to the clival recess and laterally between each lamina papyracea.

Devascularization

With the use of EEA we have been able to gain circumferential access to lesions and their blood supply early in the case, obviating the need for embolization in the majority of cases. The EEA is ideally suited to provide exposure to the base of the tumor, facilitating surgical ligation/cauterization of the feeding vessels before tumor dissection is performed. Anteriorly based meningiomas provide an excellent example of this technique because the anterior and posterior ethmoidal arteries as well as the dural base feeders can be coagulated at the start of the exposure, removing a significant portion of the vascular supply to the tumor. In addition, we commonly identify an arterial feeder arising from the distal portion of the paraclinoid carotid at the level of the opticocarotid recess, which is coagulated. When dealing with the posterior ethmoidal artery it is important to prevent the proximal stump from retracting into the orbit. This can be responsible for a retrobulbar hematoma. To provide further devascularization, the exposed dura is then coagulated.

Dural Opening

Being cautious not to transgress the prechiasmatic cisterns, the dura is opened in a cruciate fashion with the sickle knife and then endoscopic scissors. It should be emphasized that the dura should be opened in stages because an extensive dural opening could allow normal brain to herniate through the defect and obscure visualization. The extent of the dural opening is marked by the anterior margin of the lesion and its brain interface. If this interface is not seen, further bone and dura removal should be done at this point.

Intradural Dissection

The principles of endoneurosurgical dissection have already been discussed and include a systematic extracapsular dissection, which in this case extends through the parachiasmatic cisterns to identify the critical neurovascular structures.

To identify the optic nerve, first locate the paraclinoid carotid as it emerges intradurally at the level of the mOCR **(Fig. 4–4A).** Following the carotid, the optic nerve will be located slightly superiorly. Tumor can be separated from the optic nerve, with circumferential extracapsular dissection leading to the chiasm and infundibulum **(Fig. 4–4B).** At this point the extracapsular circumferential dissection continues to expose the anterior communicating artery (AcomA), and then the contralateral A_1, optic nerve, infundibulum, and carotid **(Fig. 4–4C).** Safe extracapsular dissection should only be undertaken when the tumor capsule is thin enough to allow for gentle traction with no more than a 4 or 6 French suction. The thinned capsule will allow the arachnoid bands of the parachiasmatic cisterns to be on enough tension to facilitate sharp dissection **(Fig. 4–4D).**

Prior to coagulation of the capsule, there are several additional critical anatomical structures that should specifically be identified and dissected. The infundibulum can be adherent to the posterior margin of the capsule and can be easily damaged during coagulation of the base of the tumor at the tuberculum–sellar junction. The infundibulum should be identified prior to bipolaring in this region. As discussed previously, there are several small subchiasmatic perforators that can be draped around the circumference of the tumor. If there is adequate debulking and mobilization of the tumor these perforators can usually be spared. Branches from the perforators that feed the tumor can be isolated, coagulated, and then sectioned. Lastly, during the parachiasmatic dissection, it is critical to identify the Acom, and also the recurrent artery of Huebner, which can be draped over the superior surface of the tumor **(Fig. 4–4C).**

Transcribriform Approach

Extradural Approach

This module extends the previous exposure rostrally to the level of the crista galli. Access can also be gained to the back wall of the frontal sinus via the frontoethmoidal recess. The exposure utilizes the general bilateral exposure and the transplanum module. To initiate the transcribriform approach the anterior attachment of the posterior

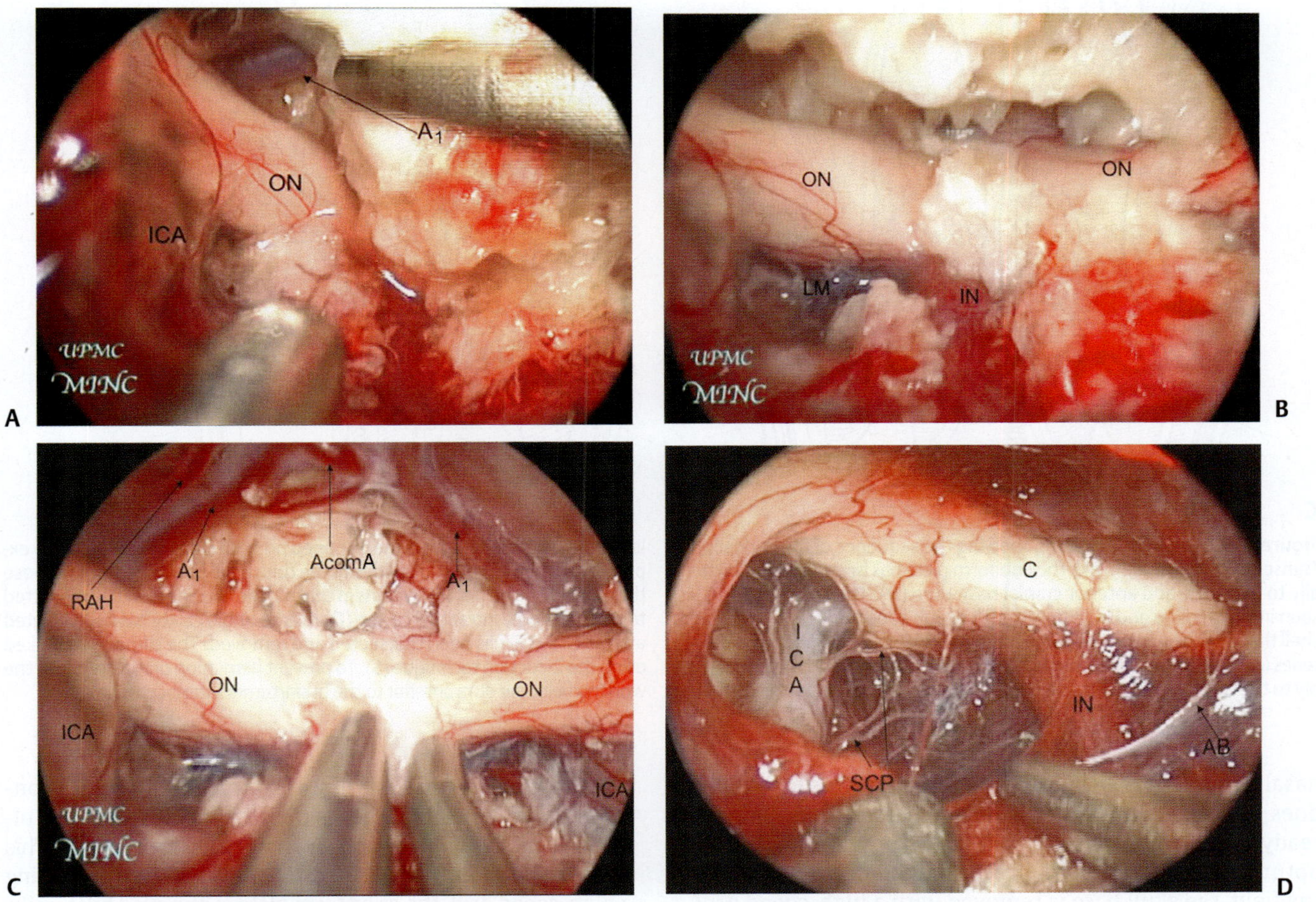

Figure 4–4 (A,B) Initial exposure of the optic nerve, carotid, and A_1. ICA, internal carotid artery; ON, optic nerve; A_1, first segment of right anterior cerebral artery; IN, infundibulum; LM, membrane of Liliequist. **(C)** Exposure of the anterior communicating artery complex. AcomA, anterior communicating artery; RAH, recurrent artery of Huebner. **(D)** Final exposure demonstrating arachnoid band (AB) dissection. C, chiasm; SCP, subchiasmatic perforators.

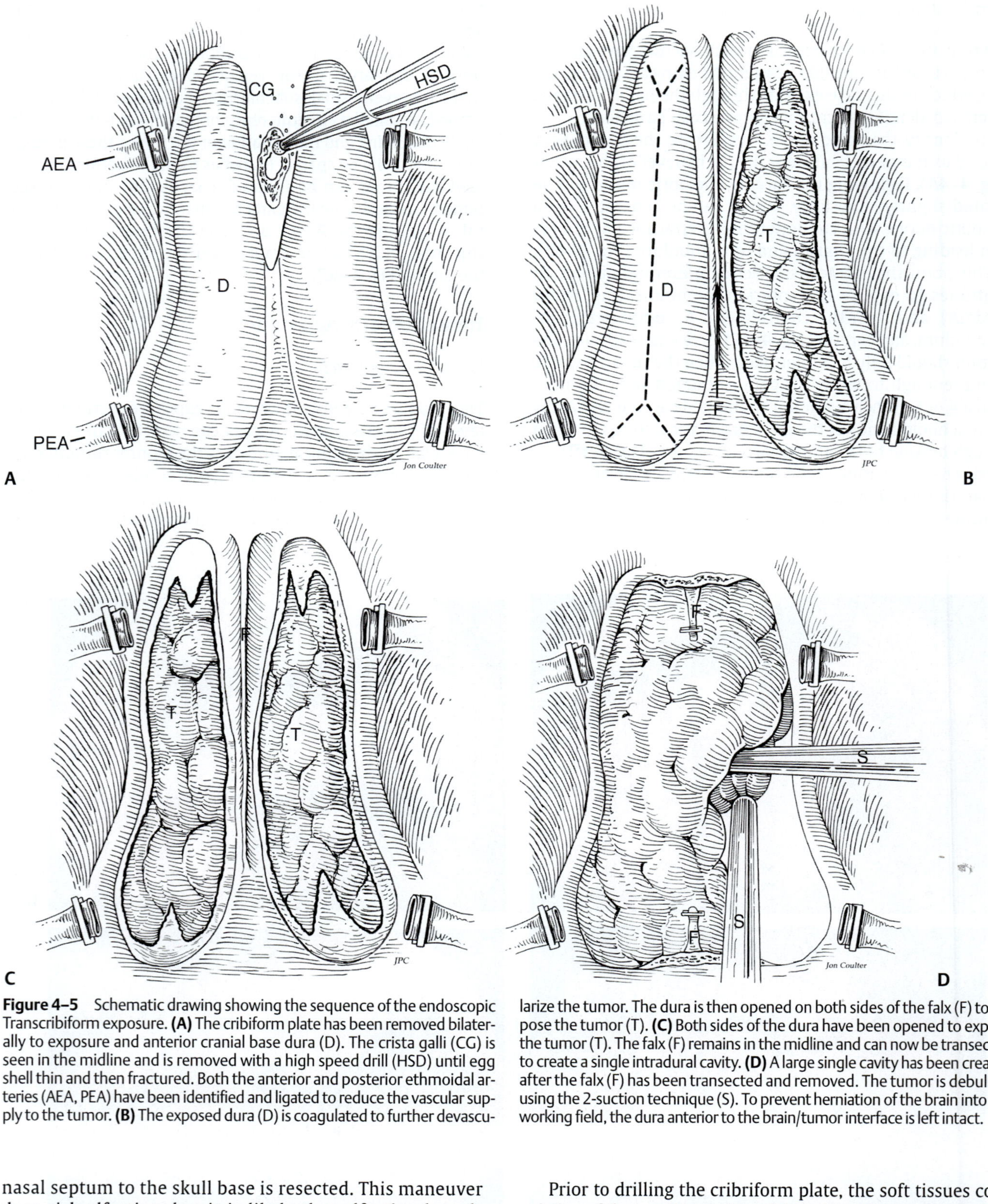

Figure 4–5 Schematic drawing showing the sequence of the endoscopic Transcribiform exposure. **(A)** The cribiform plate has been removed bilaterally to exposure and anterior cranial base dura (D). The crista galli (CG) is seen in the midline and is removed with a high speed drill (HSD) until egg shell thin and then fractured. Both the anterior and posterior ethmoidal arteries (AEA, PEA) have been identified and ligated to reduce the vascular supply to the tumor. **(B)** The exposed dura (D) is coagulated to further devascularize the tumor. The dura is then opened on both sides of the falx (F) to expose the tumor (T). **(C)** Both sides of the dura have been opened to expose the tumor (T). The falx (F) remains in the midline and can now be transected to create a single intradural cavity. **(D)** A large single cavity has been created after the falx (F) has been transected and removed. The tumor is debulked using the 2-suction technique (S). To prevent herniation of the brain into the working field, the dura anterior to the brain/tumor interface is left intact.

nasal septum to the skull base is resected. This maneuver does risk olfaction, but it is likely that olfaction has already been compromised by the pathology in question. To optimize visualization by preventing blood running into the field, the skull base is removed with a high-speed drill from a rostral to caudal direction. To promote further tumor devascularization the anterior ethmoidal artery is identified and sacrificed.

Prior to drilling the cribriform plate, the soft tissues consisting of the small branches of the ethmoidal arteries and olfactory fimbriae, which enter the crista galli, are resected. This tissue removal further aids in tumor devascularization. Using a high-speed drill, the cribriform plate is removed bilaterally, leaving the crista galli in the midline **(Fig. 4–5A)**. The crista galli can extend for a variable depth into the intracranial cavity and can be particularly prominent in the case of olfactory groove meningiomas with secondary hyperostosis. The crista galli is removed by additionally drilling until it becomes eggshell thin, then fracturing and removing it using circumferential dissection. At this point a large single cavity in the anterior skull base is created. As the entire exposed dura is coagulated, the tumor is further devascularized. At this point, the anterior falcine artery remains as the primary residual blood supply to the tumor along with any cortical vessels that have been parasitized from the anterior circulation.

Intradural Dissection

The dura, which has already been coagulated, is opened on both sides of the falx **(Fig. 4–5B)**. The midline, which still has tumor vascularization, is kept intact at this point. Depending on the tumor consistency, internal debulking is sequentially performed on each side of the falx using the two-suction technique or the ultrasonic aspirator **(Fig. 4–5B)**. Shortly, the feeding vessels arising from the anterior falcine artery can be identified along the free edge of the falx bilaterally. These vessels are coagulated along with the falx and the falx is transected to create a single intradural cavity **(Fig. 4–5C,D)**. The remainder of the tumor is debulked starting in the center. To prevent herniation of the brain into the working field, the dura anterior to the brain/tumor interface is left intact.

It is not uncommon to encounter subpial brain invasion of the tumor into the overlying cortex during the extracapsular dissection of large tumors. This will require sharp dissection of small pial vessels **(Fig. 4–6A)**. The subpial invasion is addressed using a 4 French suction and fine endoneurosurgical bipolars under low heat. The subpial dissection proceeds along the superior pole of the tumor to the level of the interhemispheric fissure (IHF). During this dissection, extreme caution should be used to identify vessels such as the A_2 segments of the anterior cerebral artery and the frontopolar artery, which can be draped over the surface **(Fig. 4–6B)**. The identification of the optic nerves and the Acom greatly facilitates the extracapsular dissection of the A_2 segments along the IHF from a preferred proximal to distal direction **(Fig. 4–6B)**. It is very useful to establish this proximal control during the vascular dissection along the tumor capsule interface. To provide the necessary visualization of the most anterior and rostral portions of the dissection, we have found that the 70 degree endoscope is invaluable. To maximize visualization and facilitate the use of instruments, it is often preferable to invert the position of the endoscope and the suction within the nares at this point, so that the endoscope is placed in the 6 o'clock position rather than its normal 12 o'clock position.

Once the internal debulking has allowed for the capsule to be mobile, we have found it very useful to proceed toward the inferior pole of the tumor at the parasellar space. Dissection in this region will allow access to the parasellar cistern and the identification of several key neurovascular landmarks that have been described in the transplanum section. For exceptionally large tumors, we have found that staged tumor removal may be an excellent option.

Reconstruction for Expanded Anterior Base Modules

Reconstruction of the dura is necessary to prevent a postoperative CSF leak and subsequent meningitis. A variety of surgical techniques and materials have been used for small and larger dural defects. The mucosa is stripped from the surrounding bone prior to repair. Inlay and onlay fascial grafts are placed with excess graft material overlapping the surrounding bone. It is possible to suture the onlay graft to the exposed dura in some cases. Abdominal fat autograft is used to cover the grafts, and fibrin glue is used to hold the grafts in place and promote healing. As already discussed, a no. 10 Foley catheter balloon can be inflated to provide pressure in holding the grafts in place and removed on day 5. In cases without the use of the Foley balloon, Silastic splints can be placed to prevent synechiae between the nasal septum and turbinates.

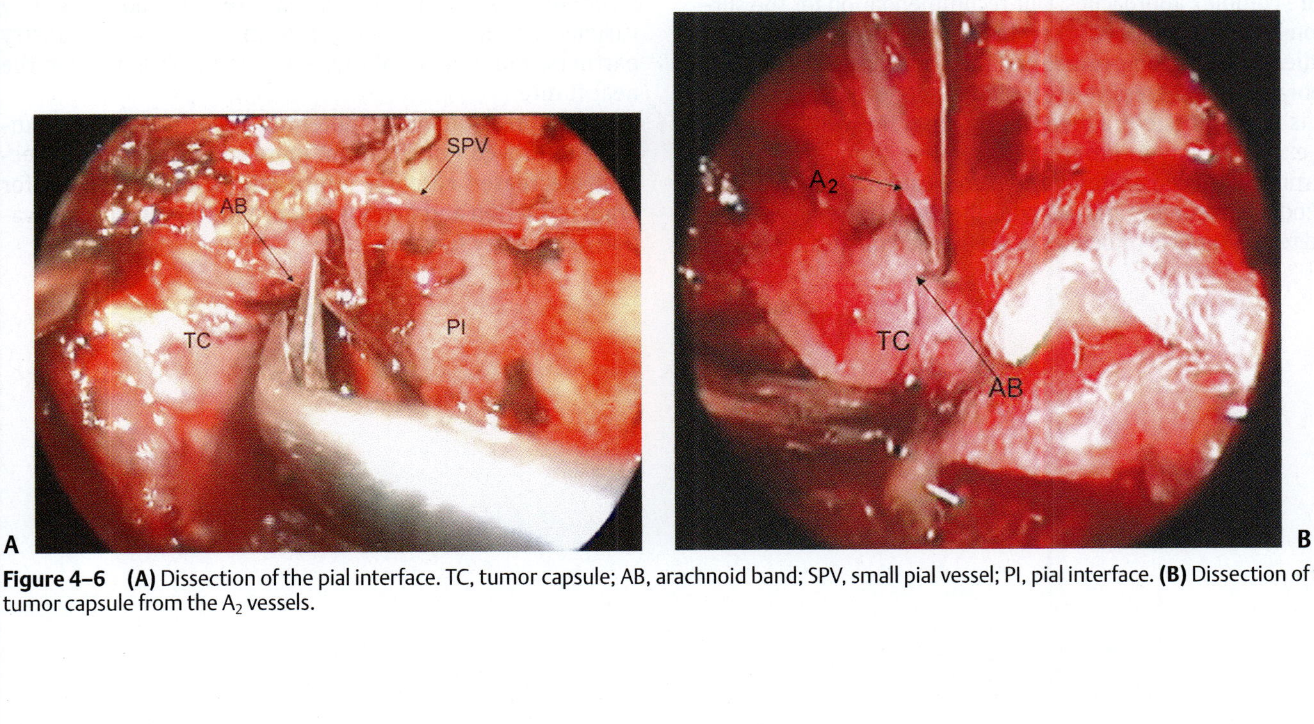

Figure 4–6 **(A)** Dissection of the pial interface. TC, tumor capsule; AB, arachnoid band; SPV, small pial vessel; PI, pial interface. **(B)** Dissection of the tumor capsule from the A_2 vessels.

◆ Postoperative Management

Until the packing is removed the patients are maintained on antibiotic prophylaxis, which begins in the operating room preoperatively. The packing and nasal splints or balloons are removed at the same time around postoperative day 5. Although lumbar spinal drains are not used routinely, they may be inserted in the operating room for large dural defects when repair of a postoperative CSF leak is necessary and in suspected cases of benign intracranial hypertension.

At the removal of nasal packing, the patients are placed on a saline nasal spray or irrigation for nasal hygiene and reduction in crusting. The patients are seen by the endoscopic surgeon every few weeks for several weeks until healing is complete. During these visits, endoscopic debridement of nasal crusts is accomplished. All patients are cautioned to avoid activities that cause a Valsalva maneuver (coughing, sneezing, nose blowing, physical exertion, etc.), which results in elevated intracranial pressure and may contribute to a CSF leak. If a patient presents with concern regarding CSF leakage, they undergo an endoscopic examination and any fluid is sent for testing to confirm the presence of β-2 transferrin.

◆ Discussion

We have presented our modular approach and demonstrated that the EEA can be used to access the sellar and anterior skull base regions. The EEA starts at the sphenoid sinus and extends rostrally and caudally in a modular fashion based on the tumor extent.

Complication avoidance by strict adherence to endoscopic principles and detailed knowledge of the skull base anatomy has been stressed. Our approach is based on a progressive learning curve that is developed systematically as one progresses through each module. The surgeon will acquire increasing experience with endoscopic skills, skull-based anatomy, and endoscopic instrumentation, as well as, establish the teamwork and coordination necessary to perform more complex approaches. Our recommendation for the surgeon beginning endonasal endoscopy would be to attend a dedicated endoscopic course and then practice in the cadaver laboratory. A progressive escalation of surgical case complexity is key. If possible, a mentorship program would provide an excellent way to progress in the case complexity while learning advanced anatomy and complication avoidance.

Endoneurosurgery has adapted the anatomical knowledge and tested surgical principles of skull-based microsurgery and endoscopic surgery to form the modular approaches we have presented. Through close collaboration with industry, there have been significant technological advances that have facilitated the development of endoneurosurgical techniques. endoneurosurgery is a team effort with collaboration between the otolaryngologists and neurosurgeons working in concert to develop an understanding of the relevant anatomy and acquire the surgical skills to undertake more complex cases. EEA done as a team results in significant advantages by having a second surgeon to maintain the endoscopic view in cases of an emergency, such as a vascular injury, and on a routine basis provides the dynamic endoscopic adjustment to ensure optimal visualization and avoiding contact with the surgical instruments. In addition, the issue of "copilot surgery" by having a second surgical opinion has been proven to be invaluable.

We strongly encourage surgeons to begin with level I procedures that include pituitary tumors and CSF leak repairs to gain the endoscopic skills, understand the skull base anatomy from an endoscopic view, and develop coordination and teamwork with the second surgeon. The level II procedures include the expanded approaches to the clival and paraclival region that are exclusively extradural (these are not discussed in this chapter). Many of the anterior skull base approaches that have been detailed here represent level III approaches (intradural dissection without subpial invasion and vascular adherence to the tumor capsule) and level IV (intradural dissection with subpial invasion and vascular adherence to the tumor capsule). Further expansion into more advanced level III and IV procedures will require significant further training and dedication from the surgical team. Many surgeons may wish to restrict their practices to level I and II procedures.

The ongoing problem with reconstruction represents a major worldwide focus, and it is anticipated that improvements in biomaterials will provide the answer in the near future. Our current technique has undergone significant evolution from inlay grafts, to balloon stenting, suturing of onlay grafts, and the development of local pedicle flaps and distant free flaps. The technical advances of reconstruction and of other limitations are being addressed by various endoneurosurgical groups in concert with industry partners, and unique solutions should be obtainable in the near future.

Our impression on the potential benefits of the EEA include improved visualization; more complete tumor resection; decreased cerebral injury due to reduced need for brain retraction and manipulation, and improved preservation of pituitary function.

Section II

Intraventricular Tumors

5

Endoscopic Approaches for Intraventricular Brain Tumors

Mark M. Souweidane

Endoscopic surgery for intraventricular brain tumors is a logical application of endoscopic technology. Because of the central and deep location of intraventricular brain tumors, conventional neurosurgical approaches have a relative increase in potential morbidity. Auspiciously, the location of intraventricular tumors being within a cerebrospinal fluid (CSF)-containing interface affords excellent light and image transmission, a requisite for endoscopic surgery. In addition, the inherent benefits of minimally invasive techniques, including reduced surgical time, improved cosmetic results, shortened hospital stay, and reduced cost, also factor into the appeal of neurosurgical endoscopy for patients with intraventricular tumors. The general approach toward the patient with an intraventricular brain tumor is described, with a special emphasis on patient selection and operative technique. The particular details are then elaborated upon for endoscopic tumor biopsy, endoscopic colloid cyst resection, and endoscopic removal of solid tumors.

◆ Patient Selection

Although endoscopic tumor biopsy or resection should always be considered as a therapeutic alternative for patients with intraventricular brain tumors, not all patients are adequate candidates. All therapeutic candidates should have symptoms attributable to the lesion or should have a realistic expectation of disease progression. Incidental lesions within the intraventricular compartment are diagnosed with some regularity, given the sensitivity of magnetic resonance imaging (MRI). Logically, some patients found to have small asymptomatic lesions with no alteration in the CSF circulation could justifiably be observed using serial imaging **(Fig. 5–1).** Examples of such an approach would include individuals that do not have hydrocephalus but are found to have subependymal nodules in the context of tuberous sclerosis complex (TSC) or those patients with a relatively small asymptomatic colloid cyst.

For those individuals deemed to require surgical therapy, the advantage of using neuroendoscopy for an intraventricular brain tumor is predicated upon the pathological considerations, the intended goal of surgery, and the expected need for further surgery. Incumbent in this consideration is an educated prediction of the possible pathological diagnosis. Factors including patient age, medical history, associated diseases, general physical examination, and radiographic characteristics will typically suggest certain pathological diagnoses. Thus, in patients in whom the expected disease will be treated primarily with nonsurgical means, examples including primary central nervous system (CNS) germ cell tumors, primary CNS lymphoma, metastatic cancer, and hypothalamic/chiasmatic astrocytomas, endoscopic tumor biopsy rather than a primary resection can offer a distinct benefit by avoiding a more extensive intracranial procedure. Alternatively, an endoscopic biopsy would not be recommended in situations where biopsy would not predictably obviate the need for an open microsurgical resection. Included in this latter category are patients with a clinical and radiographic suggestion of a choroid plexus tumor, ependymoma, or meningioma **(Fig. 5–2).**

Several features pertaining to the morphology and position of the intraventricular tumor should be taken into account when considering a primary endoscopic procedure. The size of the lesion, the composition of the tumor, and the relationship with the ependymal surface are important features that need to be carefully assessed on the preoperative imaging studies. Tumors greater than 2 cm, although amenable to biopsy, present an obstacle to total endoscopic removal due to inadequate compatible instrumentation. Heavily calcified lesions predictably limit a total endoscopic removal given the reliance on suction-aspiration as the primary means for volumetric reduction. Computed tomography (CT) can be valuable in distinguishing between tumors that are compact and calcified compared with tumors that are less cellular and friable **(Fig. 5–3).** The relationship of the tumor to the ependymal surface needs to be critically reviewed using preoperative MRI. Lesions that arise within the ventricular compartment or have a significant exophytic component into the ventricle are easily distinguished at the time of ventriculoscopy. However, tumors that are subjacent to the ependymal surface with no overt exophytic component can prove to be surprisingly difficult to identify at the time of ventriculoscopy **(Fig. 5–4).** A smooth and intact ependymal surface covering such tumors not only reduces the diagnostic yield due to sampling error but also creates a scenario where juxtaposed vascular or neural structures cannot be adequately visualized. This feature is very relevant for intrinsic tumors at the rostral mesencephalon and inferior diencephalon.

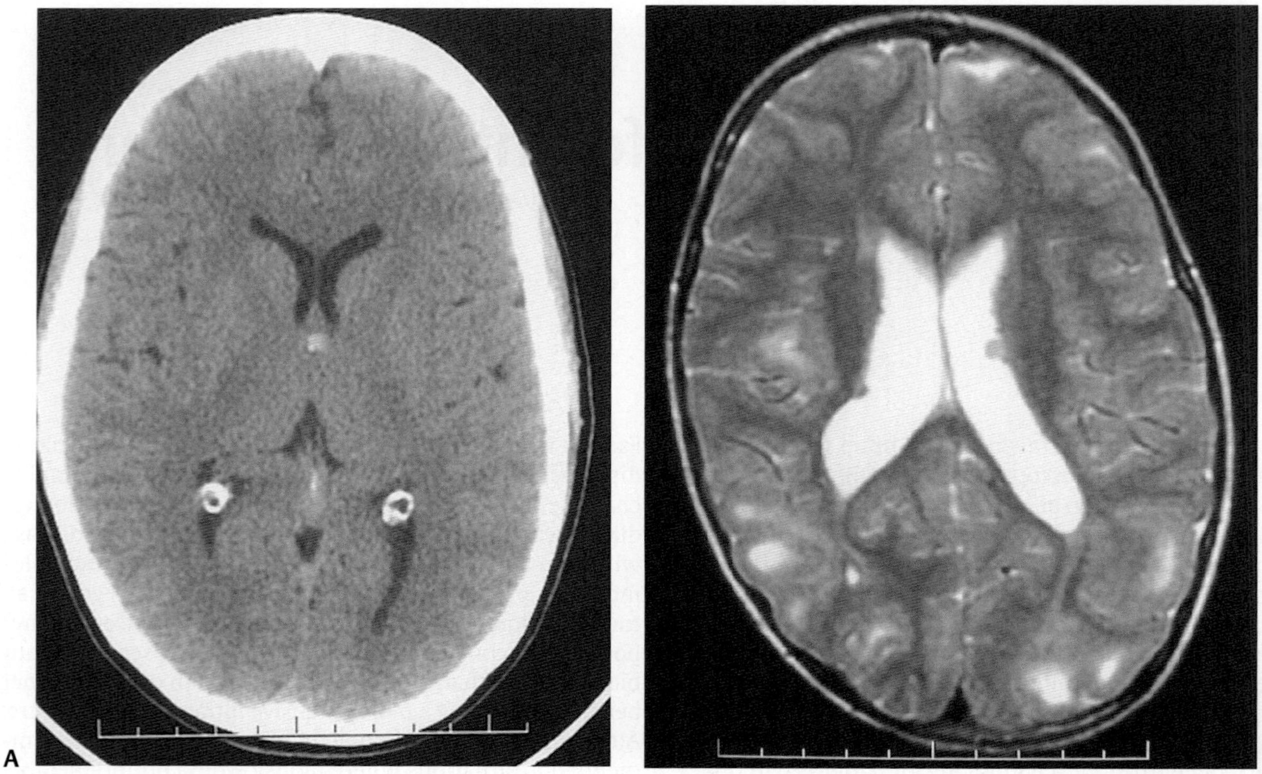

Figure 5–1 Representative images of patients with asymptomatic intraventricular lesions who were not offered endoscopic intervention. **(A)** Typical noncontrast computed tomography of the brain in an individual with an incidental colloid cyst and **(B)** T2-weighted axial magnetic resonance imaging and of a child with tuberous sclerosis complex.

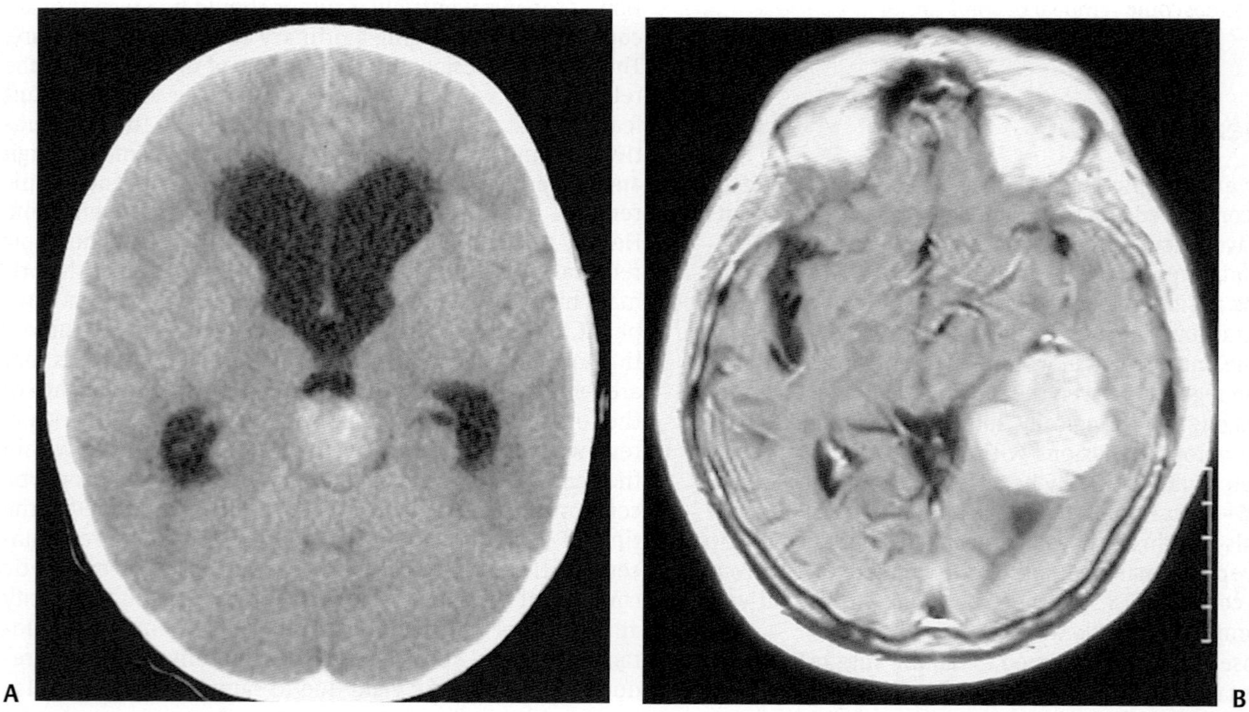

Figure 5–2 Patient selection for endoscopic tumor surgery is guided by the ability to predict probable tumor type. **(A)** A noncontrast computed tomographic scan of the brain of an 8-year-old boy with ocular symptoms and diabetes insipidus suggested a germ cell tumor. The hyperdense mass situated at the posterior third ventricle was confirmed as a pure germinoma using a right frontal endoscopic biopsy. He was spared a craniotomy and was subsequently treated with neoadjuvant chemotherapy and irradiation. **(B)** A contrast-enhanced axial magnetic resonance image of a 46-year-old female is highly suggestive of an intraventricular meningioma. The patient was not offered endoscopic biopsy but instead underwent a craniotomy and total excision of a meningioma.

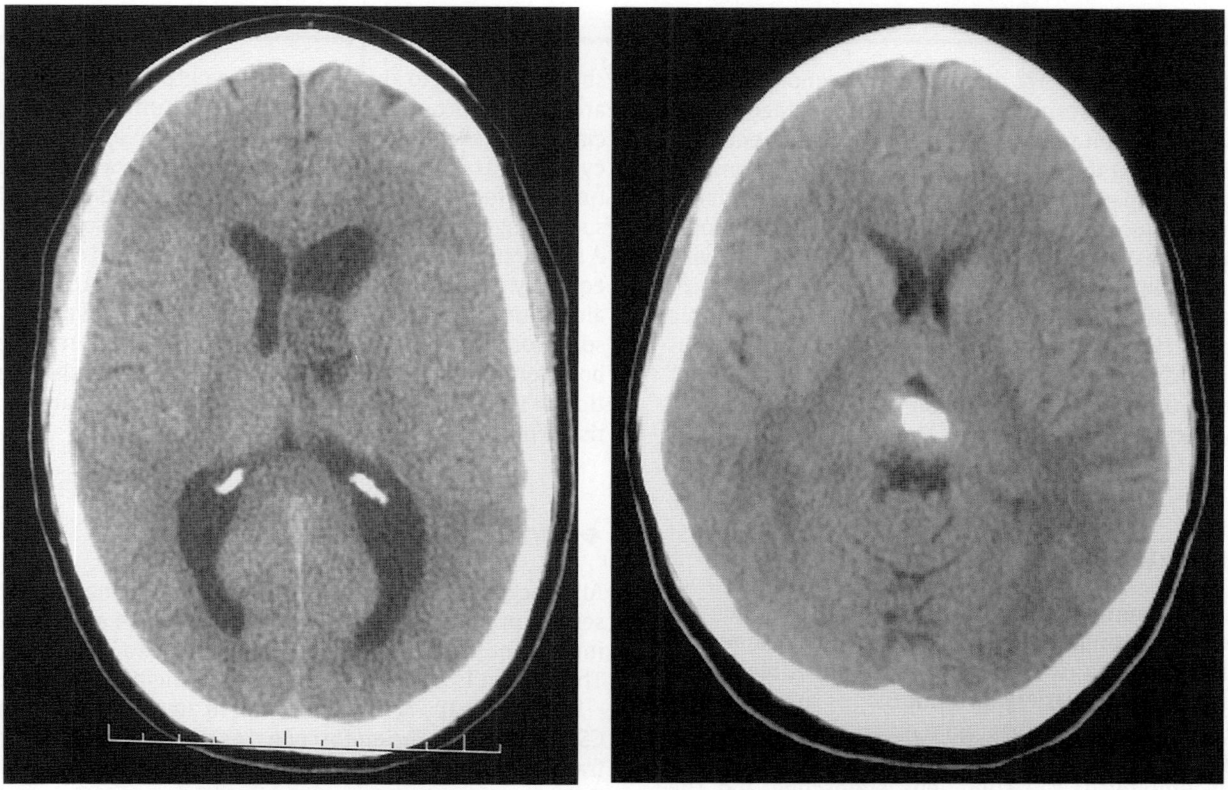

A

B

Figure 5–3 The use of computed tomography (CT) for estimating the tumor composition is exemplified by **(A)** a hypodense lesion situated at the foramen of Monro and **(B)** a hyperdense, calcified tumor of the pineal region. Because aspiration serves as the primary means for endoscopic tumor removal, hypodensity on CT and lack of calcification are appealing preoperative features when considering the option of endoscopic tumor removal.

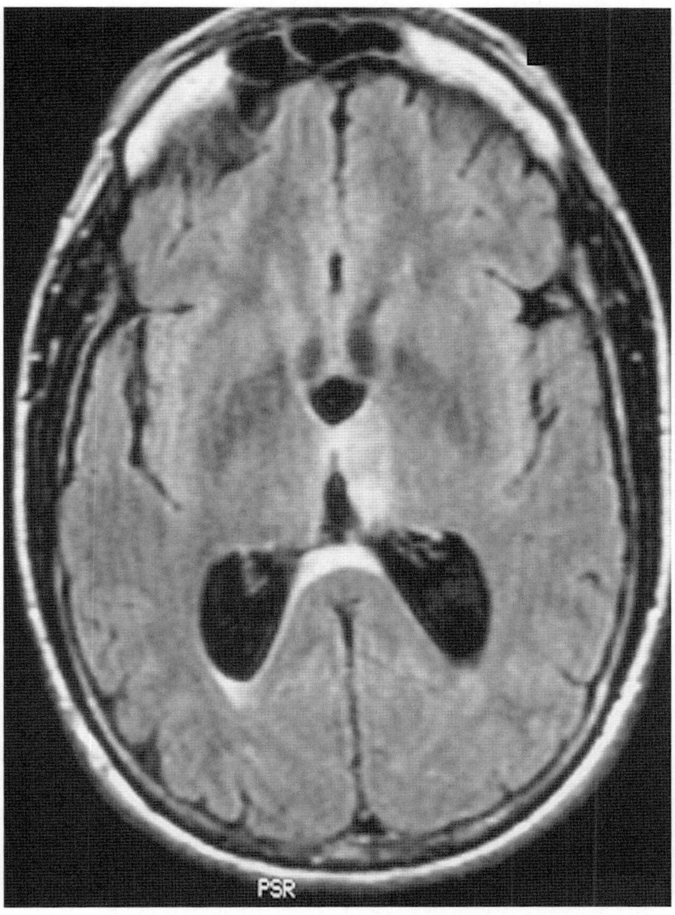

Figure 5–4 Axial FLAIR (fluid-attenuated inversion recovery) image of an infiltrative tumor of the left hypothalamus. The ipsilateral wall of the third ventricle is minimally displaced and there exists no overt exophytic tumor mass in the ventricular system. At the time of ventriculoscopy, this particular tumor would be covered by ependyma and an optimal site of biopsy would be difficult to establish.

In addition to procedures directed at the tumor mass, endoscopic approaches can offer significant advantages in patients with concomitant hydrocephalus. Many patients will benefit by treating the tumor manifestations of noncommunicating or compartmentalized hydrocephalus through the use of endoscopic third ventriculostomy (ETV) or endoscopic septostomy, respectively. A common misconception with regard to patient selection is that those individuals with small ventricles are not adequate candidates for endoscopic tumor surgery. However, as will be discussed here, the absence of hydrocephalus does not preclude the option of endoscopic techniques if appropriate experience and technological integration are available.

◆ Equipment

The essential components of an endoscopic armamentarium include an endoscope, a high-resolution camera, a bright light source, a video monitor, and compatible instrumentation. A wide variety of endoscopes are currently available that satisfy the essential requirements of intracranial endoscopy. Two major categories of endoscopes are currently employed: the solid lens endoscope and the fiberoptic endoscope. The former offers superior image resolution, is reusable, and is nonmalleable. These endoscopes are typically available having varying angles of view with reference to the scope axis (0, 30, 70, and 120 degrees). Alternatively, the fiberoptic endoscope has less image clarity, is disposable, and can be designed to have stearable capacity. The image resolution of fiberoptic endoscopes is directly dependent upon the number of fiberoptic components within the scope.

The critical technological advancement allowing for neurosurgical applications has been the reduction in equipment size. The diameter of the endoscope can vary widely. Most rigid lens systems measure between 3 mm and 6.5 mm in diameter. This variance is usually a function of the required versatility of compatible instrumentation. The author currently utilizes the MINOP system (B. Braun Aesculap, Tuttlingen, Germany) consisting of 0 and 30 degree angled scopes. The endoscopes are used through a 6-mm operating sheath having a 2-mm straight working channel, two 1 mm angled working channels, and one irrigating portal. Ideally, a dedicated neuroendoscopic arsenal would include a variety of endoscopes, each being applied for a specific procedure. In actuality, most surgeons favor one type of endoscope given the types of procedures being performed, budgetary constraints, and familiarity with the equipment.

Compatible instrumentation expands the potential of endoscopic neurosurgery beyond diagnostic purposes to include therapeutic intervention. Biopsy forceps are an integral component of endoscopic tumor management. Whether for tissue sampling, cyst fenestration, or tissue dissection, the biopsy forceps is a versatile and important endoscopic instrument. Either insulated unipolar or bipolar devices offer the ability to achieve hemostasis through coagulation. The power requirements for these devices is less than that needed for conventional means of coagulation due to the smaller surface area of the endoscopic instrument, and care should be taken to always adjust the output source. Scissors are also important for intraventricular tumor work, especially for resection of solid tumors or the creation of tumor cyst fenestrations. Suction catheters serve a very useful function for aspirating the contents of colloid cysts or for suctioning parenchymal components of friable solid tumors. A self-regulated, 6 French pediatric endotracheal suction adequately serves this purpose. The neodymium:yttrium-aluminum-garnet (Nd:YAG) laser has been advocated by some for tissue ablation and tumor removal. A 3 French embolectomy catheter, in addition to being used for the dilatation of fenestration sites, is also used for the separation of tissue planes and tamponade for hemorrhage.

◆ Preoperative Preparation

All procedures are performed using general anesthesia. No seizure prophylaxis is utilized. All patients are administered intravenous antibiotic prophylaxis prior to skin incision. The patient is positioned supine with the head elevated to ~30 degrees above the horizontal in an effort to minimize CSF egress from the endoscope. For procedures integrating frameless stereotaxy, the patient's skull is secured with pin fixation, otherwise a horseshoe head frame is sufficient.

◆ Surgical Technique

General

Trajectory planning is critical for successful and safe endoscopic tumor procedures. Most important is selecting an entry site that offers the most direct intraventricular, linear route to the target **(Fig. 5–5).** This principle avoids undue torque on the cortical and ependymal surfaces. Lesions situated in the anterior third ventricle or frontal horn of the lateral ventricles are best approached using a standard coronal bur hole and a 0 degree angled endoscope. However, an anterior precoronal entry site using a 30 degree angled scope directed posteriorly is critical for lesions situated in the posterior third ventricle or pineal region. Because this relatively anterior entry site can lie in front of the hairline, a forehead crease can be used for the approach. If a forehead crease is necessary, a cosmetic closure using autologous cranioplasty from harvested bone chips and meticulous skin closure can be very acceptable **(Fig. 5–6).** With respect to laterality, most entries are placed on the nondominant side. Exceptions to this recommendation include (1) unilateral hypothalamic lesions, which are best targeted using a contralateral approach, and (2) in the presence of significant ventricular asymmetry, the preference is to utilize the side with the greater ventricular size. The optimal location of the bur hole can be more ambiguous if simultaneous procedures are intended. The patient with noncommunicating hydrocephalus from a pineal region tumor requiring both an ETV and tumor biopsy depicts such a scenario. The optimal entry site for the tumor biopsy is precoronal, whereas a coronal site is better employed for the ETV. Although some have advocated multiple bur holes in such a situation, a single bur hole midway between these entry sites is the author's preference. Using interchangeable

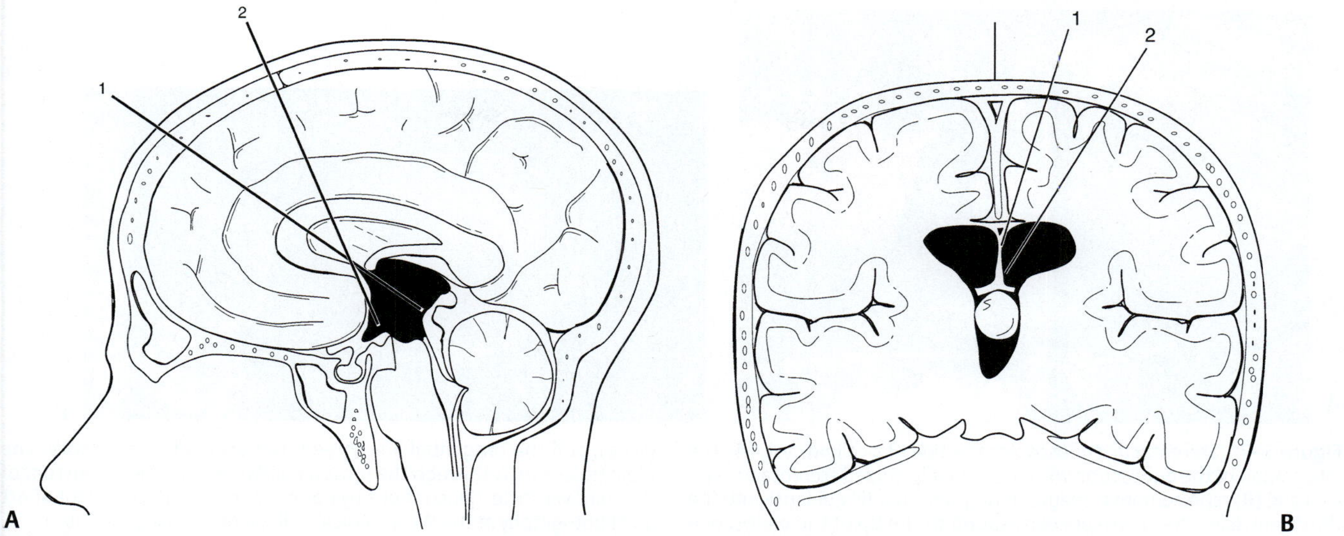

Figure 5–5 Different trajectories for endoscopic biopsy depending upon the tumor location and presence of compartmentalized hydrocephalus. **(A)** Posterior lesions require a precoronal entry site (1), whereas for lesions situated anterior to the massa intermedia, a standard coronal trajectory (2) can be used. **(B)** an entry site 4 to 6 cm from midline (2) is preferred over a standard parasagittal entry (1) when performing a simultaneous endoscopic septostomy. (Illustrations by permission of the Department of Art and Photography at the Weill Medical College of Coraell University.)

endoscopes, the 0 degree lens is used for the ETV followed by the 30 degree lens directed posterior for the tumor biopsy. Similarly, when an endoscopic septostomy is simultaneously required due to compartmentalized hydrocephalus, a bur hole 4 to 6 cm lateral to the midline is advantageous in reducing a tangential approach toward the septum pellucidum. Once the bur hole is created, it is helpful to create a conical shape to the outside of the bur hole using a high-speed drill.

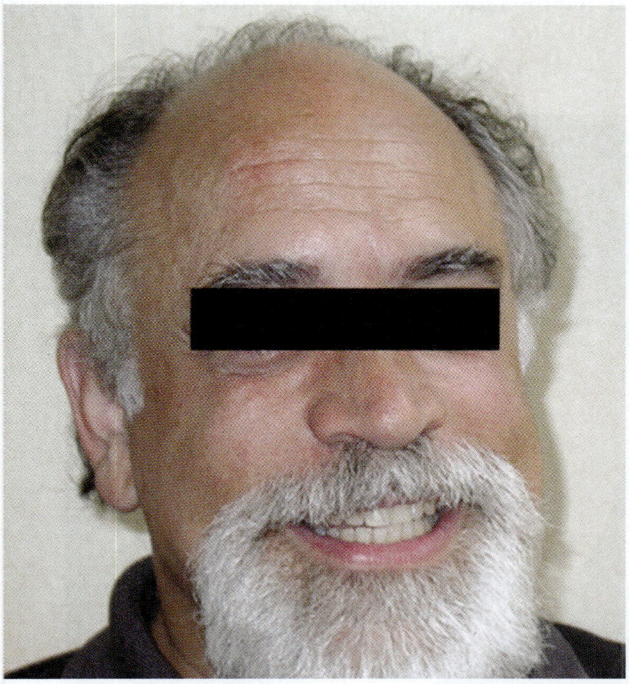

Figure 5–6 Image of a man who underwent a right frontal endoscopic removal of a third ventricular ependymoma. The precoronal entry site was accessed through a forehead crease. Cosmetic closure consisted of autologous cranioplasty and a meticulous skin closure. (Reproduced with permission from Thieme Medical Publishers Inc.)

This simple maneuver allows greater variability in the trajectory and maneuverability of the scope.

There exists an inherent and understandable sentiment that endoscopic surgery for intraventricular tumors should be limited to patients with hydrocephalus. However, with appropriate imaging, navigational assistance, and technical modifications, patients without ventriculomegaly can safely undergo endoscopic tumor biopsy or resection but with a different technical approach. First, a reliance on navigational aids for successful access to the ventricular compartment is recommended. Most frameless stereotactic systems afford integration with endoscopic equipment for real-time, triplanar navigational planning **(Fig. 5–7).** This adjunct minimizes repeated attempts at ventricular cannulation and hence reduces the potential for intraventricular hemorrhage and visual obscuration. Further, the initial ventricular cannulation is usually accomplished using a catheter rather than the operative sheath owing to the smaller caliber. If indicated, CSF is then collected for cytological and biochemical analysis prior to any tissue manipulation. Once an intraventricular position is confirmed, continuous irrigation is begun to maintain a clear medium of image transmission, for enhancing hemostasis, and to maintain ventricular patency. Lactated Ringer's solution warmed to 37°C is preferred. A simple manual syringe system or an automated pump can provide an irrigation system. Commonly employed is an irrigating bipolar apparatus. Regardless of the irrigation method, it is critical that a constant purge be employed to avoid overinsufflating the ventricular system and elevating the intracranial pressure. The simplest method for accomplishing this involves maintaining patency of a portal separate from the working channel or using a system in which the diameter of the sheath is greater than the endoscope. During this process, constant awareness of the patient's hemodynamic status is necessary.

Once ventriculoscopy begins, normal anatomical landmarks including the choroid plexus, venous tributaries,

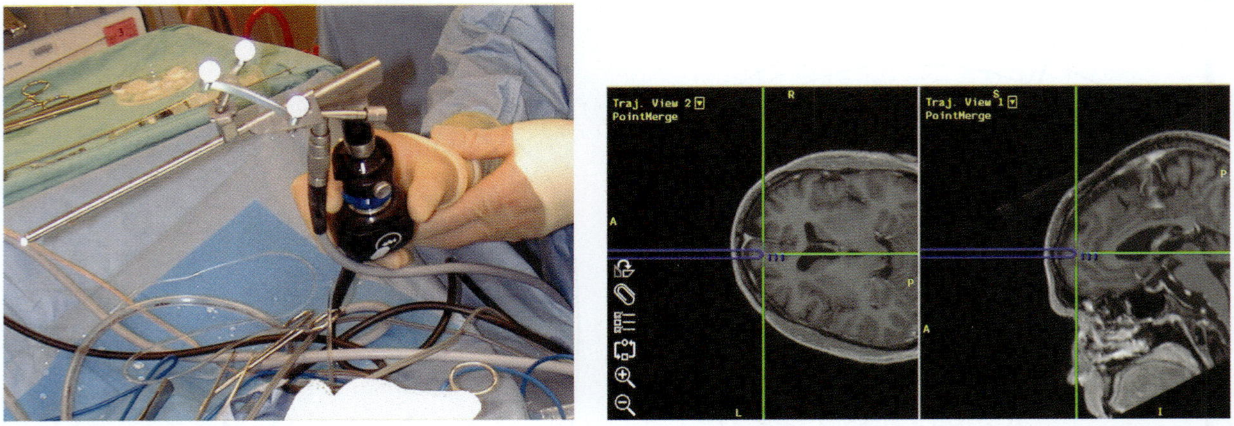

A B

Figure 5–7 Stereotactic endoscopic resection of a colloid cyst. **(A)** The integration of the endoscope with the optically guided stereotactic system and **(B)** representative images during stereotactic guidance into the third ventricle. The crosshairs correspond to the tip of the endoscope (blue), and the tangential line (green) represents the trajectory. The ideal trajectory is through the foramen of Monro parallel to the roof of the third ventricle. (Illustrations by permission of the Department of Art and Photography at the Weill Medical College of Cornell University.)

foramen of Monro, and septum pellucidum are used to establish appropriate lateralization and orientation **(Fig. 5–8)**.

Tumor Biopsy

Endoscopic biopsy has become a well-established method for sampling intraventricular brain tumors. Following ventriculoscopy, the technique of endoscopic biopsy is summarized as follows. Once the lesion is identified, a regional inspection of the ventricular surface should be conducted. The tumor surface is inspected to select an optimal site of sampling. With direct visualization of the tumor surface vascular structures can be avoided. Cupped biopsy forceps are used for tissue sampling **(Fig. 5–9)**. Given the limited sample size, coagulation of the tumor surface is intentionally avoided prior to biopsy to avoid any thermal artifact in pathological interpretation. Depending upon the firmness of the tumor surface, sharp dissection can be used to create a conduit into the tumor substance. Otherwise, direct insertion of the biopsy forceps in a closed position followed by mild rotation and sampling is most commonly employed. Once pathological tissue is confirmed with frozen section, one additional sample is collected for permanent fixation. The degree of sampling is primarily dictated by the hemorrhagic nature of the lesion. Thus, with relatively avascular lesions, multiple samples are safely taken, thereby maximizing the pathological interpretation. Following adequate tissue sampling,

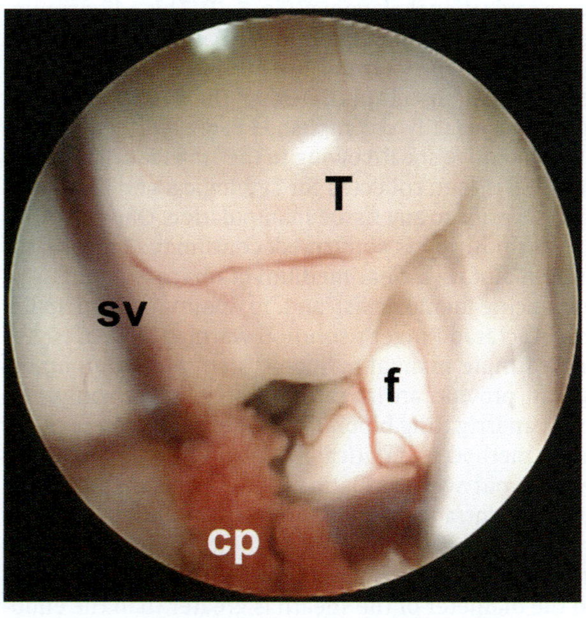

Figure 5–8 Intraoperative view using a solid lens endoscope. A right-sided intraventricular dysembryoplastic neuroepithelial tumor (T) is clearly visualized. The surrounding structures, including the septal vein (sv), the fornix (f), and choroid plexus (cp) are used for orientation. (Reproduced with permission from Thieme Medical Publishers Inc.)

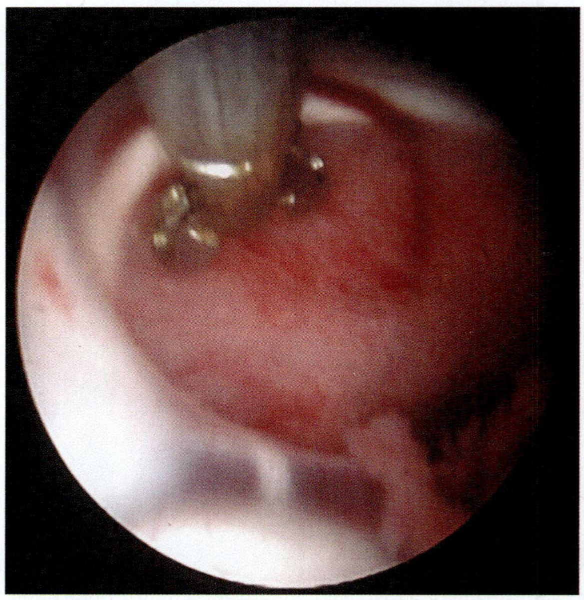

Figure 5–9 An intraoperative view transmitted through a fiberoptic endoscope during endoscopic tumor biopsy. A tumor obstructing the right foramen of Monro is clearly distinguished from the surrounding ependymal surface, the choroid plexus, and the venous tributaries.

hemostasis is achieved using directed irrigation, diathermy, or balloon tamponade. Most hemorrhage is of no clinical significance and is controlled with irrigation. If visual clarity is lost during this portion of the procedure, it is recommended that the endoscope be removed from the ventricular compartment and irrigation be conducted via a standard ventricular catheter. Once CSF return becomes clear, then reinspection and biopsy if necessary can be performed.

Colloid Cyst Resection

The colloid cyst truly lends itself to endoscopic removal given the primarily cystic composition. Numerous publications have established the merits and success of using the minimally invasive, endoscopic approach for what has always been traditionally considered a challenging microsurgical procedure. Expectedly, the success of endoscopic colloid cyst removal is heavily dependent upon the surgeon's experience and the technique. It is the author's practice to use a precoronal entry site that is established with the aid of stereotaxy. This relatively anterior entry site for endoscopic colloid cyst resection is mandatory in avoiding torque upon the structures surrounding the foramen of Monro, specifically the fornix and thalamostriate vein. The operating sheath coupled to a stereotactic navigational system is used in selecting a trajectory as tangential to the undersurface of the roof of the third ventricle as possible. The 30 degree endoscope is then inserted into the sheath and rotated until the view is directed toward the roof of the third ventricle **(Fig. 5–10).** Clear visualization of the tumor cyst should be apparent at this time, although on some occasions the choroid plexus needs to be cleared using bipolar coagulation **(Fig. 5–11).** The cyst wall is then generously coagulated with bipolar diathermy. Sharp dissection is used to incise the cyst wall. A suction tube is then placed within the cyst and aspiration is gently applied. Caution needs to be utilized in applying intraventricular suction. Specifically, only when the lumen of the catheter is fully imbedded within the target tissue should suction be applied. This simple practice avoids a rapid evacuation of CSF. Cyst contents, although highly varied, can be tenacious, thus requiring blunt dissection and repeated manipulations of the suction catheter. Once the contents have been emptied, the cyst wall is thoroughly coagulated using bipolar diathermy. The cyst wall can then be dissected away from the roof of the third ventricle primarily using a rotational or spreading maneuver of the grasping forceps. Remnants of the cyst, if adherent to venous tributaries, are not forcibly removed, but rather managed with bipolar coagulation. In extracting large fragments of tumor tissue, it is sometimes necessary to remove the entire endoscope and sheath due to the relative mismatch between the tumor fragment and the working channel. Once tumor extirpation is complete, inspection of the third ventricle is performed to ensure that there are no viable tumor remnants or occlusion of the aqueduct by tumor debris or hematoma.

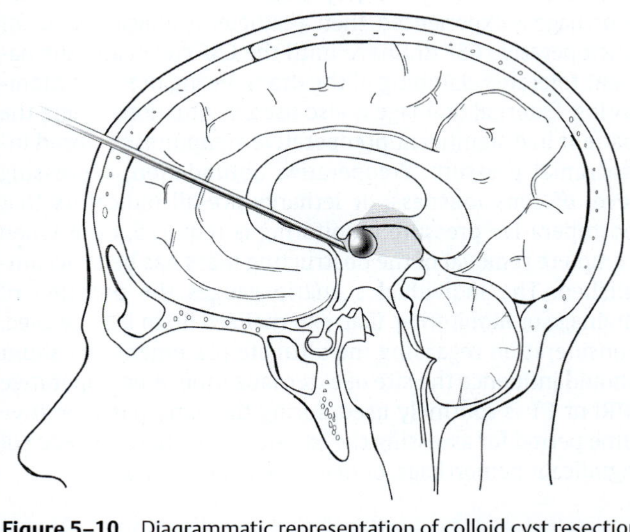

Figure 5–10 Diagrammatic representation of colloid cyst resection using a precoronal entry site and a 30 degree angled endoscope directed posterior. Using this method, a clear view (shaded area) of the roof of the third ventricle and site of colloid cyst attachment is achieved. (Illustration by permission of the Department of Art and Photography at the Weill Medical College of Coraell University)

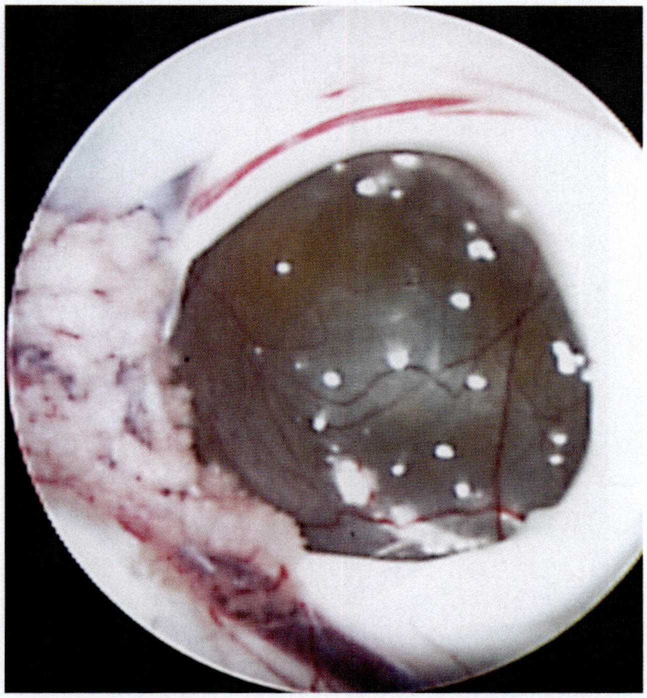

Figure 5–11 Operative view of a colloid cyst obliterating the right foramen of Monro. (Reproduced with permission from Thieme Medical Publishers Inc.)

Solid Tumor Resection

When used in appropriate candidates, the endoscopic removal of solid tumors can be very rewarding and clearly offers a distinct advantage to the patient **(Fig. 5–12).** Solid tumor removal, although a logical application of endoscopic techniques, is somewhat limited due to the inadequacy of compatible instrumentation and the small caliber of current endoscopic portals. The use of piecemeal removal using cupped biopsy forceps entails prolonged operative times, even for relatively small tumors. Instead, the resection of solid tumors is principally achieved through the use of aspiration with a variable, self-regulated suction catheter. Unlike the endoscopic tumor biopsy technique, generous

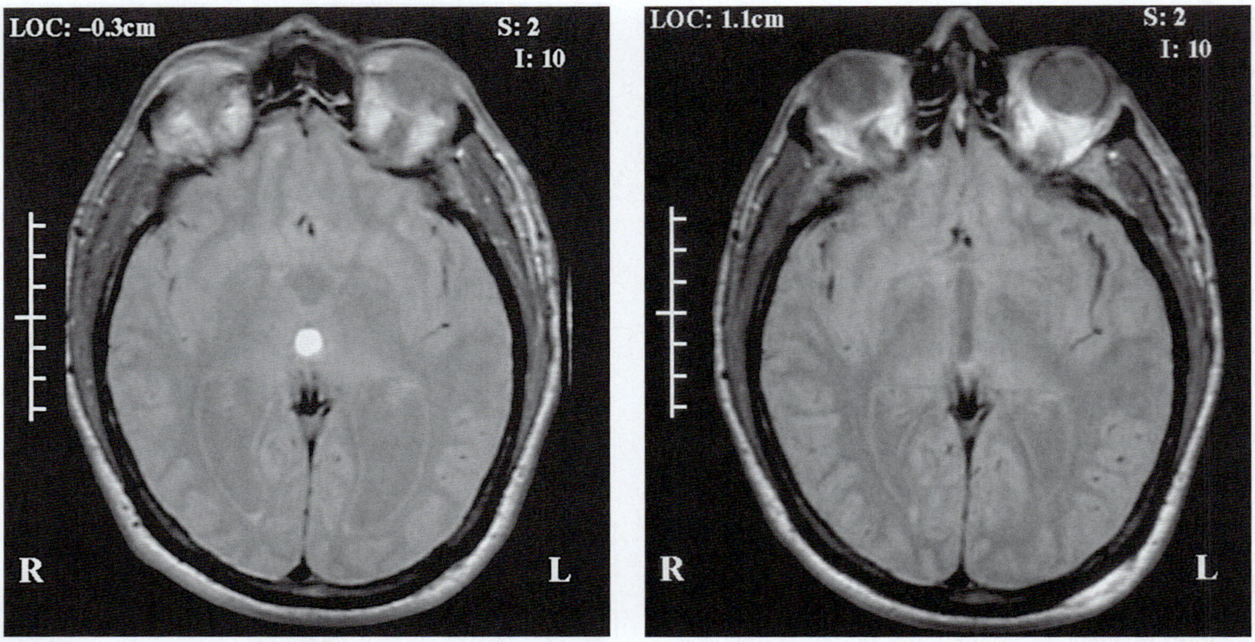

A B

Figure 5–12 **(A)** Preoperative and **(B)** postoperative axial magnetic resonance imaging scans (FLAIR sequences) from a patient treated with endoscopic resection of a low-grade glioneuronal tumor. The tumor was completely resected using endoscopic aspiration and the patient did not require further cerebrospinal fluid diversionary procedures. (Reproduced with permission from Thieme Medical Publishers Inc.)

coagulation of the tumor surface precedes any tumor manipulation or attempted removal. Scissors are helpful to incise the capsule or tumor surface. Through this incision, a suction catheter is inserted into the mass and the self-regulated fenestration is then occluded. Again, aspiration is only applied once the catheter tip is firmly and completely imbedded within the tumor tissue. Frequent manipulations of the suction catheter consisting of rotation and small back-and-forth motions assist in tissue removal. Following volumetric reduction of the tumor mass, the biopsy forceps can be used to spread the tumor surface away from juxtaposed ependyma or vessels. Separated remnants are then removed using a similar technique of bipolar coagulation and aspiration.

Obviously, the success of such a procedure is dependent upon the tumor size, tissue composition, and the ability to define an interface between the tumor and subjacent white matter. This latter objective is guided primarily upon visual inspection and differing tissue consistency. In an effort to enhance tumor removal some authors have advocated the use of multiple entry sites to accommodate additional instrumentation. However, the use of multiple endoscopes becomes technically burdensome and begins to negate the concept of minimally invasive. The feasibility of endoscopic removal of solid tumors within the ventricular system would logically be expected to improve with the advent of compatible instrumentation designed for tissue ablation, such as an ultrasonic aspirator.

◆ Postoperative Management

Ventricular drainage for monitoring intracranial pressure is used on an individual basis depending upon the degree of intraventricular hemorrhage and preoperative symptoms. Thus, if at the time of surgery moderate intraventricular hemorrhage is experienced, then a catheter is typically used for postoperative CSF drainage until the CSF clears and the patient tolerates clamping of the drain during pressure monitoring. External drainage is also used in situations where the patient had significant preoperative symptoms of raised intracranial pressure. Preoperative obtundation, decreasing level of consciousness, or lethargy are all indicators that postoperative pressure monitoring is required, even when complete removal of the obstructing mass has been accomplished. The individual scenario gauges the duration of drainage or monitoring. If an externalized drain is to be used, consideration regarding the ultimate placement of a shunt should influence the site of externalization. A postoperative MRI or CT is routinely used during the early postoperative time period for assessing the extent of resection, evidence of significant hemorrhage, or degree of hydrocephalus.

◆ Summary

Endoscopic surgery for intraventricular brain tumors has burgeoned over the past decade to a field with clearly defined surgical indications, dedicated instrumentation, and general acceptance by the neurosurgical community. Patient selection requires a thorough understanding of neuro-oncological principles and the limitations of neuroendoscopic methods. Endoscopic tumor biopsy and colloid cyst resection have been shown to be highly successful while affording significant advantages over conventional neurosurgical techniques. Endoscopic excision of solid intraventricular tumors, although feasible, remains challenging due to technical limitations. Intraoperative guidance contributes greatly toward a safer and more efficacious procedure and should be considered as an integral adjunct in patients undergoing endoscopic neurosurgery for third ventricular brain tumors or in patients without hydrocephalus. The potential of endoscopic surgery for intraventricular brain tumors is expected to expand with technological advancements in compatible instrumentation.

6

Surgical Approaches to Tumors of the Third Ventricle

Kevin C. Yao and Frederick F. Lang

Tumors arising within the third ventricle are challenging to remove surgically because the third ventricle is located within the center of the brain, and it is surrounded by vital neural and vascular structures, injury to which can have devastating consequences. In terms of complexity, a distinction should be made between tumors that grow secondarily into the third ventricle but are also within the lateral ventricle, and primary third ventricular tumors that are located entirely within the ventricle. Because the *secondary* tumors create their own surgical corridor into the third ventricle, these tumors are easier to resect than *primary* third-ventricular tumors, for which the surgeon must create the corridor into the ventricle. These latter corridors are generally narrow and usually require dissection near critical neural and vascular structures. This chapter describes the surgical corridors that can be used to remove primary third-ventricular tumors.

Because the third ventricle has a roof, an anterior wall, and a posterior wall, one can enter the third ventricle from above, from the front, or from behind **(Fig. 6–1)**. Although the third ventricle has a floor that can be opened from within during third ventriculostomy procedures or during tumor resection, primary tumors are generally not accessible from below (i.e., through the floor). In addition, posterior approaches are usually considered as pertaining to pineal region tumors and are not discussed here (see Chapter 24 for approaches to the pineal region). This chapter focuses on the superior and anterior-inferior approaches, specifically the transforaminal, transchoroidal, and lamina terminalis approaches to the third ventricle. The authors have found that mastering these approaches permits removal of most lesions within the third ventricle.

In addition, because the third ventricle is a midline cavity that lies in the center of the brain, operations on tumors found here can be considered to involve two stages. In the initial or approach stage, the surgeon obtains access to either the anterior or superior wall of the ventricle using a variety of approaches **(Table 6–1)**. In the second, or entry stage, the surgeon dissects through a specific corridor to the third ventricle and removes the tumor. Mastery of the initial stage is thus a prerequisite for mastery of the second stage. This chapter emphasizes the nuances of the second stage and assumes that the reader has some familiarity with the first stages of the operations described.

◆ Anatomy

The anatomy of the third ventricle has been extensively reviewed, and for details the reader is referred to these excellent works. Here we emphasize various features of the third ventricle that are important for the surgical approaches described.

For the superior approaches, the important structures from the surgeon's perspective are those encountered when the third ventricle is viewed from within the body of the lateral ventricle. Most anteriorly is the foramen of Monro, which is the natural conduit for passage of cerebrospinal fluid (CSF) from the lateral ventricle to the third ventricle. This foramen is an obvious corridor into the third ventricle, but under physiological conditions it is small, measuring from 3 to 7 mm in diameter. The choroid plexus is an important landmark that extends around the thalamus in the choroidal fissure, through the foramen of Monro, and into the roof of the third ventricle. The choroid plexus acts as a guide that can be followed to the foramen of Monro. In the body of the lateral ventricle, the choroid plexus lies between the thalamus and the fornix. Along the thalamus and fornix are small ridges, called teniae, to which the tela choroidea, the membrane in which the choroid plexus arises, is attached. The line of tenia on the thalamic side is called the tenia thalami or tenia choroidea, and that on the forniceal side is called the tenia fornicis. Because the thalamus comprises the lateral wall of the third ventricle behind the foramen, and the fornix is the most superior structure of the roof of the third ventricle, the choroidal fissure is a potential corridor from the body of the lateral ventricle into the third ventricle. Use of this corridor does not disrupt any neural structures. Dissection along the tenia fornicis leads under the fornix and into the roof of the ventricle. The roof of the third ventricle is composed of four layers: the fornix, two layers of tela choroidea, and blood vessels between the sheets of tela choroidea. The body of the fornix forms the anterior part of the roof, and the crura and hippocampal commissure of the fornix form the posterior part, so that the choroidal fissure becomes more lateral toward the back of the ventricle. The telae choroidea are thin membranes derived from the pia mater and are interconnected by loose trabeculae. The CSF space between the two layers of tela is the velum interpositum, in which are found the internal cerebral veins and the medial posterior choroidal arteries. The internal cerebral veins begin at the level of the foramen of Monro by the union of the septal vein and the thalamostriate vein

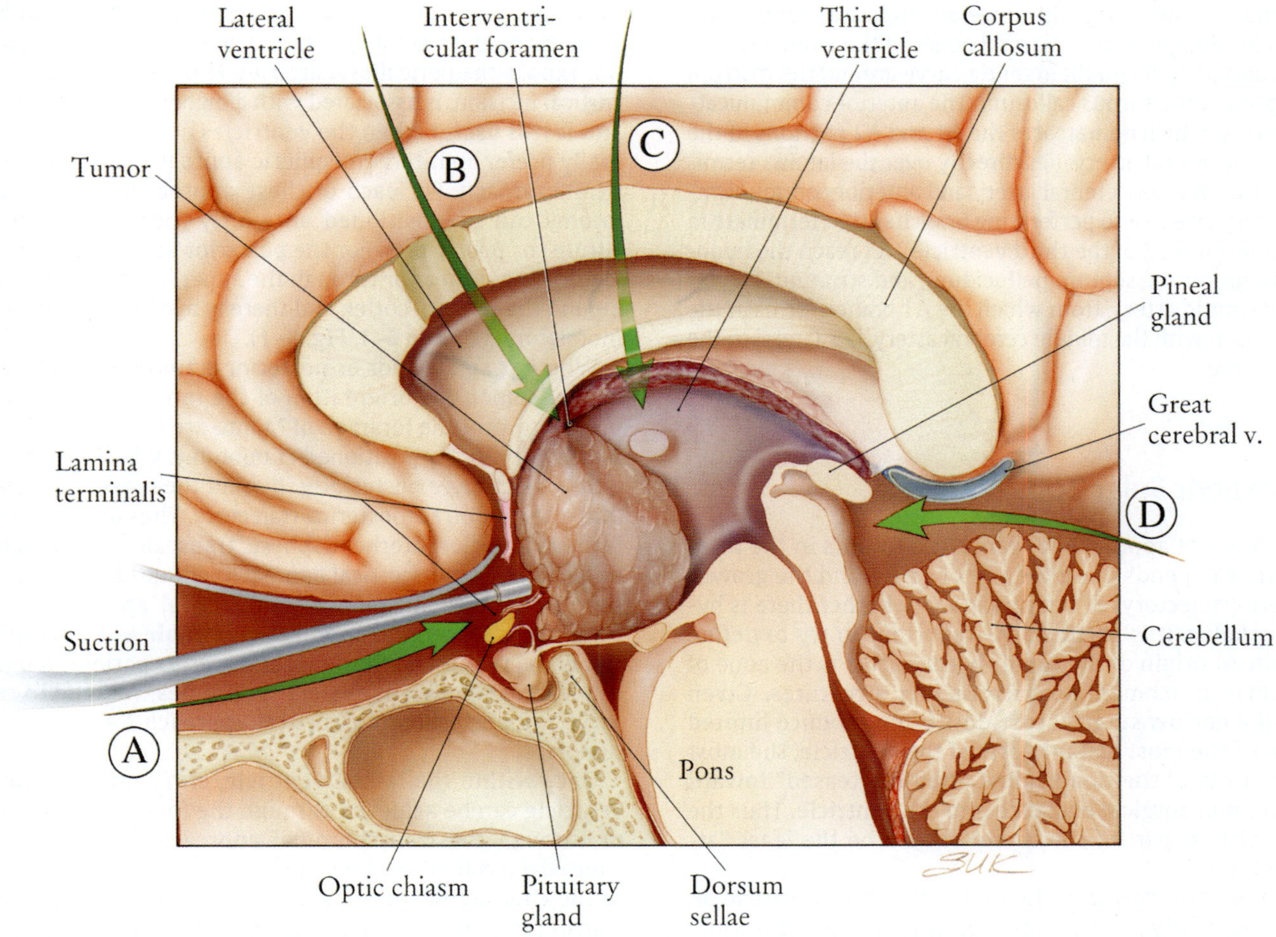

Figure 6–1 Artist's depiction of the various approaches to the third ventricle. **(A)** Anterior-inferior approaches are primarily through the lamina terminalis. The approach to the lamina terminalis can be either via a unilateral or bilateral subfrontal approach. Others have suggested an interhemispheric approach. Superior approaches can be **(B)** anterior or **(C)** posterior. These approaches lead the surgeon into the lateral ventricle. Once within the lateral ventricle, the third ventricle can be entered either through **(B)** the foramen of Monro or **(C)** a transchoroidal corridor. **(D)** For posterior third ventricle tumors that occupy the pineal region, posterior approaches can be used, including the supracerebellar infratentorial approach or the occipital transtentorial approach.

and extend posteriorly to join the basal vein at its junction with the vein of Galen.

With the anterior-inferior approach, the surgeon navigates through the anterior wall of the third ventricle, which extends from the upper surface of the optic chiasm to the foramina of Monro. As viewed from a superior to inferior direction, the structures are the rostrum of the corpus callosum, the anterior commissure, the lamina terminalis, and the optic chiasm. Because the rostrum of the corpus callosum overhangs much of the anterior wall, at best only the lower two thirds of the anterior wall is visible to the surgeon. This visible part is essentially only the optic chiasm and the lamina terminalis. Thus the lamina terminalis is the membrane that defines the portion of the anterior wall of the third ventricle, spanning the 8 to 12 mm between the anterior commissure superiorly and the optic chiasm inferiorly. The lamina terminalis is a thin sheet of gray matter and pia through which an anterior-inferior approach into the third ventricle can be directed without neurological consequence. Behind the lamina terminalis is the optic recess, a small beaklike extension of the third ventricle. Posterior to the optic chiasm, forming the anterior portion of the floor of the third ventricle, are the pituitary stalk, infundibulum, and tuber cinereum. The critical vessels surrounding the lamina terminalis are the anterior cerebral arteries and anterior

Table 6–1 Approaches to the Third Ventricle

Stage 1	Stage 2
Superior Approaches	
Anterior transcortical transventricular	Transforaminal
Anterior interhemispheric transcallosal	Transchoroidal
Posterior transcortical transventricular	Transchoroidal
Posterior interhemispheric transcortical	
Anterior-Interior Approaches	
Bifrontal craniotomy: subfrontal	Translaminar
Unilateral craniotomy: subfrontal	
Interhemispheric	

communicating artery. The anterior cerebral arteries travel rostrally along the anterolateral edges of the lamina terminalis until they begin their gentle curve around the rostrum and genu of the corpus callosum. The anterior communicating artery, which demarcates the A1 and A2 portions of the anterior cerebral artery, lies directly over the lamina terminalis. The anterior cerebral artery and anterior communicating artery give rise to perforating branches that terminate in the anterior wall of the third ventricle and reach the hypothalamus, fornix, septum pellucidum, and striatum. The internal carotid artery, from which the A1 branch forms at the bifurcation with the middle cerebral artery, lies lateral to the optic nerve.

◆ Patient Selection

The choice of approach for removing tumors in the third ventricle depends upon the site of origin and the growth pattern (trajectory) of the tumor and whether there is hydrocephalus. It is particularly important to try to define the site of origin of the tumor because this is the zone of maximal attachment to surrounding structures. Given that the narrow surgical corridors often produce limited views of the most distant parts of the ventricle, the most distal areas of the tumor must often be "teased" toward the point of surgical entrance into the ventricle. Thus the most distant part of the tumor should be the least "attached" part.

Tumors originating in the roof of the third ventricle or, more generally, in the anterior-superior or posterior-superior part of the third ventricle (even if they extend to fill much of the ventricle inferiorly) can be approached from above **(Fig. 6–1, Table 6–1)**. When entering the third ventricle from above, the surgeon must first enter the body of the lateral ventricle (initial approach stage, **Table 6–1**). This can be achieved either through an interhemispheric transcallosal approach or through a transcortical approach. The advantages of the interhemispheric transcallosal approach are that cortical structures are not violated, that it can be used when the ventricles are small, and that there are multiple surgical landmarks that guide the dissection (the falx, the cingulated gyri, the pericallosal arteries, and the corpus callosum). It has the disadvantage that bridging veins to the sagittal sinus may limit exposure. The transcortical approach is not hindered by these veins, does not divide the corpus callosum, and does not expose the pericallosal arteries. However, it requires a cortical incision, is associated with a higher rate of seizures, and is less useful when the ventricles are small. We generally prefer an interhemispheric approach to a transcortical approach. For each of these approaches, the craniotomy can be positioned anteriorly (near the coronal suture) or posteriorly. For the posterior approach the trajectory begins near or through the superior parietal lobule behind the sensory cortex and thereby avoids the eloquent motor cortex **(Table 6–1, Fig. 6–1)**.

Whether an anterior or posterior craniotomy is placed depends upon the orientation of the tumor. Tumors that project toward the foramen of Monro are best approached with an anteriorly positioned craniotomy, whereas tumors that project more posteriorly (behind the massa intermedia) often require a posterior trajectory. Thus one can perform an anterior interhemispheric transcallosal approach or an anterior transcortical approach; or one can perform a posterior interhemispheric transcallosal approach or a posterior transcortical approach (see **Table 6–1**). Because the dissection through the right superior parietal lobule can lead to significant neglect syndromes, we tend to reserve the posterior transcortical approach for left-sided tumors.

Once within the lateral ventricle, entry into the third ventricle can be achieved through the foramen of Monro or through the transchoroidal approach, in which the choroidal fissure is opened lateral to the fornix and medial to the choroid plexus along the tenia fornicis. Use of the transforaminal approach depends upon the size of the foramen of Monro. Tumors that expand the foramen either directly or as a secondary result of hydrocephalus can often be resected exclusively through the foramen. This is common with colloid cysts. When the foramen is not enlarged, however, the opening into the third ventricle requires dissection through the choroidal fissure. The transchoroidal dissection, which can often begin at the foramen of Monro and extend posteriorly, allows access to the central and posterior-superior portions of the third ventricle (see later discussion). Tumors that have been resected via this approach include large colloid cysts, pilocytic astrocytomas, ependymomas, germ cell tumors, choroid plexus papillomas, and epidermoid and dermoid cysts **(Fig. 6–2)**.

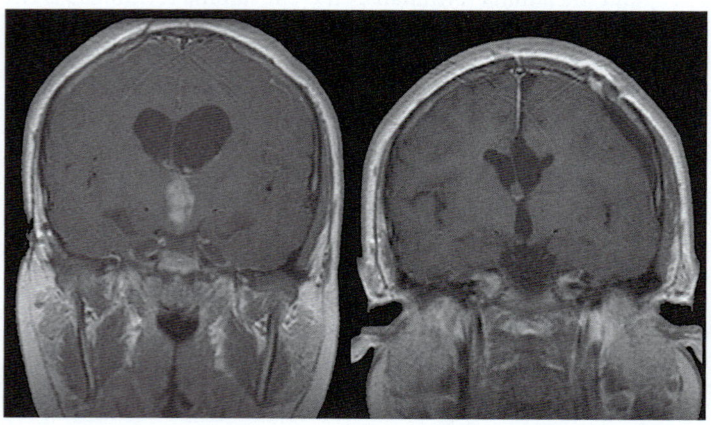

Figure 6–2 Preoperative (left) and postoperative (right) coronal T1-weighted magnetic resonance images of a primary third ventricular tumor. The foramen of Monro is not enlarged. The tumor fills the third ventricle without extension into the lateral ventricle. This lesion was removed via an interhemispheric transcallosal approach (stage 1) followed by a transchoroidal entry into the third ventricle. Histological analysis revealed a pilocytic astrocytoma.

Several surgeons have described entering the third ventricle by dissecting between the two fornices (interforniceal approach). This approach is technically difficult due to the fragile composition of the fornices and subjects the patient to bilateral injury to the fornices that invariably results in severe anterograde memory loss. Therefore, we generally do not recommend this approach except in the very rare instance in which the tumor itself has grown between the two fornices and has essentially split them apart, thus performing the dissection for the surgeon.

Tumors originating in the anterior-inferior part of the third ventricle can be approached from the front wall of the third ventricle through the lamina terminalis. The surgical corridor into the third ventricle from this approach is small, and the most superior aspect of the tumor is often difficult to see. Thus this approach is most effective for tumors that are attached to the floor of the third ventricle, typically pilocytic astrocytomas, craniopharyngiomas, and germ cell tumors **(Fig. 6–3).** Although many of these tumors can grow to be quite large, the distal portions of the tumors are often composed of cysts that are only loosely adherent, or more commonly not adherent, to the superior walls of the third ventricle. These cysts can be drained and then teased down without injuring neural structures. Thus large, superiorly projecting cysts are not a contraindication for the trans–lamina terminalis approach. It should also be noted that many suprasellar tumors extend superiorly without extension into the third ventricle **(Fig. 6–4).** In these cases, in which intraventricular approaches are obviously not needed, the ventricle is often displaced rather than filled with tumor.

The initial access to the lamina terminalis is achieved via a subfrontal approach (**Table 6–1**), which can be performed through either a unilateral or a bilateral craniotomy, with or without removal of the orbital rim(s). The advantage of the bilateral approach is that a more midline trajectory is achieved, which allows for equal access to both the left and right sides of the tumor within the third ventricle. However, this approach involves exposure of both frontal lobes, which may lead to more neurological sequelae than the unilateral approach. In contrast, the unilateral approach suffers from limited visualization of the ipsilateral ventricular wall but has the advantage that only one frontal lobe is exposed. If a

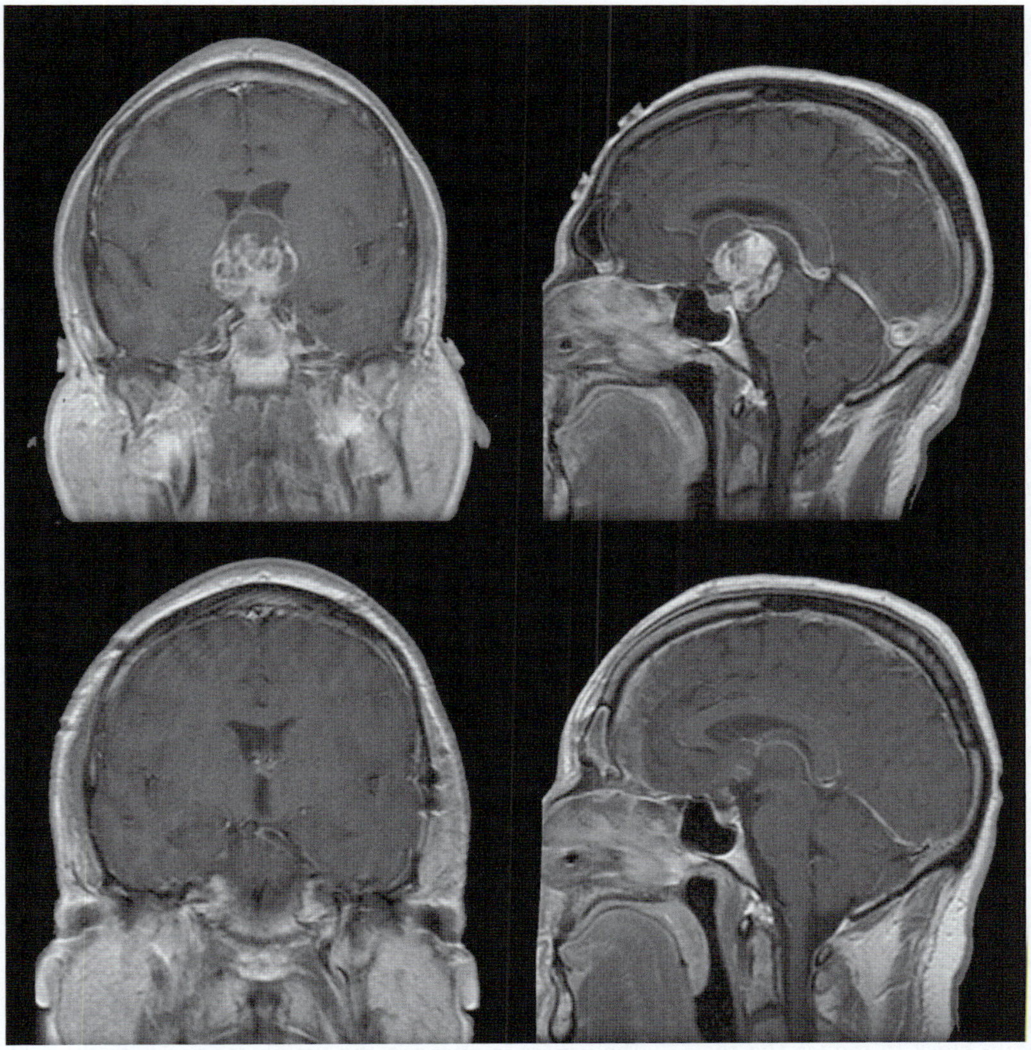

Figure 6–3 Preoperative (upper panel) and postoperative (lower panel) T1-weighted magnetic resonance images of a large third ventricular craniopharyngioma. The third ventricle is completely filled with tumor. There is no extension into the sella turcica. The tumor was removed via a unilateral subfrontal craniotomy and a translaminar approach. The cyst on the upper end was "teased" down and removed with its capsule intact. There were no postoperative deficits.

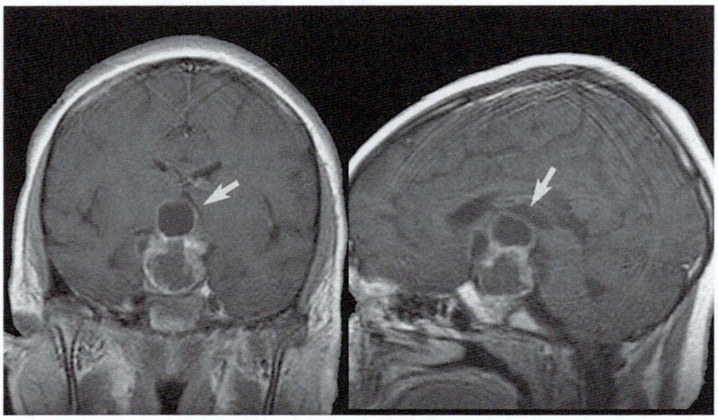

Figure 6–4 T1-weighted magnetic resonance image with contrast depicting a tumor that displaces rather than fills the third ventricle. On coronal images (left) the third ventricle is displaced laterally (arrow), and on sagittal images (right) the ventricle is displaced superiorly (arrow). The tumor does not fill the third ventricle. This tumor was removed via a frontotemporal craniotomy with splitting of the sylvian fissure. Entry into the third ventricle was not required.

unilateral approach is used, the choice between a right- or left-sided approach is determined by the extension of the tumor. Tumors projecting more to the right are exposed from the left side, whereas tumors extending more to the left are exposed from the right side. Although there is a short increase in operating time, removal of the orbital rim(s) is generally recommended because it reduces the need for brain retraction and shortens the operative distances.

◆ Preoperative Preparation

Patients with third-ventricular lesions may have obstructive hydrocephalus, demonstrable on computed tomography (CT) or magnetic resonance (MR) imaging scans. The timing of performing CSF diversion is based on the clinical status of the patient, recognizing that removal of the tumor may often resolve the hydrocephalus and avoid the need for permanent shunting. Third ventriculostomy is usually not feasible for tumors that fill the third ventricle because the lesion usually obstructs the foramen of Monro. For patients with symptomatic hydrocephalus, a preoperative external ventricular drain is placed, and definitive surgery is performed semiurgently. The operative approach and the side of the patient on which surgery will be performed must be considered prior to placing the drain. For a patient with asymptomatic hydrocephalus, an external drain is placed at the time of surgery for postoperative monitoring. For patients without hydrocephalus, we generally avoid the use of external drains, even in the postoperative period.

Patients with tumors arising in the floor of the ventricle may present with endocrine disturbance or have undetected endocrine dysfunction. In these patients, a full endocrinologic workup is warranted prior to surgery. In addition, a formal ophthalmological exam should be performed.

At the time of surgery, preoperative doses of corticosteroids and intravenous antibiotics are administered. General anesthesia is induced. Our anesthesiologists generally perform a circumferential scalp block to reduce the requirements for general anesthesia and to assist with patient awakening at the end of the operation. Large-bore intravenous lines or a central venous catheter (if preferred) are placed to facilitate medication and fluid administration. An arterial catheter is required for blood pressure monitoring and serial blood gas assessment. Sequential compression devices are placed on the patient's calves and an indwelling Foley catheter is placed for fluid management.

◆ Operative Procedure

As already stated, approaches to the third ventricle can be considered to consist of two stages (**Table 6–1**). The first stage involves reaching the wall of the third ventricle, through which access into the ventricle will be achieved, and the second stage involves establishing the corridor into the third ventricle itself and subsequent removal of the tumor. The following descriptions emphasize the second stage of the operation.

Transforaminal and Transchoroidal Approaches

The transforaminal and transchoroidal approaches require the surgeon to first gain access to the lateral ventricle from above (stage 1). Although we have used the transcortical transventricular approach when midline access is limited by bridging veins, we generally prefer the interhemispheric transcallosal approach for lesions in the third ventricle because the exposure is anatomically clear, and there is less disruption of neural structures (only the corpus callosum is divided). An anterior or posterior trajectory is chosen based on the criteria already discussed (see Patient Selection). Minor adjustments in the positioning of the craniotomy are made to avoid midline-bridging veins as determined from preoperative MR imaging studies of both brain and veins. A right anterior interhemispheric transcallosal approach is described.

Patient Position and Skin Incision

The patient is placed in the supine position with the neck flexed such that the craniotomy is at the top of the field and the proposed trajectory is comfortable to the surgeon **(Fig. 6–5A)**.

The patient's head is immobilized with a three-point skull-fixation device. The trajectory to the tumor can be accurately determined using a computer-assisted frameless stereotactic surgical system, and we recommend this adjunct for resecting all third-ventricular tumors. The scalp incision is fashioned to allow the creation of a rectangular bone flap that extends at least 4 cm from the midline to the right. In most cases, the craniotomy is 2 cm anterior and 3 cm posterior to the coronal suture.

The craniotomy is made as shown in **Fig. 6–5A,B.** The goal of the craniotomy is to expose the midline sinus. Surgical and cotton pledgets can be used to control bleeding from the superior sagittal sinus. The dura is opened to create a medially based flap that extends to the midline. The dura is reflected carefully to prevent inadvertent tearing of cortical veins and arachnoid granulations. Bridging veins between the right frontal cortex and the superior sagittal sinus are identified. Preservation of all bridging veins is a goal, but if necessary, small veins can be coagulated and sharply cut. There is typically a zone free of bridging veins in the region of the coronal suture. The dura is reflected and held in position using sutures but without applying excess tension that might inadvertently occlude the sinus. Ideally, there should be at least 3 cm of anterior-posterior distance between bridging veins to allow retractor placement for lateral frontal lobe retraction. A self-retaining retractor system (e.g., Budde Halo Retractor System [Integra, Plainsboro, NJ] or Greenberg Retractor System [Codman, Raynham, MA]) is attached to the skull-fixation device. The operating microscope is used to facilitate further dissection.

Aided by the microscope, an interhemispheric dissection to the corpus callosum is performed **(Fig. 6–5B).** Frameless stereotactic navigation clarifies the appropriate trajectory to the third-ventricular lesion. Adhesions between the right frontal lobe and falx are sharply divided. A retractor blade with an underlying rubber dam of equivalent size is inserted into the interhemispheric fissure. Continued sharp dissection of arachnoid adhesions between the falx and frontal lobe permits lateral frontal lobe retraction and progressively deeper dissection of the interhemispheric fissure to the base of the falx. The interhemispheric fissure is dissected further between the cingulate gyri. The pearly white corpus callosum marks the end of the interhemispheric fissure. The pericallosal arteries are identified. Exposure of a working space 2 to 3 cm long should be achieved in the corpus callosum.

The surgeon next dissects through the corpus callosum between the pericallosal arteries. Frameless stereotactic navigation helps guide the position of this callosal incision so that it is centered over the lesion. This incision is created in a stepwise fashion with electrocautery, sharp dissection, and gentle aspiration until the entire length of the incision reveals the grayish ventricular ependyma. The ventricular ependyma is opened sharply, and the retractors are advanced through the corpus callosum. CSF is allowed to drain, which provides increased brain relaxation and expands the surgical corridor.

Once the ventricle is entered, the surgeon must take the time to understand the orientation of the surgical field and to identify critical structures. The choroid plexus curves from laterally to medially as it sweeps anteriorly along the floor of the lateral ventricle into the foramen of Monro **(Fig. 6–5C).** Similarly, the thalamostriate vein sits laterally and courses anteromedially to enter the foramen. These structures serve as the critical orienting landmarks. The fornix is identified at the base of the septum pellucidum as it courses around the foramen. The midline septum pellucidum may be fenestrated and retracted to gain access to the opposite ventricular system.

Once oriented, the surgeon prepares to enter the third ventricle **(Fig. 6–5C).** The transforaminal route makes use of a naturally occurring corridor and should be the first choice for entry into the third ventricle. Tumors such as colloid cysts can often be seen projecting into or just below the foramen. In many cases, tumors can be resected without further dissection if the foramen is large enough. However, when the foramen is not dilated or the tumor is larger than the foraminal aperture, the opening can be increased or a separate entry into the ventricle can be achieved by a transchoroidal approach.

The transchoroidal corridor is developed on the medial side of the choroid plexus and lateral to the fornix by sharp dissection through the tenia fornicis **(Fig. 6–6).** High magnification is used, with the microscope zoomed into the field. The dissection can be facilitated by beginning at the posterior edge of the foramen of Monro and proceeding posteriorly. A 1-cm opening of the fissure usually provides a view ranging back to the aqueduct of Sylvius. The choroid plexus can be coagulated to reduce its mass and to better visualize the plane of dissection. Gentle retraction of the septum can help displace the fornix medially and provide a larger corridor.

It is safer to proceed on the medial side of the choroid plexus than on the lateral side (along the tenia thalami) because the thalamostriate vein, other veins that drain the central neural structures, and the branches of the choroidal arteries, pass through the tenia thalami. By dissecting along the tenia fornicis, these vessels are avoided and are less likely to be torn. Dissection through the choroidal fissure permits visualization of the internal cerebral veins. Further entry into the third ventricle can be achieved without sacrificing any vessels by dissecting between the two internal cerebral veins. It is possible to proceed laterally to the internal cerebral vein, but branching veins may need to be sacrificed. Small vessels from the choroidal arteries can be taken.

Dissection between the internal cerebral veins can also be facilitated by beginning at the foramen of Monro; here the thalamostriate vein can be followed until it meets the septal vein to form the internal cerebral vein. Dissection on the medial side of the thalamostriate vein leads directly to the plane between the internal cerebral veins. The point of union of these vessels relative to the foramen can be variable. If the thalamostriate vein joins the internal cerebral vein very posteriorly, a wide corridor into the third ventricle can easily be achieved. If the junction is close to the foramen, however, it may be necessary to sacrifice the anterior septal vein. This maneuver untethers the internal cerebral vein and the thalamostriate vein, opening the space between the two internal cerebral veins and thereby increasing the size of the corridor. We have found that this maneuver is safe and reduces the chance of tearing the internal cerebral vein at the junction

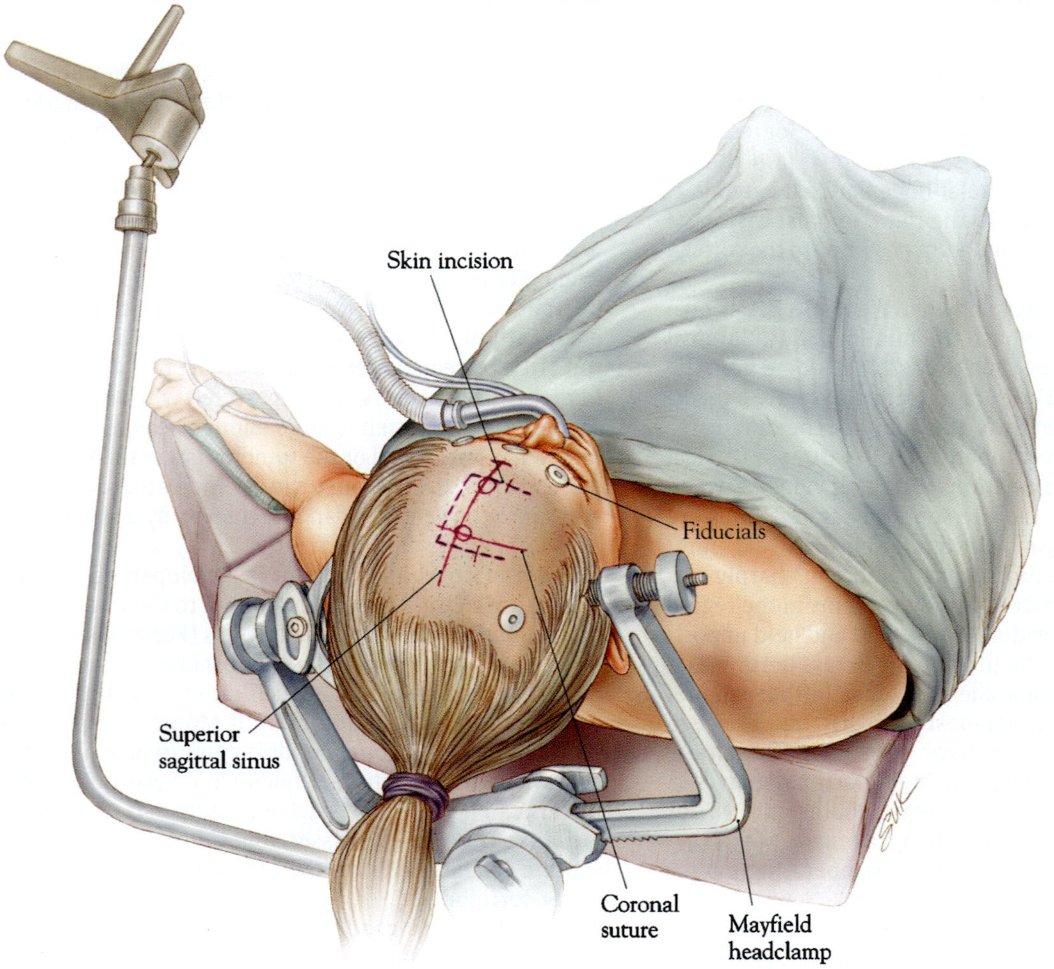

Skin incision
Fiducials
Superior
sagittal sinus
Coronal
suture
Mayfield
headclamp

A

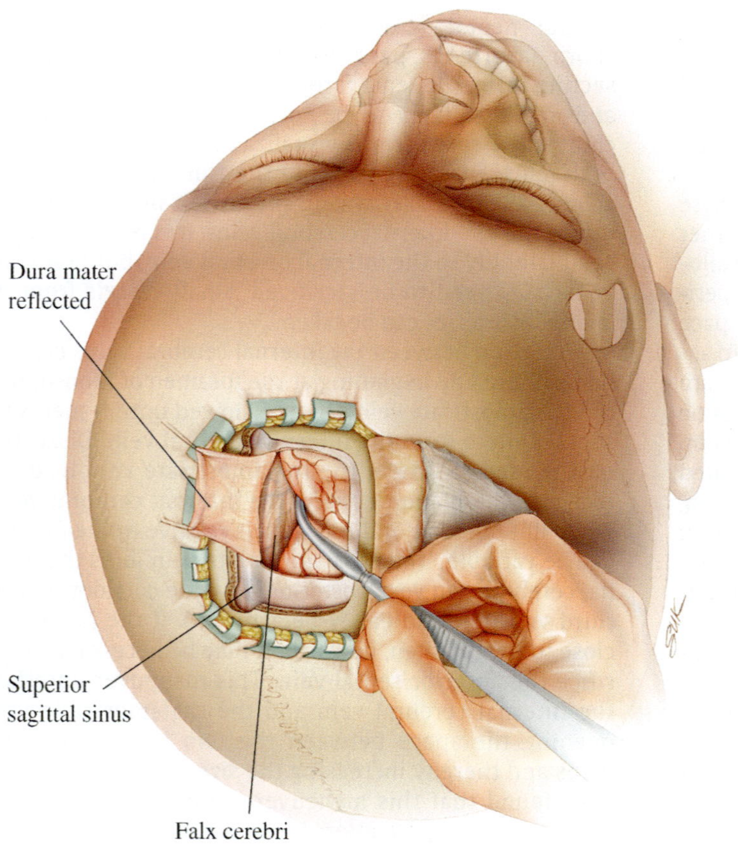

Dura mater
reflected
Superior
sagittal sinus
Falx cerebri

B

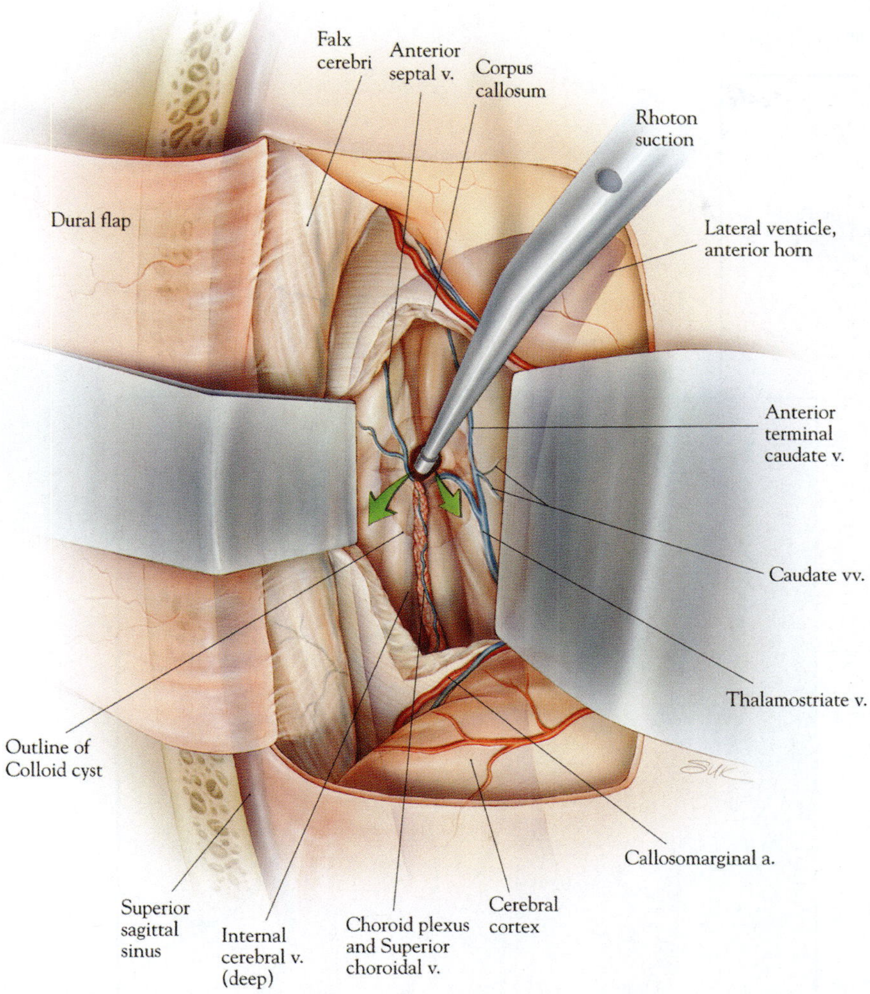

(Continued) **Figure 6–5** Artist's depiction of the anterior transcallosal interhemispheric approach and transforaminal entries into the third ventricle. **(A)** The skin incision is planned based on the coronal suture and midline sagittal sinus. The incision is based laterally. Bur holes are made on the sinus and laterally. Fiducials and the localizer for computer-assisted surgery are shown. The craniotomy is at the top of the surgical field. **(B)** The dura is flapped medially toward the sagittal sinus. The brain is gently retracted exposing the falx cerebri. Dissection down the falx continues until the cingulate gyri are divided and the corpus callosum is seen. **(C)** The divided corpus callosum is shown. The choroid plexus is a landmark to the foramen of Monro. This concludes stage 1 of the operation. The suction is within the foramen of Monro. Tumors can be removed from the third ventricle through an exposed foramen of Monro via a transforaminal approach.

with the thalamostriate vein, an untoward event that can have serious adverse effects.

Tumor Resection

Once the third ventricle has been entered, the tumor is identified and removal is performed in piecemeal fashion. To remove large tumors through the small surgical corridors afforded by the transchoroidal and transforaminal approaches, tumor material should first be removed from within the capsule (or pseudocapsule). This internal decompression and debulking facilitates tumor wall manipulation and resection. The tumor is sequentially decompressed from within and then dissected around the outer capsule. This reduces a large mass to a small mass and facilitates removal. Tumors such as colloid cysts can be reduced to small masses in this way and brought out through a mildly expanded foramen of Monro. Highly vascular tumors, such as germ cell tumors, should be dealt with in a similar fashion, and the surgeon must maintain a calm and focused demeanor, knowing that when the bleeding subsides, the tumor is usually nearly completely removed.

Because the third ventricle is a loculated structure, vessels within the center of the tumor almost invariably supply the tumor but not the surrounding neural structures and thus can be coagulated and cut to control bleeding. Vessels that are attached to the capsule can usually be preserved by sweeping them off the tumor capsule using microdissectors.

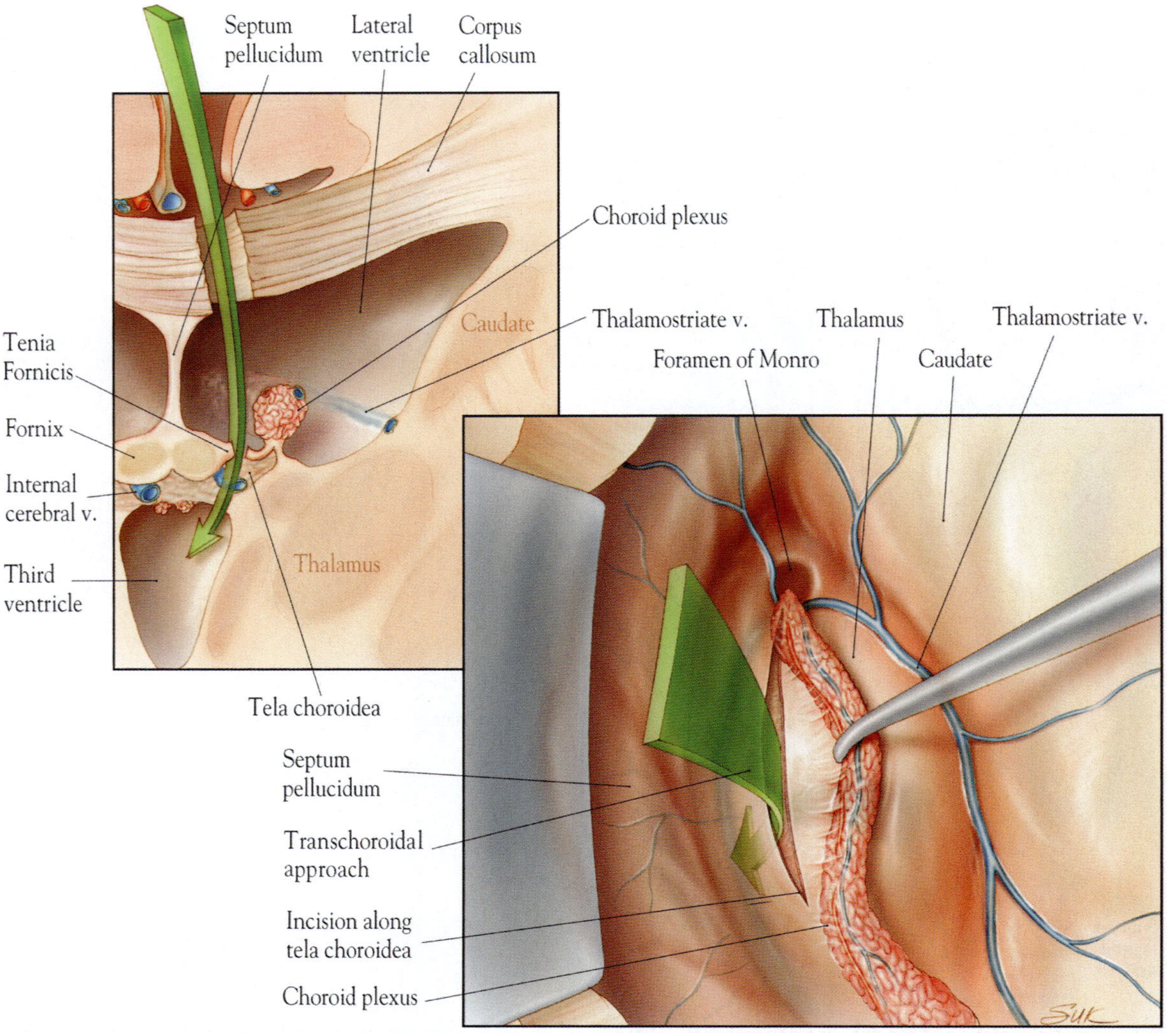

Figure 6–6 The transchoroidal approach into the third ventricle. A corridor into the third ventricle can be achieved via a transchoroidal approach when the foramen of Monro is small. Upper left shows a coronal view of interhemispheric transcallosal entry into lateral ventricle. The safest passage to the third ventricle is on the medial side of the choroid plexus (along the tenia fornicis). (Lower right) An incision is made along the tenia fornicis through the tela choroidea. The surgeon can then dissect between both internal cerebral veins to be free of any vessels. By beginning at the foramen of Monro exposure of the entire third ventricle can be achieved.

Closure

Hemostasis must be obtained meticulously prior to closure of the surgical corridor. Stepwise retractor withdrawal, evaluation of hemostasis, and application of electrocautery and hemostatic agents is mandatory. A Valsalva maneuver should be performed to test the adequacy of hemostasis. Copious irrigation aids removal of intraventricular blood or tissue debris that may subsequently obstruct CSF pathways. Excess hemostatic material may likewise obstruct CSF pathways and should be irrigated from the field prior to closure. An external ventricular drain may be left in place for management of postoperative hydrocephalus. Excess intraventricular air is removed with copious irrigation prior to closure of the dura in a watertight fashion. The skull is secured and the wound is closed in layers.

Trans–Lamina Terminalis Approach

The first part of the trans–lamina terminalis approach involves accessing and identifying the lamina terminalis. The following discussion describes the unilateral subfrontal approach. The second part of the operation involves dissection through the lamina and removal of the tumor.

Patient Positioning and Skin Incision

For the unilateral subfrontal approach, the patient is placed in the supine position with the neck extended such that the floor of the anterior cranial fossa is 30 degrees beyond vertical **(Fig. 6–7A).** The head is rotated 30 degrees away from the operative side. Three-point pin fixation helps to maintain head position and is essential for frameless

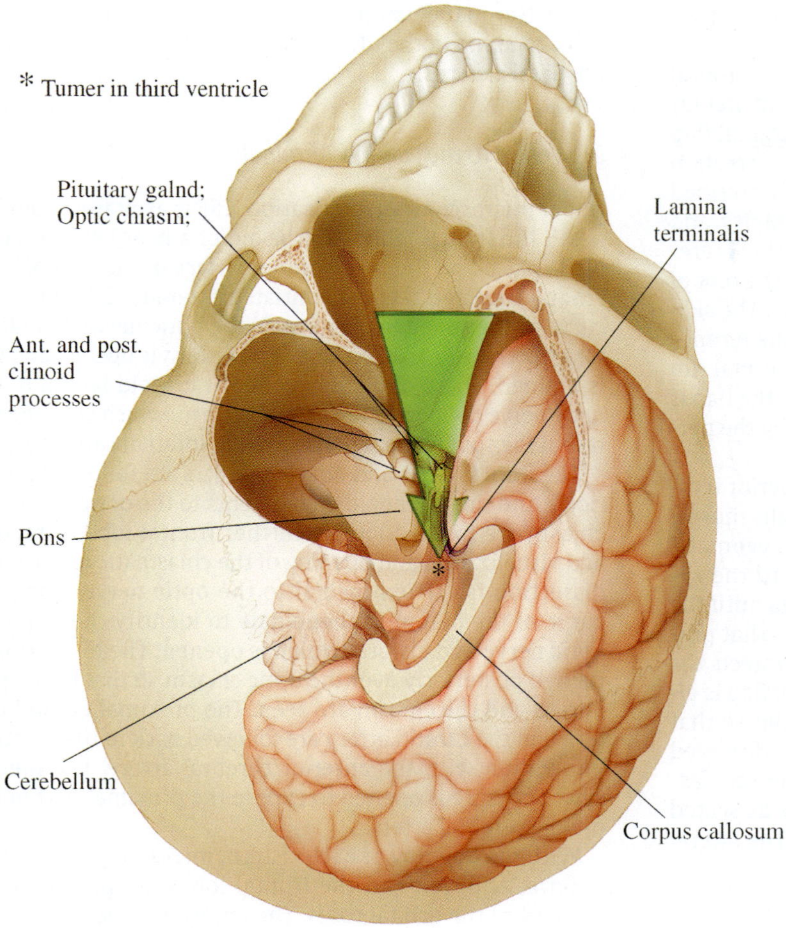

A

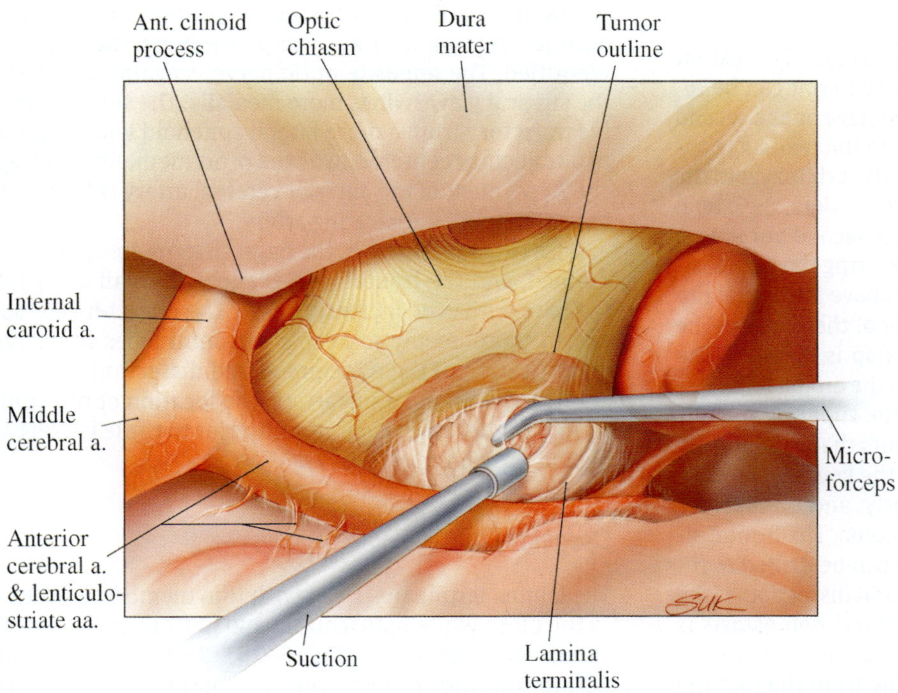

B

Figure 6–7 Artist's depiction of the unilateral subfrontal trans–laminar terminalis approach. **(A)** The lamina terminalis can be reached by performing a unilateral craniotomy that goes to the midline. Removal of the orbit is shown. This provides a unilateral subfrontal approach. **(B)** The cisterns around the carotid artery and optic nerve are opened bilaterally. The anterior cerebral artery is dissected from the optic chiasm. The lamina terminalis is posterior to the chiasm. Entry through the lamina terminalis results in entry into the third ventricle.

stereotactic navigation, which is a useful adjunct to surgical navigation.

The skin incision is designed to allow access for a frontal craniotomy with resection of the orbital roof and rim. Details of this approach, including elevation of the pericranial flap and incision of the temporalis muscle fascia for preservation of the frontalis branch of the facial nerve, are described elsewhere in this atlas (see Chapter 22 by Al-Mefty and Kadri). Briefly, a three-fourths bicoronal scalp incision is created behind the hairline, extending laterally from the root of the zygoma to the opposite superior temporal line. The skin flap is elevated in the subgaleal plane and over the temporalis muscle fascia to a finger's breadth above the orbital rim anteriorly and to the level of the keyhole laterally; the flap is reflected anteriorly over a rolled-up sponge, leaving the pericranium and temporalis fascia intact.

The pericranium is then incised along each superior temporal line, and an incision is made in the temporalis muscle fascia beginning a finger's breadth above the zygomatic process of the frontal bone and extending toward the zygoma. This incision is extended through the fascia until the temporalis muscle can be identified, a procedure that preserves the fat pad of the temporalis muscle and protects the frontalis branch of the facial nerve. The pericranial flap is elevated, and this dissection is carried into the orbit so that the periorbita (continuous with the pericranium) is dissected off the superior orbit. Laterally, the temporalis muscle fascia, which is continuous with the pericranium, is dissected off the lateral orbit to the origin of the zygoma. The lateral periorbita is freed from within the orbit.

Craniotomy and Dural Opening

A unilateral orbital craniotomy is performed. The extent of bone removal is shown in **Fig. 6–7A**. The orbit can be removed with the frontal craniotomy in one stage or as a second stage after the craniotomy is completed. In the two-stage approach, a bur hole is placed just behind the orbitozygomatic suture. This bur hole exposes the frontal fossa dura, the lateral periorbita, and the temporal fossa dura. A second bur hole is placed just medial to the medial orbit, entering the frontal sinus. Bur holes can then be placed ~4 cm above the orbital rim near the midline and anterior to the root of the zygoma. The bur holes are connected and the bone flap is elevated. The dura over the orbit is then separated from the orbital roof.

Using a chisel or reciprocating saw, the superior and lateral orbital rims are removed by bony cuts that extend from the frontal medial bur hole posteriorly, the keyhole bur hole medially, the keyhole bur hole inferiorly, and then across the inferior orbit at the origin of the zygoma. The frontal sinus is exenterated. The sphenoid ridge can be drilled to reduce the amount of bone so that intradural dissection of the basal cisterns is not obstructed. Extradural hemostasis is obtained, and dural tack-up sutures are placed. The dura is opened in curvilinear fashion, extending from the midline inferiorly along the sinus posteriorly and curving just across the sylvian fissure to expose the tip of the temporal lobe. This latter maneuver provides orientation to the sphenoid ridge to assist in the identification of the structures within the basal cisterns.

Dissection to the Lamina Terminalis

Under microscopic magnification, CSF is aspirated from beneath the frontal lobe with the aid of a handheld retractor blade placed on the lateral undersurface of the frontal lobe. Frontal lobe retraction is initiated laterally, following the curve of the sphenoid ridge until the optic nerve and olfactory tracts are visualized. The optic cistern is opened and CSF is drained. Sharp dissection of the arachnoid lateral to the optic nerve delineates the carotid cistern, which is opened to reveal the supraclinoid portion of the internal carotid artery.

The frontal lobes and olfactory tracts are followed posteriorly, and the arachnoid attachments to the optic nerve and chiasm are freed, allowing further frontal lobe retraction and visualization and opening of the chiasmatic cistern. The dissection is carried medial to the optic nerve along the curve of the planum sphenoidale to identify the opposite optic nerve and cistern, which is opened. The dissection is carried posteriorly over the optic chiasm so that both optic nerves and the chiasm are seen. The proximal carotid cistern and the carotid artery are followed back to the carotid's bifurcation with the anterior cerebral artery. The medial sylvian fissure is opened to expose the proximal part of the middle cerebral artery.

With the opening of each cistern, increasing brain relaxation is achieved and the frontal lobes fall progressively away from the orbital roofs. The anterior cerebral artery is followed medially as it courses toward the chiasm, and the anterior communicating artery overlying the chiasm is identified. The opposite optic nerve is again identified as the surgical view swings more medially. The surgeon moves his trajectory from a more lateral sphenoid wing approach to a trajectory centered over the orbit medially. The opposite A_1 segment of the anterior cerebral artery is followed to the anterior communicating artery.

With these maneuvers, the basal cisterns are sequentially drained, and the frontal lobe is allowed to fall away from the base with ever-increasing ease. The retractors are positioned more deeply to keep the frontal lobes back. With identification of the A_1 segment and dissection across the anterior communicating artery, the location of the lamina terminalis becomes clear just anterior to these vessels and behind the chiasm **(Fig. 6–7)**.

Opening of the Lamina Terminalis

The lamina terminalis is a grayish thin membrane posterior to the more white optic chiasm and in front of the anterior communicating artery **(Fig. 6–7B)**. Bulging of the tumor within the anterior third ventricle or a bluish color offers further clues to the precise location of the lamina terminalis. Opening of the lamina terminalis is performed with sharp dissection, beginning with a small incision in its center. Vessels from the anterior cerebral arteries to the chiasm and nerves must not be disrupted. The lamina is gently expanded and the junction with the optic chiasm usually becomes clearer as the lamina opens. The amount of space afforded by the translaminar approach is dictated by the relationship between the optic chiasm and the anterior communicating artery. In the setting of short optic nerves (a so-called prefixed chiasm), the translaminar space is larger than in the setting of long optic nerves (a so-called postfixed chiasm). In either case, surgical manipulation within the translaminar corridor must be gentle so that the adjacent optic tracts are not injured by excessive traction or pressure.

Similarly, vascular injury must be avoided. The anterior cerebral arteries typically run along the lateral borders of the lamina terminalis and obstruct direct visualization of its most lateral margin. The anterior communicating artery often courses across the front wall of the lamina terminalis. Consequently, manipulation of these vessels and their associated perforating vessels is often necessary and can be performed gently. Nevertheless, excessive traction and inadvertent disruption of these vessels and perforating arteries must be avoided. Gentle Gelfoam and cotton pledget tamponade rather than electrocautery is the preferred method of hemostasis around the chiasm and anterior cerebral artery complex.

Tumor Removal

To avoid excessive traction on adjacent neural and vascular structures, particularly the optic chiasm and tracts, tumor within the third ventricle is removed in piecemeal fashion. As described earlier, the internal contents of the tumor are removed to transform a large mass into a smaller mass. Tumor-related cysts are decompressed, and the tumor capsule is judiciously dissected into the lamina and removed. The patient is rotated as needed to provide sequential exposure of the tumor abutting the opposite wall of the ventricle and the ipsilateral wall. This ipsilateral wall is often difficult to visualize and may require judicious use of a mirror. Likewise, inspection of the third ventricle itself can be aided by a small mirror. Despite the small opening, many large tumors can be removed piecemeal through the lamina.

Closure

Prior to closure, meticulous hemostasis must be achieved. The dura is closed in a watertight fashion. The pericranial graft is reflected over the anterior cranial fossa floor and tacked to the underside of the dura with sutures. This graft serves to obliterate the opened and exenterated frontal sinus. The bone flap is replaced, with the orbital rim being positioned over the pericranial graft. Bur hole covers provide adequate cosmesis for bony defects in front of the hairline. The wound is closed one layer at a time.

◆ Postoperative Management

Patients are managed postoperatively in an intensive care setting. From the time of wound closure through at least the first 48 postoperative hours, normal blood pressure is maintained, with the aid of an intravenous antihypertensive infusion, if needed. The patient is kept on a regimen of normovolemic fluid management and supraphysiological steroid replacement.

All patients should undergo postoperative MR imaging within 24 to 48 hours of surgery to evaluate the extent of tumor resection and to assess any signs of potential complications, including blood in the ventricle, hydrocephalus, brain edema, or stroke. This early postoperative scan also serves as an important baseline should a change develop later **(Figs. 6–2 and 6–3)**.

Although not routine, patients may undergo placement of an external ventricular drain, which is typically positioned 3 to 5 cm above the ear for 24 to 48 hours to allow for drainage of blood-tinged CSF or surgical debris. The reservoir is raised, and drainage is monitored. Persistent elevation in intracranial pressure and CSF drainage despite elevation of the drain are criteria for shunting.

Resection of tumors of the third ventricle can lead to myriad neurological complications. Incisions through the corpus callosum are generally well tolerated but may result in disorders of interhemispheric transfer of information. Injury to the fornix, if bilateral, can result in profound memory loss. Manipulation of lesions within the walls of the third ventricle can cause hypothalamic dysfunction, including altered temperature control, disturbances of respiration, altered consciousness, and behavioral changes, all of which must be monitored carefully and treated appropriately. Patients can develop diabetes insipidus (DI), which should be managed with fluid replacement and judicious administration of desmopressin acetate (DDAVP). DI can be transient, permanent, or part of a triple-phase response, and the need for changing fluid requirements must be detected early to prevent dramatic swings in total body water content, intravascular volume, and serum osmolality.

Translaminar approaches can result in visual impairment. For midline approaches, the development of delayed neurological decline may be due to venous infarction if bridging veins were sacrificed. For transcortical approaches, the onset of new seizures is possible. Postoperative neurological deterioration may also result from intracranial hemorrhage, hydrocephalus, retraction-related brain injury, or vascular injury and infarction. CT and MR imaging with diffusion weighting can assess each of these potential complications.

Despite these potential problems, with careful preoperative planning, meticulous surgical technique, and aggressive postoperative management, the operative morbidity and mortality associated with removing third-ventricular tumors can be kept to a low frequency, and most patients should return to normal function.

7

Surgical Approaches to Intraventricular Tumors (Lateral Ventricles)

Eylem Ocal, Joachim M. Baehring, and Joseph Piepmeier

Intraventricular tumors present a difficult surgical challenge for the neurosurgeon, requiring a careful entire preoperative assessment to determine the optimal surgical approach with the best outcome and minimal morbidity. Lesions confined to the lateral ventricles are relatively rare and constitute ~1% of all intracranial tumors. A variety of tumors arise in the region; however, a majority of them are benign, including low-grade gliomas (50%), choroid plexus papillomas (20 to 25%) **(Fig. 7–1),** and meningiomas (15%) **(Fig. 7–2).** Teratomas, epidermoid, neurocytomas, and metastatic tumors are less commonly seen in the lateral ventricles.

◆ Patient Selection

Because the intraventricular space can accommodate a slowly expanding tumor, these lesions may remain unnoticed for a long time. A brain tumor should be considered in all patients with a new headache or change in quality of a chronic headache, focal neurological symptoms, or a psychiatric manifestation. The clinical presentation of lateral ventricular tumors is nonspecific and can be acute (strokelike due to intratumoral hemorrhage, pressure valve effect) or subacute (slowly progressive headache, which is typically worst upon awakening, personality changes, memory loss). Seizures are much less common than in hemispheric tumors and indicate tumor growth beyond the confines of the ventricles.

Once the tumor reaches a certain size, symptoms of cerebrospinal fluid (CSF) flow obstruction ensue. Cognitive decline or personality changes are accompanied by progressive headache and followed by nausea, vomiting, hiccoughing, yawning, and increasing somnolence. In infants, prior to

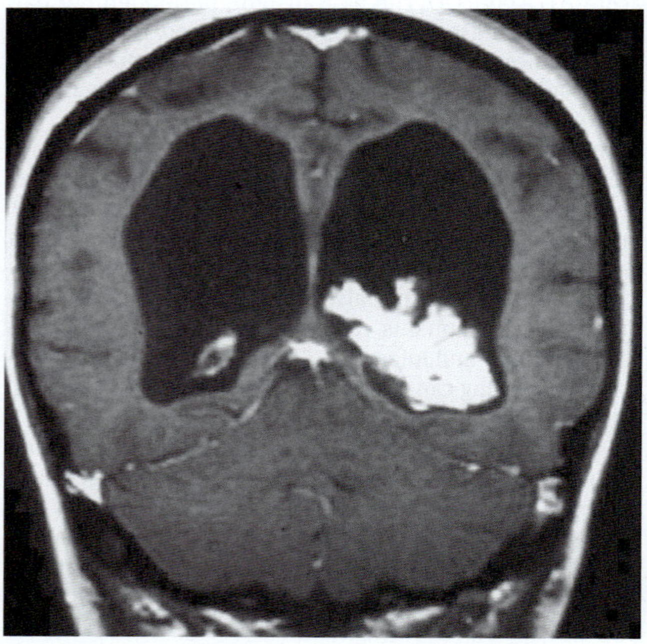

Figure 7–1 Coronal enhanced magnetic resonance imaging of a choroid plexus papilloma in the trigone of the left lateral ventricle. Note the typical frondlike projections and large ventricles.

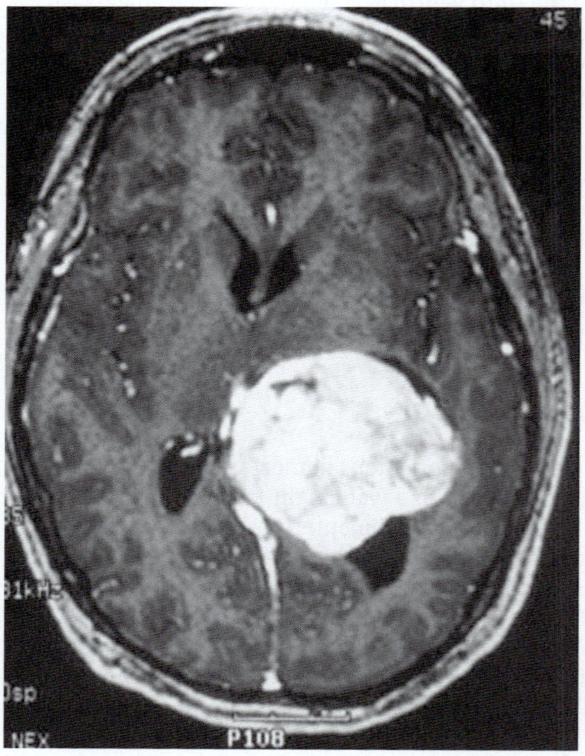

Figure 7–2 Magnetic resonance imaging of a meningioma in the posterior horn of the left lateral ventricle (axial images with dense contrast enhancement).

closure of the calvarial sutures, hydrocephalus is accompanied by enlargement of head circumference. Communicating hydrocephalus in patients with intraventricular tumors is the result of spinal fluid overproduction (choroid plexus papilloma) or decreased reabsorption.

Asymmetric hydrocephalus is observed in patients with tumors of the body and the temporal and occipital horn of the lateral ventricle. Focal neurological symptoms arise when the tumor infiltrates the adjacent commissural or projection fiber tracts. A subcortical hemiparesis results from growth into the centrum semiovale. Tumors surrounding the atrium or the occipital or temporal horn give rise to visual field defects. Infiltration of the corpus callosum is the basis for disconnection syndromes such as alexia without agraphia or transcortical dysphasias.

Infiltrative gliomas affecting the lateral ventricles are commonly amenable to stereotactic biopsy only. Surgical removal of subependymal giant cell astrocytoma is curative and indicated when progressive growth obstructs CSF flow. Of the few supratentorial intraventricular ependymomas, the majority is found within the trigone of the lateral ventricle. Complete surgical removal may be curative for the patient with a low-grade ependymoma. Subependymomas are benign, well-demarcated tumors in proximity to the ventricular system. Resection is only required when CSF obstruction occurs or the tumor enlarges. Choroid plexus papilloma is one of the most common lateral ventricular tumors in children. Resection is curative. Neurocytomas are rare tumors of neuronal origin that are typically found at the inferior septum pellucidum. Because the tumor is broadly adherent to the interventricular septum or the ventricular wall, surgical cure is accomplished in fewer than 50% of patients. However, long-term tumor control can be achieved with partial resection. Meningioma is the most common atrial mass. Complete resection is the goal. Primary lymphoma of the central nervous system is frequently found adjacent to the lateral ventricle. Primarily a medical disease, surgery is limited to stereotactic biopsy. Metastases to the choroid plexus are rare and predominantly arise from renal and lung carcinoma in adults and Wilms' tumor and retinoblastoma in children. Surgery is rarely indicated unless there is diagnostic uncertainty.

◆ Preoperative Preparation

Designing the surgery for the lateral ventricles depends on a number of variables that a neurosurgeon must consider. Preoperative neurological examination and review of the imaging studies are mandatory as in any kind of brain surgery. The location, probable histopathology, vascularity of the adjacent structures, as well as the blood supply of the lesion should be considered carefully. Standard preoperative testing with magnetic resonance imaging (MRI), including magnetic resonance angiography (MRA) and venography (MRV), can provide important information for selecting an approach. The majority of the tumors in this region are contrast enhancing and expand the ventricular space as they grow in size. The trigone is the most common site of origin, particularly for meningiomas and papillomas. Neurocytomas and gliomas are frequently located in the ventricular body. The frontal, temporal, and occipital horns are less common sites of origin. Additionally, MRA and MRV images can visualize the arterial and venous anatomy. Cerebral angiography may provide further information in particular cases such as highly vascularized choroid plexus papillomas and meningiomas.

Tumors of the lateral ventricles usually receive their blood supply from both the anterior and posterior choroidal arteries. Tortuosity, hypertrophy, or displacement of these vessels can be appreciated by preoperative angiographic studies. Careful review of the images also identifies highly vascularized tumors and permits preparation for possible intraoperative blood loss. Perioperative neurological examination, including cognitive testing, constitutes an important part of patient assessment. Recognition of preoperative deficits illustrates the importance of avoiding further injury to cortical structures and white matter tracts with impaired function. Neuropsychological tests serve as a baseline revealing memory deficits. Impaired functioning of intelligence with more profound decrease in performance IQ more than verbal IQ is characteristic and attributed to longstanding hydrocephalus in these patients.

Another important consideration is to define the patients with cross-dominance where speech and dominant handedness are controlled by opposite hemispheres. This documentation, alone, may be a contraindication for a transcallosal approach. These patients may suffer permanent language, writing, or reading deficits following surgery. A posterior callosotomy where the splenium is sectioned is also contraindicated in patients with homonymous hemianopia in the dominant hemisphere, which may lead to alexia.

◆ Operative Procedure

Because the majority of the tumors located in the ventricles are benign or low grade, surgery is usually the optimal treatment modality with curative intent. There are a variety of surgical procedures to access the lateral ventricles providing the surgeon with a range of options. Each of these options has its own complications and none is more superior to the others. These approaches may be divided into transcallosal and transcortical techniques. A combination of both can be used if appropriate, depending on the tumors size, location, blood supply, presumptive pathology, as well as the surgeon's experience.

Transcallosal Approach

The transcallosal approach is commonly utilized for lesions in the body of the lateral ventricles. Anterior callosotomy is directed to the frontal horn and the body. Anterior callosotomy is a reliable method when it is used in carefully selected patients and is limited in the amount of callosal sectioning.

Proper patient positioning should allow maximal exposure. The patient is placed supine with the head fixed in a neutral position but flexed 20 to 30 degrees from the horizontal to improve venous drainage and to help control bleeding. Some surgeons prefer to position the head laterally with the affected hemisphere facing downward. This

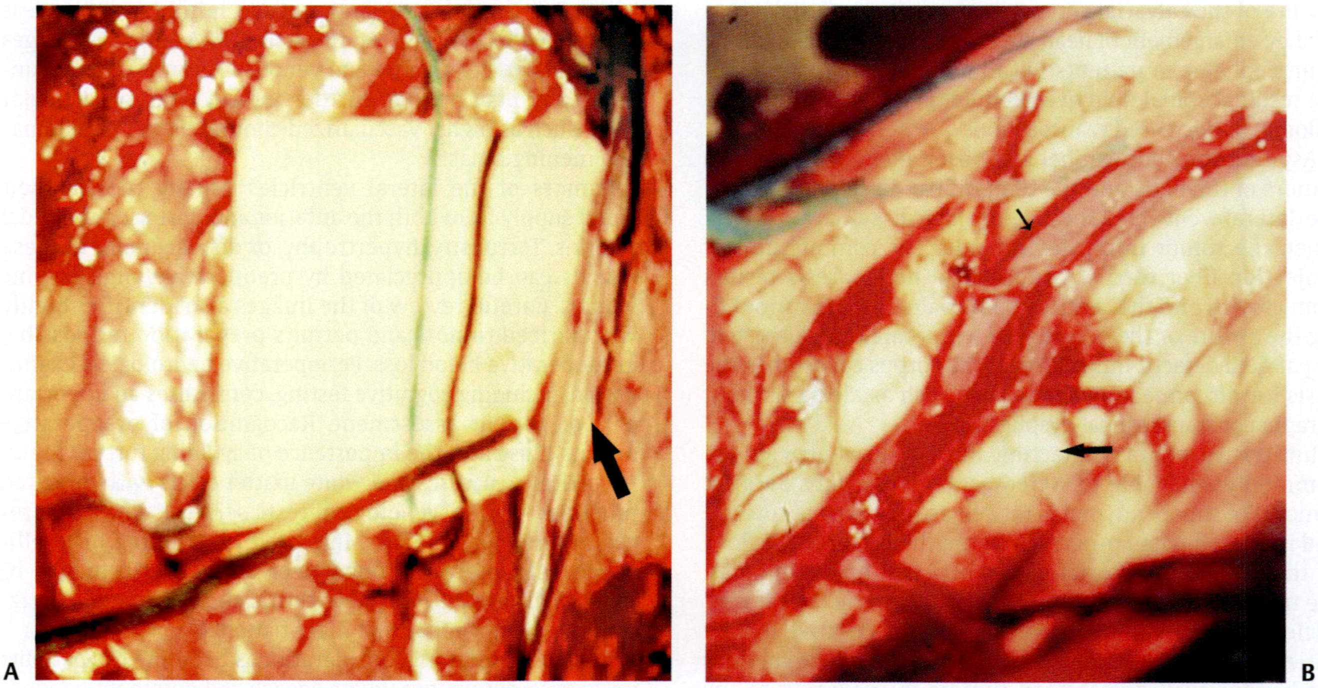

Figure 7–3 Intraoperative images from a transcallosal approach. **(A)** Splitting of the interhemispheric fissure to access the corpus callosum (arrow, falx). **(B)** Anterior cerebral arteries overlying the corpus callosum (arrow, corpus callosum; small arrow, anterior cerebral arteries).

allows gravity as a retractive force without excessive manipulation. A bicoronal or frontal horseshoe skin incision crossing the midline is used. The craniotomy is centered on the coronal suture and should extend beyond the midline over the superior sagittal sinus (SSS). Although the nondominant hemisphere is usually preferred, the side of the craniotomy in either hemisphere may be appropriate depending on the presence of midline draining veins as defined by the preoperative MRV. Prior to interhemispheric or any cortical incision, brain relaxation should be obtained with osmotic diuresis, hyperventilation, and/or CSF drainage. A ventricular catheterization is commonly used. Interhemispheric dissection starts with the aid of the surgical microscope **(Fig. 7–3A)**. A plane is maintained between the falx and the cortex. The falx is exposed to its free edge inferiorly following this falx–cortical interface. At the inferior edge of the falx, the corpus callosum and both anterior cerebral arteries are visualized **(Fig. 7–3B)**. The corpus callosum is identified by its typical whiter appearance and hypovascularity. A 1.5- to 2-cm incision is made depending on the size of the tumor, between the pericallosal arteries, and the ventricle is opened. The foramen of Monro can be found by following the thalamostriate veins and the choroid plexus. The lesion is easily identified in most cases **(Fig. 7–4)**. It is essential to maintain the boundary between the lesion and the ependyma clearly before starting and during the resection. Tumors are commonly removed piecemeal and delivered from the incision with gentle traction. Bleeding should be controlled meticulously. When

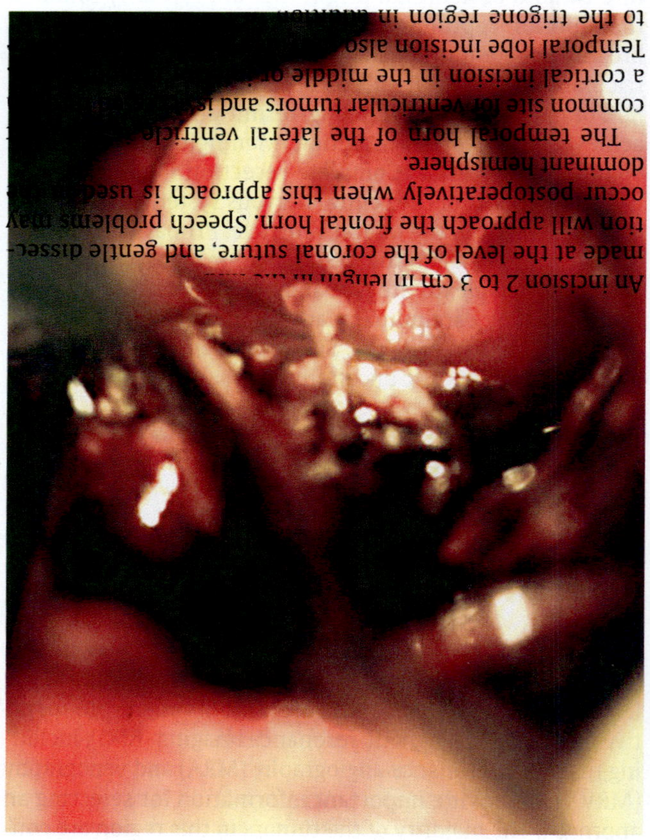

Figure 7–4 Tumors.

bleeding occurs, the foramen of Monro should be protected to prevent blood accumulation in the ventricles. The ventricles should be irrigated with warm saline at the end to remove trapped air and blood.

Transcortical Approach

Transcortical approaches are used for lesions in the temporal horns, posterior trigone, and superior frontal horn. For this purpose, the surgeon may select variable cortical incisions according to the site of the tumor. Transcortical approaches include the anterior cortical approach through the middle frontal gyrus; lateral approaches through a temporoparietal incision or middle temporal gyrus incision; and posterior approaches by way of superior parieto-occipital or occipital cortisectomies.

A middle frontal gyrus route is commonly preferred for the lesions within the superior portion of the frontal horn and also provides access to the anterior part of the body of the ventricle. The craniotomy should expose the superior and middle frontal gyri and extend to the midline. The nondominant hemisphere is preferably used for the approach. An incision 2 to 3 cm in length in the middle frontal gyrus is made at the level of the coronal suture, and gentle dissection will approach the frontal horn. Speech problems may occur postoperatively when this approach is used in the dominant hemisphere.

[illegible] approximately locates the temporal horn. Even though the temporal approach gains the shortest distance to the tumors of this region and early access to the anterior choroidal artery, postoperative neurological deficits are possible. Damage to the angular gyrus of the dominant hemisphere during a temporal approach extending to the temporoparietal junction may produce dyslexia, agraphia, acalculia, and ideomotor apraxia. Lesions in the nondominant hemisphere may impair visual memory. Additionally, incisions in this region traverse the optic radiations, causing visual field deficit. Middle temporal gyrus incision, on the other hand, may result in speech deficits.

The most common posterior transcortical approach to lateral ventricles is through the superior parietal lobule. This approach exposes the trigone and lesions within the posterior body of the lateral ventricles. For parietal approaches, the exposure should take into consideration the vein of Trolard. The cortical incision is demarcated by the postcentral sulcus anteriorly, parietooccipital sulcus posteriorly, and 3 cm away from the falx. The dissection proceeds medial to the visual fibers of the optic radiation. Postoperative complications may also include apraxia, acalculia, and impairment in visual–spatial processing.

◆ Postoperative Management

The patient should be monitored in a neurointensive care unit following intraventricular surgery. Hemorrhage, seizures, subdural hematomas due to excessive drainage of CSF, and persistent hydrocephalus may complicate the postoperative period, particularly when large tumors are removed. A CT scan should be obtained if any change occurs in the patient's neurological status. However, in our experience patients are routinely imaged on the first postoperative day.

An intraventricular catheter placed perioperatively is used to monitor intracranial pressure. In uncomplicated cases, it can be removed commonly on the second postoperative day and patients are allowed to mobilize. Patients with persistently high intracranial pressure and hydrocephalus may be candidates for shunt placement, which further improves cognitive and focal deficits.

[illegible] deficits related to each approach [illegible] evaluation of [illegible]

◆ Conclusion

With the use of advanced technology in neurosurgery, the mortality rate for intraventricular tumors has greatly decreased. However, surgery for these lesions still remains one of the most challenging topics. Adequate knowledge of the cortical and ventricular anatomy and histopathological features of the tumors helps the surgeon select the most proper surgical approach for each individual lesion. Among the broad range of options, none of the approaches is completely satisfactory or superior to others, but careful planning and preoperative evaluation are mandatory for the best outcome. Attention to detail maximizes the patient's recovery and restoring the previous level of function.

Section III

Spinal and Peripheral Nerve Tumors

8

Surgical Management of Spinal Meningiomas

Samir B. Lapsiwala and Daniel K. Resnick

Meningiomas are relatively common neoplasms, accounting for ~15% of all central nervous system tumors. Approximately 10% of meningiomas represent spinal meningiomas. Spinal meningiomas are the second most common tumor of the spinal canal located in the intradural extramedullary space. They arise from arachnoid cap cells and account for ~20% of intraspinal neoplasms. Most occur in middle life, usually after the fourth decade, and show a 10:1 preference for women. Thoracic meningiomas account for ~80% of all spinal meningiomas followed by upper cervical spine meningiomas **(Fig. 8–1)**.

◆ Patient Selection

Meningiomas are generally slow-growing, benign tumors attached to the dura. About 10% of meningiomas are both intradural and extradural or entirely extradural. The clinical

A

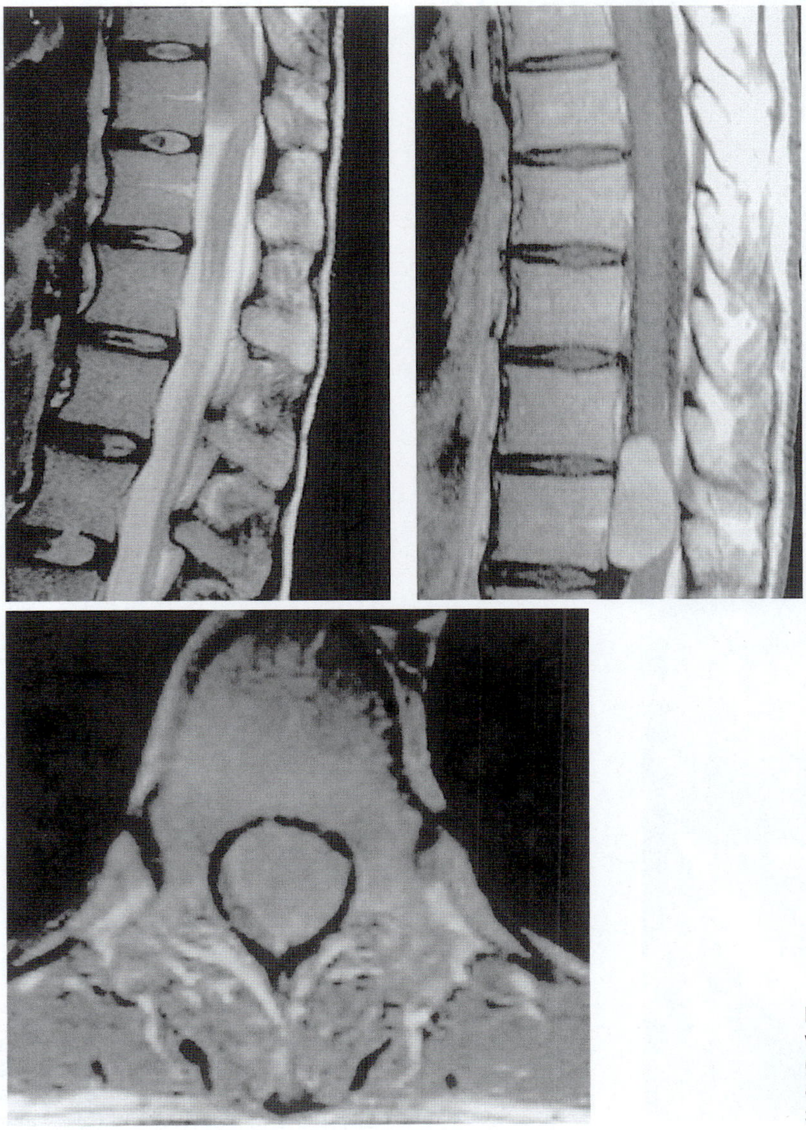

B

C

Figure 8–1 Magnetic resonance imaging of a patient with a thoracic meningioma. Sagittal T2-weighted image **(A)**, sagittal T1-weighted image with contrast **(B)**, and axial T1-weighted image without contrast **(C)** are shown.

presentation can be quite variable depending on the size and location of the tumor. Generally pain precedes the progressive neurological deficits. Tumors in the cervical region are often ventral to the cord and present with arm paresthesias, weakness, and clumsiness. Thoracic tumors tend to produce lower extremity paresthesia, stiffness, and fatigability, followed by spasticity. Weakness, if present, starts distally and the patient may also have a sensory gait ataxia due to dysfunction of posterior columns. Bowel and bladder are usually not affected until late in the clinical course. Regardless of the presenting complaint, the neurological exam at the time of diagnosis reveals long tract signs and myelopathy.

Due to a slow indolent growth pattern diagnosis is usually delayed. In 1970, Davis and Washburn reported a delay in diagnosis of greater than 6 months in 75% of patients. Recent advances in imaging technology have reduced time to diagnosis. Multiplanar imaging of the spine with magnetic resonance imaging (MRI) has become the gold standard. Typically, spinal meningiomas will appear isointense to the spinal cord on T1- and T2-weighted images and enhance intensely with gadolinium infusion **(Fig. 8–2)**. Axial MRI is very important in establishing the relationship of the tumor with the spinal cord, allowing better presurgical planning. Computed tomographic (CT) scan is very helpful in assessing the degree of tumor calcification **(Fig. 8–3).** A myelogram may show a wide dural-based mass or a complete myelographic block. MRI also helps assess the entire spinal axis in cases where there are multiple lesions. Unlike in cases of neurofibromas, plain radiographs add very little to the diagnosis.

A preoperative understanding of the relationship between the tumor, spinal cord, nerve roots, and dura is crucial. In 1925, Elsberg developed terminology to describe extramedullary intradural tumors, taking into account the nerve roots and dentate ligaments. According to Elsberg, tumors anterior to the motor roots are ventral, those between the motor roots and dentate ligaments are ventrolat-

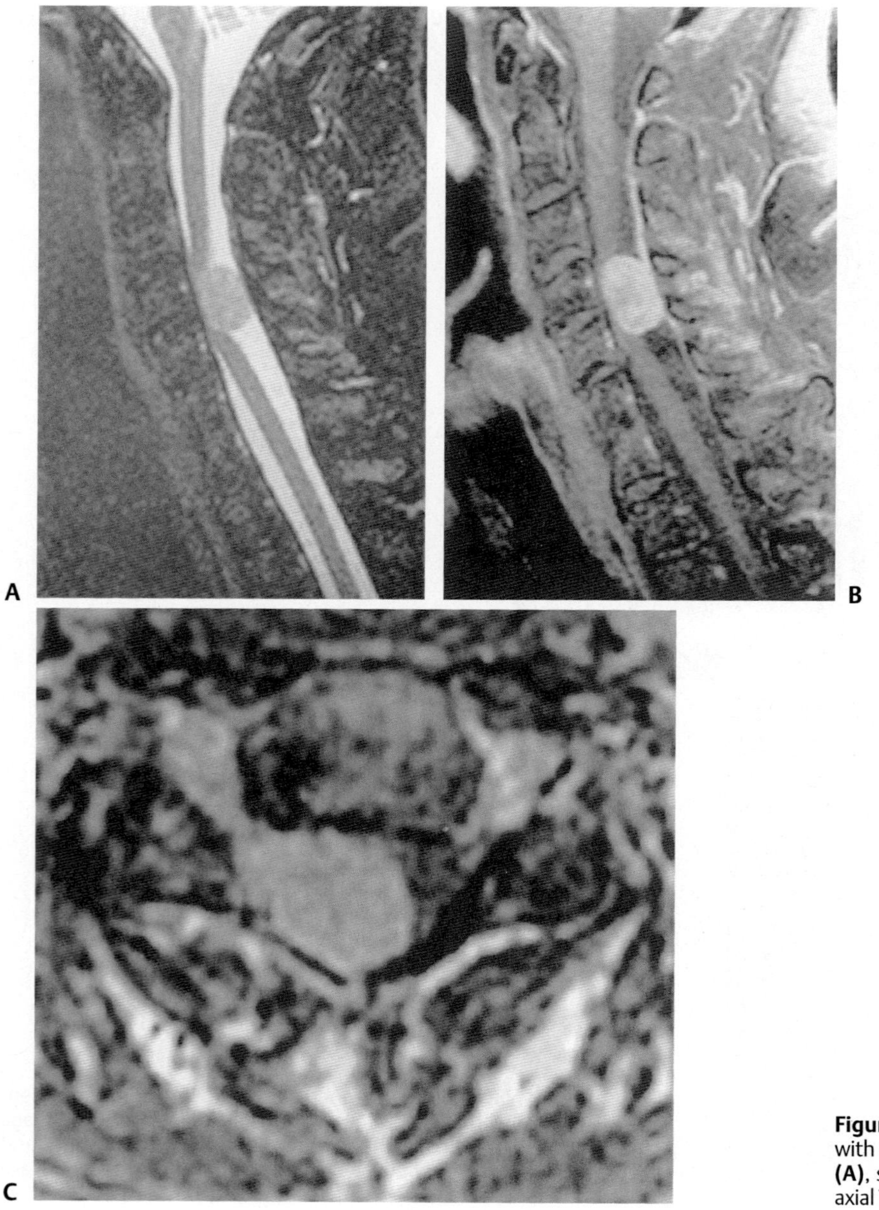

Figure 8–2 Magnetic resonance imaging of a patient with a cervical meningioma. Sagittal T2-weighted image **(A)**, sagittal T1-weighted image with contrast **(B)**, and axial T1-weighted image without contrast **(C)** are shown.

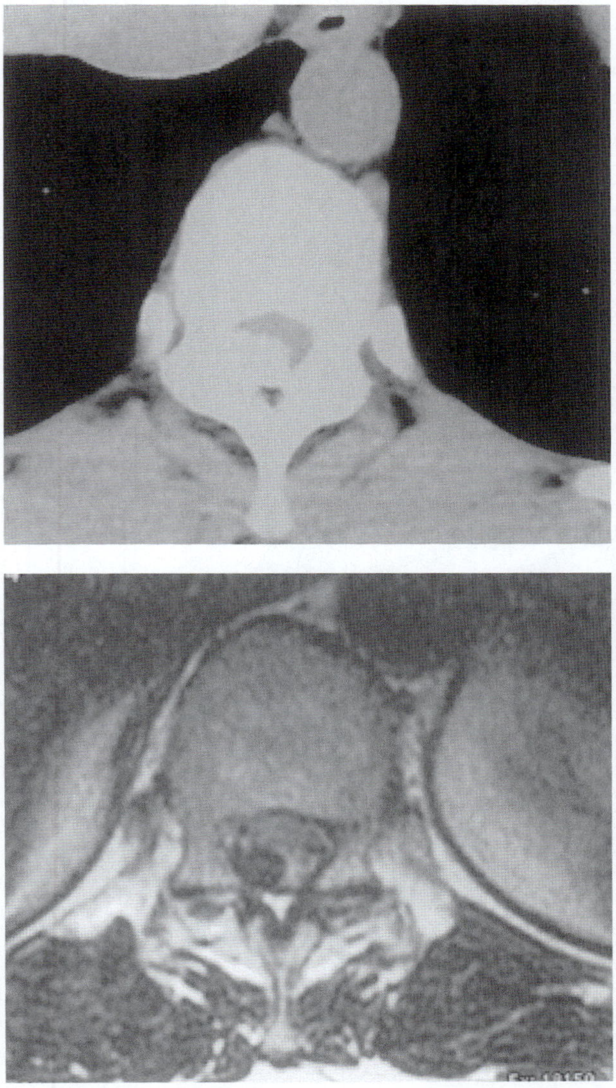

A

B

Figure 8–3 Axial computed tomographic scan **(A)** and magnetic resonance imaging **(B)** demonstrating a calcified thoracic meningioma.

eral, those between the dentate ligaments and sensory roots are dorsolateral, and those posterior to the sensory roots are dorsal. Generally tumors are classified as either dorsal or ventral based on the location of the largest tumor mass. Most spinal meningiomas arise laterally close to the nerve roots due to the high concentration of arachnoid cap cells and close proximity of the arachnoid and dura.

◆ Preoperative Preparation

The first consideration to be made once one has decided that a spinal meningioma should be resected is the avenue of approach. The goal of the surgical procedure is total removal of the lesion. With few exceptions, a posterior or posterolateral approach offers the preferred route for removal of meningiomas. The levels involved and the number of lamina that must be removed to expose the entire tumor are determined using preoperative imaging studies. One must also consider postoperative stability of the spine, especially with lesions of the cervical spine. If significant postoperative instability is anticipated, provision for a concomitant fusion should be made.

◆ Operative Procedure

Some surgeons use prophylactic high-dose corticosteroids (dexamethasone 10 mg) along with prophylactic antibiotics on call to the operating room. General anesthesia is preferred because of the need for microsurgical technique. Central venous access and arterial line are helpful adjuncts when indicated due to preexisting cardiopulmonary disease or anticipated significant blood loss. A Foley catheter and pneumatic compression stockings to both legs are placed. If electrophysiological monitoring is to be performed, scalp and extremity electrodes are placed prior to turning the patient prone. The author does not use prophylactic steroids or intraoperative monitoring for the majority of these procedures.

The operation is performed with the patient in the prone position. At the author's institution, a Jackson table is used. A standard operating room table with chest rolls can also be used. It is very important to reduce intra-abdominal pressure by allowing the abdomen to hang freely. This will reduce central venous pressures and blood loss. For selected cervical lesions, the head may be fixed in a Mayfield-Kees frame with the neck in the neutral position. Prior to scrubbing and draping, particularly for thoracic lesions, lateral or anterior-posterior radiographs are obtained to localize the level of the planned surgery. For midthoracic tumors, levels can be counted on the radiograph from either the first rib or the sacrum. In a very tall person where such a long film is not possible, fluoroscopy may be used to determine the level. It is very helpful to have preoperative plain films to make sure that the patient does not have an anatomical variant that could cause an error in localization (such as a cervical rib, lumbarized sacral vertebra, or absent twelfth rib).

Because the majority of spinal meningiomas are benign, slow-growing tumors, total resection of the tumor should be the goal of treatment. The general principle is to obtain exposure of the area of concern as well as a margin of normal anatomy in both rostral and caudal directions. In the case of a dorsally located tumor, a dorsal exposure encompassing the level of the tumor as well as a margin above and below the tumor is recommended. A midline incision is made in a cephalad to caudad direction using a scalpel. Using electrocautery Bovie, soft tissue is dissected to the fascia of the paraspinal muscles. The fascia is then incised in the same direction as the skin incision. Subperiosteal dissection of the paraspinal muscles is performed using electrocautery Bovie. Care is taken in exposing the lamina to avoid injuring the dura or neural structures. The lamina are exposed bilaterally to the level of the facet joints. Care is taken to preserve the facet joint capsule unless a concomitant fusion is planned. In the thoracic spine, the medial aspect of transverse processes should also be exposed. A laminectomy is performed. The authors prefer to use a high-speed drill with a small bur to drill troughs bilaterally at the lateral margin of the lamina. The troughs are drilled completely through with the drill or may be completed with 1- or 2-mm Kerrison punches **(Fig. 8–4)**. The

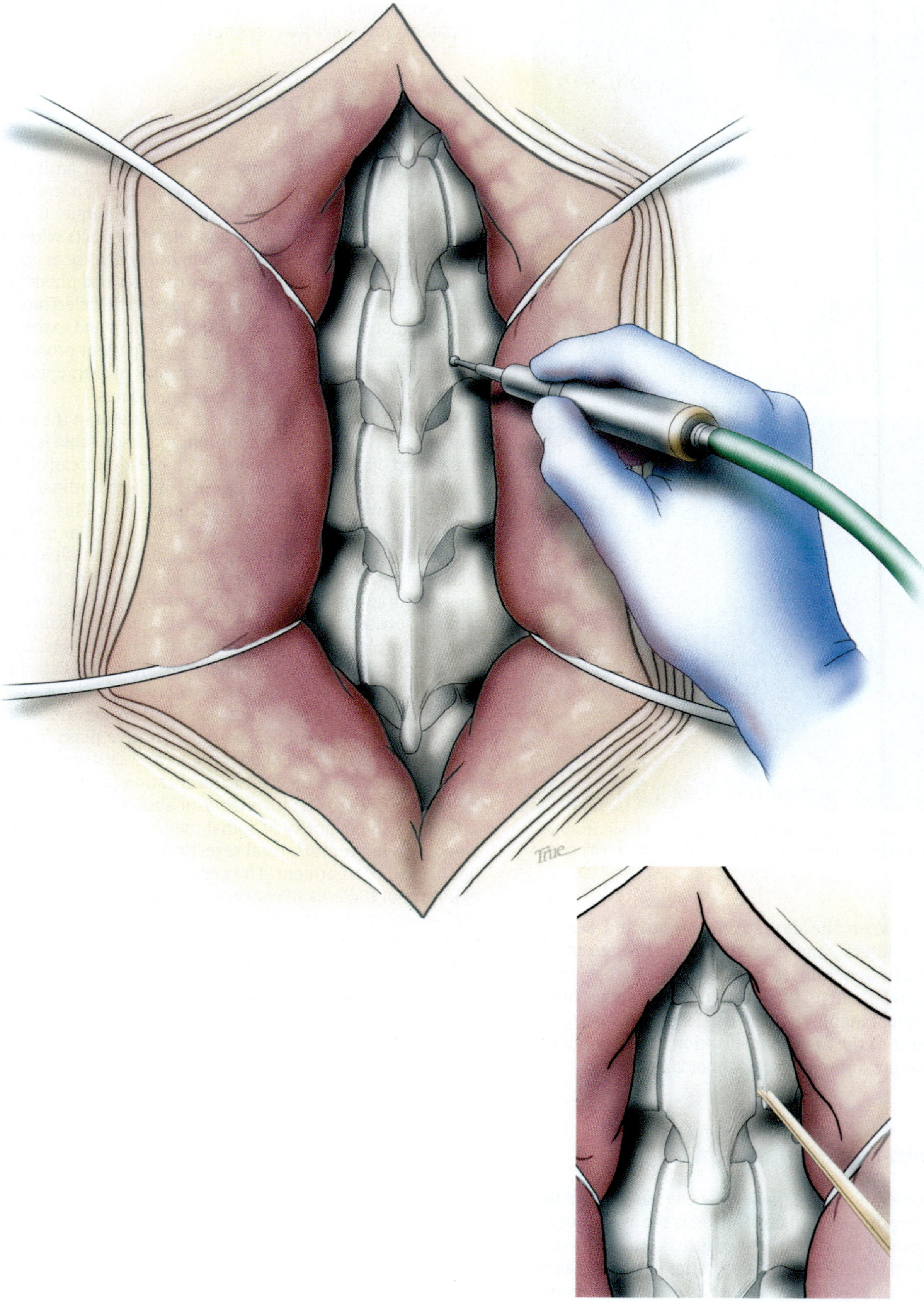

Figure 8–4 A high-speed drill with a small bur is used to drill troughs bilaterally at the lateral margin of the lamina. The troughs are drilled completely through with the drill or may be completed with 1- or 2-mm Kerrison punches (inset).

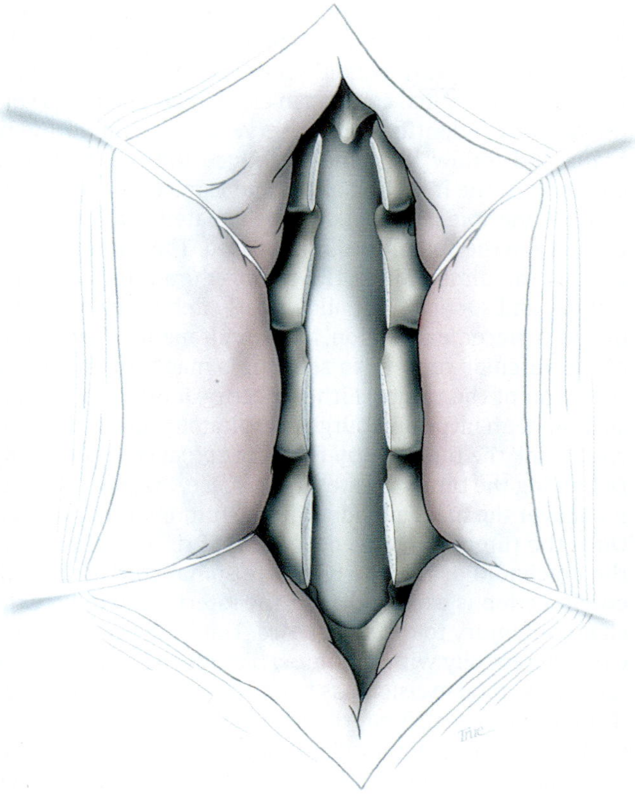

Figure 8–5 The dorsal dura is exposed after multilevel laminectomy. A faint outline of the tumor is occasionally seen through the thinned dura.

lamina and spinous process are removed en bloc. This may allow replacement of the bony arch later in the case or use of the bone as autograft if a fusion is performed **(Fig. 8–5).** Oftentimes there may be dural adhesions attached to the undersurface of the lamina; they have to be detached carefully before en bloc removal is possible. Once the dura is exposed, intraoperative ultrasound may be helpful to pinpoint the exact location of the tumor. In situations in which the tumor extends into the neural foramen, either a partial or complete facetectomy may be performed. Usually unilateral facetectomy does not lead to spinal instability. Anterolateral extension of the tumor may be dealt with through a dorsolateral approach in many cases. This situation should be anticipated preoperatively because the incision and patient position and bony removal may be somewhat different than with a standard midline approach **(Fig. 8–6).** Typically the lateral extent of dissection with a dorsal approach should be performed until pedicles are seen and the lateral aspect of the thecal sac is seen without retraction. Hemostasis is obtained with waxing of bony surfaces and coagulating the epidural venous plexus with bipolar electrocautery.

If there is an extradural component of the tumor, it can be removed using electrocautery bipolar or debulked using an ultrasonic surgical aspirator machine. Debulking the

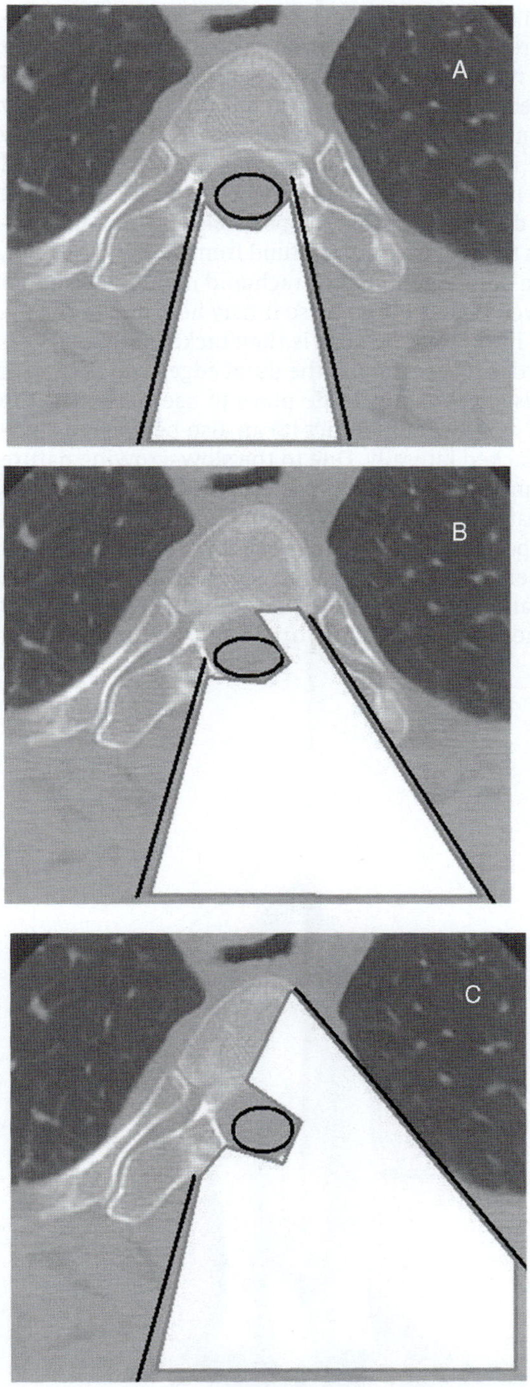

Figure 8–6 **(A)** Most spinal meningiomas are accessible through a direct dorsal approach. Many of these tumors are dorsal or dorsolateral in location. Many lateral or even ventrolateral tumors displace the spinal cord to such an extent that resection is possible with minimal or no manipulation of the spinal cord. **(B)** If a tumor is located more ventrally, a dorsolateral approach may be used such as a costotransversectomy. This requires a slightly longer incision but provides an increased avenue of exposure to the lateral and ventrolateral aspect of the spinal canal. **(C)** If a further ventral exposure is required, a lateral extracavitary approach may be considered in combination with the laminectomy. This approach provides further ventral exposure but is technically difficult and is associated with pulmonary morbidity.

extradural tumor will make it easy to manipulate the thecal sac. Care must be taken because violation of the dura by the tumor may not be appreciated. Good hemostasis should be obtained prior to opening the dura to prevent bloody drainage into the surgical field. Thin strips of surgical may be placed in the lateral gutters for hemostasis. A dorsal durotomy is made in the midline starting from a cephalad to caudad direction to avoid the possibility of caudal herniation from the release of spinal fluid from below the tumor. During the dural opening the arachnoid membrane should be preserved if possible because it may help define the tumor–cord interface. The dura is then tacked laterally. Cottonoid patties placed behind the dural edges will help with hemostasis and provide a safe place to use suction. If the arachnoid membrane is intact it can also be opened similarly and tacked laterally. Due to the slow-growing nature of these tumors the spinal cord is usually displaced from its normal anatomical position **(Fig. 8–7).** To maximize the exposure, especially in ventral meningiomas, cutting the dentate ligament will allow more retraction of the spinal cord.

Preservation of the neural structures relies upon a clear understanding of the tumor origin and its surrounding structures. The tumor is in the subdural space; however, due to the mass effect the arachnoid is stretched over the tumor and the subarachnoid space is obliterated, bringing the tumor and spinal cord pia in close apposition. It is very important to identify and preserve the arachnoid membrane and follow its plane to reduce the risk to neural elements. If the investing arachnoid is mistaken for tumor capsule, the spinal cord pia will be violated and the chance of injury to the spinal cord is increased. The authors prefer to start the dissection at the tumor–dura interface using cautery and suction. This allows early debulking of the tumor in a piecemeal fashion, and simultaneous elimination of the vascular supply. No attempt is made for an en bloc resection of the tumor. Either electrocautery bipolar and suction or an ultrasonic surgical aspirator is used to debulk and shrink the tumor away from the spinal cord **(Fig. 8–8).** Debulking the tumor creates more space, making it easy to maneuver the mass and identify the tumor–cord interface. Once the tumor is reduced to a rim of tissue adherent to the arachnoid or pia overlying the spinal cord, sharp microdissection is used to dissect the interface to reduce the chance of injury to the spinal cord. This plane is developed circumferentially with continued piecemeal tumor removal until gross total excision has been accomplished **(Fig. 8–9).** If the tumor is calcified, then careful use of a high-speed drill with a small diamond bit may be useful. The authors have not had to resort to this, however, because even calcified fragments may be sharply dissected along the arachnoid planes. If used, drilling should be limited to areas away from the spinal cord because vibrations and heat from the drilling can induce injury. **Fig. 8–10** shows an intraoperative view both before and after the tumor is removed.

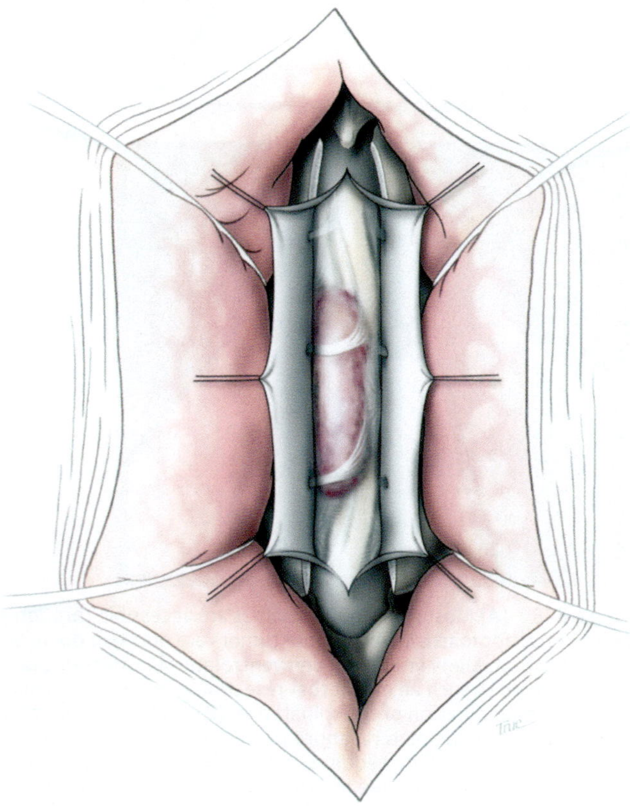

Figure 8–7 After the dura is opened and tacked up, the tumor is seen through the arachnoid displacing the nerve roots and the spinal cord.

Some difference of opinion exists as to treatment of dural attachment of the tumor. Some surgeons advocate electrocauterization of the dura, whereas others have advocated a more aggressive approach and resection of the involved dura. Overall, treatment of the dural attachment should be individualized depending on patient age, location of the tumor, and the technical feasibility of dural repair. If a tumor is ventral to the spinal cord then it may be technically very challenging to safely resect the dura and suture in the graft. If the dura is not adequately closed there is a risk of postoperative spinal fluid leakage and formation of a pseudomeningocele. In an older patient with a ventrolateral tumor, the potential benefit of dural resection must be weighed against the potential for increased morbidity. In general, the authors tend to be more aggressive in younger patients and in patients with dorsally located tumors. As seen in **Table 8–1,** 14% to 26% of patients included in several recent series were able to be treated with dural resection.

When dura is resected a dural patch is recommended rather than a primary closure of the dura. Some of the choices for the dural patch include dorsal paraspinal muscle fascia, autograft of the patient's fascia lata, Gore-Tex, bovine pericardium, and cadaveric fascia lata. The authors prefer to use the paraspinal muscle fascia when the defect

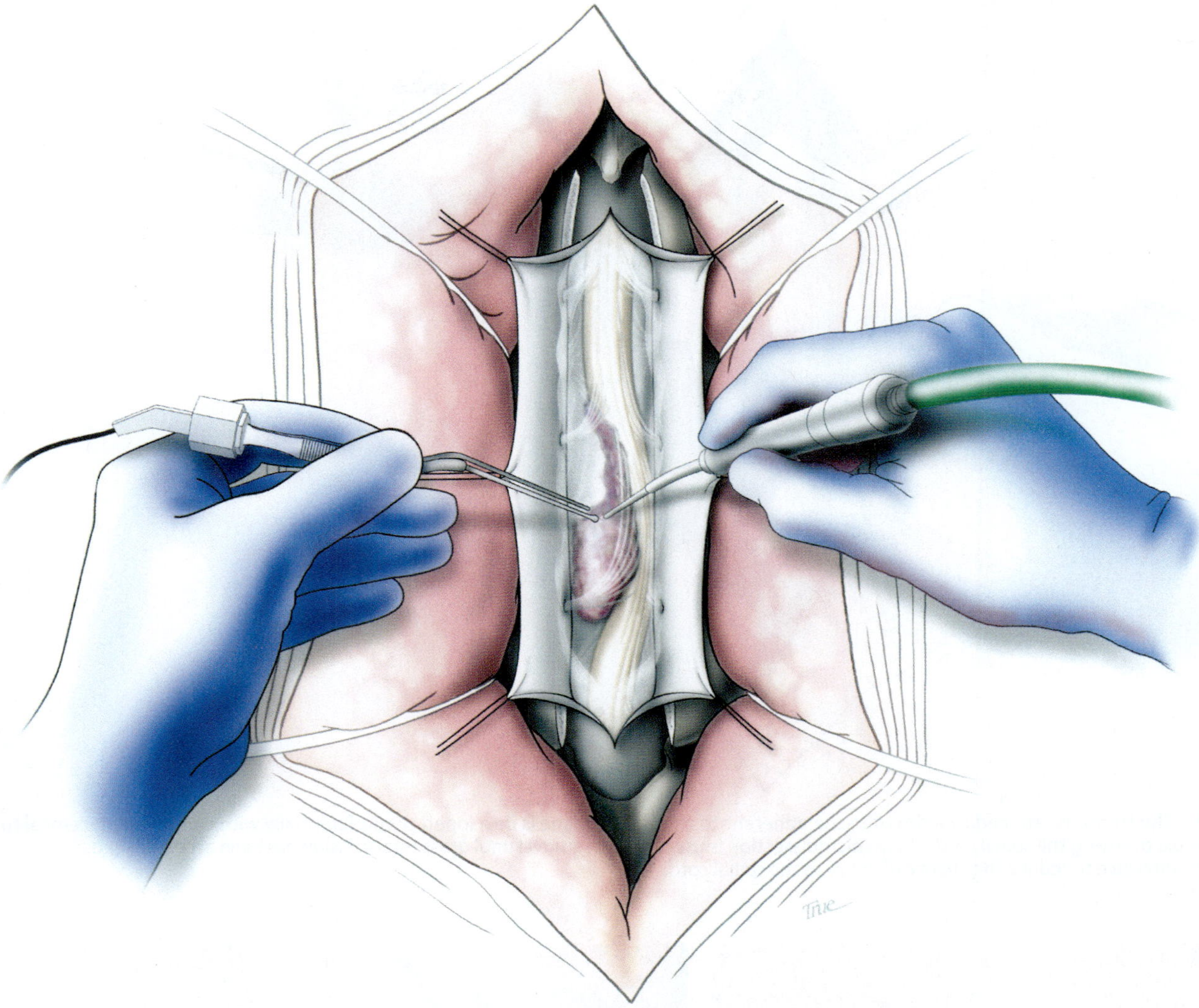

Figure 8–8 Either electrocautery bipolar and suction or an ultrasonic surgical aspirator is used to debulk and shrink the tumor away from the spinal cord. Debulking the tumor creates more space, making it easy to maneuver the mass and identify the tumor–cord interface. Initial debulking should be done away from the spinal cord and within the tumor's capsule.

is small or cadaveric fascia lata if the defect is large. Large paraspinal fascia grafts are impractical because their harvest will inhibit facile closure of the paraspinal fascia, the most important layer of the wound closure. Although it is possible to harvest autograft fascia lata from a patient in the prone position, it is generally difficult and may be impossible with the patient positioned on a frame-based support such as the Jackson table. If it is anticipated that a large piece of autograft tissue will be required, harvesting of the fascia lata is probably best performed as a separate procedure prior to prone positioning. The dura is closed with a 4–0 Neurolon with a running simple stitch. If the lamina were removed en bloc then they can be reattached to the spine using a microplate and screw system **(Fig. 8–11)**. The wound is closed in multiple layers in the standard fashion.

◆ Postoperative Management

The results obtained through surgical resection of spinal meningiomas depend upon the extent of tumor resection, the incidence of perioperative complications, and the degree of neurological compromise seen prior to surgery. The extent of resection depends on the location and physical characteristics of the tumor. Heavily calcified tumors are difficult to remove piecemeal and generally are more adherent to the dura, making them difficult to remove. Ventrally located meningiomas also present a challenge to resect because they tend to displace the spinal cord and nerve root dorsally. In 1999 Klekamp and Samii reported that only 53% of en plaque meningiomas were completely resected compared with 97% of encapsulated meningiomas. Such factors may result in incomplete tumor resection. As

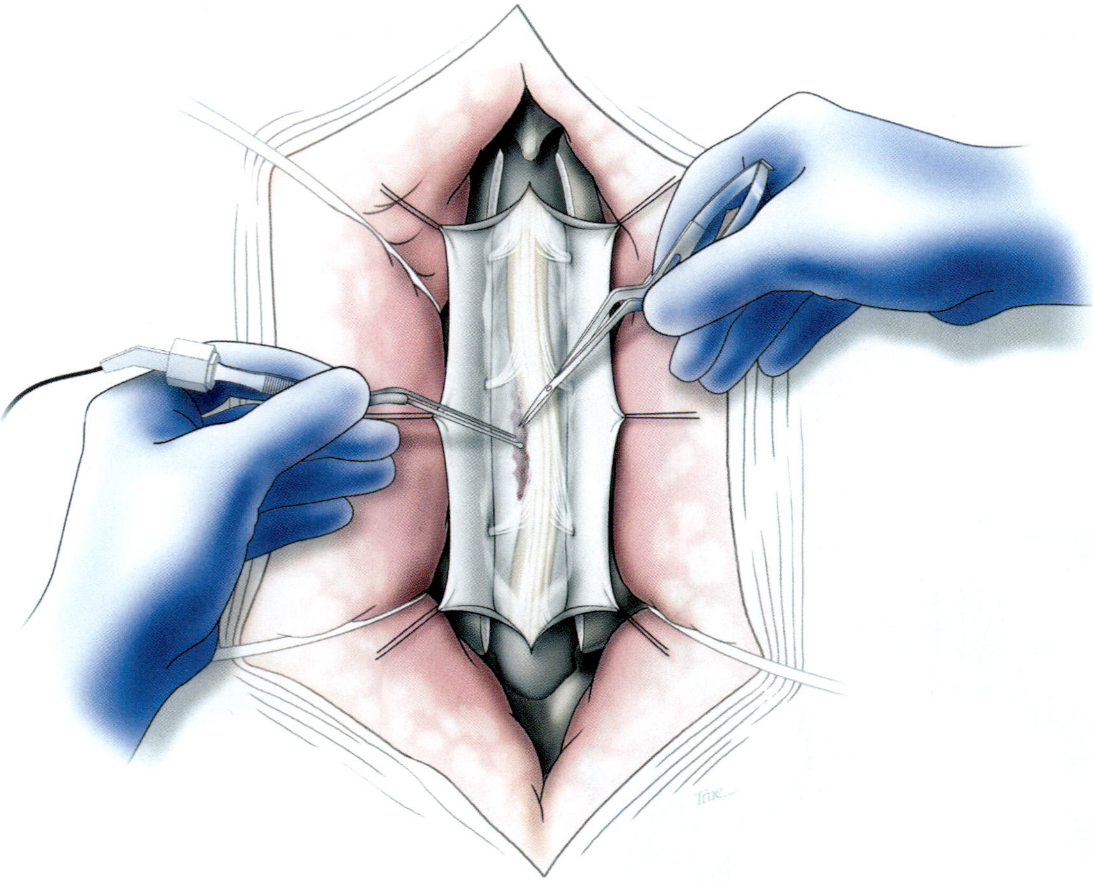

Figure 8–9 The tumor is reduced to a rim of tissue adherent to the arachnoid or pia overlying the spinal cord. Sharp microdissection is used to dissect the interface to reduce the chance of injury to the spinal cord. This plane is developed circumferentially with continued piecemeal tumor removal until gross total excision has been accomplished.

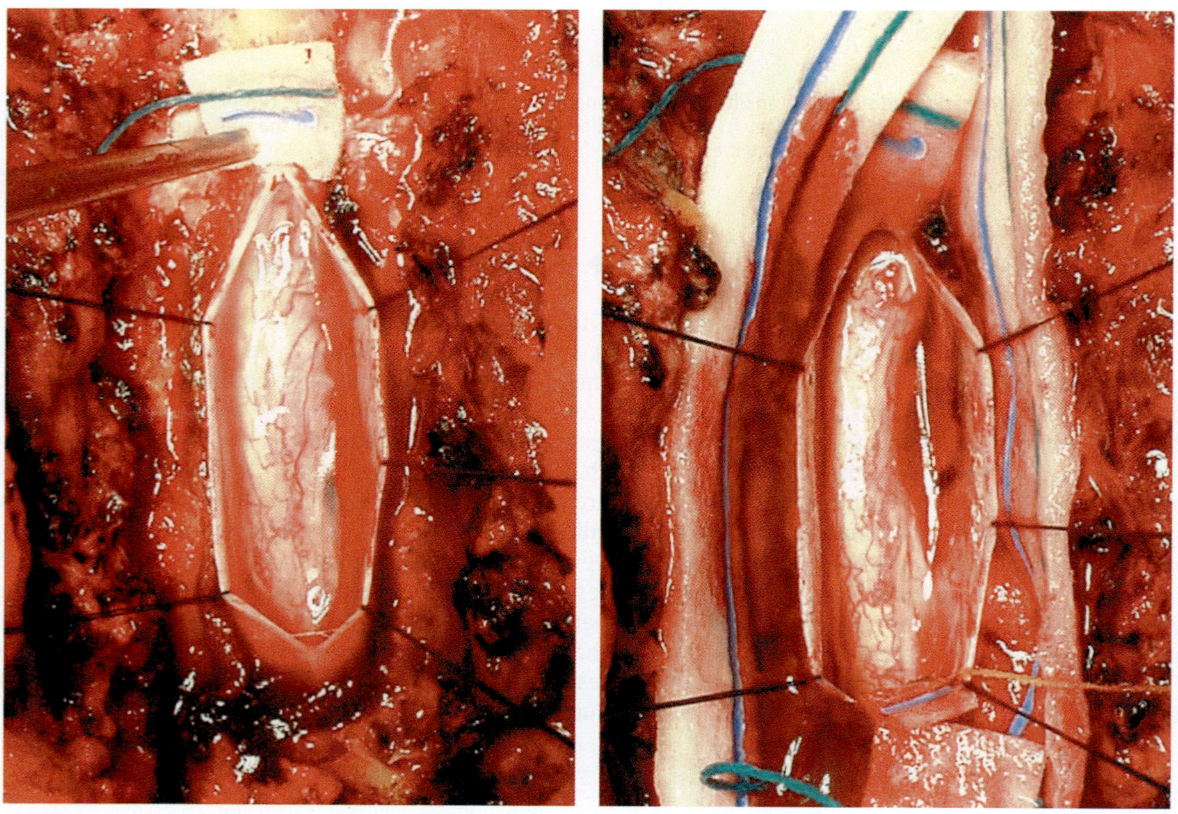

A B

Figure 8–10 Intraoperative view of the tumor before **(A)** and after **(B)** it has been removed.

Table 8–1 Dural Treatment

Series and Year	Dural Resection (%)	Dural Coagulation (%)
Solero et al, 1989	14	86
Roux et al, 1996	15	85
King et al, 1998	26	74

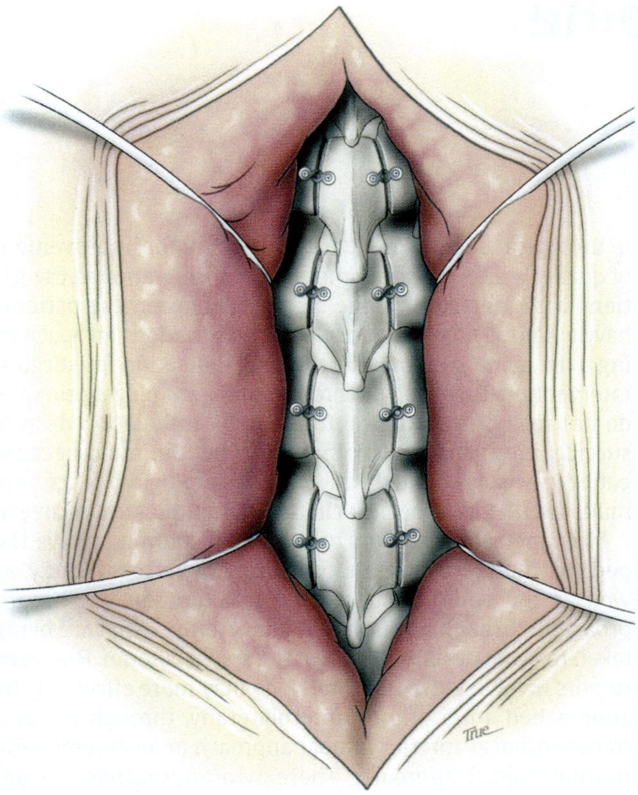

Figure 8–11 Reattaching the lamina and spinous process to the spine using a microplate and screw system.

seen in **Table 8–2,** gross total resection ranges from 82 to 99% of patients.

Improvement in neurological symptoms is the rule rather than the exception. As reported in **Table 8–2,** very few patients deteriorate postoperatively. In 1988 Ciappetta reviewed 22 cases of spinal meningioma with severe motor deficits. The motor deficits were graded according to a modified version of the scale proposed by Levy et al in 1982. Grade IV was given to patients with only toe movements and muscular contractions and grade V to paraplegics. All 10 grade IV patients were able to walk normally within a year of surgical treatment, whereas only 50% of the grade V patients (12 cases) recovered, but not completely. Surgical morbidity and mortality are also generally very low. As reported in **Table 8–2,** surgical mortality ranges from 0 to 3%. Reported causes of death are due to pulmonary embolism, aspiration pneumonia, myocardial infarction, or stroke. Other complications include postoperative cerebrospinal fluid leakage and wound infection.

The rate of recurrence ranges from 1.3 to 14.7% **(Table 8–2).** There is a higher rate of recurrence in en plaque or infiltrating meningiomas and partially resected meningiomas. It is more difficult to obtain a complete resection if a tumor has already recurred. Predictors of poor outcome include elderly age, profound neurological deficits, long duration of symptoms, subtotal removal of tumor, and extradural tumor extension.

◆ Conclusion

Spinal meningiomas are neoplasms with a particularly favorable outcome with surgery. Recurrence is rare, with very few patients having postoperative deterioration. Complex surgical approaches are not always necessary for complete resection of tumors, even for ventrally located tumors. Excision of dura is not always necessary to obtain a low recurrence rate.

Table 8–2 Outcome

Author and Year	Number of Patients	Gross Total Resection (%)	Outcome (%)		Complications (%)			Recurrence (%)
			Improved/ Stable	Deteriorated	Mortality	CSF Leak	Wound Infection	
Levy et al, 1982	97	82	100	0	1	3	1	3.1
Solero et al, 1989	174	97	90	10	1	1	1	6.4
Roux et al 1996	54	93	98	2	0	0	1	3.7
King et al, 1998	78	99	96	4	1	4	0	1.3
Klekamp et al, 1999	117	89	NR	NR	2	4	1	14.7
Gezen et al, 2000	36	97	97	3	3	3	6	5.6

CSF, cerebrospinal fluid; NR, not reported.

9

Surgical Management of Spinal Metastatic Tumors: The Anterior Lumbar Approach and the Lateral Retroperitoneal Approach to the Thoracolumbar Spine

Kurt Eichholz, Timothy Ryken, and William Sharp

Metastatic lesions to the vertebral column present a unique challenge for the spine surgeon. Multiple factors are taken into account when considering surgical intervention for the patient with metastatic spinal disease. These factors include the location and aggressiveness of the primary tumor, prognosis and life expectancy of the patient, symptoms, the presence of neurological deficit, the level of the spinal metastatic tumor involvement, the presence of comorbidities, and the patient's overall ability to undergo surgery. In addition, the surgeon and the patient must have a clear understanding of the goals of surgery, which may differ significantly from performing the same procedure for a patient with other clinical conditions such as degenerative spinal disease.

The goal of surgical intervention in the treatment of spinal metastases differs when compared with the treatment of spinal degenerative processes. The goal of surgery in the treatment of degenerative processes most often entails decompression of neural elements and, when necessary, stabilization of the spinal column. Treatment of metastatic lesions of the spinal column also involves neural decompression; however, due to the often extensive involvement of metastatic disease, instability is a more frequent consequence of aggressive surgical intervention, and therefore the maintenance of long-term stabilization is a significant consideration. The determination of the surgical approach is based upon several factors, including tumor location, the number of spinal levels involved, and the type and length of instrumentation to be used for stabilization. Several studies have indicated that surgical intervention may not improve long-term survival (Ryken et al, 2003). Therefore the indication for surgery frequently involves maintenance of the patient's quality of life and neurological function, or at the very least, prevention of the progression of neurological deficit. Maintenance of ambulation and bladder control are important factors for consideration in determining whether surgical intervention is indicated.

◆ Patient Selection

The patient who presents for consideration of surgical intervention for spinal metastatic disease often has complaints of pain, with or without spinal instability, as well as progressive neurological deficit. The reduction of pain for improvement of quality of life can be an important consideration in the patient with metastatic spine disease because these patients have a limited life expectancy. In some situations incapacitating axial spine pain may be the only indication for surgical intervention. Patients who present with paraplegia generally do not regain neurological function or ambulation despite surgical intervention. This should be kept in mind because patients who are treated early, when neurological deficits are mild, usually have the best chance for neurological recovery.

Most metastatic tumors of the spinal column involve the pedicle, the costovertebral junction, the vertebral body, as well as the epidural space. Epidural tumors may be approached through a standard laminectomy, with care being taken to avoid destabilization of the spinal column. However, tumors involving the vertebral body may more effectively be approached anteriorly or anterolaterally, through either a transperitoneal anterior lumbar approach or an anterolateral retroperitoneal approach. These two approaches are described in detail in the following sections.

◆ Preoperative Preparation

The anterior transperitoneal lumbar approach has been employed most often in conjunction with anterior lumbar interbody fusion, most frequently in the setting of degenerative disease. This approach can also be effective in the setting of metastatic disease when the lower lumbar segments (L4 and L5) are involved. The presence of the great vessels (aorta, inferior vena cava, and their branches), can complicate approaches above the level of L4. We have typically employed a team approach for these procedures, with a vascular surgeon assisting with the approach to help minimize injury to the major vessels, which appears to be the major concern for morbidity in this situation.

The anterolateral retroperitoneal approach is generally utilized when performing a corpectomy between T12 and L4. The bulk of the iliopsoas muscle usually prevents the surgeon from using this approach when an L5 corpectomy is required. When considering a corpectomy above T12, a transthoracic approach is usually required. As with the anterior transperitoneal exposure, we utilize a team effort combined with general or vascular surgery, although any surgeon familiar with the approach can gain this exposure satisfactorily.

◆ Operative Procedure

Anterior Transperitoneal Lumbar Approach

When an anterior transperitoneal approach is elected, the incision is made from the symphysis pubis inferiorly to the umbilicus superiorly **(Fig. 9–1).** If necessary, the incision can be extended around and above the umbilicus to obtain more exposure superiorly. A standard laparotomy is performed, with care being taken to avoid injury of the urinary bladder or ureters. A table-mounted Omni-style retractor is useful to facilitate exposure. Once the small bowel is retracted cephalad and to the right, the retroperitoneum is exposed, overlying the bifurcation of the great vessels.

The retroperitoneum should be lifted anteriorly with forceps and incised sharply with a Church or Metzenbaum scissors, or with an electrocautery, taking care not to damage the great vessels beneath. The sympathetic hypogastric plexus lies between the sacrum and the retroperitoneum. Damage to this nerve plexus can cause retrograde ejaculation postoperatively and electrocautery should be used with discretion in this area to minimize injury.

The level of the bifurcation of the aorta and vena cava is of significant importance in this approach. Preoperatively, the surgeon should determine the level of the bifurcation of the great vessels because limitation with retraction of these structures often impedes adequate exposure of the adjacent vertebral bodies. Injury to the thin walls of the venous structures is of particular concern given the amount of instrumentation typically involved with these procedures. The bifurcation of the vena cava can be as superior as the L4 vertebral body or as inferior as the S1 vertebral body, but generally is located at the L4–L5 interspace. Access to the L4 vertebral body sometimes requires the mobilization of the vena cave or iliac veins. A vein or spring retractor can be useful in retracting these vessels laterally while performing the corpectomy and may require alternating the direction of dissection from side to side.

In the setting of a spinal metastasis involving the L5 vertebral body, a complete L5 corpectomy can usually be performed with minimal vessel retraction **(Fig. 9–2).** It is preferable to remove the vertebral body with rongeurs to prevent seeding of tumor cells to the peritoneal cavity. Use of a high-speed air drill may cause dispersion of bone dust or fragments containing tumor cells. The corpectomy defect can then be replaced by femoral allograft or carbon fiber cages, which can be packed with autograft obtained from the iliac crest, or allograft material **(Fig. 9–3).**

Some anterior interbody cages are specifically designed for corpectomy applications. These cages have threaded holes for screws that attach to the posterior instrumentation in cases using combined anterior and posterior instrumentation.

Closure of the incision is in routine fashion for laparotomies.

Anterolateral Retroperitoneal Approach

A left-sided approach is most commonly selected due to the left-sided location of the aorta, which is less fragile than the vena cava and therefore less prone to injury and blood loss. The location of the liver can also complicate retraction with a right-sided approach. The patient should be positioned in the left lateral decubitus position (right side down), with either a slight break in the table or a roll under or just above the iliac crest **(Fig. 9–4).** The surgeon must make sure that

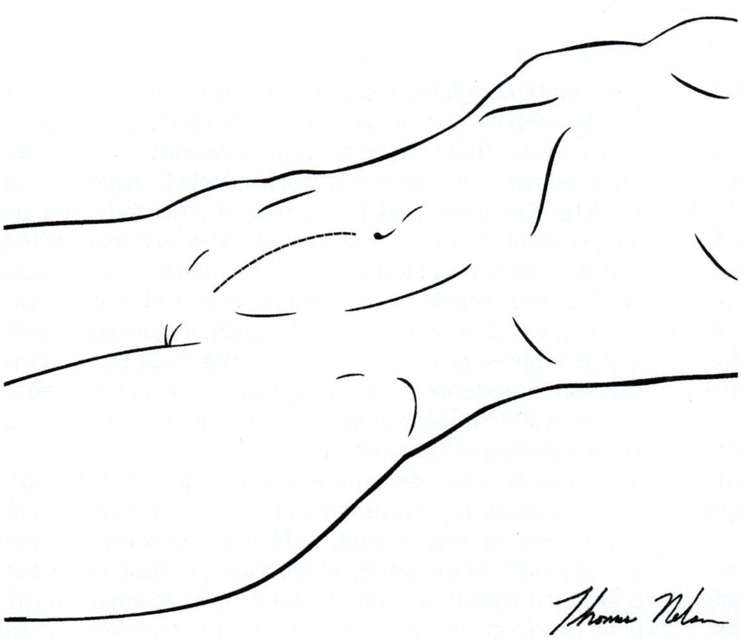

Figure 9–1 The skin incision for the anterior transperitoneal approach to the lumbar spine.

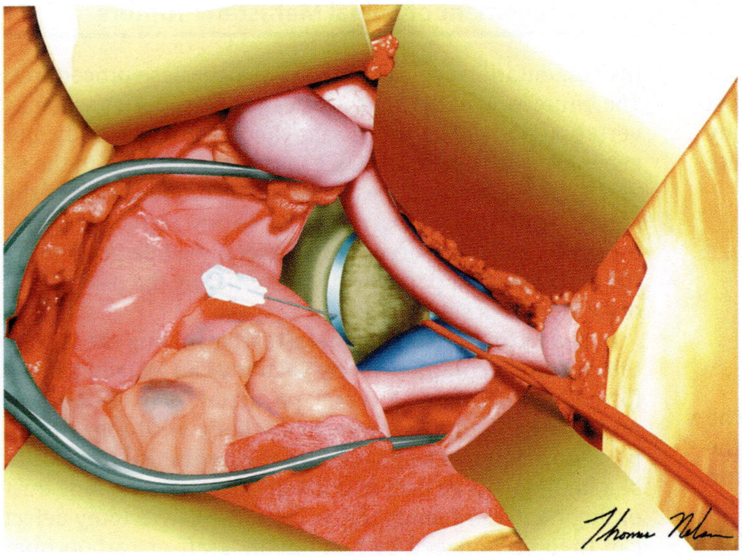

Figure 9–2 Operative exposure of the anterior lumbosacral junction through an anterior transperitoneal approach. The spinal needle is in the L5–S1 disk space, just below the bifurcation of the aorta and vena cava.

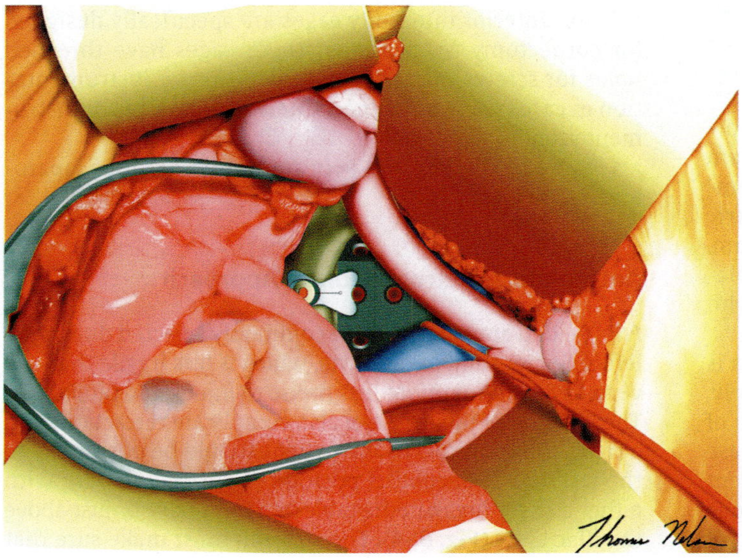

Figure 9–3 Anterior instrumentation after an L5 corpectomy. A carbon fiber cage is in place in the corpectomy defect, with a staple at the superior aspect of S1, to prevent anterior displacement of the graft.

the break or roll is not too generous because too much of an angle will cause the spine to be fused in a right lateral bending posture. The incision is made starting posteriorly, ~3 in. posterior to the midaxillary line. The incision should generally parallel the orientation of the ribs, ending just at the lateral aspect of the rectus abdominis muscle and requires adjustment depending on the level of approach required. Preoperative fluoroscopic views are helpful in assuring the appropriate location of the incision. Successive layers of the external oblique, internal oblique, and transversus abdominis muscles are then incised sharply in the line of the incision and should be reapproximated in layers upon closure.

After the abdominal musculature is transected, the transversalis fascia is incised, allowing entrance into the retroperitoneum. At this point, the psoas muscle is visualized, attached to the lateral aspect of the spinal column. The psoas is then retracted posteriorly to expose the anterior aspect of the vertebral column. The ureter is usually located along the anterior aspect of the psoas muscle, and care should be taken when dissecting and mobilizing in this area to avoid injury. The ureter may be safely retracted anteriorly with the contents of the peritoneal cavity. These can be retracted anteriorly with a table-mounted retractor system or with a handheld C-shaped ribbon retractor. The psoas muscle is retracted posteriorly, and attempts should be made to avoid division because many of the nerves of the lumbar plexus traverse the substance of the muscle. The psoas should be retracted enough to allow visualization of the pedicle, which is the key landmark for corpectomy and decompression of the central canal **(Fig. 9–5).** Decompression and corpectomy proceed in similar fashion to the anterior approach attempting to limit the need for high-speed drills to avoid scattering of tumor-laden tissue.

Once satisfactory decompression is achieved **(Fig. 9–6),** several options for reconstruction can be considered when performing an anterolateral lumbar corpectomy through this approach. In the setting of metastatic disease, bone that is afflicted with tumor should not be used to augment the bony construct, as is often done when this approach is used

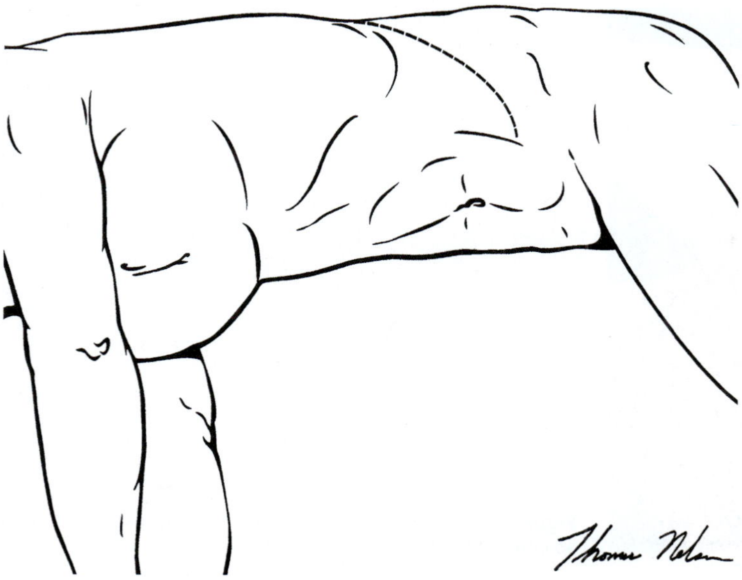

Figure 9–4 The skin incision for a lateral retroperitoneal approach to the lumbar spine. The incision starts superiorly at the lower costal margin and extends to the lateral aspect of the rectus abdominis.

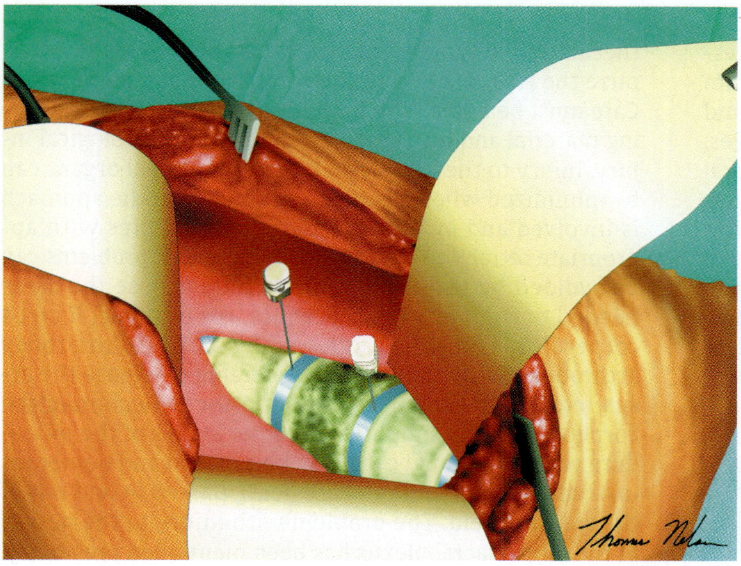

Figure 9–5 The exposure of the lumbar spine through a lateral retroperitoneal approach. Spinal needles are located above and below the L3 vertebral body, which is infiltrated with tumor.

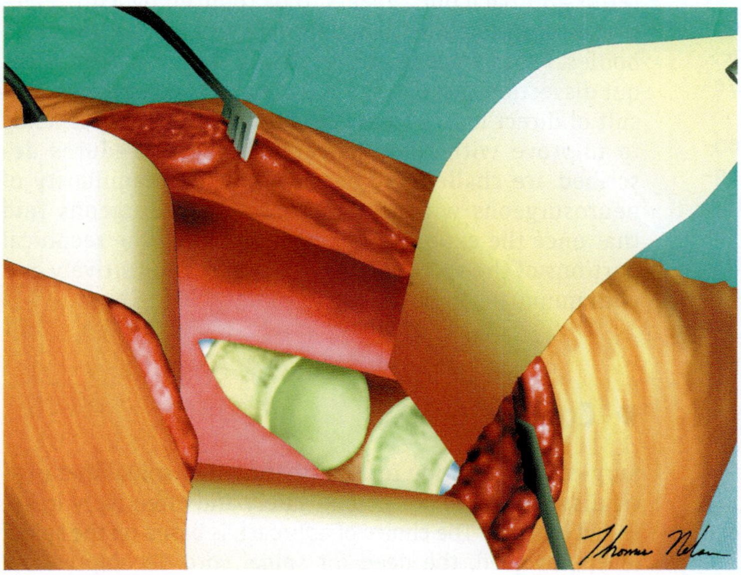

Figure 9–6 The operative field after L3 corpectomy through a lateral retroperitoneal approach.

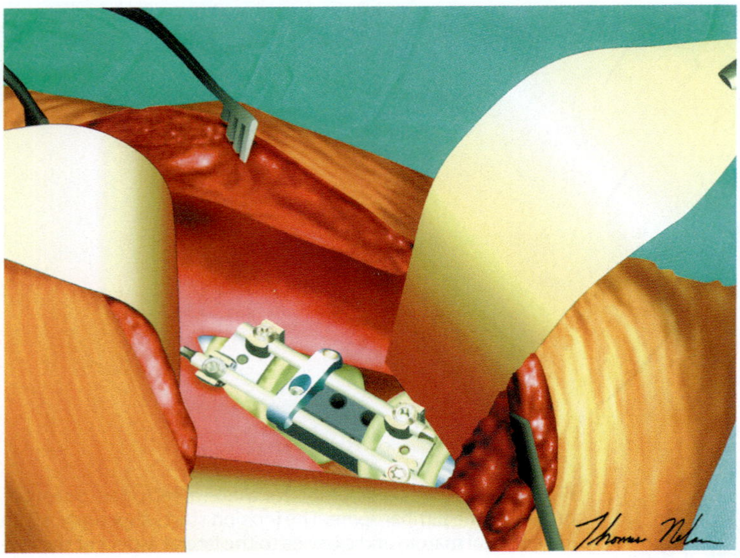

Figure 9–7 A carbon fiber cage and dual rod instrumentation spanning an L3 corpectomy defect.

to treat thoracolumbar burst fractures. If autograft is necessary, a rib may be harvested, or bone can be harvested from the iliac crest. These autografts may be morcellized and used in conjunction with carbon-fiber or titanium cages, which are sized to the corpectomy defect. Cadaveric femoral allograft is another option. If there is a paucity of autograft bone, bone graft extender can be used in conjunction with these devices. The bone graft is supplemented with instrumentation, most often with either a dual rod construct **(Fig. 9–7)** or one of several lateral plating systems, which may afford a lower profile than the dual rod and screw constructs.

◆ Postoperative Management

Generally a nasogastric tube is useful to assist with the management of postoperative ileus, which is more common with the anterior approach and is atypical for standard posterior spinal surgery. A similar amount of postoperative pain control is required when compared with posterior approaches, and the role of postoperative bracing remains at the discretion of the surgeon.

Postoperative care of the patient with the anterior transperitoneal approach is similar to that of the patient with the anterolateral approach, although the degree of postoperative ileus may be less and a nasogastric tube is not usually required. If the thoracic cavity is entered, a chest tube is necessary. Bracing is again at the discretion of the surgeon because no convincing studies either for or against it are available for guidance.

The risks of these approaches include neurological injury, injury to the major vessels, injury to the nerves of the lumbosacral plexus, as well as injury to the intra-abdominal organs. The risk of neurological injury is related to the degree of spinal instability and the amount of neural decompression that is required. In general these two approaches allow good control in the approach to the thecal sac and good visualization, which helps to minimize the risk of injury to the spinal cord and nerve roots. Care must be taken with both insertion of interbody grafting material and instrumentation to avoid neurological injury. Injury to the vessels and intra-abdominal organs can be minimized when a surgeon familiar with the approach is involved and by protection of the structures with appropriate retraction devices. Many potential problems can be avoided by taking the time to fully expose the areas needed to complete the procedure. For example, if an L4 corpectomy is planned followed by an L3–L5 interbody arthrodesis with plating, it is preferable to expose the areas required for instrumentation prior to beginning the corpectomy. This simplifies the later stages of the procedure when the spinal cord may be exposed and numerous instruments and implants are being passed in and out of the surgical field. The problem with injury to the nerves of the lumbosacral plexus has been mentioned previously. Retrograde ejaculation remains a potential risk of the anterior approach but appears to be reduced by using electrocautery judiciously in clearing the anterior vertebral bodies. Psoas weakness is relatively common even without dissection through the muscle and is most likely a result of direct injury from retraction. Fortunately it tends to improve with time. In general, the procedures described are challenging because of the unfamiliarity of neurosurgeons with the approach. Most surgeons find that once the exposure has been obtained the technical portions of the spinal procedure progress intuitively and with minimal complication.

◆ Conclusion

Surgical intervention for the treatment of spinal metastatic disease can be performed safely and effectively in selected patients. The choice of approach is based on the spinal levels involved, the need for spinal cord decompression, and the presumed degree of spinal instability. The anterior transperitoneal approach to L4 to the sacrum and the anterolateral retroperitoneal approach for T12 to L4 have been highlighted in this section. Many variations are available and the need for multiple staged approaches for extensive reconstruction may be required in some situations. The overriding goal of surgical intervention is to improve or maintain the patient's quality of life. Surgical decompression and stabilization alone is not likely to prolong survival in the patient with spinal metastases unless it assists with maintaining neurological function. Therefore it is important that both the surgeon and the patient have a clear understanding of the goals of surgical intervention.

10

Surgical Management of Peripheral Nerve Tumors

Joseph Wiley, Asis Kumar Bhattacharyya, and Abhijit Guha

Peripheral nerve tumors (PNTs) are infrequently encountered soft tissue lesions that are usually associated with the extremities and subcutaneous space, but in fact can occur in visceral cavities in close proximity to any organ of the body, thereby leading to a myriad of presentations. Rarity of these tumors and uncertainty of their cell of origin have precluded the development of an all-encompassing classification. A simplified classification is presented in **Table 10–1,** which, although excluding several rare pathological subtypes, serves well in management of most PNTs. Like any organ system, PNTs can be divided into benign or malignant. Tumors may arise not only from the Schwann cells, which gives rise to the most common schwannomas and neurofibromas, but from the variety of cells or their cells of origin that are found in normal nerves.

Table 10–1 Classification of Peripheral Nerve Tumors

Benign	Malignant
Schwannoma	Primary
Typical	Malignant peripheral nerve sheath tumor
Atypical	Primary central nervous system lymphoma
Ancient	Ganglioneuroblastoma
Psammomatous melanotic	Secondary
Cellular	Local spread
Benign epithelioid	Pancoast tumor
Neuroblastoma-like	Soft tissue sarcoma
Plexiform	Intraneural metastasis
Neurofibroma	Tumorlike lesions
Dermal	Ganglion cyst
Subcutaneous	Desmoids
Plexiform	Traumatic neuroma
Perineuroma	Inflammatory
Palisaded encapsulated neuroma	Pseudotumor
Neurothekoma (nerve sheath myxoma)	Leprosy
Ganglioneuroma	Radiation neuritis
Hemangioma	
Angiomatosis of peripheral nerve	
Meningioma	
Lipoma	

◆ Patient Selection

A focused history should be directed toward the onset, duration, and growth alterations of the mass. Presence or absence of neurological and nonneurological symptoms such as pain, numbness, and weakness and any associated systemic complaints suggestive of an underlying cancer is of importance. A family history suggestive of neurofibromatosis type 1 (NF-1) or NF-2 or other predisposition syndromes is of special importance because almost half of all PNTs are linked with these syndromes. The physical exam should be directed toward the mass, including comments on whether the mass is firm versus soft, pulsatile versus nonpulsatile, mobile versus adhered to the soft tissues, and, if mobile whether it moves perpendicular to but not along the long axis of a known peripheral nerve, which is highly suggestive of a PNT. Although the majority of PNTs will not have any fixed sensory or motor deficits on presentation, the presence or absence of a Tinel's sign may give a clue toward nerve of origin or one that is juxtaposed to the PNT. The physical examination is not complete without examination of local structures such as vessels and joints that may be compressed by the PNT, and a systemic examination with a focus on absence or presence of clinical signs associated with NF-1, NF-2, or the much rarer schwannomatosis predisposition syndromes, as listed in **Table 10–2.**

Only a subset of patients suspected to have a PNT require surgical intervention. A long-standing slowly growing mass, with magnetic resonance imaging (MRI) features suggestive of a schwannoma in an elderly or medically compromised patient is best left alone, if minimally symptomatic. Multiple dermal or plexiform neurofibromas in an NF-1 patient are best watched, unless local compressive symptoms are seen or malignant conversion in the latter is suspected. If surgery is warranted, the preoperative goals (total excision versus subtotal debulking versus biopsy) and associated risks must be thoroughly discussed with the patient. Microneurosurgical techniques, intraoperative magnification, and electrophysiological monitoring are essential prerequisites.

Table 10–2 Clinical Diagnostic Criteria for Neurofibromatosis 1 and 2 and Schwannomatosis

Neurofibromatosis Type 1

Two or more of the following:

1. Six or more of café au lait macules of over 5 mm greatest diameter in prepubertal individuals or over 15 mm in postpubertal individuals
2. Two or more neurofibromas of any type or one plexiform neurofibroma
3. Freckling in axillary or inguinal regions
4. Optic nerve glioma
5. Two or more Lisch nodules
6. A distinct osseous lesion such as a sphenoid dysplasia or thinning of the long bone cortex with or without pseudarthrosis
7. A first-degree relative (parent, sibling, or offspring) with neurofibromatosis type 1 by the above criteria

Neurofibromatosis Type 2

Definitive

Bilateral vestibular schwannomas or a family history of neurofibromatosis type 2 (first-degree relative) and either:

1. Unilateral vestibular schwannoma diagnosed at age less than 30 years *or*
2. Any two of the following: meningioma, glioma, schwannoma, juvenile posterior subcapsular lenticular opacities/juvenile cortical cataract

Presumptive or Probable Neurofibromatosis Type 2

1. Unilateral vestibular schwannoma at age less than 30 years plus one of the following: meningioma, glioma, schwannoma, juvenile posterior subcapsular lenticular opacities/juvenile cortical cataract
2. Multiple meningiomas (two or more) plus unilateral vestibular schwannoma at age less than 30 years or one of the following: meningioma, glioma, schwannoma, juvenile posterior subcapsular lenticular opacities/juvenile cortical cataract

Schwannomatosis

Definitive

1. Two or more pathologically proved schwannomas *plus*
2. Lack of radiographic evidences of vestibular nerve tumors, at the age more than 18 years

Presumptive or probable schwannomatosis

1. Two or more pathologically proved schwannomas, without symptoms of eighth nerve dysfunction, at age more than 30 years *or*
2. Two or more pathologically proved schwannomas in an anatomically limited distribution (single limb or segment of the spine), without symptoms of eighth nerve dysfunction, at any age

◆ Preoperative Preparation

Preoperative electrophysiological examination is not routine because it does not contribute to the diagnosis or add any information to that obtained from the history, physical examination, and radiological workup. In terms of radiological evaluation, MRI is best; however, occasionally computed tomographic (CT) scans are helpful, especially to demonstrate remodeling of adjacent bony structures such as the neural foramina or spinal canal. There are no pathognomonic MRI features for PNTs and the various subtypes, though some features are highly suggestive. For example, a well-circumscribed elliptical or spherical tumor, with low T1 and high T2 signal and homogeneous contrast enhancement, is highly suggestive of schwannoma **(Fig. 10–1A).** Demonstration of the nerves of origin or exit and displaced "passerby" fascicles around the capsule are also suggestive of schwannoma and its typical extrafascicular growth. In contrast, neurofibromas appear as fusiform or multinodular masses with an intrafascicular growth pattern **(Fig. 10–1B).** Of diagnostic note, a PNT in the context of an NF-1 patient will most certainly be a neurofibroma versus an NF-2 patient, who likely harbors a schwannoma. Lipoma and ganglion cyst can usually be diagnosed by characteristic MR signals **(Fig. 10–1C,D).** PNTs may be nonhomogeneously enhancing, indicating intratumoral hemorrhage, necrosis, or cystic degeneration; however, corelationship with these MRI features and malignancy is poor. In fact, there are no definitive radiological features of a malignant peripheral nerve sheath tumor (MPNST), a diagnosis mainly suspected on rapid clinical and radiological growth, progressive neurological deterioration, and most importantly pain. Use of fluorodeoxyglucose positron emission tomography (^{18}FDG PET) scanning is of potential promise in distinguishing MPNST from benign PNTs, though further clinical verification is required.

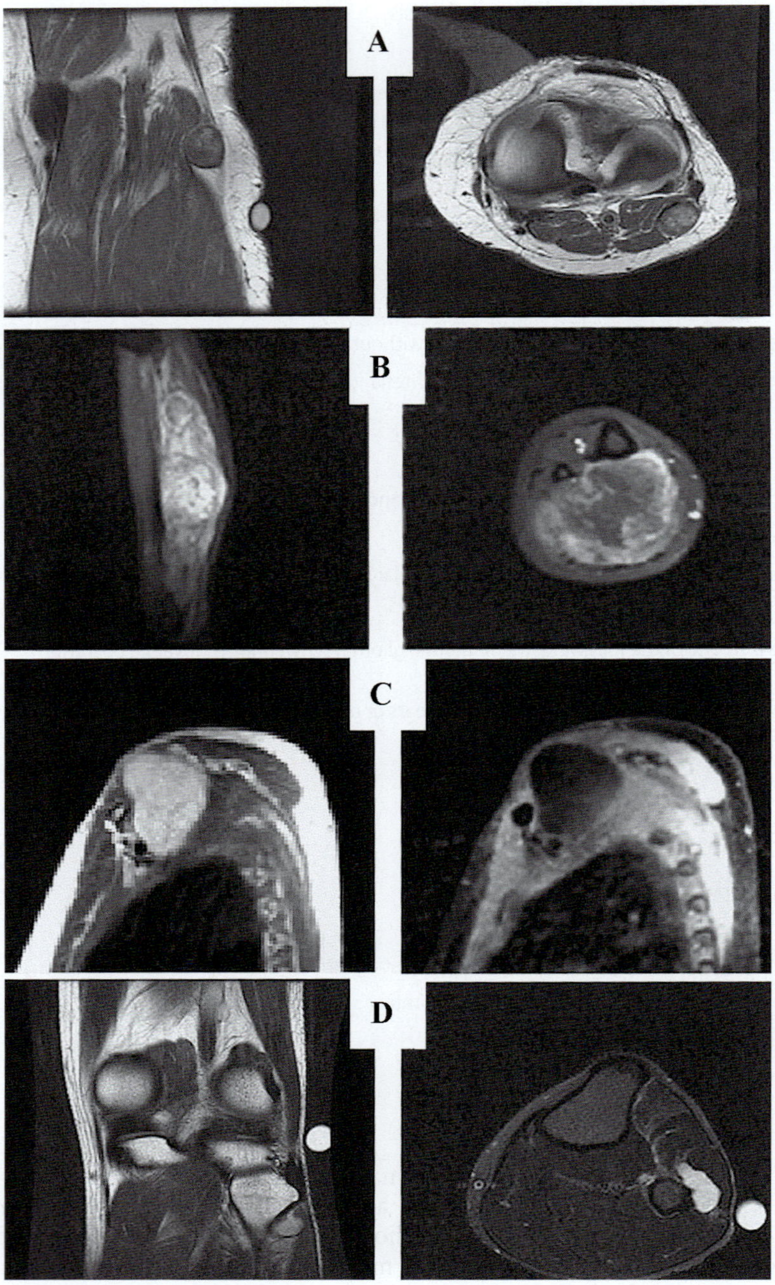

Figure 10–1 Magnetic resonance imaging of peripheral nerve tumors. **(A)** Sagittal and axial gadolinium-enhanced T1-weighted images of a schwannoma arising from the common peroneal nerve in the popliteal fossa. Note the well-circumscribed spherical nature of the tumor, typical of a schwannoma. **(B)** Sagittal and axial gadolinium-enhanced T1-weighted images of a plexiform neurofibroma in a neurofibromatosis type 1 patient. Note the fusiform, nondiscrete, and heterogeneously enhancing nature of the neurofibroma, which cannot radiologically be distinguished from one that has undergone malignant conversion. **(C)** Sagittal nonenhanced T1-weighted (left) and fat suppression images (right) of a typical lipoma in the infraclavicular space. Lipomas can be diagnosed clinically and with these typical radiological characteristics. The extraneural component of the lipoma can be removed safely, whereas the intraneural component is best left intact with decompression of any associated entrapment point. **(D)** Coronal and axial T2-weighted images of a ganglion cyst arising from the tibula-fibula joint and causing extrinsic compression of the common peroneal nerve.

◆ Operative Procedure

The affected limb should be positioned and draped to allow evaluation of the distal muscles supplied by the relevant nerve or audible electromyographic (EMG) electrodes inserted into those muscles, and the incision should be long enough to expose the proximal and distal normal nerve **(Fig. 10–2A).** Anesthesia should be without neuromuscular paralysis to allow intraoperative electrophysiological evaluation.

Exposure commences with isolation of the proximal and distal segments of the nerve of origin, which are encircled in vessel loops and electrophysiologically confirmed **(Fig. 10–2B)**. If the PNT is near a natural entrapment point, such as the carpal tunnel or fibular head, prophylactic release of the nerve traversing through these regions should be undertaken to defray delayed entrapment syndromes. Next, gross and microscopical examination of the PNT, supplemented by electrophysiological mapping for functional passerby fascicles, which may be splayed across the tumor capsule, are then undertaken **(Fig. 10–2C)**. An area devoid of any fascicles and one that is electrically silent, hence representing only tumor, is then chosen to obtain a quick section to be interpreted by an experienced neuropathologist. If the microscopical and pathological diagnosis is of a schwannoma, then total removal is to be expected, whereas subtotal but radical debulking can be accomplished with neurofibromas.

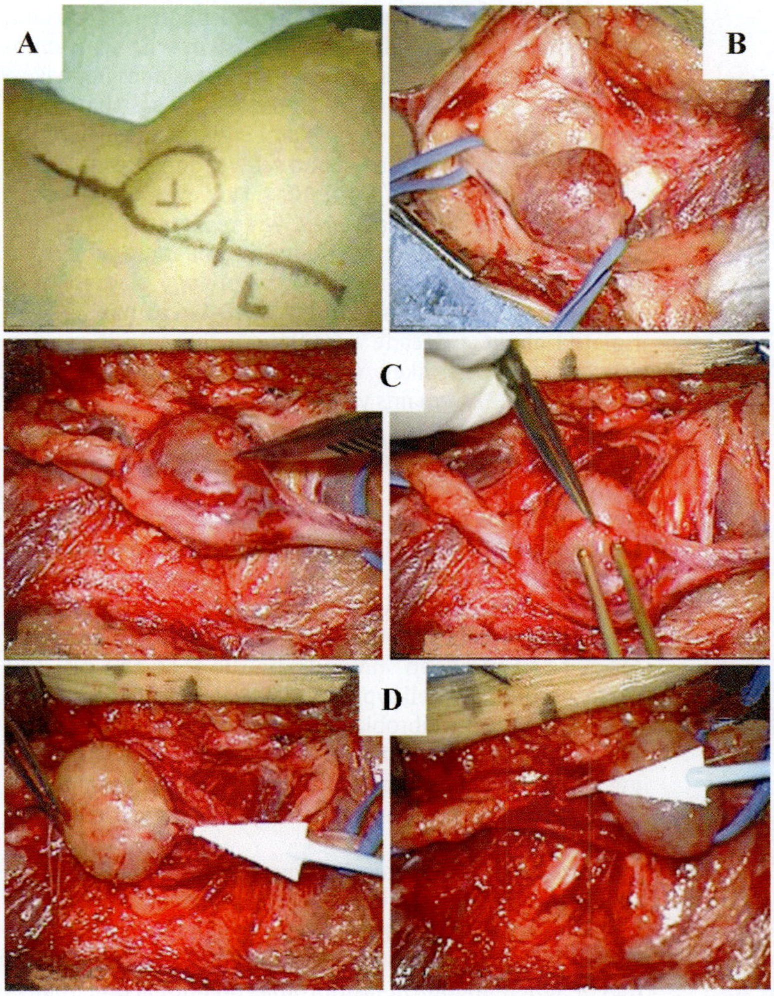

Figure 10–2 Intraoperative points of management of peripheral nerve tumors. **(A)** Planning of the skin incision for safe removal should extend proximal and distal to the tumor mass itself and any associated natural entrapment point, such as the fascial bands of the anterior compartment during the course of the common peroneal nerve at the knee. **(B)** Isolation of the proximal and distal poles of the tumor. **(C)** Splaying of thinned-out passerby fascicles along the tumor capsule, visualized by microscopy and confirmed by electrophysiological stimulation. **(D)** Microneurosurgical techniques and electrophysiological monitoring to isolate the nerve of origin and exit, allowing safe removal of the tumor and preservation of the passerby fascicles.

Often the exact differentiation of the PNT subtype cannot be made on the quick section, requiring use of good clinical judgment to maximize tumor removal with minimal deficits. The majority of small to medium-sized PNTs can be removed in total, though removal of larger tumors or those adjacent to vital structures such as the spinal canal may first require intratumoral decompression by ultrasonic aspirator, followed by resection of the capsule from adjacent functioning neural and nonneural structures. Nerve grafts after resection of PNTs are rarely required if good clinical judgment and microneurosurgical principles are used. The management of MPNST is considered separately because the oncological objectives are somewhat different than the more common benign schwannomas and neurofibromas. Similarly, intraoperative management goals and strategies also differ between some of the more rare PNT subtypes and will be discussed in each section.

Schwannoma

Schwannomas are the most common PNTs in adults, with most incidentally diagnosed as slowly growing solitary tumors in middle-aged patients, without any gender predilection. Malignant transformation of a typical schwannoma does not occur, with only a small risk in some of the atypical varieties listed in **Table 10–1.** Paraspinal, retroperitoneal, and mediastinal schwannomas, presenting as space-occupying lesions, though of similar biology to the typical PNT schwannoma, present with unique local issues and will not be discussed further in this chapter. Microscopically, a typical schwannoma consists of alternating areas of cellular Antoni-A and loosely arranged Antoni-B regions with palisading organization of nuclei, termed Verocay bodies. The cells are spindle shaped with indistinct cytoplasm and elongated nuclei with blunt-point ends. Immunohistochemically they demonstrate S-100 and Leu-7 positivity and epithelial membrane antigen (EMA) negativity, with absence of intratumoral axons a key point to differentiate them from neurofibromas **(Fig. 10–3A).** Electron microscopy, seldom required, demonstrates Schwann cell composition characterized by a completely surrounding basal lamina.

Atypical variants of schwannomas include ancient, psammomatous melanotic, cellular, benign epithelioid, neuroblastoma-like, and plexiform schwannomas. The term *ancient* denotes aging and degenerated appearance in histology, which is characterized by cyst formation, stromal edema,

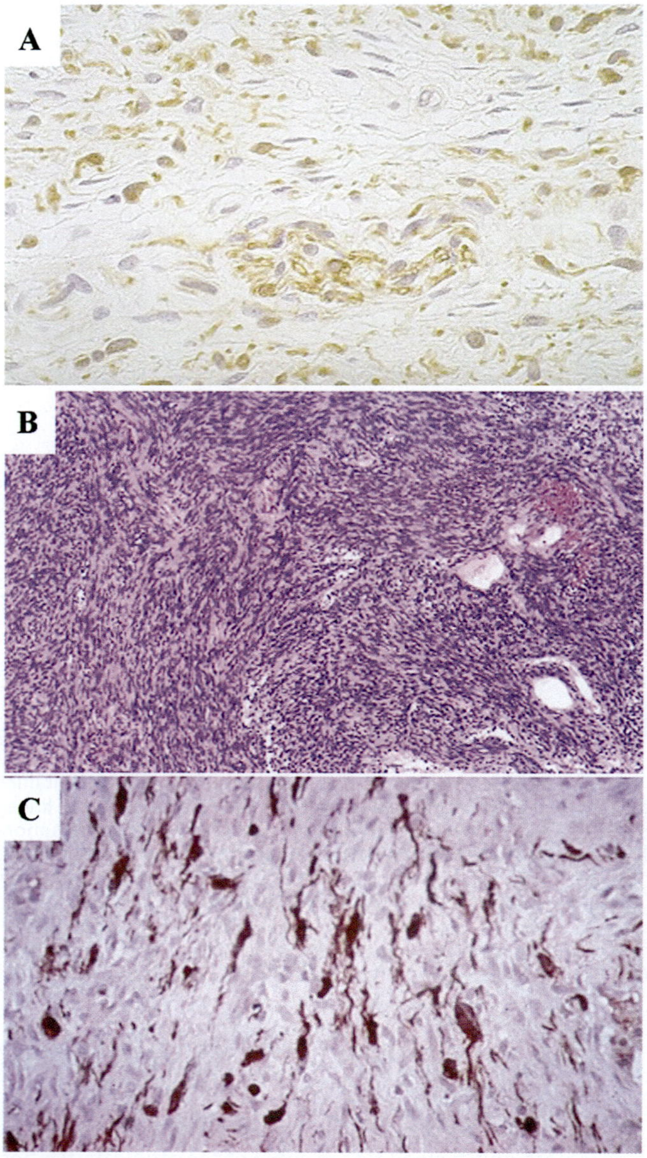

Figure 10–3 **(A)** Pathology of S-100 +'ve Schwann cells of a schwannoma. **(B)** Hypercellularity on Hematoxylin and Eosin of a cellular but benign schwannoma, which is sometimes mistaken for a malignant peripheral nerve sheath tumor. **(C)** A typical neurofibroma with loose myxoid architecture containing several cellular elements, including the transformed Schwann cells and axons, consistent with the intrafascicular growth.

xanthomatous changes, and fibrosis. Although totally benign, rapid growth and inhomogeneous contrast enhancement may falsely suggest malignancy. Psammomatous melanotic schwannomas packed with melanin and lamellated calcospherules may occur sporadically or as a part of Carney's syndrome. Cellular schwannoma **(Fig. 10–3B)** is another neuropathological challenge, which may histologically mimic malignancy though has less mitotic figures than the usual MPNST. Benign epithelioid schwannoma is characterized by epithelioid cells arranged in cords or nests with occasional features of degenerative changes. Neuroblastoma-like schwannoma, a very rare atypical variant, composed of a giant rosette, may histologically simulate neuroblastoma. Plexiform schwannoma are a rare morphological variant, which may occur sporadically, with NF-2 or with schwannomatosis, but unlike plexiform neurofibromas does not have a propensity for malignant transformation. Less than 5% of schwannomas arise in the context of either of these two predisposition syndromes, NF-2 and schwannomatosis, as peer clinical criteria listed in **Table 10–1.** However, one needs to be aware of these rare patients, where observation rather than multiple radical interventions may be more prudent in most circumstances. The molecular biology of these syndromes is slowly evolving, with the NF-2 gene having been isolated about a decade ago, though the culprit gene in schwannomatosis, likely a neighbor of the NF-2 gene on chromosome 22, remains yet to be located.

Neurofibroma

Neurofibromas may arise sporadically or, as in half of patients, as part of NF-1. Histologically, neurofibromas consist of elongated wavy interlacing hyperchromatic cells with spindle-shaped nuclei in a disorderly, loose myxoid background with collagenous fibrils **(Fig. 10–3C).** The transformed cell has been shown to be the Schwann cell, but there are multiple cell types in a typical neurofibroma such as perineural cells, fibroblasts, lymphocytes, and mast cells. Intratumoral presence of axons is a cardinal and distinguishing feature of neurofibromas compared with schwannomas and is the main reason that attempts at radical resection may lead to deficits.

There are at least three subtypes of this tumor: dermal, subcutaneous, and plexiform neurofibromas, which vary in their biology and clinical behavior, though in all, the underlying transformed cell is the Schwann cell. For example, dermal or subcutaneous neurofibromas do not become malignant and hence removal should be rare and restricted to those lesions, which are being abraded or causing gross cosmetic issues. Plexiform neurofibromas can occur sporadically and thus are not pathognomonic of the diagnosis of NF-1 in isolation of other clinical signs, unlike bilateral vestibular schwannomas for NF-2. They have a predominantly intrafascicular diffuse growth pattern along multiple branches of more proximal nerves, leading to a "string of onion" appearance. The wrongly used term *elephantiasis*, which is somewhat offensive to NF-1 patients, is associated with a very large PNF and accompanying massive soft tissue growth. Plexiform neurofibromas can occur anywhere in the body and may be present at birth, with a majority manifesting within the first decade of life followed by persistent slow growth throughout life, sometimes accentuated during early childhood, puberty, pregnancy, and, rarely, after traumatic intratumoral hemorrhage.

Spontaneous onset of unremitting pain, especially if documented by increased radiological growth, is suggestive of malignant transformation of a plexiform neurofibroma. This risk is ~3 to 5% of NF-1 patients and perhaps a cumulative lifetime risk as high as 10%. Surgical indications for plexiform neurofibromas are therefore for cosmesis, pain, progressive enlargement of size causing pressure effect on adjacent structures, increasing neurological deficit, and suspected malignant transformation. The aim of surgery is to debulk the lesion with preservation of nerve function, which is often possible despite intrafascicular growth, with microscopy and nerve stimulation intraoperatively.

Other Benign Peripheral Nerve Tumors

Perineurioma

These benign, solitary, circumscribed tumors of perineural cell origin clinically mimic schwannomas. Immunohistochemically they are positive for EMA and negative for S-100, Leu-7, and neurofilament staining.

Palisaded Encapsulated Neuroma

These benign, solitary, dome-shaped tumors most commonly affect the face of middle-aged persons. Immunohistochemistry reveals that they are composed of Schwann cells, perineural cells, and small axons.

Neurothekoma

These are benign tumors mainly affecting the face, neck, shoulder, and arm of young women and are of two subtypes: myxomatous and cellular. Immunohistochemistry suggests that the myxomatous subtype is of Schwann cell origin, with the cellular subtype occasionally having atypical histological futures.

Lipoma

These lesions arise from adipocytes and fibrofatty tissues and infiltrate adjacent nerves. They typically affect the median nerve and present with carpal tunnel syndrome and macrodactyly. MRI **(Fig. 10–1C),** is characteristic and most of the time intervention is not warranted unless progressive neurological symptoms occur. The treatment, if indicated due to progressive symptoms or growth, depends on whether the lipoma is intrinsic or extrinsic to the nerve bundle. If intrinsic, attempts at removal of the lipoma from the nerve fascicles may lead to neurological deficits and hence surgery should be restricted to release of the entrapment or, at most, biopsy of the lesion.

Benign Tumor-Like Lesions of the Peripheral Nerves

Ganglion Cyst

Ganglion cysts, arising from joint or tendon sheaths, lead to extraneural compression and even after resection may recur **(Fig. 10–1D).** They are most frequently located around the wrist, knee, elbow, and hip joints. Surgical treatment is aimed at removal of the cyst from the nerve as well as the joint capsule to prevent recurrence as demonstrated in **(Fig. 10–4)**. The cyst is isolated from the adjacent nerve **(Fig. 10–4A),** which is often the common peroneal nerve adjacent to the tibula-fibula joint. Next, the cyst is resected in total, including extirpation from the joint capsule itself **(Fig. 10–4B,C)**. Rare

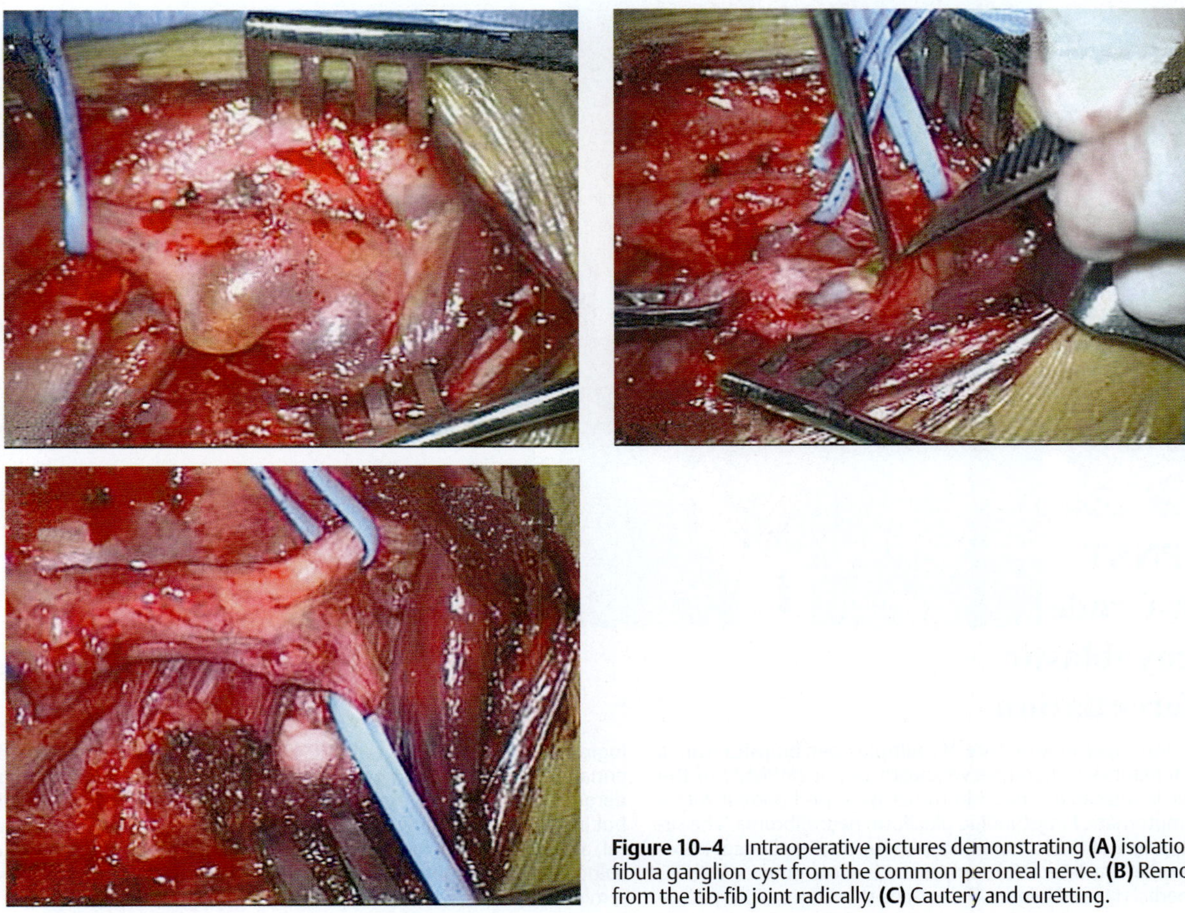

A B C

Figure 10–4 Intraoperative pictures demonstrating **(A)** isolation of the tibula-fibula ganglion cyst from the common peroneal nerve. **(B)** Removal of the cyst from the tib-fib joint radically. **(C)** Cautery and curetting.

intraneural ganglion cysts may arise like their extraneural counterparts and subsequently track along the sheath of small articular nerves into their final destinations.

Desmoids

These locally aggressive tumors of fascial and musculoaponeurotic structures may arise from supraclavicular fossa of the chest wall and invade the brachial plexus. Although gross total removal is the goal, the aim should be maximum surgical removal with minimal neurological morbidity, which is challenging due to their invasive and infiltrative growth pattern. Many centers advocate postoperative radiotherapy to reduce recurrence, but radiation-induced neuritis prompts others to keep it reserved for recurrent disease after reoperation.

Peripheral Nerve Pseudotumor

These lesions result from chronic inflammatory cell infiltration of the peripheral nerve, such as in leprosy, requiring conservative microsurgical resection with neural sparing and appropriate systemic medical therapy.

Malignant Peripheral Nerve Tumors

Primary Malignant Peripheral Nerve Sheath Tumors

These tumors account for ~3 to 10% of all soft tissue sarcomas, with half representing malignant transformation of a preexisting plexiform neurofibroma in an NF-1 patient **(Fig. 10–5).** Progressive enlargement, increasing neurological deficit, and especially incapacitating pain are suggestive

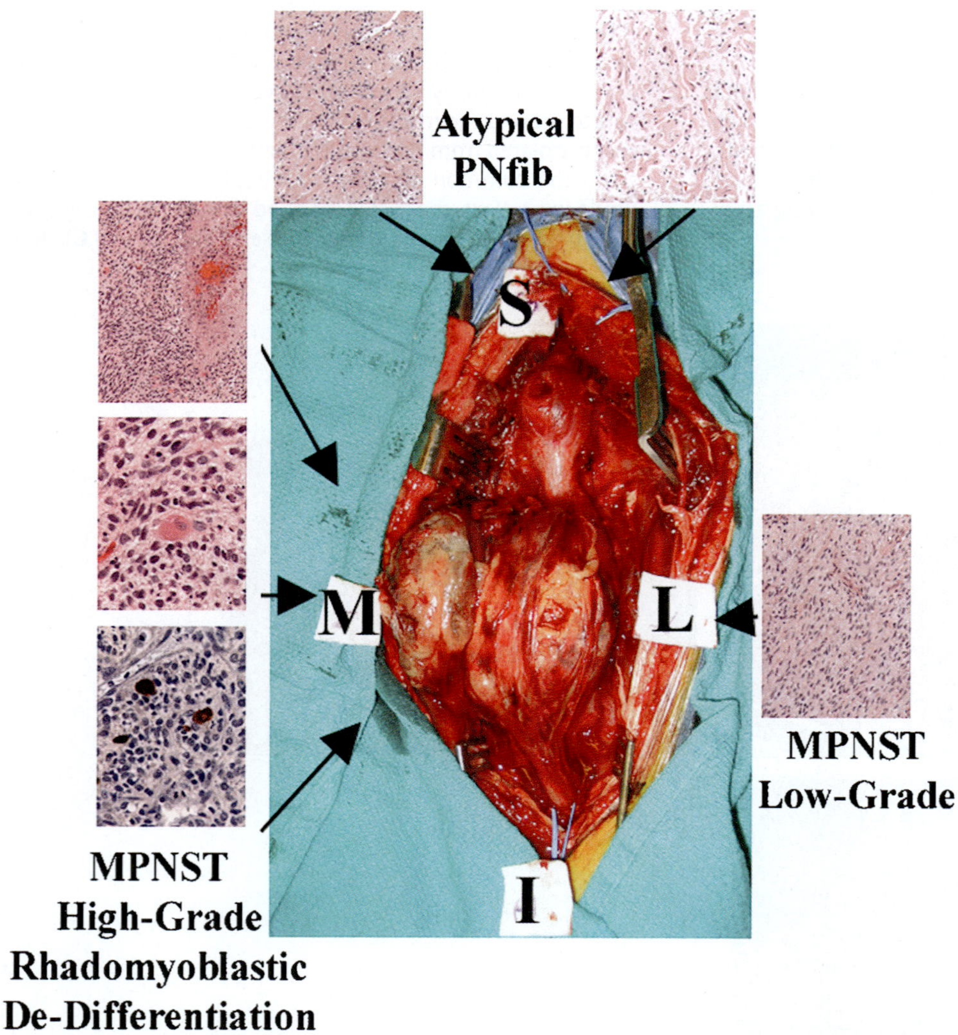

Figure 10–5 Intraoperative picture of multiple open biopsies from a suspected malignant peripheral nerve sheath tumor (MPNST) of the posttibial nerve in the calf of a neurofibromatosis type 1 patient with a previously asymptomatic longstanding plexiform neurofibroma. The superior (S) component of the tumors is atypical but not malignant plexiform neurofibroma. The lateral (L) component is a low-grade 1 MPNST, whereas the medial (M) and inferior (I) sections show aggressive pathological features of a high-grade MPNST with rhabdomyoblastic dedifferentiation. After confirmation of the diagnosis of MPNST, the patient undergoes a metastatic survey, preoperative radiation, followed by radical but limb-salvaging surgery, which includes the nerve proximal and distal, adjacent muscle, fascia, and compartmental blood vessels. The oncological goal is to obtain tumor-free margins and thereby minimize systemic metastasis, the main cause of mortality.

of malignant transformation of a preexisting plexiform neurofibroma. MRI is the investigation of choice, though it cannot distinguish between other PNTs or soft tissue sarcomas with certainty. Nonhomogeneous contrast enhancement, necrosis, and hemorrhage are only suggestive but not confirmatory. Classification of MPNST is based on those used for the much more common soft tissue sarcomas, from grade 1 to 3, depending on the number of mitotic figures and degree of nuclear and cellular atypia.

The ideal management of a rare MPNST remains problematic, with our institute recommending a multidisciplinary management strategy. Clinical suspicion is followed by biopsy, which we recommend to be a four-quadrant open biopsy rather than fine needle or percutaneous biopsy, to maximize retrieval of representative tissue for a thorough pathological examination with minimal morbidity and pain to the patient. An MPNST can be heterogeneous, especially those arising from preexisting plexiform neurofibromas, as demonstrated in **Fig. 10–5.** Some regions, such as the top of this MPNST, harbor atypical but benign pathological features of a plexiform neurofibroma. Other regions, such as the middle or lateral components, represent sarcomatous transformation of varying degrees, from low-grade to a highly malignant dedifferentiated MPNST. This heterogeneity is another reason for advocating open four-quadrant biopsy to adequately sample the tumor.

The implication of the pathology, once confirmed, and the proposed management strategy, need thorough discussion with the patient because the objective is not to spare the nerve but rather that of oncological local control, with obtaining tumor-free margins. We undertake a metastasis survey with CT/MRI of the chest and abdomen, preoperative radiation in many but not all cases, and then follow with definitive oncological surgery. As mentioned, the goal of the surgery is to achieve an en bloc removal with tumor-free margins, even at the cost of major nerves and adjacent soft tissue structures, hence requiring collaboration with orthopedic oncology colleagues and physio- and occupational therapists. Nerve grafting is not considered because more proximal nerves are not amenable to reinnervate with grafting, adjuvant radiation therapy, and the natural history of MPNST is often not long enough for effective reinnervation.

◆ Postoperative Management

Adverse prognostic factors include: large size (>5 cm), higher tumor grade, advanced histology, non-tumor-free surgical margin, and association of NF-1. The use of pre- or postoperative chemotherapy, which mainly has involved Adriamycin, is controversial as is radiation therapy in MPNST. Large-scale randomized studies to address some of these issues on treatment options and evaluation of novel biological therapies are extremely hard to achieve, given the small numbers of these patients, which are often managed despoutside of a multidisciplinary academic center. Systemic spread, especially pulmonary metastasis, is the terminal event and, despite of limited efficacy, chemotherapy is usually tried. The 5-year survival rate of MPNST is worse than other soft tissue sarcomas and is generally ~34 to 51%, with our management strategy resulting in a 64% 5 year survival.

Secondary Intraneural Metastasis

Only a few cases of intraneural metastasis from breast carcinoma, malignant melanoma, and carcinoid have been described so far. The diagnostic dilemma resides in intraneural invasion versus radiation neuritis in the context of prior breast cancer or lung cancer patients treated with radiation, presenting with brachial plexopathy. In these cases, MRI cannot distinguish the two pathologies, which on surgery may both be present, leading to the progressive neurological deterioration.

Secondary Pancoast Tumor

Primary carcinomas in the apex of the lung involving or abutting the lower elements of the brachial plexus warrant a combined neurosurgical and thoracic surgical procedure to obtain radical tumor removal. Radiation followed by surgery results in 15 to 50% 5-year survival in these patients. A supraclavicular exposure combined with sternotomy provides an open exposure to the great vessels, brachial plexus, and intrathoracic contents to facilitate resection.

Secondary Radiation-Induced Plexopathy

Immediate or delayed-onset radiation-induced brachial plexopathy occurs in 1.5 to 35% of breast carcinoma patients and differentiation from recurrence or metastasis is often difficult as previously discussed. Different surgical procedures including neurolysis, omentoplasty, and muscle pedicle flap have been attempted with variable results. The surgical objective is to obtain pathology to rule in or out tumor recurrence and undertake limited neurolysis to help alleviate some of the neuropathic pain, which is often the most disabling symptom. Restoration of motor function, which is often lost in the intrinsics of the hand supplied by lower trunk elements, is not feasible.

◆ Conclusion

Peripheral nerve tumors are rare and present with a myriad of clinical manifestations. A thorough history, physical examination, and radiological examination combined with sound clinical judgment, provides the best avenue for optimal management. A family history for predisposition syndromes associated with PNTs is essential, with many of these patients not requiring surgical intervention, just regular clinical and radiological follow-up. Similarly, the optimal management of certain PNTs, based on our current knowledge of their likely biological behavior, may also be nonsurgical follow-up. However, when surgical intervention is indicated, proper microneurosurgical techniques combined with intraoperative electrophysiological evaluation should render minimal added neurological morbidity in most cases of

PNTs. The exception is the management of MPNST, where staged surgery is advocated. The first stage is pathological confirmation with open sampling from multiple regions of the suspected tumor. After confirmation, the objective of the second procedure is to obtain tumor-free margins, which can usually be accomplished with a radical but limb-salvaging procedure. Despite these management strategies, PNTs can cause significant morbidity and in some cases, especially MPNSTs, significant mortality. This requires increased understanding of the molecular biology of these tumors, with the objectives of defining better diagnostic, prognostic, and biological therapeutic strategies.

11

Surgical Management of Spinal Schwannomas

Joshua Medow and Gregory Trost

Spinal schwannomas are relatively common tumors, representing between 20 and 30% of all spinal neoplasms. Most schwannomas occur without association with neurofibromatosis type 1 (von Recklinghausen's disease). Treatment for these spinal tumors is diverse and sometimes controversial. Consequently treatment options are considered anecdotal. This chapter reviews the available literature and describes the pathology, management strategies, and a few surgical approaches for the treatment of patients with spinal schwannomas.

◆ Patient Selection

General Considerations

Schwannomas are neoplasms derived from the peripheral nerve sheath and are composed entirely of Schwann cells. They are characteristically benign masses that may slowly recur if they are not completely resected. Spinal schwannomas are intradural extramedullary lesions that preferentially affect sensory nerve roots over motor nerve roots. They usually develop at the root entry zone (REZ) where there is a transition between oligodendrocytes of the central nervous system (CNS) and Schwann cells of the peripheral nervous system. This differs from extraspinal schwannomas, which can arise from sensory, motor, or autonomic nerves.

In general, schwannomas are more easily removed than neurofibromas because they arise in a single nerve fascicle and displace the nerve eccentrically. Conversely, neurofibromas involve the nerve circumferentially, investing in the nerve in fusiform fashion. The size of some schwannomas may preclude the ability to visualize the nerve fibers because they are stretched across the surface of the mass, making resection more complicated. This resultant stretch may cause the nerve to become very attenuated over time. Schwannomas rarely undergo malignant degeneration.

Macroscopically, schwannomas appear as firm, well-circumscribed, encapsulated, globular masses that can have multiple nodules. They are typically solid and tan on the cut surface. Older schwannomas may have a prominent lobulated surface and cystic, xanthomatous, and hemorrhagic changes that occur with increasing age of the mass. This is classically referred to as ancient change. These larger, longstanding lesions may erode surrounding bone and become adherent to adjacent structures without infiltrating them. Schwannomas usually have an excellent blood supply, and entering the capsule often results in a fair amount of bleeding.

Imaging

There are many adjunctive studies that can be performed to help arrive at the diagnosis of a spinal schwannoma; however, a detailed history and physical examination remain the gold standard for determining and treating disease successfully. There may be a discrepancy between the percentage of patients demonstrating changes on imaging studies and the symptoms (if any) that they present with. Consequently, it is imperative that the physician considers the patient's condition when reviewing radiographs. This section will briefly mention the current studies available to address diseases of the spine.

Plain Film X-Rays

The earliest imaging modality, x-ray images still provide substantial information to the physician. Oblique x-rays image the neural foramina fairly well and can often demonstrate changes in configuration that may indicate the presence of a mass lesion. Spinal schwannomas may demonstrate erosion of the bony confines of the neural foramen through which they pass and sclerosis of the foraminal margins. Depending on the size of the lesion, damage to the vertebral body may be present as well. Spinal alignment must also be noted to help assess for instability.

Myelography

Computed tomographic (CT) myelography is the gold standard imaging study for assessing cord and root compression, with magnetic resonance imaging (MRI) running a close second because of its ability to display detailed anatomy.

Computed Tomography

CT of the spine is an axial compilation of x-ray lines, from multiple angles, that provides exceptional anatomy of the bone and soft tissues in cross-section. These images can demonstrate fractures/dislocations, degenerative/sclerotic changes of the bone, and, with reconstruction, abnormal alignment of the vertebrae. Today's CT scanners can also provide limited visualization of the dura and spinal cord within the spinal canal delineating compression of the cord by mass lesions or stenosis. Measurements of canal diameter can be performed more accurately with CT than with plain film x-rays. The details regarding nerve root and spinal cord compression are limited, however, unless a contrast medium such as Omnipaque (Amersham Health, Princeton, NJ) is injected intravenously. Injection can also be performed intrathecally and the result viewed as a postmyelogram CT, where a contrast void indicates the location of compression.

Magnetic Resonance Imaging

MRI provides excellent resolution of anatomy in multiple planes. Using algorithms similar to those in CT, MR images can be reconstructed with great detail. Soft tissues such as the spinal cord, ligaments, fat, and vascular structures are visualized exceptionally well, whereas bone is less clearly defined. Inflammation within the bone, such as that seen in acute fractures, is fairly well imaged. The spinal cord and its position within the canal as well as the neural foramina and their contents are well demonstrated. Spinal schwannomas are typically neutral on T1 MRI and enhance considerably with IV contrast because of their significant vascularity. On a T2 MRI sequence, schwannomas usually appear as solid masses but may induce a variable amount of edema in surrounding structures **(Fig. 11–1).** The noninvasive nature of the MRI and its exceptional resolution of anatomical structure have made it the imaging study of choice for assessing spinal pathology.

Nonoperative treatment is sometimes effective during the acute symptomatic phase. It is imperative that the patient who is undergoing nonoperative treatment return to the clinic for frequent evaluation to ensure that there is no progression of symptoms. Although conservative management may relieve pain, radiculopathy and myelopathy symptoms can continue to progress with evidence of sensory or motor deterioration or both. These symptoms may progress rapidly or insidiously. It is the physician's responsibility to address the need for operative intervention early before the deficits become permanent.

In asymptomatic patients, small size, peripheral location, and advanced age may warrant careful observation rather than surgery. Conservative management is always accompanied by periodic imaging. We typically reimage our patients that are followed conservatively with MRI at 6 months and then every year thereafter.

Surgical intervention is generally indicated for those patients with a large, enlarging, or centrally displaced tumor and in patients that have either or both intractable pain and progressive neurological symptoms in the presence of a documented mass lesion. Pain relief and resolution or reduction of neurological deficits can be expected in the vast majority of patients if managed appropriately. The prognosis for patients with myelopathy is the most variable.

The use of somatosensory evoked potentials (SSEPs) should be guided by the type of deficit that may result. As long as resection does not risk any additional damage to the spinal cord, the use of SSEPs in these patients is probably not indicated. Concern often arises when nerve roots that contribute to the cervical or lumbosacral plexi are involved because injury to these nerves will often result in a motor deficit. There are no clear guidelines as to the use of SSEPs during surgical resection of spinal schwannomas, and it is up to the surgeon's judgment whether to utilize them.

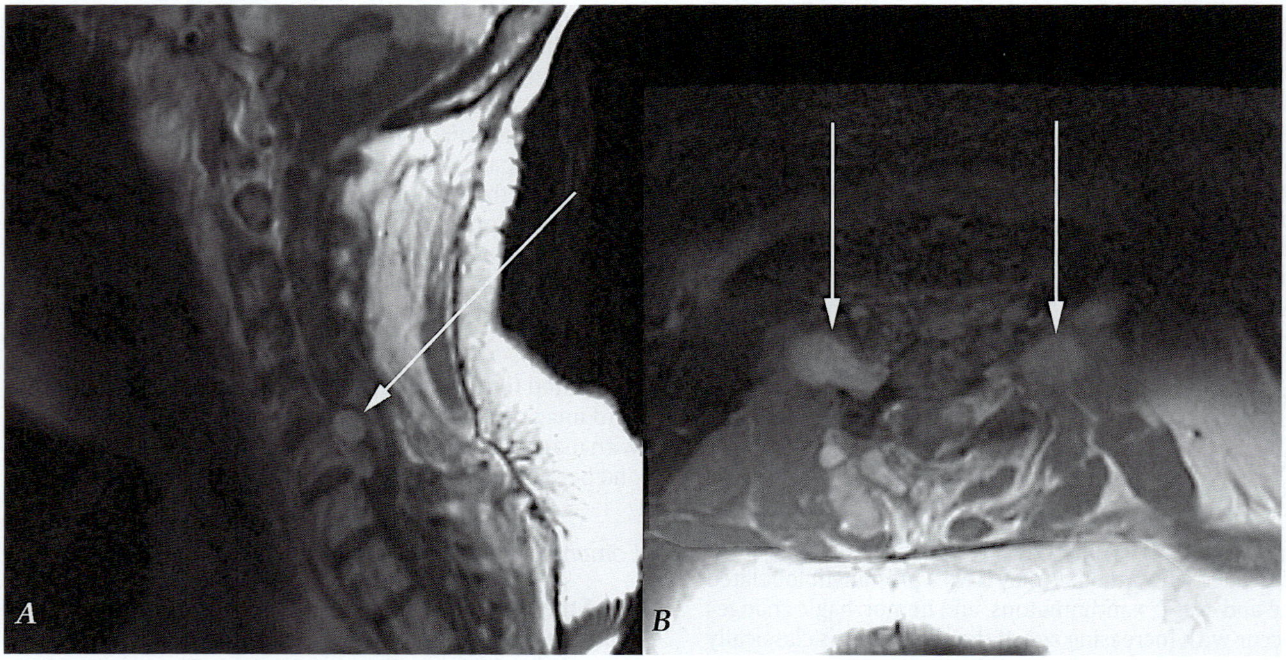

Figure 11–1 Composite contrast-enhanced magnetic resonance imaging of the cervical spine. **(A)** Sagittal image showing an intradural extramedullary schwannoma (arrow) as it approaches the C5–C6 neural foramen. **(B)** Axial image revealing two dumbbell-shaped schwannomas (arrows) extending through the neural foramina bilaterally.

◆ Indications for Choice of Surgical Approach

The surgical approach to the resection of spinal schwannomas is primarily guided by the location and size of the tumor. Following is a brief synopsis of three different types of approaches and their indications. In many circumstances schwannomas develop on sensory nerve roots, and the sensory portion of the nerve root can usually be resected if necessary. Other times the nerve is not functional at all. More rarely, the schwannoma involves a functional motor root. In most cases schwannomas can be resected en bloc with a clear margin of the nerve.

The criteria for choosing the appropriate operative approach are variable and should be based on both the patient's symptoms and adjunctive study findings. Surgery is basically categorized by the direction of the approach (anterior versus posterior, medial versus lateral) and the need for internal fixation, if so desired. Posterior approaches are designed to access the posterior elements of the spine **(Fig. 11–2).** The

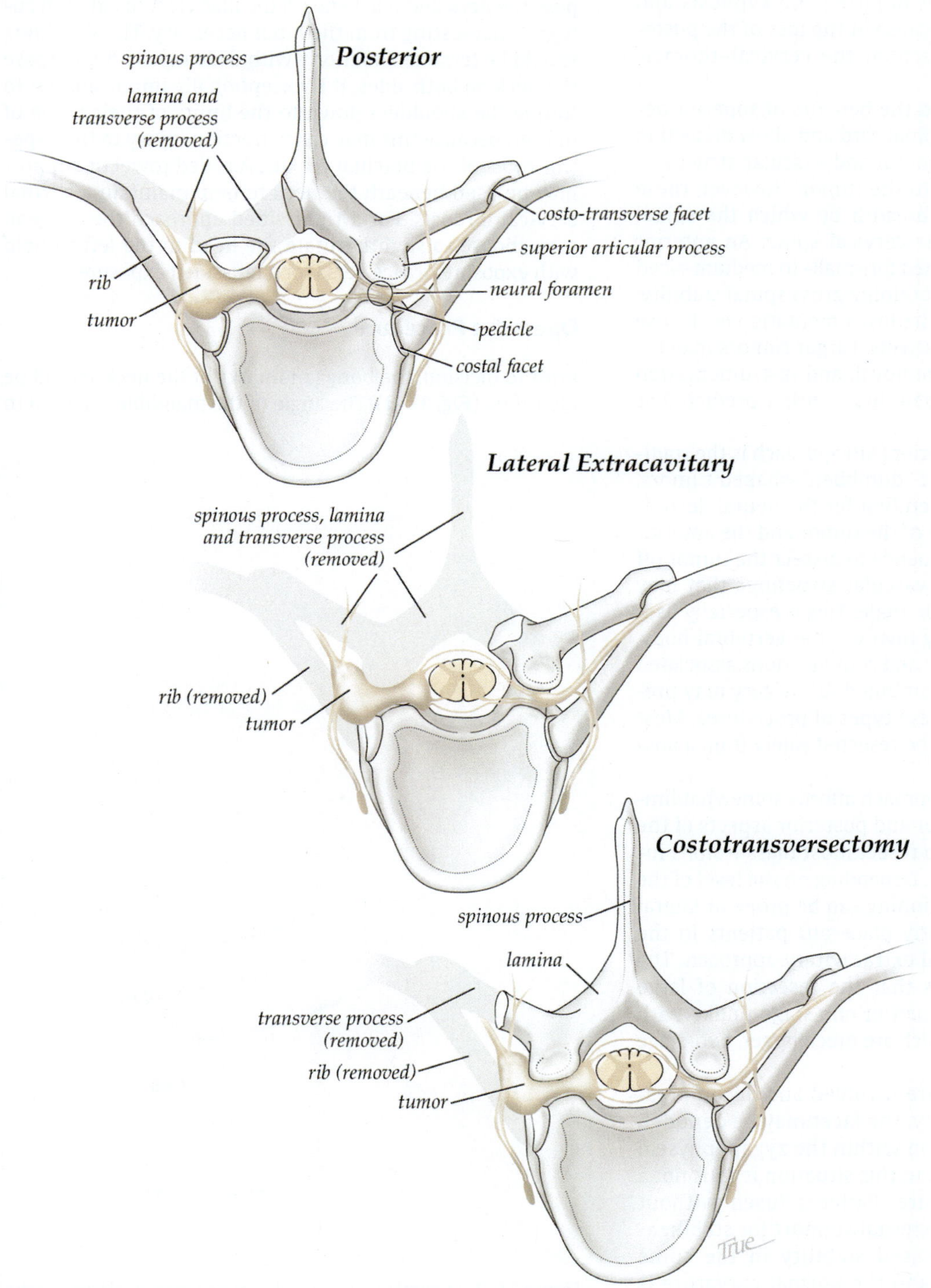

Figure 11–2 Bone removal performed during posterior and lateral approaches to the thoracic spine.

choice of a posterior decompressive procedure depends on the patient's clinical presentation and the extent of tumor involvement. Laminectomies are typically performed on patients who have large intradural or high cervical masses. The neural foramina can be exposed posteriorly and as such can be successfully decompressed from this direction. Combined posterior laminectomy and foraminotomy procedures are often effective if the patient presents with a combined myeloradiculopathy. With larger resections, concerns arise regarding the stability of the cervical spine as a consequence of facet damage. Additionally, posterior procedures can result in iatrogenic kyphosis and late degenerative disease because of the loss of the posterior tension band, particularly at the cervical–thoracic junction.

Anterior approaches afford the benefits of superior decompression of the ventral spinal cord and allow dissection of a mass lesion off of the neural and vascular structures that are normally adherent to the tumor. However, these approaches have a limited breadth by which the spinal canal can be accessed in the cervical spine. An anterior foraminotomy can be performed for small- to medium-sized foraminal tumors while maintaining gross spinal stability. This procedure does not require instrumentation or the use of a cervical collar postoperatively. Larger tumors may require more extensive bone removal, and instrumentation may become necessary if instability is either predicted or observed intraoperatively.

A combined anterior–posterior (AP) approach is the traditional method of resection of "dumbbell"-shaped tumors. The posterior approach is used first for the neural decompression and initial resection of the tumor and the anterior approach is then used in sequence to dissect the tumor off of the adherent neural and vascular structures that may not be visible from a posterior angle. This is especially useful if the tumor significantly involves the vertebral body. The prolonged operative time and complications associated with multiple wounds in a combined AP surgery may preclude some patients from these types of procedures. Most schwannomas, however, can be resected solely from a posterior approach.

The lateral extracavitary approach affords somewhat limited exposure of both anterior and posterior aspects of the spine that is often enough to resect most mass lesions involving the spinal nerve roots. Depending on the level of the spine involved, patient positioning can be prone or lateral decubitis. We most frequently place our patients in the prone position for the lateral extracavitary approach. The benefit of this procedure is that the resection of large masses can often be performed in one stage unlike with combined AP approaches, which are much larger, two-stage procedures.

If the facet components are involved and decompression and fusion are necessary, the facet may be denuded of cartilage to promote fusion within the zygapophyseal joint itself. The use of a graft in this situation is thus not a prerequisite of the procedure. Patients fused without graft material rarely need external support for stabilization. Fusion provides increased stability in the spine if the bone heals correctly and the normal curvature is maintained.

◆ Anterior Approaches to the Cervical Spine

Preoperative Preparation

Patient positioning, as with all surgical approaches, is critical when performing surgery on the cervical spine. The use of tongs for traction and SSEPs should be considered if the patient's spine is unstable or if there is evidence of position-dependent neurological compromise. A bolster roll should be placed between the scapulae longitudinally to help expose the neck and one beneath the iliac crest to aid with autograft harvesting from the hip if necessary. The shoulders should be retracted inferiorly with wide tape to help expose the neck on both sides. It is exceptionally important not to torque the shoulders down to the limits of their range of motion because this may cause traction injury to the superior roots of the brachial plexus. A rolled towel or support may be used beneath the neck to help maintain a normal cervical lordosis. For a right-sided approach the surgeon may choose to slightly rotate the head to the left to help with exposure or vice versa for a left-sided exposure.

Operative Procedure

Prior to incision, the bony landmarks of the neck should be identified **(Fig. 11–3)**. The angle of the mandible is lateral to

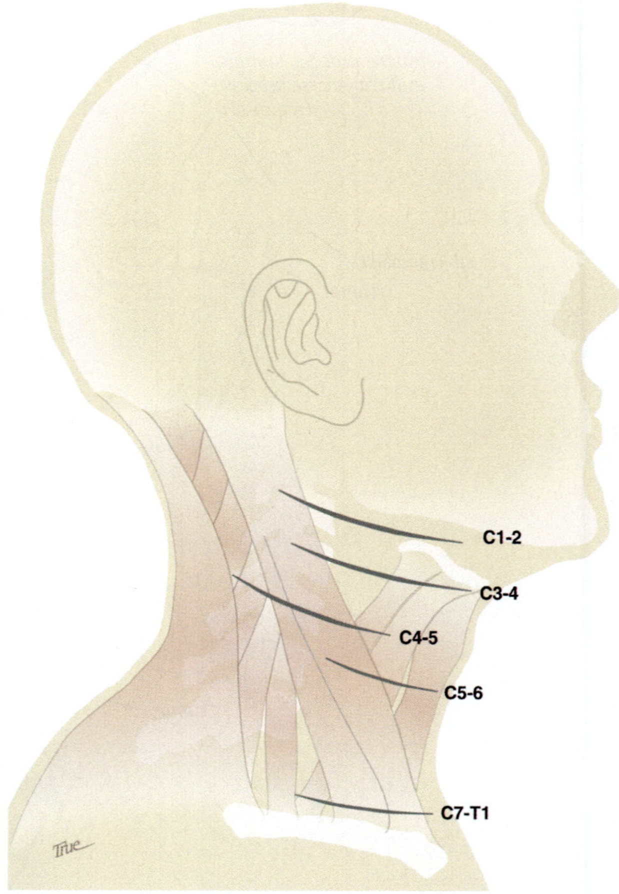

Figure 11–3 Typical incisions used to access individual levels of the cervical spine anteriorly.

C2–C3, the hyoid bone traverses anterior to the cervical spine at C3, as does the thyroid cartilage at C4, and the cricoid cartilage at C6. The carotid tubercle can be used to help identify the C5–C6 interspace. These landmarks become especially important for transverse incisions where the exposure offers a limited view of the structures within the operative field.

The cervical spine can be approached anteriorly from the right or left sides. Although many surgeons are right handed and prefer to operate on the patient's right side, some surgeons prefer a left-sided approach. This is because of the predictability of the left recurrent laryngeal nerve as it tracks through the carotid sheath and enters the thorax, looping under the aorta before ascending back into the neck adjacent to the trachea and esophagus. The right recurrent laryngeal nerve has a more inconsistent course. It passes beneath the subclavian artery and enters the tracheoesophageal groove at a more rostral level than on the left side. Consequently it can readily be injured, especially during an approach to C6–C7.

The incision for a single-level anterior approach to the cervical spine is best performed for cosmetic purposes by a transverse incision, preferably in a natural crease of the skin. The patient should be prepped in the appropriate sterile fashion and the choice of incision should be marked on the neck prior to draping.

The incision is made with the scalpel down to the platysma and is followed by electrocautery for hemostasis. The platysma is then incised in line with its fibers in a rostral-caudal fashion to facilitate deep retraction. Blunt dissection is then used to identify the anterior plane between the sternocleidomastoid and the carotid sheath laterally, and the trachea, esophagus, and strap muscles medially.

The carotid artery is identified during the approach to ensure its integrity. The thyroid vasculature may be visualized anterior to the cervical spine and can be ligated during the exposure. The omohyoid, although a useful landmark, may obstruct the operative field rostrally if exposing the C2–C4 levels and can be retracted or divided if necessary. Care is taken to protect the esophagus, which is retracted to the side opposite the exposure. The loose, middle cervical layer fascia that bridges the sternocleidomastoid and the strap muscles of the larynx is then dissected to reveal the anterior portion of the cervical spine.

The prevertebral fascia is opened using electrocautery and blunt dissection, revealing the anterior aspect of the vertebral bodies. The longus colli muscle is then dissected with either or both electrocautery and a Cobb periosteal elevator to facilitate the placement of retractors. Care is taken to avoid the sympathetic chain located at the lateral surface of this muscle. Adequate retraction is attained when the uncovertebral joints are noted. Adjustable retractors are then placed in transverse and cranial-caudal fashion, respectively. Again, care is taken to protect the esophagus and carotid sheath against trauma from the retractor devices.

One or two spinal needles can be inserted into the disk spaces suspected to be the levels that need repair and a cross-table, lateral C-spine radiograph is obtained to confirm position. The film is then examined and if the location is correct, the needle is removed while it is marked with electrocautery. If the patient is obese or has large shoulders and the inferior cervical vertebrae cannot be visualized, the second spinal needle can be placed into a rostral disk space that is not in need of repair. Its location can be confirmed radiographically, and the disk spaces between the rostral and caudal spinal needles can be carefully counted to determine the location of the caudal needle.

At this point the surgical microscope is brought into the field. The longus colli muscle ipsilateral to the pathology is resected medially to expose the transverse processes of the two vertebrae at the level of the affected nerve root or segment. The vertebral arteries enter the transverse foramina at C6 in 90% of the population after proceeding anterior to the transverse process at C7. Because there is some variability in the course of the vertebral artery, dissection of the longus colli should involve careful observation but does not require purposeful exposure of the vertebral artery unless operating at the C6–C7 level. Additionally, the surgeon should be aware of the proximity of the cervical sympathetic ganglia, which can be injured during dissection of the longus colli, especially if it is not subperiosteally dissected.

The dissection should reveal the uncovertebral joint between the transverse processes **(Fig. 11–4);** however, severe spondylosis may obscure this landmark. A high-speed drill is then used to bur a 6- × 8-mm hole through the uncovertebral joint under the modest protection of an angled guide used to protect the vertebral artery from the moving bit. The surgeon maintains careful attention to the location of the vertebral artery so that a thin layer of cortical bone is left attached to the ligamentous tissue surrounding the artery at its medial aspect. A slight medial angle to the drill is applied as the course of the hole proceeds posteriorly to the posterior longitudinal ligament (PLL). The thin posterolateral remnant of the uncinate process is freed from the adjacent ligamentous tissue and removed carefully via curettage, revealing the transverse artery. Meticulous drilling of posterior osteophytes is continued as the trajectory of the drill crosses the midline and is angled toward the opposite margin of the spinal cord. The PLL is then incised and resected to the origin of the contralateral nerve root to effectively decompress the spinal cord and ipsilateral nerve root.

Many times the tumor is large enough that a portion and possibly all of the vertebral body may need to be removed to adequately expose the mass lesion in its entirety. If only a small portion of the vertebral body needs to be removed, a hemicorpectomy can be performed. Once the exposure is complete, resection of the tumor is performed.

Meticulous hemostasis is imperative prior to closure of the wound. If the wound continues to ooze excessively despite reasonable measures, a drain may be placed to prevent the formation of a large hematoma. Thrombin-soaked Gelfoam is often instrumental in these situations. The middle cervical fascia is closed with 2–0 Vicryl or other absorbable suture, thereby approximating the sternocleidomastoid and strap muscles over the carotid sheath. The platysma and subcutaneous regions are then closed independently with a similar 2–0 or 3–0 absorbable suture and technique. The skin is approximated in a subcuticular fashion or with surgical glue. A dressing is then applied over the wound and a hard cervical collar is fitted around the patient's neck if indicated.

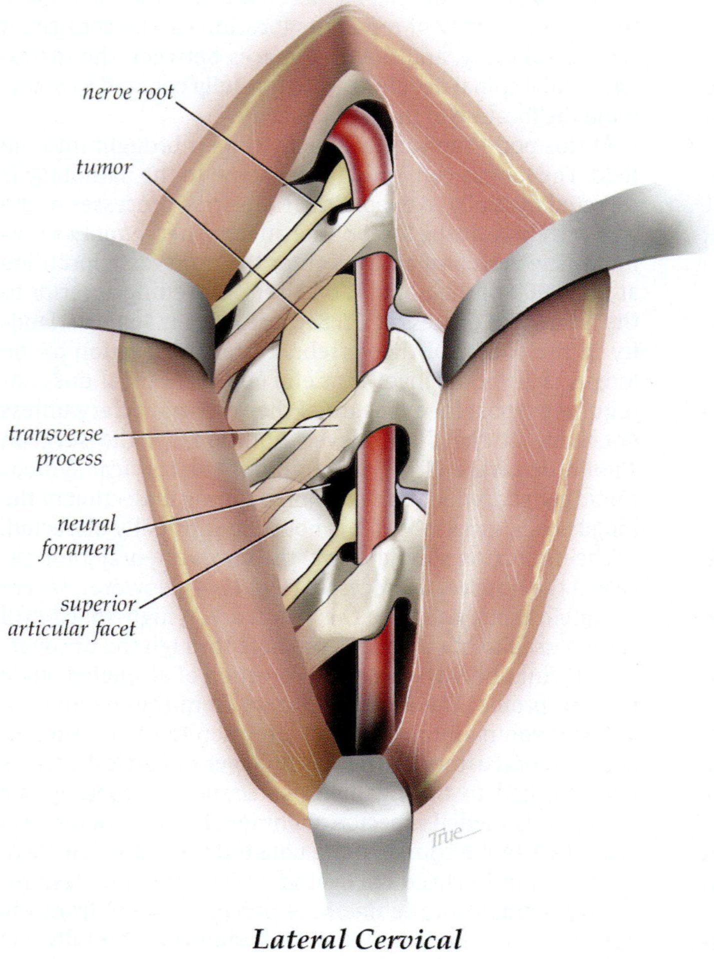

Figure 11–4 Anterolateral view of the cervical spine after surgical exposure.

If iliac crest autograft is used, the overlying fascia is approximated with 2–0 Vicryl or similar absorbable suture and the subcutaneous layer is similarly closed with 3–0 suture. The skin edges are either stapled together or sutured with 4–0 nylon.

◆ Posterior Approaches to the Spine

Preoperative Preparation

Positioning the patient for a posterior cervical procedure can be performed in three fashions with variations on each. The prone/ "Concorde" position involves putting the patient in a three-pin headholder with the patient's neck placed in flexion and the operative table in reverse Trendelenburg so that the operative field is parallel to the floor. For the lateral decubitus/ "park bench" position patients lie on their side with the head propped so that the spine is parallel to the floor. This position is best employed in parascapular approaches.

The sitting position offers the surgeon a more straightforward view of the upright contour of the cervical spine and allows the anesthesiologist ready access to the patient's airway. During the procedure, the surgeon should notice a reduction in venous congestion as opposed to prone positioning. The greatest risk associated with the sitting position is air embolism because the atrium of the heart lies below the operative field. This risk, however, is small, primarily because there are no large venous structures capable of drawing in air at a rate that could rapidly cause catastrophic airlock. To help prevent the complications of air embolism during seated procedures, the patient should have a precordial Doppler in place and the patient's end tidal CO_2 should be closely monitored. A central venous catheter should also be positioned in the superiormost portion of the right atrium to evacuate any air that is detected should air embolization occur.

Operative Procedure

A midline incision provides improved exposure of the spine bilaterally. The spinous processes are palpated. Oftentimes, one or two spinal needles are placed through the prepped skin superficial to the spinous process(es) thought to be part of the target vertebrae. A lateral spine x-ray is obtained.

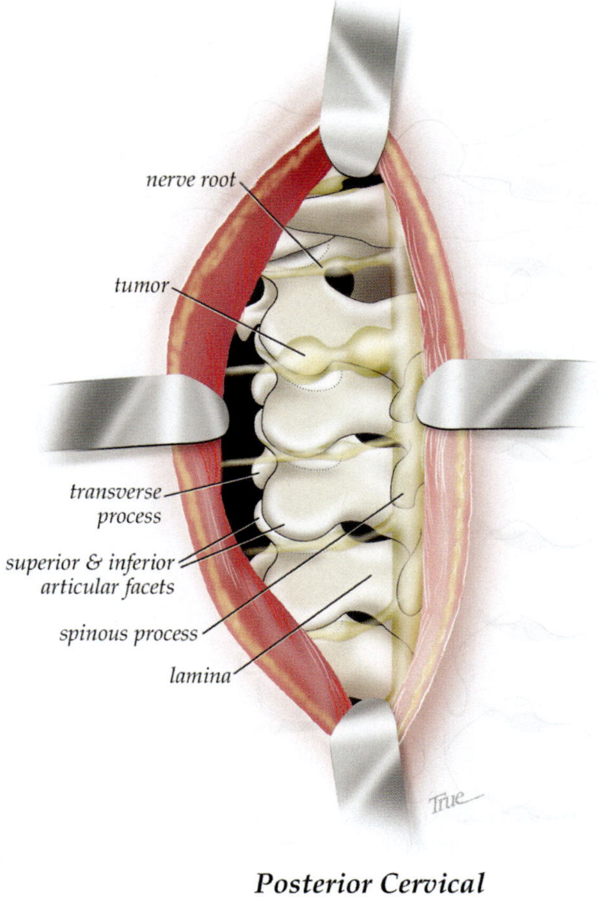

Figure 11–5 Surgical exposure of the posterolateral aspect of the cervical spine prior to laminectomy.

The needles are removed and the skin marked where they were present. Position is confirmed and the incision is adjusted accordingly. The overlying subcutaneous tissue is dissected sharply with electrocautery and the fascia is divided either bilaterally or unilaterally over the affected side. A marker such as a clamp is placed on the spinous process and a second cross table x-ray is performed. Once position is confirmed, dissection is continued subperiosteally to the expose the entire facet. The paraspinous muscles are retracted **(Figs. 11–5 to 11–8).** The lamina can be removed with Kerrison punches, a Leksell rongeur, or a high-speed drill. To prevent against iatrogenic injury to the cervical or thoracic spinal cord, instruments should not be placed beneath the lamina until adequate exposure is attained because the compressed spinal cord is often unforgiving. The ligamentum flavum can be removed in a separate step or with the bone. Many surgeons find that a one-step process of removing bone and ligament together makes the removal of the ligamentum flavum easier. Oftentimes a high-speed drill is used to grind down the lamina. The ligamentum flavum and interspinous ligament are transected at the rostral and caudal extents of the decompression, and the lamina are removed. A small Kerrison punch can then be used to carefully detach the ligamentum flavum from its lateral borders. A Penfield or other blunt probe may prove useful in the careful dissection of the ligamentum flavum off of the underlying thecal sac. With the major portion of the lamina removed, attention is turned toward resection of the remaining portion of the lamina laterally. In the cervical spine, resection with Kerrison punches should not exceed the medial third of the facet joint without planning to perform a fusion because significant instability will likely result. A wide unilateral decompression in the lumbar spine (more than half of the facet) to expose the mass lesion is often permitted but may result in instability requiring fusion. A wide unilateral decompression in the thoracic spine to expose the mass lesion is often permitted without resulting in any significant instability. A foraminotomy is performed simultaneously with the lateral laminectomy to completely decompress the structures within the neural foramen. Tumor resection is then performed. Before closure, a blunt probe is positioned within the foramen to ensure adequate decompression.

Meticulous hemostasis is imperative. If the wound continues to ooze excessively despite reasonable measures, a drain may be placed to prevent the formation of a large hematoma. Thrombin-soaked Gelfoam is often instrumental in these situations. The fascia is closed with 2–0 Vicryl or other absorbable suture, often in interrupted fashion. The subcutaneous regions are then closed independently with a similar 2–0 or 3–0 absorbable suture. The skin can be approximated in subcuticular fashion but because wounds of the posterior neck may have more difficulty healing secondary to tension and the moist folds of skin, many surgeons

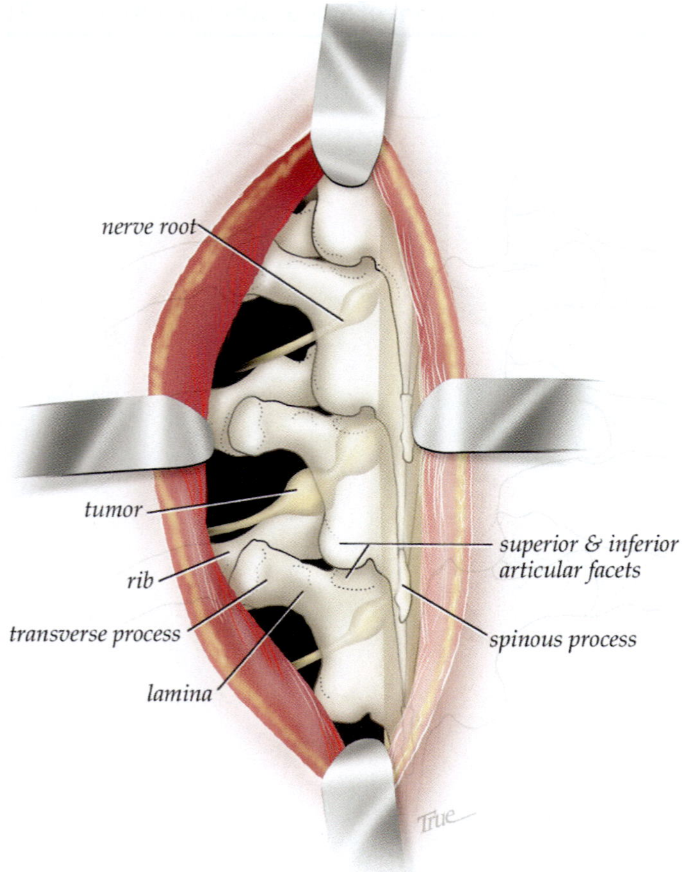

Posterior Thoracic

Figure 11–6 Surgical exposure of the posterolateral aspect of the thoracic spine prior to laminectomy.

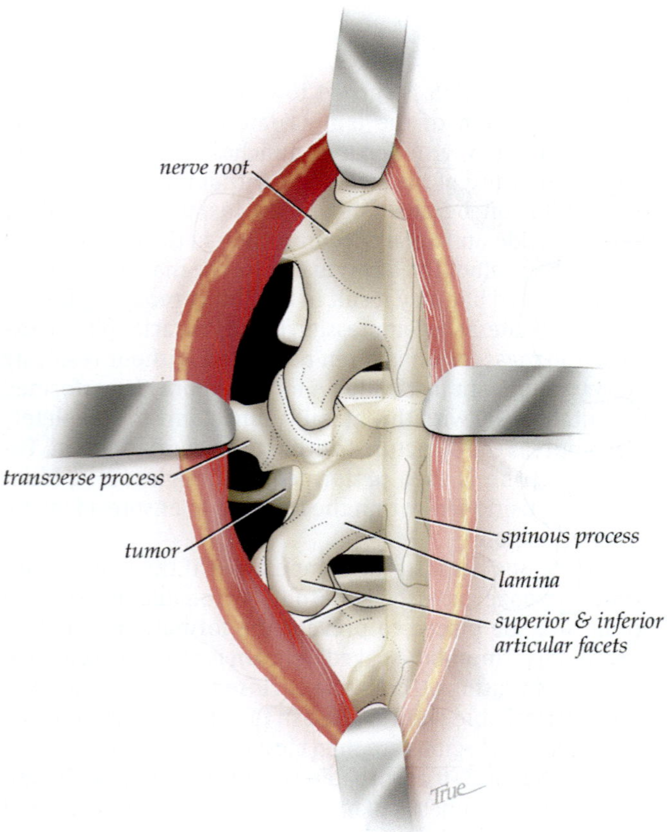

Posterior Lumbar

Figure 11–7 Surgical exposure of the posterolateral aspect of the lumbar spine prior to laminectomy.

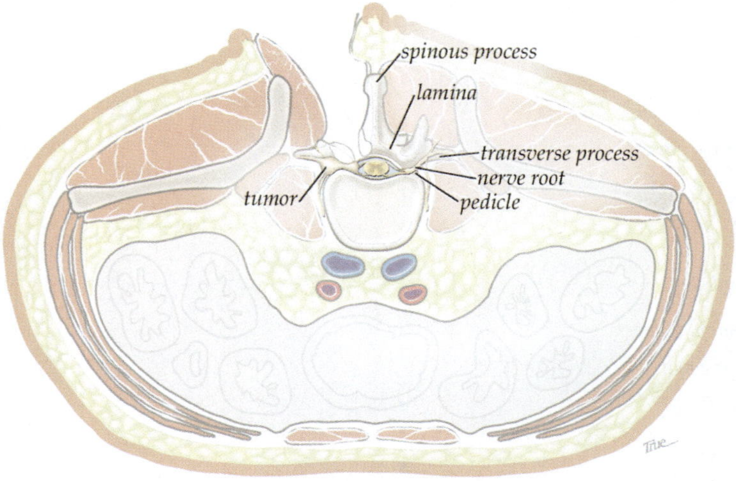

Figure 11–8 Axial view of the surgical exposure used during a laminectomy for tumor resection.

prefer to close with a nonabsorbable suture that can be removed 10 days later. A dressing is then applied over the wound and an orthotic device is applied if necessary.

◆ The Lateral Extracavitary Approach

Combined anteroposterior approaches to the spine are often necessary to completely resect spinal nerve tumors. The anatomy of the thoracic spine affords a reasonable view of both aspects via a single retropleural, lateral approach. Often this is performed via a lateral extracavitary approach (Capener) or a modified version of this approach known as the transparaspinal approach (Michelsen). Both approaches offer consistent access from T3 to L2.

Preoperative Preparation and Operative Procedure

The patient is positioned either prone or on a bean bag in the lateral decubitus position with the operative side up and the lower extremity slightly flexed at the hip. Lesions at T3 and T4 should be approached via a medial parascapular approach. T5–T10 should be approached along the superior border of the rib of the affected level. T11–L2 lesions should be approached via an incision that extends along the rib of the level above because of the caudal direction of the ribs of the inferior thoracic spine. All incisions should extend from 4 cm off of the midline to the dorsal axillary line. The rib is subperiosteally dissected free from the costotransverse ligament laterally along the entire length of the incision. It is removed with heavy shears and the bone surfaces are waxed for hemostasis. The remainder of the rib bed medially is carefully resected to protect the parietal pleura, which is adherent to the endothoracic fascia above T10. The neural and vascular structures are also contained within the endothoracic fascia. The endothoracic fascia is continuous with the rib periosteum. As long as the fascial plane remains intact, it is incised with the rib head, and at this point the endothoracic fascia is bluntly dissected away from the pleura with a peanut sponge clamp. Blunt pleural dissection is continued off of the rib head, and the vertebral body and disk space are exposed laterally to their ventralmost aspect **(Fig. 11–9).** Electrocautery is used to divide the endothoracic fascia to the vertebrae, sacrificing the sympathetic chain. Ultimately, the proximal rib is removed when the muscular and ligamentous attachments to the rib are divided. The periosteum is then stripped away from the vertebral body and the pedicle is exposed and then defined with curettage **(Fig. 11–10).** The pedicle can be removed with a high-speed drill or with a Kerrison punch. From T10 to L2, the endothoracic fascia is absent and is anatomically replaced by the diaphragm. The diaphragm's dorsal aspect is elevated off of the inner surfaces of the rib origins. The result is exposure of retropleural and retroperitoneal spaces. The psoas muscle must be elevated at L1 and L2 to provide adequate exposure. With the exposure complete, tumor resection can begin by completely removing the bony architecture that comprises the neural foramen resulting in exposure of the anterior and posterior aspects of the nerve root and lateral aspect of the spinal cord. The tumor can then be resected cleanly.

Closure consists of reapproximating the endothoracic fascia or the diaphragm to the psoas and quadratus muscles with 0-Vicryl or other heavy absorbable suture. A chest tube is placed only if the pleura and lung parenchyma are separated or if the pleura cannot be closed in airtight fashion. Meticulous hemostasis is imperative prior to closure of the wound. The deep dermal and subcutaneous regions are then closed independently with a similar 2–0 or 3–0 absorbable suture in inverted and interrupted fashion. The skin is approximated in subcuticular fashion or with surgical glue. A dressing is then applied over the wound. If indicated a thoraco-lumbar sacral orthosis (TLSO) can be fitted once the chest tube is removed. Oftentimes the chest tube (if present) can be removed on the first postoperative day.

Intraspinal Tumor Resection

We employ SSEP monitoring and direct stimulation during tumor resection. The plane between the tumor and the dura is defined sharply with microscissors, microdissectors, and

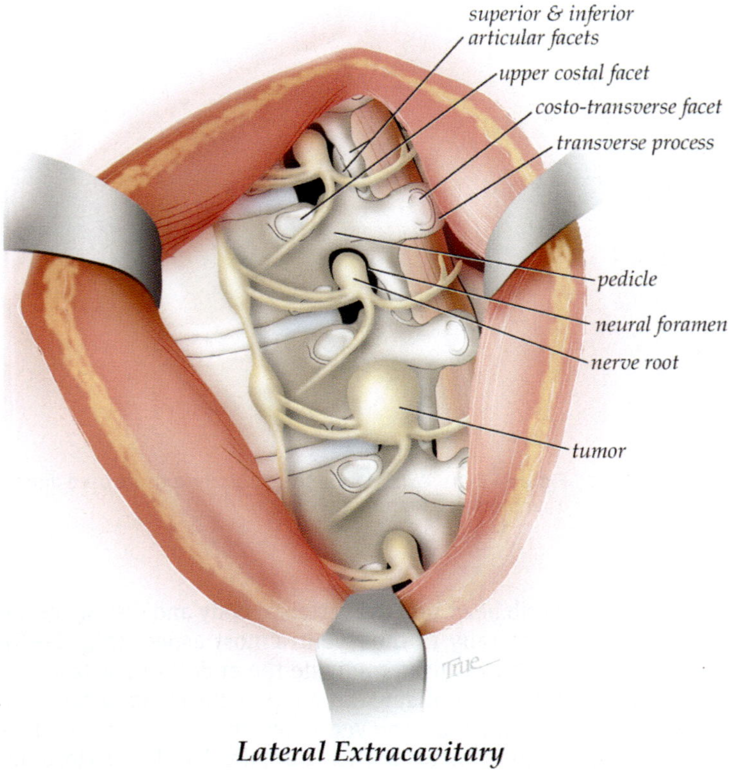

Figure 11–9 Operative field during a lateral extracavitary approach.

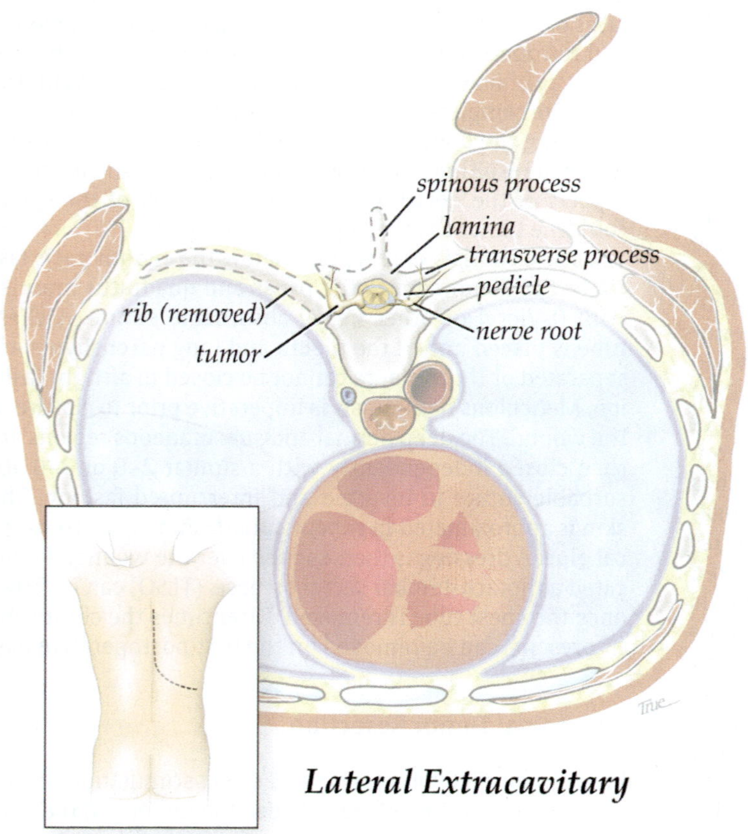

Figure 11–10 Axial view of the surgical exposure used during a lateral extracavitary approach for tumor resection.

bipolar electrocautery. Only minimal retraction is permitted when resecting the mass in the cervical or thoracic spine, whereas in the lumbar spine, more liberal manipulation is considered safe. If the tumor enters the spinal dura, the dura is opened permitting exposure of the entire mass. Once the initial survey of the neural structures and tumor border is complete, resection of the tumor can begin. With larger tumors or with tumors that have significant extension into the spinal canal, internal debulking may be required. This permits gentile retraction of the tumor, which then facilitates the use of microdissectors to peel the tumor capsule off of the adherent neural structures. Some nerve roots will be severely attenuated and may not be able to be safely preserved with resection. In this situation, the capsule (where the flattened root is located) should be stimulated. If the retained root has motor function a small residual tumor burden must be left because a motor deficit is rarely worth complete resection. The exception is in the thoracic spine where loss of a single motor root is often unnoticeable. More often than not, however, the tumor stems from a sensory root, and a sensory deficit in a radicular distribution is usually well tolerated. Furthermore, as progressive compression of the nerve from tumor growth occurs, sensation in that dermatome may shift to alternate sensory pathways.

Extracanalicular Tumor Resection

At this point the intracanalicular and intraspinal portions of the tumor should have been resected. The extracanalicular portion of the tumor is internally debulked in a similar fashion as with the intraspinal portion (with ultrasonic aspiration, suction, bipolar electrocautery) while maintaining the integrity of the tumor capsule to protect the neural and vascular structures deep to it. Once internally debulked, the capsule is surrounded with microcottonoid patties and is mobilized from the nerve with microdissectors and microscissors. Usually a direct posterior or posterior view from a lateral extracavitary approach produces the greatest view of the tumor and adjacent neural structures. Thus it is easiest and safest to leave the anterior dissection for last.

◆ Postoperative Management

Perioperative complications in the surgical treatment of spinal schwannomas are an infrequent but inevitable occurrence. Appropriate patient selection, careful planning, and intraoperative attention to detail will help improve overall patient outcome. This section outlines the morbidity and management strategies employed when complications occur.

◆ Complications

Complications of Anterior Approaches to the Cervical Spine

The most common complications after anterior approaches to the cervical spine are sore throat and dysphagia. They typically resolve with time and may or may not be associated with swelling in the soft tissue of the neck. Care must be taken however to observe these changes closely because an enlarging hematoma may be the source of the problem. Evaluate the neck by palpating for a mass, skin tension, or tracheal deviation. If tracheal deviation exists and upper respiratory issues arise, open the incision immediately to release pressure, intubate the patient, and explore the wound emergently to locate the source of the hemorrhage. The cervical sympathetic ganglion can be injured if the longus colli is not subperiosteally dissected. This results in ipsilateral ptosis, miosis, and anhydrosis (Horner's syndrome).

Injury to the vertebral artery occurs in 0.3% of anterior cervical approaches with deep dissection, foraminotomy, graft, or instrumentation placement. To help prevent such injury, excessive lateral dissection should be avoided. If hemorrhage occurs as a result of vertebral artery injury, the first measure should involve packing the hemorrhage. The risks of packing a vertebral artery disruption without exploration are hemorrhage, pseudoaneurysm, arterial thrombosis, or arteriovenous fistula. Often, dissection of the proximal and distal portions of the tissue surrounding the artery followed by either ligation or direct repair is necessary. Postoperative angiography and embolization may be required.

Complications of Posterior Approaches to the Spine

Positioning the patient seems relatively benign, but complications from poor head and shoulder placement not only compromise exposure but can also have devastating consequences. If the patient's eyes are unprotected from pressure in the prone position, the central retinal artery can cease to flow and the resulting thrombosis can lead to blindness. Excessive retraction of the shoulders to provide for improved exposure may lead to stretch injuries of the superior roots of the brachial plexus.

Complications of the Lateral Extracavitary Approach

Complications of the lateral extracavitary approach include hemothorax, pneumothorax, and direct lung parenchymal injury. This is often noted intraoperatively and is best treated by a 32F chest tube to help remove fluid buildup and air that can occur.

In the upper thoracic spine, the aorta is noted on the left side and can be injured if not properly mobilized. Vascular surgery should be contacted for the repair but a nonabsorbable monofilament such as a Prolene suture is typically used in simple running fashion. During a right-sided exposure in the lower thoracic spine and upper lumbar spine, injury to the vena cava and liver can occur. Again, hemostasis is imperative and the appropriate surgical specialty should be notified to help with the repair.

Bone Graft and Instrumentation Complications

Pseudarthrosis that is asymptomatic does not require surgical intervention; however, unsatisfactory outcomes are known to occur when pain persists. If the anterior hardware should become loose, it must be revised immediately to prevent against catastrophic injury to the esophagus.

The anterior extrusion of bone graft occurs more frequently after multilevel procedures but can occur in single-level procedures as well. Surgical intervention is required if the patient develops radicular pain or dysphagia or if there is loss of alignment.

Graft fractures can also occur in instrumented and noninstrumented fusions. If there is no spinal canal or neural foramina compromise resulting in myelopathy or radiculopathy, the fusion should be observed with AP and lateral x-rays of the spine at regular intervals, as with asymptomatic pseudarthroses, to insure proper healing.

Graft Harvest Complications

Graft harvest complications can result in significant morbidity and include chronic pain syndromes, hematoma, infection, ilium fracture, pelvic instability, muscle weakness with gait instability, poor cosmesis, peritoneal perforation, hernia, visceral injury, nerve damage, and vascular compromise. Limiting the posterior incision less than 8 cm from the posterior-superior iliac spine decreases the risk of injury to the superior cluneal nerve and subsequent numbness or dysesthetic pain over the buttock that can be either temporary or permanent. Keeping the anterior incision 2 cm from the anterior-superior iliac spine avoids injury to the sartorius muscle, inguinal ligament, and lateral femoral cutaneous nerve, an injury that can result in either or both acute and chronic pain and numbness over the thigh. Ilioinguinal nerve injury occurs often as a result of retraction while exposing the anterior ilium. This results in groin numbness. Injury to the superior gluteal artery as it exits the sciatic notch can occur through a posterior incision and may result in significant hemorrhage and an arteriovenous fistula. Herniation and damage to the abdominal contents is best prevented by ensuring approximation of the transversalis aponeurosis and the external oblique muscles. Hip abductor weakness results in a gluteal gait. Ileum fracture can be caused by sartorius and rectus femoris muscle contraction and is treated with crutch-assisted ambulation. Cosmesis is improved by reconstructing the iliac crest either with a trapdoor technique or by removing bone through a subcrestal window. The drawback to this approach is that a tricortical graft cannot be obtained.

Cerebrospinal Fluid Leakage

Cerebrospinal fluid (CSF) leakage can be incredibly difficult to stop if the dural opening is not clean. Repair can be performed either primarily or with a patch of fascia lata or Gore-Tex using 6–0 Prolene or another, fine, nonabsorbable suture. Fibrin glue may then be applied over the repair site. Collagen-based dural substitutes can be used as well. Postoperative insertion of a lumbar drain for 3 to 4 days is sometimes indicated. Permanent lumboperitoneal shunting is reserved as a last recourse when CSF continues to accumulate in soft tissue spaces. Posterior approaches may be associated with a decreased complication rate.

Infection

Risk factors for infection are prolonged operative time, multiple incisions, diabetes, malnutrition, alcoholism, illicit drug abuse, systemic disease, autoimmune diseases including rheumatoid arthritis, immunocompromised state, malignancy, hemoglobinopathies, poor dental health, obesity, and poor hygiene.

Wound infections can be superficial or can extend deep beneath the fascia and involve the graft and hardware if present. Erythrocyte sedimentation rate (ESR) and C-reactive protein (CRP) levels are not ultimately specific for infection but can be used to monitor the effectiveness of treatment. The CRP can remain elevated during the first 2 to 14 days postprocedure, and interpretation can yield mixed results. However, because CRP levels normalize earlier than ESR levels, they are a better diagnostic aid for early postoperative infection. Regardless, clinical correlation is necessary, including incisional erythema, drainage, and fever. A white blood cell count (WBC) with differential is very useful but again can remain high in the immediate postoperative period and if steroids are used. Also, elderly and immunocompromised patients may not have an elevation in their WBC, making this laboratory value somewhat ambiguous in these populations.

If debridement is necessary, well-fixed graft and instrumentation should be left in place to promote fusion. Avoid wound packing when possible. A 6-week course of intravenous antibiotics tailored to the bacteria infecting the wound is necessary with either or both ESR and CRP levels tested every week to assess treatment effectiveness.

CSF leakage can result in meningitis if not appropriately closed intraoperatively. If a leak is noted postoperatively, antibiotics and a lumbar drain may be indicated.

Although an unlikely complication, epidural abscess can occur and is usually accompanied by fever, elevated WBC level, cervicalgia, and a wide range of neurological symptoms from radicular pain to quadriparesis. MRI is the imaging study of choice. Treatment involves debridement of all necrotic material. Prognosis is dependent on the treatment course and time to diagnosis.

◆ Conclusion

Spinal schwannomas are slow-growing, benign neoplasms that are often completely resectable. As with many surgically treatable diseases, careful planning and intraoperative attention to detail can lead to excellent results.

Section IV

Malignant Brain Tumors

12

Balloon-Catheter Brachytherapy for Malignant Brain Tumors

Stephen B. Tatter

The GliaSite Radiation Therapy System (RTS) (Cytyc Corporation, Marlborough, Massachusetts) is one of a handful of new treatments approved for malignant gliomas in the past 20 years. It consists of an inflatable balloon catheter that is placed in the resection cavity at the time of an otherwise-indicated tumor debulking. Low-dose-rate internal radiation (brachytherapy) is delivered with an aqueous solution of organically bound Iotrex, 125_{I}, (Cytyc Corporation, Marlborough, MA) continuously over 3 to 5 days. The device offers significant quality of life and ease of use advantages over older methods of delivering brachytherapy. Thus the device can be used at centers where traditional brain brachytherapy has been impractical. Initial clinical use demonstrates excellent conformance of brain to the semirigid spherical balloon placed in the resection cavity, allowing a high radiation dose to be delivered to the volume at greatest risk of recurrence.

◆ Patient Selection

Patients with brain tumors less than 6 cm in maximum diameter can be considered for brachytherapy because the postresection brain tends to conform to the inflated, semirigid, approximately spherical GliaSite balloon. Ideally a radiographically complete resection of the enhancing portion of the tumor is feasible without producing an expected, unacceptable neurological deficit. For patients in whom complete resection of the enhancing tumor is not possible, radical subtotal excision with any residual enhancing disease encompassed within the radiation dose prescription volume is the goal. In practice this makes patients with more than a centimeter of residual enhancing tumor after maximal safe resection poor candidates for this modality. Patients who have had a previous lobectomy or in whom lobectomy is anticipated are often GliaSite RTS candidates even when the anticipated resection cavity is much larger than 5 cm because the catheter's semirigid tether can easily be used to pull the balloon against the resection cavity wall, leaving the distal dura and skull untreated.

◆ Operative Procedure and Postoperative Management

The GliaSite catheter is a silicon, variable-volume balloon catheter that functions as a subcutaneous brachytherapy applicator **(Fig. 12–1)**. The distal, balloon aspect of the catheter is implanted in the cavity that remains following brain tumor resection, and the proximal aspect, which consists of a standard injection port, is brought through a bur hole and secured to the surface of the skull with magnetic resonance imaging (MRI)-compatible screws.

After surgical resection patients are implanted with a 2-, 3-, or 4-cm diameter GliaSite **(Fig. 12–2)**. The size closest to but smaller than the smallest diameter of the resection cavity generally proves to be optimal. When used for brain metastases smaller sizes than calculated from preresection scans are the rule. A frozen section or smear-prep diagnosis consistent with malignant brain tumor may be advantageous before implantation. The balloon can be inflated intraoperatively to identify the most appropriate fill volume and verify proper placement within the cavity.

The infusion port is positioned beneath the scalp in the position determined to be optimum by the operating surgeon. Optimal positioning of the balloon for delivering dose to the desired postresection volume using the semirigid portion of the catheter closest to the balloon is the primary determinant of placement of the right-angle catheter anchor and of the port. Other considerations include ease of access and removal (e.g., the catheter can often be placed so that the deflated GliaSite can be removed through a small incision or by reopening only a portion of the original incision) **(Fig. 12–3)**. Maximizing distance from the incision and from weight-bearing scalp may decrease the chance of erosion through the skin or local irritation.

Postoperatively, fluids are cycled into and out of the catheter by percutaneously accessing the infusion port with an infusion set with a noncoring needle. Intraoperatively or postoperatively the GliaSite balloon is filled to the desired treatment volume with saline alone or with a mixture of saline and 10 to 20% (v/v) iodinated contrast dye. A gadolinium unenhanced and enhanced MRI scan is obtained with

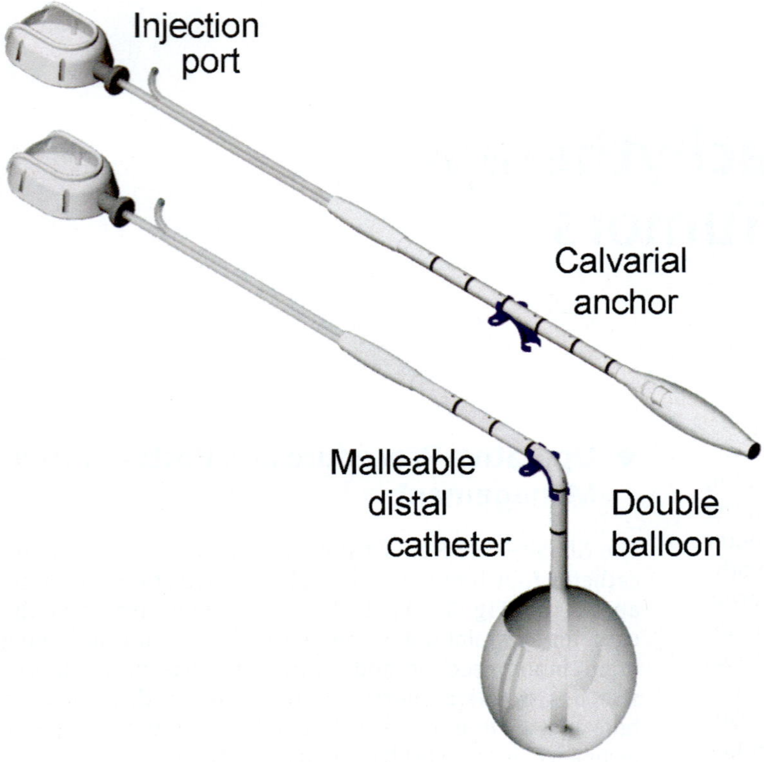

Figure 12–1 The GliaSite catheter. (Courtesy of Cytyc Corporation and affiliates, Marlborough, Massachusetts.)

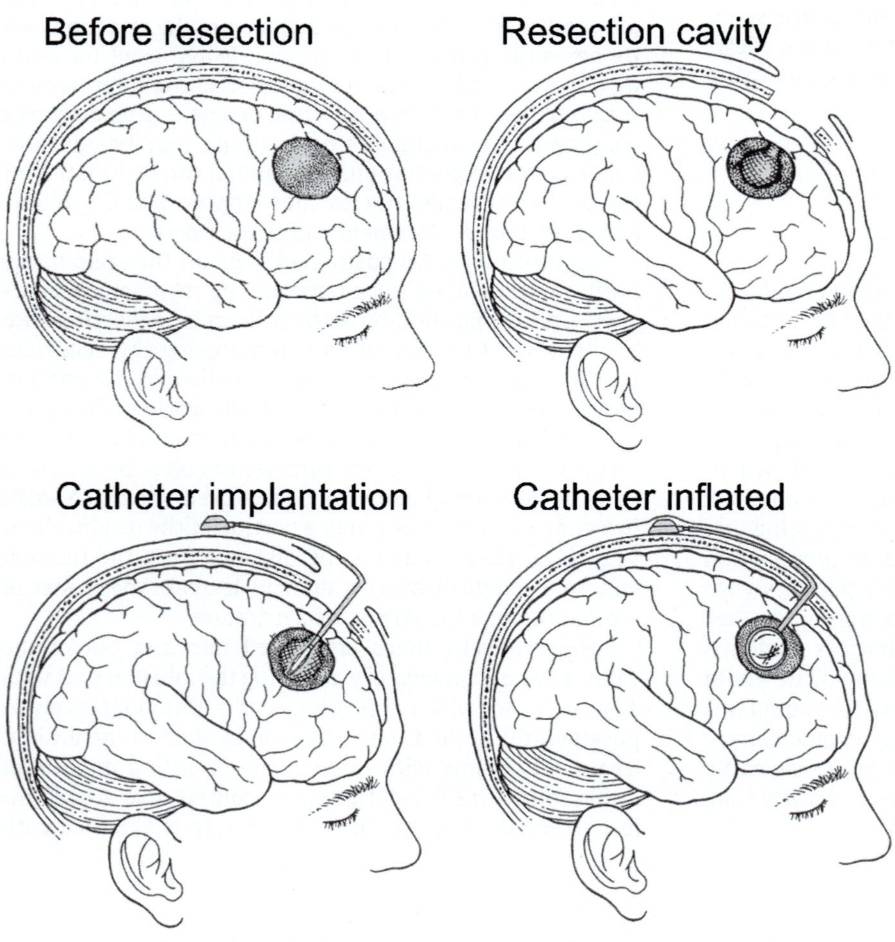

Figure 12–2 GliaSite procedure. (Courtesy of Cytyc Corporation and affiliates, Marlborough, Massachusetts.)

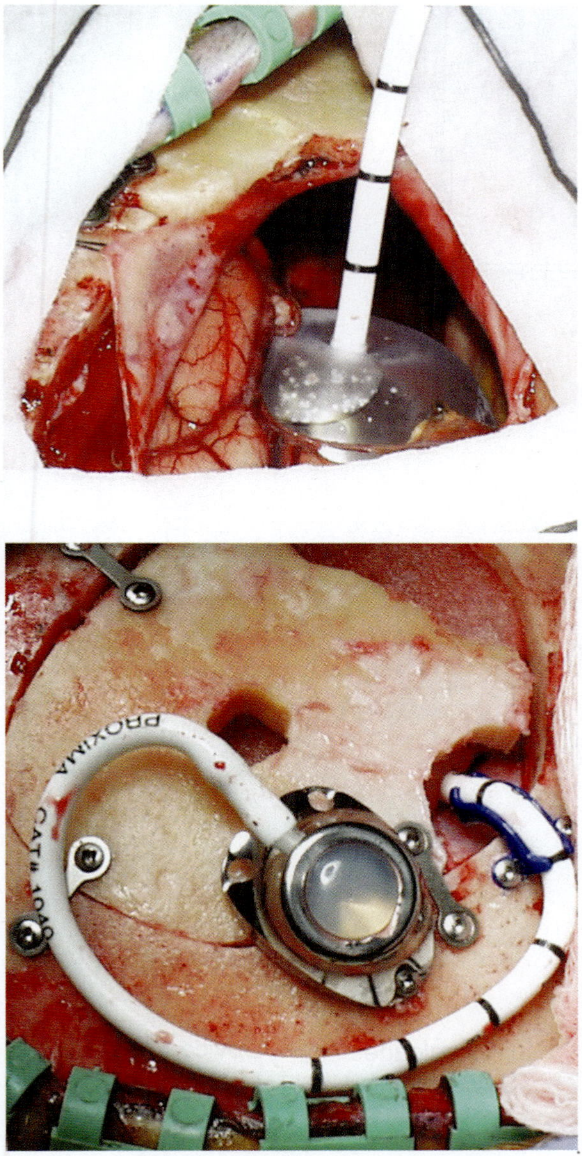

Figure 12–3 GliaSite catheter positioning.

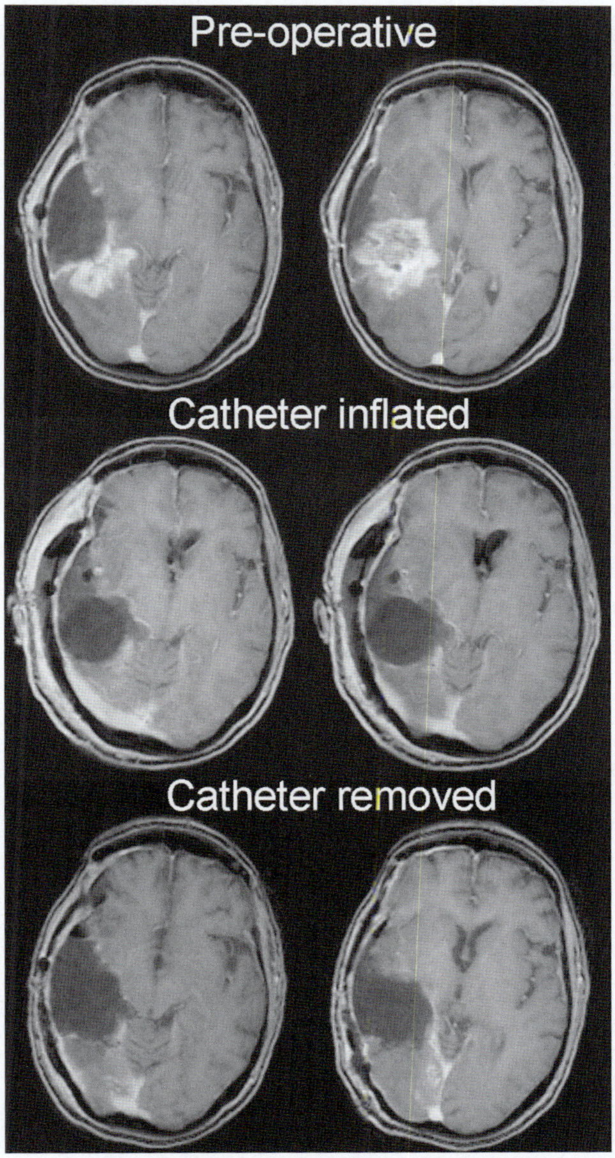

Figure 12–4 Axial, postgadolinium magnetic resonance images. Note that the balloon can be positioned using the semirigid tether, so that it is held against the desired treatment volume.

the device fully inflated. This MRI is used for dose planning **(Fig. 12–4).** Orthogonal skull x-rays can be obtained before the MRI scan, allowing comparison with pretreatment x-rays to exclude the possibility of device migration **(Fig. 12–5).**

Prescription doses are written by a licensed user (radiation oncology or nuclear medicine), and fill volumes and dwell times are obtained from look-up tables (nomograms). Doses from 40 to 60 Gy at 0.5 to 1 cm from the balloon surface have been used with previously radiated, recurrent, malignant gliomas without the need for high rates of reoperation for radiation necrosis. Rates of radiation necrosis have been somewhat higher at the upper end of this dose range when the GliaSite RTS has been used to treat metastasis resection cavities. Twenty-four hours before brachytherapy, patients began using potassium iodide (SSKI) or Lugol's solution to block the thyroid. Thyroid blocking is continued until 24 hours after the Iotrex was removed from the device.

Just before initiating brachytherapy the balloon location may be reconfirmed with orthogonal x-rays. Brachytherapy is initiated by removing the iodinated contrast and replacing it with Iotrex and saline **(Fig. 12–6)** in the amount (quantity of radioactivity) specified by the nomogram for the prescribed dose and appropriate balloon size. Care must be taken to avoid mixing a radiographic contrast agent with the radioactive Iotrex because absorption of radioactivity by the contrast will significantly reduce the effective dose. Studies show that a small fraction of the afterloaded radioactivity is expected to diffuse through the balloon during brachytherapy. This is excreted in the urine, which should be handled as radioactive waste. Radiation safety measurements (exposure rates) are made and limitations regarding visitor and staff exposure determined. After completion of the prescribed brachytherapy, the Iotrex and saline solution is retrieved using an infusion set, followed by two to three

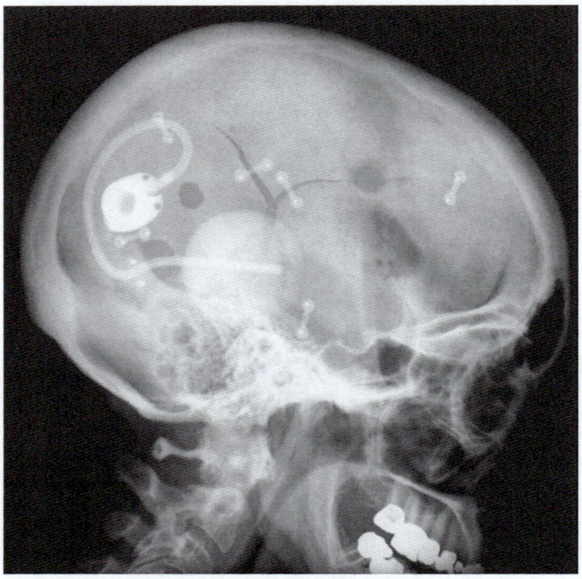

Figure 12–5 Lateral skull x-ray. Roentgenograms conveniently exclude device migration before the initiation of brachytherapy.

flushes of the catheter with 4 to 5 mL of saline to reduce the residual radioactivity in the device. The GliaSite RTS can then be removed surgically at the discretion of the treating physician and the patient.

◆ Discussion

The arguments for delivering additional local radiation to malignant brain tumors without necessitating a high rate of reoperation for radiation necrosis are compelling but not yet overwhelming. They include:

- Radiation is by far the most effective treatment for malignant glioma but presumably due to increasing normal tissue injury there is no net benefit achieved by delivering additional fractionated, external-beam, radiation dose.
- Global control cannot be achieved without achieving local control. 80 to 90% of recurrences are within 2 cm of the resection cavity margin.
- There is a dose response for seed-based brachytherapy in the local control of malignant gliomas. Due to the inhomogeneity of radiation dose delivered by seed-based techniques reported rates of reoperation for radiation necrosis are 26 to 64%. This suggests that there is little room for further refinement of the older technology. It may also explain why seed-based brachytherapy has frequently but not uniformly been found to be beneficial.
- Another more subtle argument is that the rarely observed long-term survival of patients with malignant gliomas is likely at least in part achieved by activating host (presumably immune) defenses. Most of these patients have had multiple recurrences and have undergone multimodal therapy before achieving long-term remission. Among current long-term survivors many have had seed-based brachytherapy. Some have had bacterial infections that may have led to more efficient immune activation. Local tumor killing with radiation has the benefit of allowing tumor antigens to be presented to the immune system, which might sometimes result in recognition of the glioma cells as malignant.

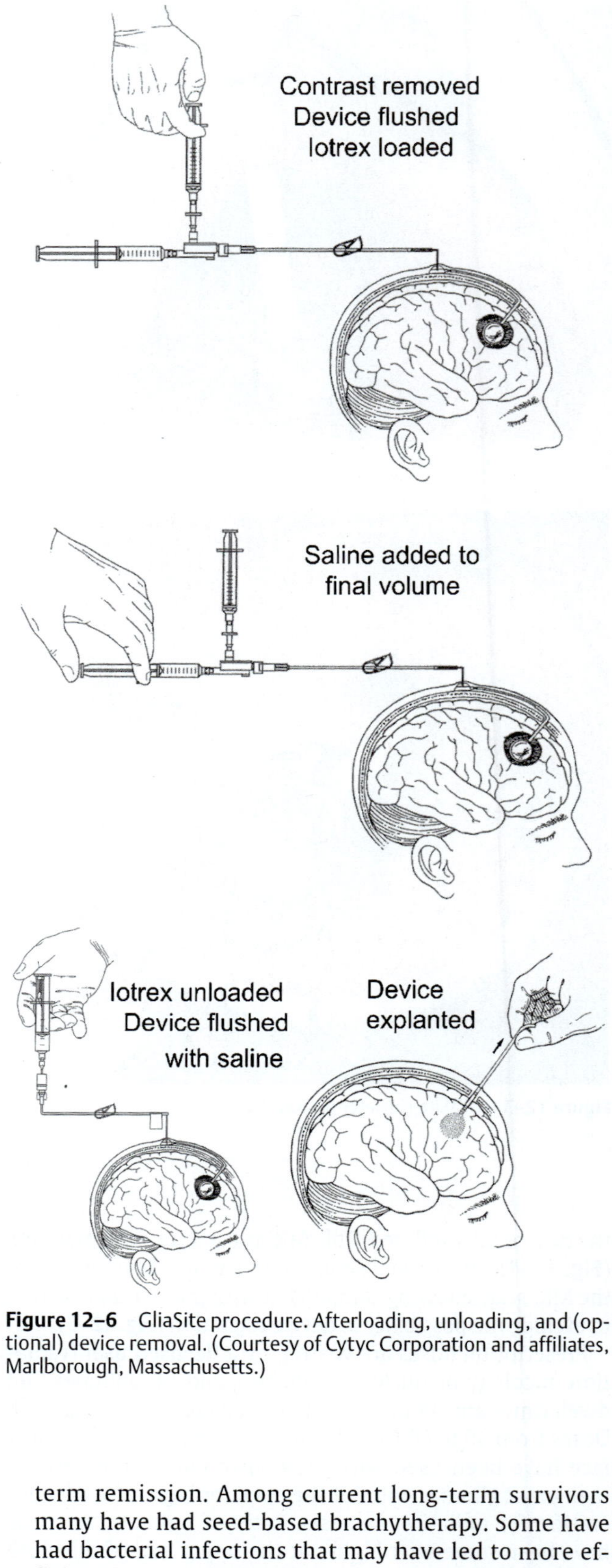

Figure 12–6 GliaSite procedure. Afterloading, unloading, and (optional) device removal. (Courtesy of Cytyc Corporation and affiliates, Marlborough, Massachusetts.)

- The case for use of the GliaSite RTS for metastases to avoid or delay whole brain radiation can be compelling for those who have seen patients die of radiation-induced dementia in the setting of tumor remission. However. as for many treatments used in neurosurgical practice, evidence-based data supporting routine use of brachytherapy for malignant brain tumors is lacking.

The GliaSite RTS offers the potential to improve quality of life during treatment by avoiding the need for external hardware. Although Food and Drug Administration approval is based on device performance and safety data and the historically documented benefit of brachytherapy, the GliaSite RTS also offers potential efficacy advantages. Chief among these is the potential for quantitatively studying and optimizing dose. This possibility is unique to the GliaSite RTS among brachytherapy modalities because the catheter functions as a single-point source of radiation, eliminating spatial distribution of radiation sources as a dependent variable that cannot be studied and optimized.

In summary, the GliaSite RTS performs safely and efficiently in initial clinical use. Brain conformance to the device after malignant brain tumor resection is excellent, allowing delivery of a readily quantifiable radiation dose to the tissue at highest risk for recurrence. This device preserves quality of life better than older brachytherapy techniques. It provides an attractive option for patients with newly diagnosed, metastatic, and recurrent brain tumors for whom standard external radiation techniques are likely to provide insufficient radiation doses or to produce unacceptable toxicity.

13

Intraoperative Magnetic Resonance Imaging for Brain Tumor Resection

Marvin Bergsneider and Linda M. Liau

Advances in neuroimaging have radically changed the practice of neurosurgery. The advantage of having the ability to accurately locate intracranial lesions in the operating room using frameless stereotactic neuronavigation systems has resulted in a worldwide adoption of this technology. However, standard neuronavigation systems have an inherent limitation; because the dataset used is based on preoperative imaging, the information becomes outdated once brain shift occurs. Intraoperative magnetic resonance imaging (iMRI) systems, which were introduced over a decade ago, are a relatively new technological approach for this long-standing problem in neurosurgery.

The introduction of an MRI scanner as a part of the operating room (OR) theater holds the potential of addressing surgery-induced brain shift but also introduces unique challenges due to the proximity of a powerful magnet and standard ferromagnetic instruments. The configuration and physical dimensions of the scanner can impose limitations with regard to patient body and head positioning. In addition, the interpretation of acquired images, obtained during the course of an operation, can be confounded by either or both surgery-induced brain edema and unaccustomed contrast agent dynamics.

In the context of an atlas of neurosurgical procedures, this brief description of surgical preparation and technique will be unique to the currently available iMRI configuration and therefore may become quickly outmoded as the technology rapidly evolves. Because it is primarily the limitations of current iMRI configurations that dictate patient selection, a significant portion of this chapter focuses on these limitations. Despite such limitations, however, the availability of intraoperative imaging is highly desirable for properly selected cases.

◆ Currently Available Intraoperative Magnetic Resonance Imaging Configurations

There have been several iMRI configurations manufactured over the last decade, each with specific advantages and disadvantages. Although this chapter focuses on the Siemens's 1.5T high-field iMRI system (Brain SUITE iMRI, BrainLAB Inc., Heimstetten, Germany) a brief description of other available iMRI configurations is given to provide context and perspective.

Interventional Stationary ("Double Donut") Intraoperative Magnetic Resonance Imaging

The operative field is directly within the center of the iMRI magnetic field. The neurosurgeon works directly within the magnetic field. These iMRI scanners (General Electric Medical Systems, Milwaukee, Wisconsin) typically are vertically oriented open magnets with a narrow opening just wide enough for only the surgeon and patient. As a result, the scrub nurse and surgical assistants stand behind the surgeon, away from the surgical field. The open configuration limits the magnets to low-field strength units (0.3 to 0.5 T). The greatest advantage to within-field surgery iMRI is the ability to obtain intraoperative images at any time during the course of the operation without having to significantly interrupt the procedure. All surgical instrumentation, including the surgical microscope, monitors, and anesthesia equipment, must be nonferromagnetic and MR compatible.

Compact Mobile Intraoperative Magnetic Resonance Imaging ("MRI Fluoroscope")

This approach utilizes a very low field strength MRI unit that is stored and shielded at the base of an operating room table. The magnet is available to be positioned whenever necessary by raising the unit (ODIN Medical Technologies, Yokneam, Israel). Updated neuronavigation is available using an infrared remote control device. The currently available 0.12 T units allow only a limited field of view (16 × 11 cm) with significantly lower resolution compared with diagnostic MRI scanners.

Low-Field Open Intraoperative Magnetic Resonance Imaging

Vertical-gap ("lateral aperture"), open MRI units (Hitachi Medical Systems, Twinsburg, OH) have also been used for intraoperative neurosurgical imaging **(Fig. 13–1A).** These consist of low-field (0.2 to 0.3 T) horizontally open magnet systems that were designed primarily for diagnostic and interventional radiological procedures but modified with specific features for intraoperative use (e.g., rotating operating table, radiofrequency (RF) coil, and ceramic MRI-compatible headholder). These stationary, "shared-resource" open iMRI configurations were intended to limit the expenses required for having a completely dedicated iMRI operating theater with fully MRI-compatible

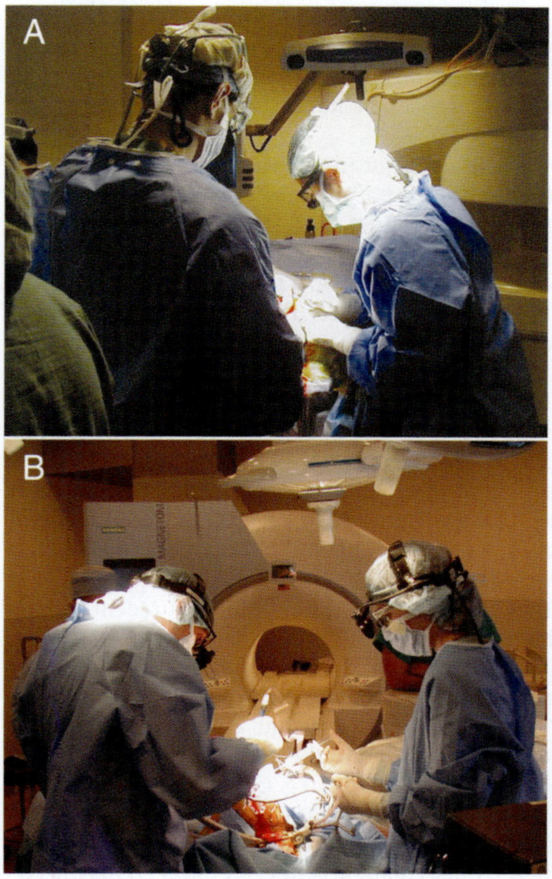

Figure 13–1 Photographs of fully functional intraoperative magnetic resonance imaging (MRI) operating room configurations. **(A)** Siemens 0.2-T Open iMR suite, with a vertical-field open MRI system. Surgery is performed in the fringe field, where the weak magnetic field (<5 gauss) does not interfere with standard operating room instruments and equipment. **(B)** Siemens 1.5-T Sonata iMR suite. Again, surgery is performed in the fringe field (<5 gauss), safely away from the scanner. For intraoperative scanning, the motorized surgical table must first pivot, then link with the scanner gantry to be slid into the short-bore magnet. Note that standard neuronavigational capability (VectorVision, BrainLAB, Inc., Heimstetter, Germany) is possible within both low-field (0.2-T) and high-field (1.5-T) intraoperative iMRI suites.

instruments while still providing much better image quality than that obtained using the very low field, compact mobile iMRI units. The disadvantages of this scanner design, however, are the low-field (0.2 to 0.3 T) image quality compared with the optimal levels obtained by the high-field (1.5 T) iMRI units and the need to transport patients into and out of the magnet during surgery, which may increase the risks of infection.

High-Field Mobile "Crane" Intraoperative Magnetic Resonance Imaging

A mobile 1.5T MRI unit (iSPACE, IMRIS, Winnipeg, Canada) is suspended from a ceiling-mounted railing system and moved from room to room as needed. With this approach, the MRI scanner can be moved between different iMRI suites or situated in an intermediate diagnostic suite. As a result, the scanner "down time" is minimized. An advantage of this system is that the overhead sliding magnet design keeps the patient immobile. Standard surgical instruments and equipment can be used safely when not scanning. Disadvantages of this system are its rather cumbersome design and the structural requirements required to accommodate the heavy weight of this mobile ceiling-mounted unit.

High-Field Stationary Intraoperative Magnetic Resonance Imaging

In a dedicated iMRI suite, the MRI unit is situated adjacent to the operative field in the same room. The MRI-compatible OR bed is moved into the magnet whenever imaging is desired. The dedicated same-room iMRI suite arrangement (Brain SUITE) integrates a Siemens 1.5 T superconducting, ultrashort, large-bore magnet, diagnostic MRI scanner (MAGNETON Sonata, Siemens Medical Solutions, Erlangen, Germany) that is permanently situated in a completely RF-shielded OR. The MRI scanner is ~1.5 m from a specially designed rotating MRI-compatible OR table **(Fig. 13–1B)**, which enables the placement of the patient out of the 5 gauss safety line during surgery so that standard neurosurgical operations can be performed using standard instruments. The MAGNETON Sonata is a high-performance neurodiagnostic unit that can rapidly acquire routine high-resolution diagnostic imaging protocols **(Fig. 13–2)**, plus specialized sequences such as MR

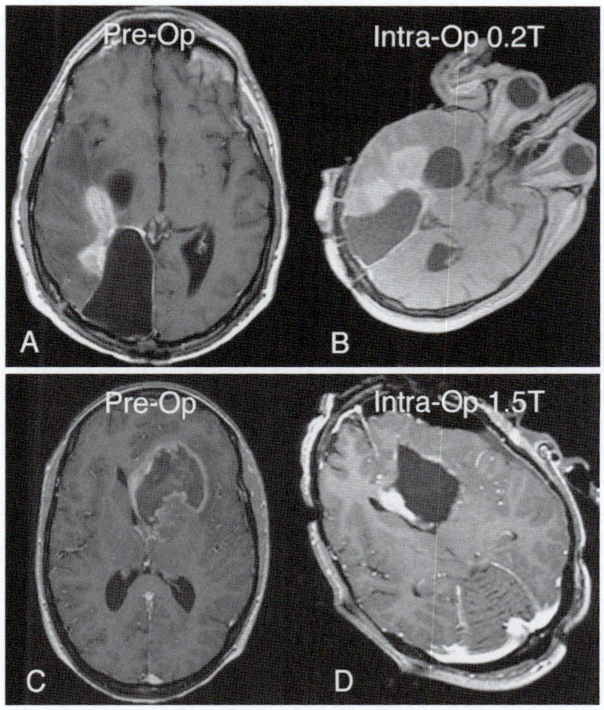

Figure 13–2 Comparison of low-field (0.2-T) and high-field (1.5-T) strength intraoperative magnetic resonance images (MRI). Upper row: **(A)** Preoperative contrast-enhanced T1-weighted MRI from a diagnostic 1.5-T MRI scanner and **(B)** intraoperative image from the Siemens 0.2-T Open iMRI scanner. Note the diminished but generally adequate resolution and quality of the low-field intraoperative image. Lower row: **(C)** Preoperative contrast-enhanced MRI studies from a diagnostic 1.5-T MRI unit and **(D)** intraoperative contrast-enhanced image from the Siemens Sonata 1.5-T iMRI scanner. These images are similarly acquired T1-weighted spoiled gradient-recalled (SPGR) sequences after the administration of contrast (gadolinium). The resolution of the intraoperative image is comparable to that of the preoperative diagnostic study and identifies the residual tumor adjacent to the septum pellucidum.

angiography (MRA), diffusion-weighted tensor imaging (DTI), magnetic resonance spectroscopy (MRS), and functional magnetic resonance imaging (fMRI).

◆ Patient Selection

Currently, there are no evidence-based guidelines delineating the neurosurgical indications for iMRI. The "indications" for its use have evolved over time and are still in a continuing process of evolution. This technology has been shown to be a useful modality in brain tumor surgery and biopsies of intracranial lesions. It is particularly useful in low-grade gliomas, pituitary adenomas, and certain pediatric tumors. Its indications in spinal surgery, epilepsy resections, and functional interventional techniques are still evolving.

Intraoperative magnetic resonance neuroimaging is useful in (1) compensating for intraoperative brain shift, (2) monitoring intraoperative brain events/complications, (3) improving extent of tumor resections, and (4) providing more accurate localization of deep brain lesions for minimally invasive techniques. Thus the criteria for patient selection should be based on determining procedures where these considerations are felt to be important.

For instance, patients with intracranial neoplasms may be considered for iMRI when there is a clinical desire to obtain a "radical" resection and intraoperative brain shift will limit the usefulness of standard frameless stereotaxis based on preoperatively acquired MR images. In practice, this particularly relates to the removal of tumors where there might be a linkage between extent of surgical resection and time to tumor recurrence, such as in low-grade gliomas and pituitary adenomas. In this setting, the main clinical utility of intraoperative imaging is the detection of residual lesions. Therefore, consideration for use of iMRI should be given to patients in whom there is a rationale for image-complete "gross total" resection and there is a reasonable chance that residual lesion will be left behind if standard neurosurgical procedures (without near real-time iMRI) are used. In our experience, the latter criterion relates to larger neoplastic lesions (>20 cm^3 volume) in which brain shift will limit the usefulness of standard frameless stereotaxic neuronavigation systems. In addition, iMRI should be considered for lesions in which it can be anticipated that the tumor–brain interface will be difficult to ascertain (e.g., low-grade gliomas) and for deeply situated lesions in which a minimally invasive approach is utilized (e.g., biopsy).

On occasion, there is a conflict between the desire to utilize the iMRI technology and methodological restrictions limiting its use. Although iMRI technology might be conceptually useful for all intracranial operations, in practice, the current limitations of the technology still restrict its use to a select subset of neurosurgical procedures and patients.

For some MRI configurations, there are several significant technical issues that must be taken into account for patient selection. For instance, the Siemens Sonata 1.5T scanner has a cylindrical bore that is 60 cm in diameter **(Fig. 13–3A).** As shown in **Fig. 13–3B,** the transport/operating table effectively reduces the cylindrical bore size of the Sonata scanner from 60 to 45 cm. As a result, adult patients cannot be placed in the lateral position, thereby practically eliminating cerebellar pontine angle (CPA) operations and increasing the difficulty of posterior temporal, subtemporal, and parietal-occipital approaches. The patient's body can be modestly turned using bumps, when necessary. Large patients with very broad shoulders may not fit into the center of the MRI bore, even in the straight supine position. In addition, the transport table has a 125 kg weight limit. A newer-generation iMRI unit recently introduced, the Siemens MAGNETON Egpnee, with a 70-cm bore diameter, will help expand patient positioning options in the future.

Other technical limitations that are important for patient selection are related to the configuration of the MRI-compatible head fixation device. Currently, the head fixation device used in the Sonata iMRI Brain Suite allows four-pin rigid head fixation **(Fig. 13–3C,D)**. The pin bolts arise from a semicircular glass fiber–reinforced plastic cradle whose base rests atop the common system circular polarized RF coil docking support. As shown in **Fig. 13–3E,** the cranial portion of the RF coil base extends more than 15 cm beyond the vertex of the head. The cranial-caudal position of the ring base has three fixed positions. The pins are aligned on an arc that only allows one degree of motion (right-left tilt). The internal diameter of the head-holder ring is fixed and cannot accommodate very large heads.

Because of the limited degrees of motion of the MRI-compatible head fixation device (and the limitation of patient body positioning as already described), positioning the patient's head for parietal and posterior temporal lesions is sometimes suboptimal. As shown in **Fig. 13–3D,** the prone position is possible. Occipital lesions can be approached via the prone position, but at added risk due to the very limited access by the anesthesiologist to the endotracheal (ET) tube due to the RF base apparatus. Newer-generation MRI-compatible operating tables and head-fixation devices are currently under development, which, it is hoped, will overcome many of these patient selection limitations in the future.

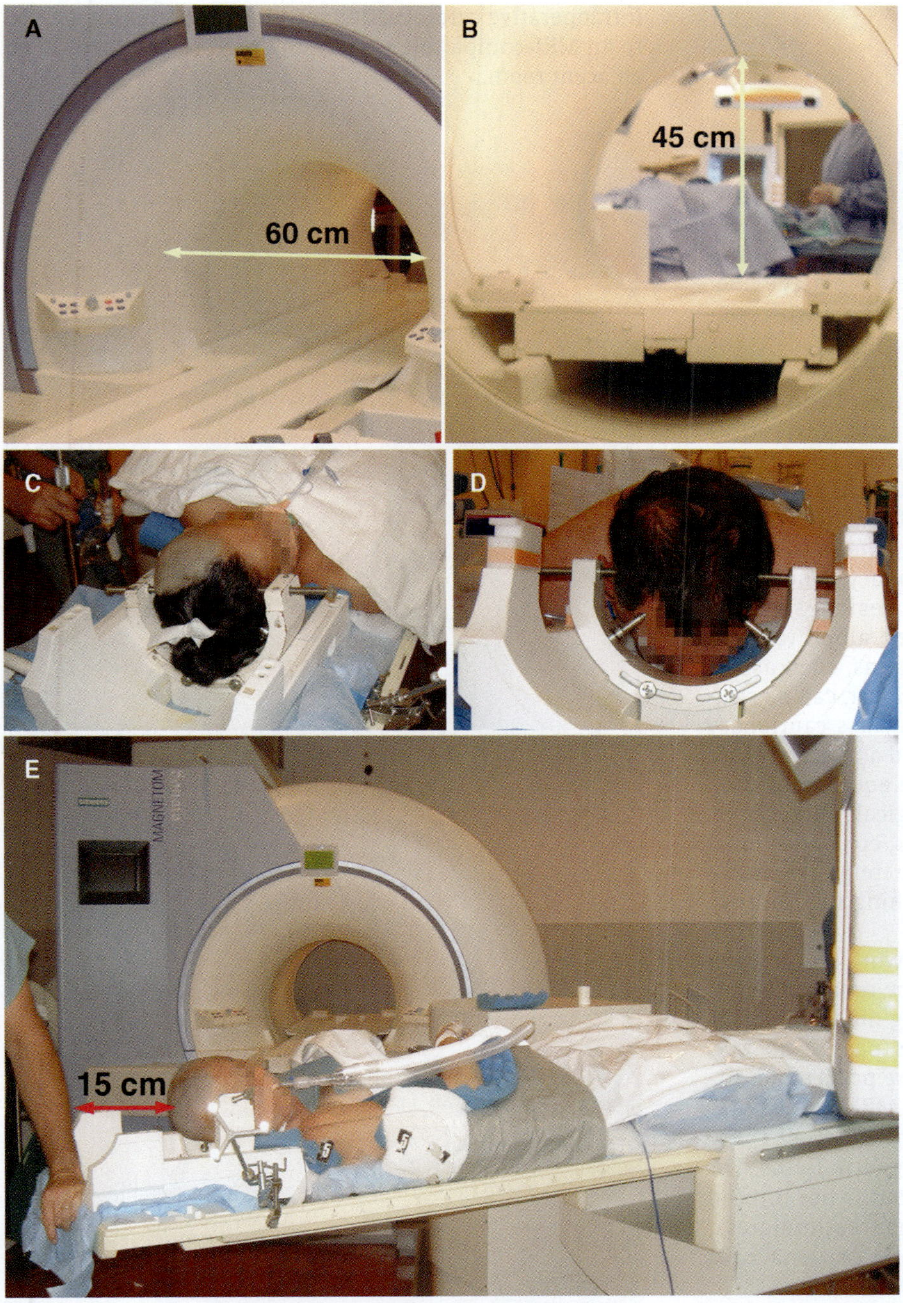

Figure 13–3 Technical limitations for patient selection. **(A)** The maximal bore diameter (arrow) of the Siemens Sonata iMRI unit is 60 cm. **(B)** Due to the presence of the transport/operating table, the effective vertical bore diameter (arrow) is reduced to ~45 cm. **(C,D)** The magnetic resonance imaging (MRI)-compatible head fixation device currently utilizes four fixed pins and allows for a limited degree of possible angles of rotation. **(E)** Note that the semicircle fixation ring sits well away (~15 cm) from the head of the bed.

◆ Preoperative Preparation

Intraoperative Magnetic Resonance Imaging Safety Precautions

A major concern for the use of iMRI for neurosurgery is safety—for both the patient and the OR personnel. The magnetic forces generated can cause objects to easily penetrate clothing and the human body. To increase awareness of the dangers related to the magnetic field, the floor of any iMRI operating suite should be marked with concentric color-coded regions signifying various magnetic field strengths **(Fig. 13–4A)**. An inner "red" zone has a 5 gauss (0.5 mTesla) strength at its perimeter and is considered the region in which no magnetically susceptible objects should enter ("exclusion zone"). Operating room personnel are able to stand and work in this region, although potentially with increased risk from airborne objects attracted to the magnet, if ferromagnetic items are carelessly handled. The yellow, "cautionary zone" has a 2 gauss (0.2 mTesla) perimeter. In this region, standard operating room instruments can be used, albeit with increased caution and vigilance. Large items, such as the surgical microscope and ultrasonic aspirator, can be situated in the outermost region of the 2 gauss cautionary zone. The outer green zone is considered a relatively safe region. For larger non-MRI-compatible equipment with wheels at the base (such as the surgical microscope, frameless stereotaxis unit, monitor carts, etc.), additional measures are taken to ensure that these items are secure (such as setting wheel brakes and leashing the items to wall brackets).

All operating room personnel who work in (or even enter) the iMRI operating suite should be required to undergo an MRI safety in-service training module. Verifiable certification that the person has passed an MRI safety test should be standard procedure prior to admittance into the iMRI suite. As with all MRI studies, patients must be questioned to determine whether there are any contraindications to large magnetic fields. For neurosurgical patients, this includes (but is not limited to) implants such as pacemakers, neurostimulators, older aneurysm clips, and certain inferior vena cava (IVC) filters.

Anesthesia Considerations

There are several important anesthesia-related safety issues. Special MRI-compatible anesthesia machines are needed because the anesthesiologist needs to work within the high-field-strength red zone **(Fig. 13–4A)**. Invasive monitors, such as esophageal temperature probes, must be MRI-compatible or be removed prior to rotating the patient into the scanner. It is critical that all conducting wires (such as electrocardiogram leads) be channeled in a parallel manner so as to avoid heat-generating loops **(Fig. 13–4B)**. Conducting loops may cause severe burns due to inductive currents generated by the RF coil. One unresolved safety issue pertains to the lack of commercially available MRI-compatible defibrillators. Patients requiring emergent intraoperative cardioversion must be expeditiously moved to an MRI-compatible gurney and then resuscitated in an adjacent room.

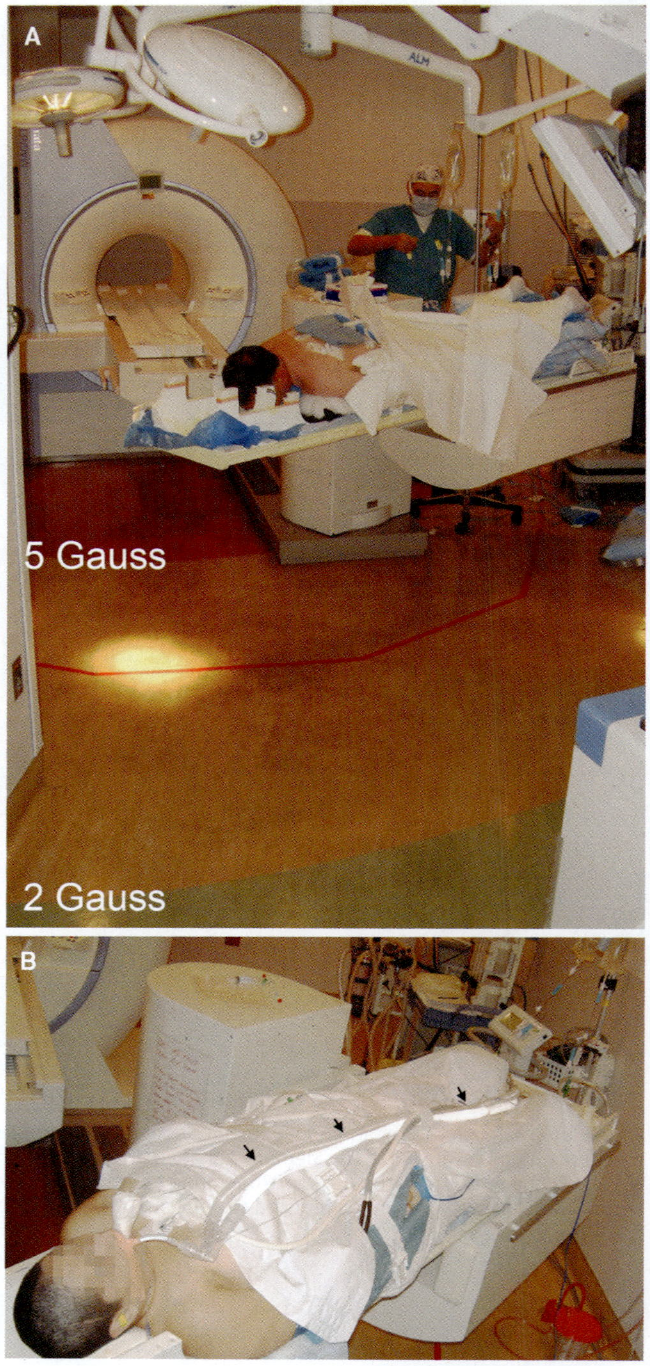

Figure 13–4 Safety considerations. **(A)** The floor of the intraoperative magnetic resonance imaging (iMRI) suite is color coded. The red tile inner region is the "exclusion zone" with an outer perimeter at the 5 gauss line. The yellow tile area ("cautionary zone") has an outer perimeter at the 2 gauss line. Ferromagnetic instruments can be used with caution in this "fringe field" zone. The green tiled region is the "safe zone" and poses minimal risk. **(B)** Anesthesia wires and tubing must be carefully arranged in a parallel fashion (arrows) to avoid heat-conducting loops. Any loop configurations can cause serious skin burns during iMRI scanning.

◆ Operative Procedure

Patient Positioning and Draping

Prior to positioning a patient in any iMRI operating suite, the MRI bore area must be terminally cleaned using hospital OR guidelines. Patients are typically placed supine and can be modestly turned with bumps, when necessary. As mentioned earlier, full lateral and sitting positions are generally not possible due to the current configurations of the iMRI suite.

After the patient's head has been fixated in the headholder, plastic drapes (3M 1010 drapes, 3M Corporation, St. Paul, Minnesota) are applied to cover the face and the ET tube to keep the adhesive Ioban (3M Corporation) drape from sticking to the ET tube **(Fig. 13–5A).** This allows easy access to the ET tube at all times. Following registration of the frameless stereotaxic system, the desired scalp region is shaved of hair and prepared with Betadine solution. A special clear Ioban drape (Steri Drape Ioban 2, Cat. # 6619, 3M Corporation, St. Paul, Minnesota) is then applied **(Fig. 13–5A)** to the surgical site. This large Ioban drape has an integral fluid collection bag and clear plastic perimeter that covers a large surface area. The clear plastic portion is then configured so that the electrical connection points for the MRI coil can be accessed by easily puncturing the plastic with the sterile RF coil supports/connectors. The excessive clear plastic draping from the Steri Drape Ioban 2 can then be cut and the edges taped to the side of the OR bed in such a way as not to interfere with the movement of the bed on the gantry of the MRI table. The MRI-compatible semicircular support rings **(Fig. 13–5B)** are then attached to the headholder, again puncturing the clear portion of the Steri Drape Ioban 2. These support rings (1) allow an anchoring point for "snake" retraction arms, (2) function as a wrist support for surgeon comfort and stability, and (3) provide a surface on which to affix a standard "split" drape **(Fig. 13–5C).** This latter drape provides the large sterile field that covers the edge of the operating table that may have been rendered nonsterile by the taping of the plastic draping. Lastly, small adhesive drapes can be placed at the perimeter of the surgical skin site, thereby covering and providing a protective barrier to the surrounding hair and face.

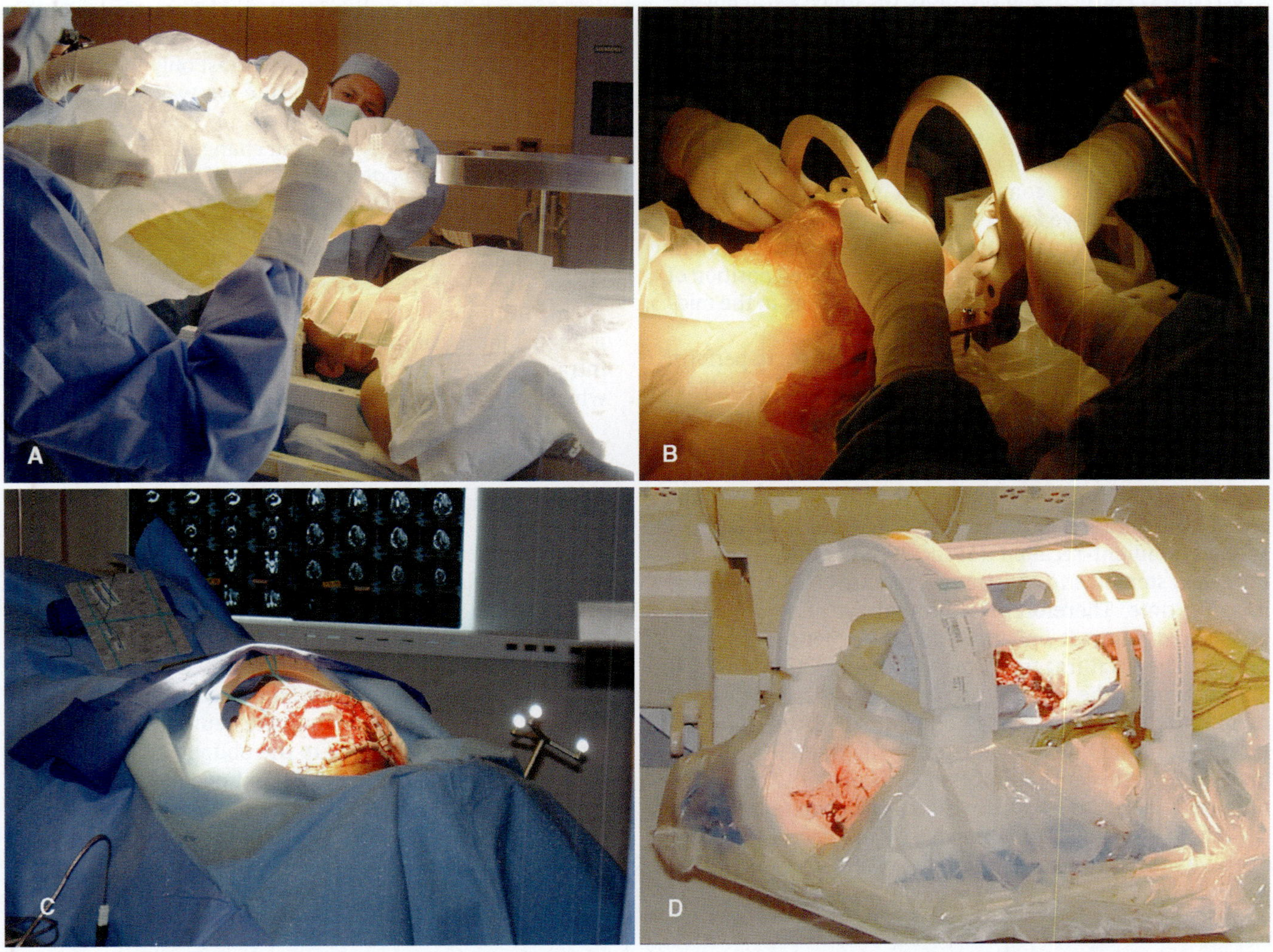

Figure 13–5 Patient positioning and draping. **(A)** After placing a plastic covering to protect the endotracheal tube from the adhesive draping, a large sterile Ioban drape is placed. **(B)** A magnetic resonance imaging–compatible support ring is secured, allowing placement of titanium fishhooks and brain retractors. **(C)** The support ring also functions as a platform onto which a "tear-off" split drape can be applied to create a large sterile field. **(D)** With removal of the split drape, the clear, sterile plastic draping applied underneath allows for the easy placement of the sterile radiofrequency head coil.

The importance of applying the split drape adhesive portion to the support rings is that when an intraoperative scan is desired, this "tear-off" drape can be easily removed. The underlying combination of Ioban, plastic draping, and paper drapes remains sterile; and there is immediate and unobstructed access to the sterile potions of the RF coil connection points. The sterile RF coil is then snapped on to the connection points **(Fig. 13–5D)**, and a sterile towel placed over the coil frame prior to rotating the patient into the MRI scanner. After a thorough survey is performed to confirm that no ferromagnetic instruments or objects are present, the iMRI OR bed is carefully rotated to the MRI gantry base. Following completion of the MR imaging study, the OR bed is repositioned back to the "fringe field" (past the 5 gauss line) and the RF coil removed. A new split drape is then easily applied, and the operation continued without significant interruption.

Intraoperative Imaging Considerations

Choice of Imaging Sequences

Intraoperative imaging differs from routine diagnostic imaging in many important ways. First, the patient's head is nearly always turned, and therefore the images will not appear as standard axial, coronal, and sagittal views **(Fig. 13–6)**. If frameless stereotactic reregistration is to be performed, it is essential that the imaging be performed with no correction for obliqueness (analogous to the requirement of orthogonal imaging when using a Leksell frame-based system). However, MR images in which the head is turned **(Fig. 13–6B,C)** may be difficult to compare with preoperative studies **(Fig. 13–6A)**. We have found that it is not always straightforward to locate residual tumor simply based on two-dimensional (2-D) images, particularly given the skewed position of the patient's head during intraoperative scanning in the middle of a procedure.

The choice of intraoperative imaging sequences to perform must consider several factors. For T1-weighted, T2-weighted, and fluid attenuated inversion recovery (FLAIR) images, each MRI scan requires 3 to 5 minutes. For updating registration of frameless stereotaxis, thinner-slice volumetric imaging (no skip) is desirable. This volumetric imaging, however, increases the duration of the scan. A volumetric T1-weighted spoiled gradient-recalled (SPGR) echo study, used for frameless stereotactic registration, requires ~18 minutes of imaging time. Therefore, if a limited set of axial T1, T2, FLAIR, and contrast-enhanced SPGR sequences are performed, the total imaging time will take ~30 minutes. If one then adds the time to prepare the patient for movement into the scanner, repositioning the bed, redraping after the scan, and finally reregistering the frameless stereotaxis system, this entire process can easily add another 45 minutes to each case. Because there is a desire to minimize the length of the operation (lower risk of infection, prevent deep venous thrombosis, etc.), every attempt should be made to (1) limit the number of intraoperative scans, and (2) select only MRI sequences that are essential for continuation of the operation. If a fiducial system is used for intraoperative neuronavigational reregistration purposes, it is important that the field of view of the MRI encompass the fiducial markers **(Fig. 13–6B)**.

Interpretation of Intraoperative Images

During surgery, delayed contrast enhancement at the resection margins may occur following an initial dose of intravenous contrast. With standard diagnostic imaging, T1-weighted scans are typically begun immediately following the rapid bolus injection of gadolinium. Contrast enhancement of structures within the brain, however, persists for a prolonged period with a dynamic time course that peaks hours after injection. This relatively long interstitial half-life has several implications with regard to intraoperative imaging. First, if contrast were to be given immediately prior to the craniotomy, then the degree of residual enhancement would have to be assessed prior to giving a second contrast dose. This may be difficult on T1-weighted imaging if there is acute hemorrhage in the resection cavity. Second, for the same reasons noted earlier, it may not be practical to obtain multiple contrast-enhanced intraoperative studies. We ordinarily administer intravenous contrast only for the crucial intraoperative scan at which time we want to assess for residual tumor.

In addition, surgically induced changes in imaging characteristics may be a potential source of error with intraoperative MR imaging. Additional areas of contrast enhancement may appear following surgical breakdown of the blood–brain barrier (BBB), leading to "contrast leakage." "Blossoming" of T2 changes, presumably secondary to edema from surgical brain trauma, may occur as well. Thus it important to compare the imaging characteristics of the intraoperative scan with those of the preoperative MRI when interpreting the extent of surgical resection.

Frameless Stereotaxy and Neuronavigational Reregistration Techniques

In our experience, one of the greatest benefits of iMRI is the ability to update the frameless stereotaxis tool during the course of the operation. Even the act of opening the dura mater can result in >10 mm shifts of cortical structures **(Fig. 13–7)**, rendering the imaging based on preoperative data unreliable in many cases. Simply acquiring an intraoperative image without updating the neuronavigational system is of limited value due to the oblique angles inherent with patient head positions. Without updated neuronavigation, it is difficult to confidently localize residual tumor deep within the resection cavity based on studying the 2-D MR images alone.

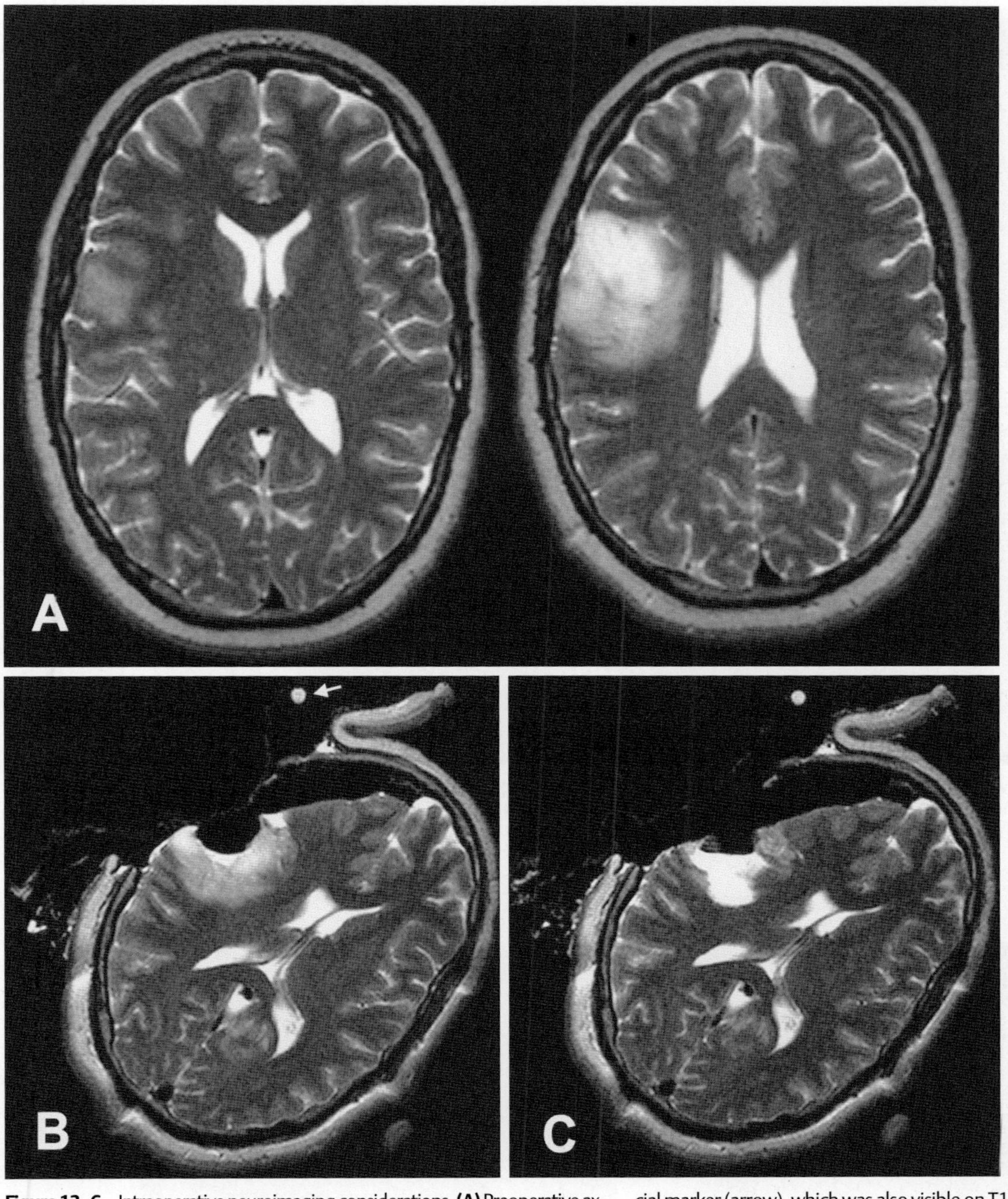

Figure 13–6 Intraoperative neuroimaging considerations. **(A)** Preoperative axial T2-weighted magnetic resonance images (MRI) of a 24-year-old patient with a right frontal low-grade astrocytoma (World Health Organization grade II). **(B)** Intraoperative T2-weighted MRI during tumor resection demonstrates the fiducial marker (arrow), which was also visible on T1-weighted images. Note that the skewed rotation of the head and the large degree of brain shift that has occurred do not allow direct comparison with the preoperative images. **(C)** Intraoperative MRI after near complete tumor removal.

The methods used for reregistration vary from system to system. We have successfully utilized a bone-fixated fiducial system (Stryker Leibinger Inc., Freiburg, Germany) in which five noncoplanar, sterile, mineral oil–filled spheres are temporarily inserted around the craniotomy opening for a landmark-point image-guided registration **(Fig. 13–8)**. Semiautomated reregistration techniques are currently under development. For instance, future configurations of the

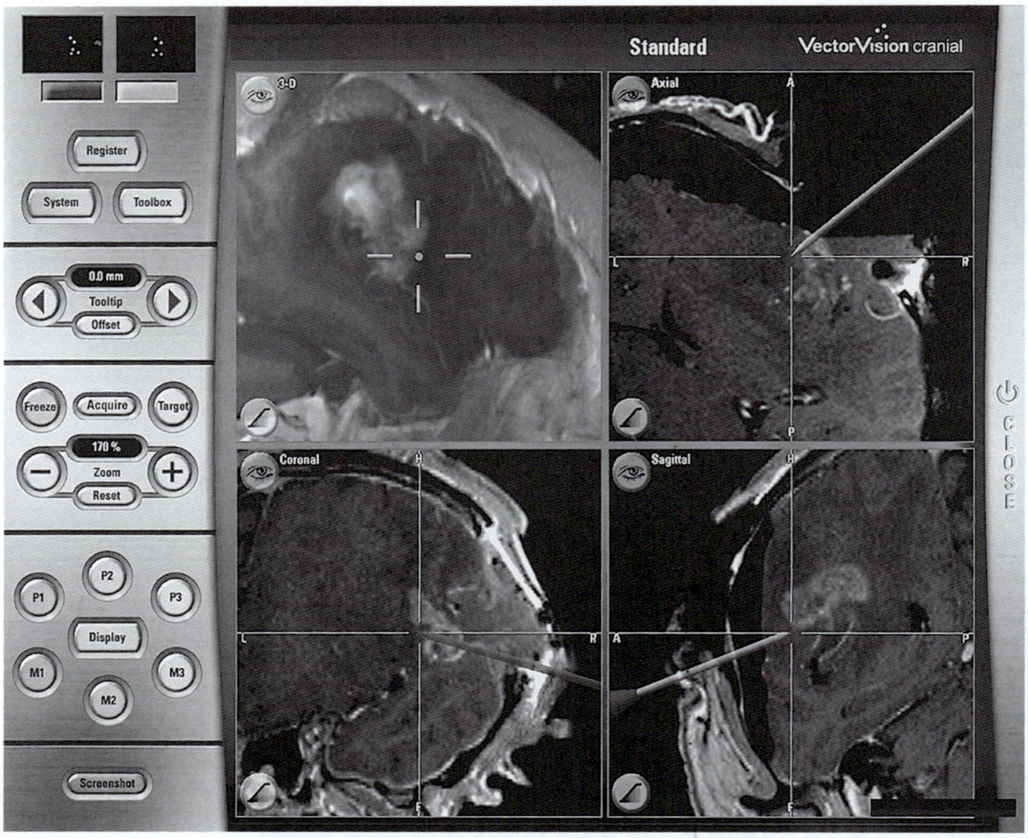

Figure 13–7 Intraoperative screen capture image taken from the VectorVision neuronavigation monitor (BrainLAB, Inc., Heimstetten, Germany) demonstrating the virtual pointer identifying the contrast-enhancing tumor margin. Note the degree of brain shift (right upper image) that would not have been apparent had the preoperative image dataset still been used.

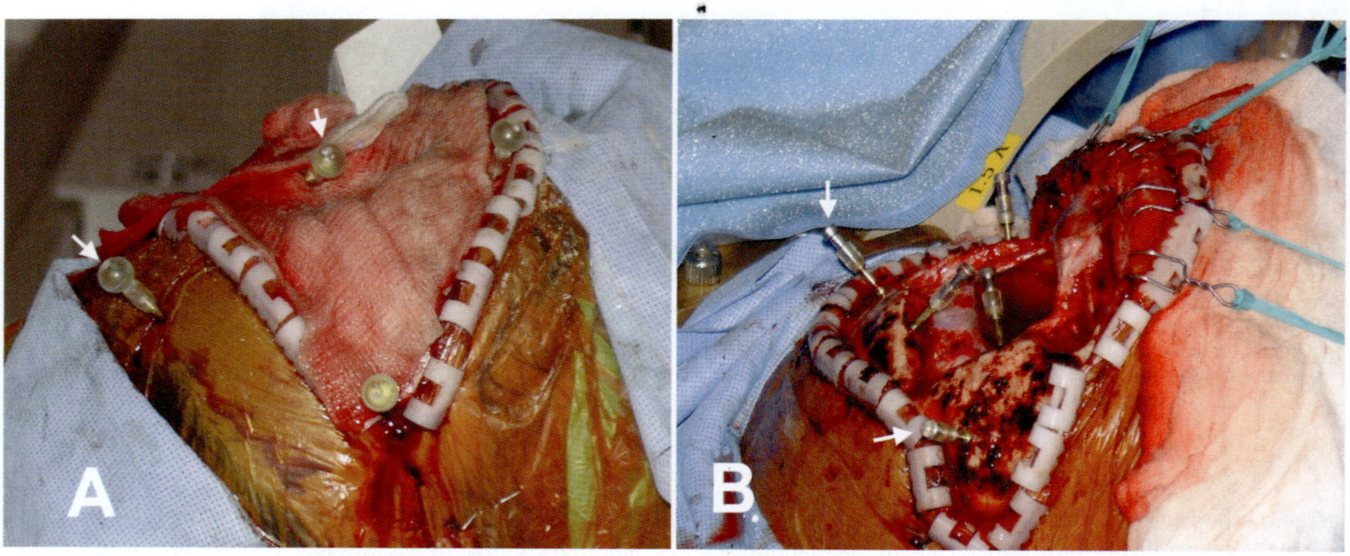

Figure 13–8 Fiducial system used for updated intraoperative neuronavigational registration of frameless stereotaxis. **(A)** Five mineral oil-filled fiducial spheres (arrows) are positioned onto temporary bone-fixated nonferromagnetic titanium screws. **(B)** After updated intraoperative magnetic resonance imaging (iMRI), the fiducial spheres are replaced by conical divots corresponding to the center of each sphere (Stryker Leibinger Inc. Freiburg, Germany). These divots serve as intraoperative fiducial markers for the image-guidance pointer (arrows). Because all components are sterile, a very accurate, fiducial-based reregistration routine can be used during surgery for updated frameless stereotaxis in conjunction with real-time iMRI.

BrainSUITE iMRI setup will allow rapid reregistration based on fiducials permanently anchored to the MRI-compatible headholder.

◆ Postoperative Management

Mobilization of the patient during surgery into and out of the iMRI increases operating time and may potentially increase the risks to patient sterility. Because of the theoretical increased risk of infection, we typically give our patients an extra 24-hour course of prophylactic perioperative antibiotics. The remainder of the postoperative management following iMRI-guided surgery is standard.

◆ Summary

Intraoperative MRI is a relatively new technology that has promise in improving the surgical outcome for a variety of neurosurgical disorders. For cases in which uncertainty increases as the brain shift–induced error of preoperative image–based neuronavigation becomes greater, the ability to update the neuronavigation system with a near-real-time image database is highly beneficial. For the dedicated iMRI operating suite configurations, many technical and design challenges still await solutions. Currently, no single intraoperative MRI configuration is clearly advantageous for all neurosurgical indications and procedures. Factors such as feasibility, safety, patient selection, and cost will play important roles in the future adaptation of this technological advancement.

14

Stereotactic Resection of Malignant Brain Tumors

Andrew E. Sloan

Approximately 17,600 primary and malignant brain tumors are diagnosed every year in American adults, and primary brain tumors are the most common solid tumor in children. Surgery continues to play a critical role in the diagnosis and treatment of these patients. Modern stereotactic surgical techniques have markedly improved the safety and efficacy of both diagnostic and therapeutic surgical procedures, and have become the mainstay of clinical treatment. Significant debulking of tumor mass can markedly improve local control, survival, time to recurrence, quality of life, and the patient's tolerance for other therapeutic modalities such as radiation and chemotherapy. Moreover, the advent of molecularly targeted drugs has also accentuated the role of surgery in obtaining a definitive tissue diagnosis even for unresectable tumors. A methodological approach to stereotactic resection of malignant brain tumors can be divided into four processes: patient selection, preoperative planning, execution of the plan, and postoperative and long-term care.

◆ Patient Selection

Patient selection and formulation of the appropriate diagnostic strategy are among the most important factors in achieving a good outcome. Management options include medical management with steroids, chemotherapy, radiotherapy, stereotactic radiosurgery, and surgical resection. A patient's medical condition should be thoroughly reviewed prior to surgery because it pertains not only to the risk of surgery but also the choice of procedure. The patient must be informed about the goals of the various surgical approaches and their potential risks. Careful consideration must be given to the relative merits of each option with respect to both tumor factors and patient factors. Patient factors include the nature of the disease, overall prognosis, medical condition, and extent of systemic disease. Tumor factors include the size and location of the lesion(s), prior treatment, the need for future systemic treatment, and the wishes of the patient and family.

The goals of surgery are threefold: diagnosis, relief of mass effect, and local control. Stereotactic biopsy may facilitate diagnosis and should be considered if there is uncertainty about the presence of malignancy. However, in most cases, if surgery is being considered, biopsy and surgical resection can be done in the same procedure if the pathologist confirms the diagnosis by frozen section. The advantage of surgical resection is the immediate relief of mass effect, which usually allows for the rapid relief of symptoms, weaning of steroids, and greater tolerance for adjunctive therapies such as chemotherapy or radiotherapy. The advent of readily available user-friendly stereotactic systems enables the surgeon to resect one or more lesions simultaneously while minimizing operative time and morbidity.

The indications for surgical resection vary somewhat for primary and metastatic brain tumors. For patients with primary brain tumors, the indications for surgical resection are relief of mass effect and significant debulking of a well-defined tumor mass. Because there is little oncological benefit of resection versus biopsy unless more than 90% of the tumor mass is resected, resection of lesions that are poorly circumscribed or in eloquent areas may not be indicated unless required for immediate relief of symptomatic mass effect. In addition, primary central nervous system (CNS) lymphoma and germinomas are exquisitely sensitive to chemotherapy and radiation and are usually treated nonsurgically.

For patients with metastatic brain tumors, one must consider the extent of systemic disease, life expectancy, and quality of life as well as the size, location, and number of intracranial lesions. Increasingly, surgical resection of large or symptomatic brain metastasis is staged with other modalities such as whole brain radiation and stereotactic radiosurgery for the treatment of small or minimally symptomatic disease. Patients being considered for surgical resection should have controlled systemic disease and a life expectancy of at least 3 months, and should lack medical and neurological contraindications. Patients who do not meet these criteria are usually managed with radiotherapy and steroids with or without chemotherapy.

◆ Preoperative Preparation

A general medical workup consisting of chest x-ray, electrocardiogram (EKG), baseline metabolic profile, complete blood count, prothrombin time/partial thromboplastin time, and urinalysis is routinely obtained preoperatively for patients over 40 years of age, patients with a history of cardiopulmonary disease, blood dyscrasias, or systemic metastasis, or patients who have had medical complications following the use of chemotherapy. An endocrine workup is also indicated for lesions in the region of the sella turcica or hypothalamus. Anticonvulsants may be administered preoperatively if the patient has seizures or if the surgeon feels that the patient is at high risk for developing them. Decadron is prescribed for control of symptomatic edema, but an effort is made to wean the patient to 8 to 16 mg/d after the initial loading dose, if this is tolerated. The use of mannitol or Lasix to control mass effect preoperatively is avoided in nonemergent cases.

◆ Image Acquisition

Most current stereotactic systems are compatible with both computed tomography (CT) and magnetic resonance imaging (MRI). Despite issues of image distortion, MRI provides superior resolution of surgical anatomy; location of vessels; and intratumoral heterogeneity such as hematoma, cysts, necrosis, and edema; and is the modality of choice for patients with intraparenchymal disease. Conversely, CT provides superior resolution of bony pathology, which may be important for treatment of skull base lesions.

Depending on the availability and convenience, we typically obtain an MRI either the evening before or the morning of surgery. Ten self-adhesive skin fiducials are placed on bony landmarks in standardized locations around the perimeter of the head. The region over the temporalis muscle is subject to movement during registration, and the inferior occipital and suboccipital region are often distorted by the patient's supine position during imaging; thus placement of fiducials in these regions is avoided. Two to four additional fiducials are often placed around the region of interest, where precision is paramount.

After placing the patient in a neutral position in the scanner, we obtain continuous 2-mm slices without intervening segments from the vertex to the foramen magnum using T1-weighted images with gadolinium and T2-weighted paradigms. Typically, T1-weighted imaging $\pm$ Gd is most useful, but occasionally, T2-weighted images, flair images, or CT is also helpful in individual patients. When radiation necrosis is part of the differential diagnosis, MRI spectroscopy (MRS) or positron emission tomography (PET) imaging with various isotopes may also be fused with preoperative functional MRI (fMRI) to guide resection. The latter (fMRI) is useful for patients with an intracranial lesion in or near the eloquent cortex, even if awake intraoperative mapping is utilized. Diffusion tensor imaging (DTI) indicates the position of individual fiber tracts and may also be useful during resection. These images are immediately downloaded to the computer workstation in the operative suite. Prior to beginning the surgery, the trajectory and approach are planned. Whereas conventional technique stresses using the *shortest* approach, stereotactic techniques allow the surgeon to use the *safest* approach, regardless of length.

◆ Operative Procedure

Anesthetic Considerations

Close cooperation between the anesthesiologist and the neurosurgeon is essential to facilitate the operation. Important anesthetic considerations that must be addressed prior to surgery include whether to perform the procedure with the patient awake or under general anesthesia, and the need for hyperventilation and diuresis. Arterial line, pulse oximetry, and EKG are continuously monitored intraoperatively. Foley catheterization is routinely employed when the procedure is likely to last longer than 2 hours, and central lines are employed when working near the posterior aspect of the superior sagittal sinus, for well-vascularized neoplasms, when cardiac monitoring is required, or due to a paucity of peripheral vessels. Thigh-high compression stockings and pulsatile boots are always employed.

Modern mapping techniques enable the accurate identification of motor and sensory regions in patients under general anesthesia, provided that their preoperative deficit is mild to moderate, with power of at least 4-/5, and minimal sensory deficits. Accordingly, general anesthesia is preferred for most patients with minimal to moderate motor and sensory deficits and with lesions outside language regions. Language function, however, can only be assessed in awake patients. Accordingly, awake craniotomies should be considered for resection of lesions in the eloquent cortex in patients with language deficits or more severe motor or sensory deficits, provided that the patient is cooperative and has sufficiently intact language function to accurately map. After the patient has been positioned on the operating room table, a mixture of lidocaine (0.5%) and Marcaine (0.25%) with epinephrine (1:200,000) is mixed using sodium bicarbonate as a buffer. This is used to block the ascending branches of the trigeminal and/or occipital nerves prior to placing the Mayfield headholder. A propofol (Diprivan) drip facilitates mild sedation during opening and closing, while facilitating maximum cooperation during mapping and resection phases. A laryngeal masked airway (LMA) may also be employed depending on the patient and the preferences of the anesthesiologist. We employ a neuropsychologist to assist with intraoperative language mapping in patients undergoing awake craniotomies.

Hyperventilation and diuresis help decrease intracranial pressure (ICP) and have become standard practice in neuroanesthesiology. However, these techniques also distort brain anatomy and decrease the accuracy of stereotaxis relative to the preoperative MRI. Careful consideration must be given to the size and location of the lesions(s) relative to eloquent regions of the brain and the angle of the surgical approach. The depth and consistency of the lesion must also be considered. For lesions that are superficial and easily accessible, we prefer to minimize hyperventilation by keeping the patient normocarbic (pCO_2 38 to 40 mm Hg) and to avoid diuresis. For patients with increased ICP secondary to deep lesions with significant mass effect or edema, some degree of brain relaxation is usually advisable. This is particularly true when resecting soft, cystic, or infiltrating tumors, visualization of which may be facilitated by moderate brain relaxation. We prefer to hyperventilate to keep pCO2 no lower than 30 mm Hg and to use Lasix diuresis for any additional brain relaxation required.

◆ Surgical Procedure

The preparation that occurs prior to skin incision is often as important to outcome as the technical skill of the surgeon. This is particularly true in stereotactic procedures. Optimizing the configuration of the operating room, as well as the positioning, registration, planning, and mapping of the patient, are essential to success.

Operating Room Configuration

The operating room configuration will vary according to the position of the patient and the location of the lesion(s), and consideration is given to optimize the patient's safety and the surgeon's convenience. The anesthesiologist must have access to the airway as well as arterial and venous access. For awake craniotomies, it is helpful to establish a "corridor" through which the patient and anesthesiologist or neurophysiologists responsible for monitoring can visualize one another. This is obviously critical for language mapping or techniques involving visual identification.

The surgeon must have unimpeded access to the region of interest, a clear line of sight to both the stereotactic and ultrasound monitors by rotation of the eyes alone (without turning the head or trunk), and easy access to the scrub nurse and the first assistant. For a right-handed surgeon performing right-sided craniotomies in the supine, lateral, or prone position, we prefer to have the anesthesiologist on the left at the level of the patient's trunk. The stereotactic camera is placed at the surgeon's left at approximately the level of the patient's nose, but somewhat superior to the patient's head. Tilting the camera diagonally may help decrease interference with its "line of sight." The viewing screens for the stereotactic and ultrasound devices are positioned below the camera at the level of the surgeon's head and tilted toward the surgeon. Finally, the scrub nurse is elevated on a Phalen table on the surgeon's right above the patient, at the level of the trunk **(Fig. 14–1)**. For infrared-based systems, the microscope must be positioned such that it does not interfere with the line of sight of the infrared camera (even when under the microscope) or with the surgeon's access to the scrub nurse or first assistant. This will vary according to the type of microscope and whether it is floor or ceiling mounted. However, it is usually placed over the surgeon's left or right shoulder. The position of the stereotactic computer is less critical but can be positioned to the left of the monitors if the surgeon requires access to it during the procedure. The setup for a left-sided craniotomy is nearly a mirror image of this configuration.

Patient Positioning

The primary consideration in patient positioning is optimal visualization of the lesion and the regions of eloquent cortex at risk during the procedure. In the case of superficial lesions, these are positioned at the superiormost point of the cranium. The head is tilted such that the surgeon's field of view will be along the axis of the desired approach. This is particularly important for deep lesions. Such positioning helps minimize the loss of cerebrospinal fluid (CSF), preserving the accuracy of the stereotactic technique. Ideally, positioning will also allow bleeding to drain away from the resection cavity, but this consideration is less crucial. When working near the major venous sinuses, one must also consider the risk of air embolism if the operative site is above or below the level of the heart.

Additional considerations include maximum patient comfort and safety to avoid abrasions or stretch or compression injuries to the patient. Accordingly, for awake craniotomies, after the patient is in optimal positioning on the table, padding and any necessary immobilization are accomplished prior to sedation. When the procedure is performed under general anesthesia, the surgical team positions the patient, with particular attention to the face, neck, extremities, and genitals. In general, the neck is maintained in a neutral position ± 15 degrees, and the hips and knees are slightly flexed. The patient is secured to the table with 3 in. cloth tape, taking care to avoid pressure points. The Mayfield headholder is also secured to prevent premature release.

Registration

Registration allows the computer to localize the virtual map of the patient's cranium acquired during the imaging step within the three-dimensional space of the operating room. The importance of precision cannot be overemphasized because registration is probably the greatest contributor to the accuracy of the stereotactic procedure itself. The first step is calibration, which generally involves touching the wand or pointer to a fixed standardized object to identify the position and characteristic of the device to the system. Many systems allow the surgeon to identify the stereotactic camera's field of view during this step. If the patient's head or

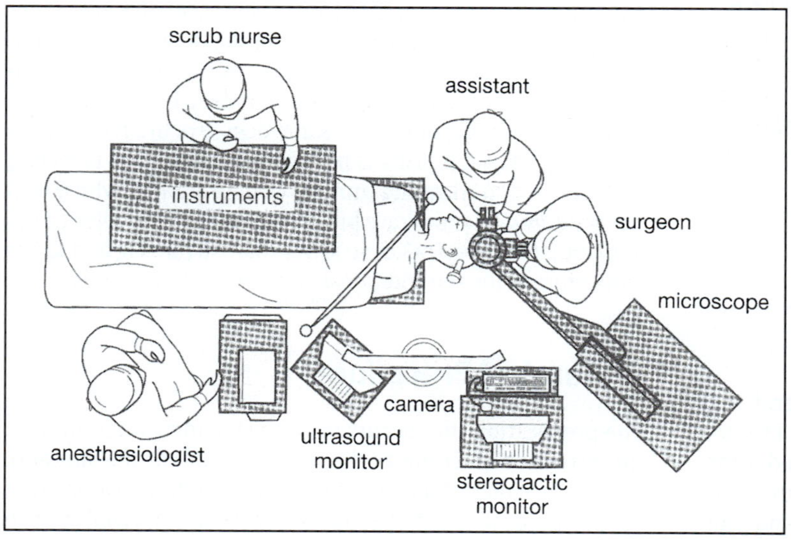

Figure 14–1 Optimum configuration of the operating room. The anesthesiologist has access to the patient's airway at all times. The surgeon has access to the region of interest, and a clear line of sight to both the ultrasound and stereotactic monitors, which can also be visualized by rotating the eyes. The scrub nurse and the first assistant are within easy reach of the surgeon. There is also an uninterrupted line of sight between the stereotactic probe and the stereotactic camera. (From Sloan AE, Perez-De La Torre R, Diaz FG. Stereotactic Resection of Brain Metastasis, Neurosurgery Operative Atlas (AANS). AANS 2000 with permission.)

the pointer is not within this region, the camera should be adjusted accordingly.

Next, registration of the patient's head is performed by sequentially touching the center of the fiducial markers. This is best done in a standardized order, proceeding circumferentially around the head. Care should be taken to minimize any pressure or traction applied to the fiducials. Although this step only requires four points, accuracy is improved by entering additional points around the perimeter of the head. Any fiducials that appear to have moved or been displaced during positioning or by the Mayfield headholder should be discarded to optimize the fit. If the error in the computer's "best fit" paradigm is greater than 2 mm, this step should be repeated. If the registration is acceptable, the resulting imaging transformation is tested by touching the wand to various regions around the perimeter of the head to test for accuracy. Regions at the perimeter, and those with the most complex three-dimensional structure, such as the tip of the nose, medial and lateral canthi of the eyes, and the scalp at the vertex and each pole, are preferred. If tracking of the head on the computer screen does not correspond to the patient's actual anatomy, the registration process is repeated.

Surgical Planning

Stereotactic technology is not a substitute for good surgical planning. The basic approach as well as the identification of vascular structures and regions of the brain at risk are based on conventional imaging obtained at the time of the decision to operate. The advantage of the stereotactic approach is that it allows the surgeon to rehearse and fine-tune this preliminary plan, and to more precisely determine important spatial relationships, to minimize any uncertainty in the operating room. Once the images are acquired, the surgeon can precisely determine the locations of the lesion(s) relative to the critical intracranial structures. The best possible trajectory to optimize resection at each phase of the operation can be determined, while dissection or retraction of the surrounding brain is minimized. A "virtual" operation can be performed using the computer monitor by advancing the plane of resection slice by slice along the various trajectories that the surgeon might employ, while noting the position of the various vessels, sulci, or gyri that will be encountered and adjusting the trajectory as required. The projection of the critical trajectories required is then outlined on the scalp. The craniotomy required to achieve this composite exposure is then outlined. This generally extends 5 to 10 mm outside the projection of the tumor itself to account for shift and rotation. In some instances, additional exposure is required for mapping purposes, especially in language regions. However, one should avoid crossing the transverse sinus or the posterior two thirds of the superior sagittal sinus unless absolutely required.

The skin incision necessary to achieve the exposure is then drawn on the scalp. Linear incisions are preferred, but in the parasagittal region above the ear, a "lazy S" or trapdoor incision is sometimes advantageous. Little or no shaving is usually required. The hairline is marked, and every effort is made to place the incision behind it. When shaving is required, a 5 to 10 mm margin on either side of the skin incision is marked with a surgical marking pen. Patients with especially thick hair or poor hygiene may necessitate additional shaving. The head is then prepped with Betadine solution or DuraPrep and painted in the conventional fashion. The operative field is then covered with clear Steri-drape, whereas the outlying regions are covered with cloth or paper drapes.

Skin Incision and Craniotomy

The early steps of the procedure are performed under loupe magnification. A no. 10 blade is used to make the scalp incision to the level of the fascia. Hemostasis is achieved with Raney clips and bipolar coagulation. The Bovie is not used on the scalp. In the temporal and suboccipital regions, where there is thick underlying muscle, the fascia is incised with a no. 10 blade prior to cutting the muscle with the Bovie. The scalp and muscle layers are not separated. Subperiosteal dissection is performed with a Langenbeck elevator, and the scalp flap is retracted with fishhooks or a self-retaining retractor **(Fig. 14–2).**

A high-speed drill with M3 surgical tool is used to create a bur hole. This is placed as strategically as possible to visualize important landmarks, such as major sinuses, using this highly controlled technique. Once the structures are visualized, the surgeon can proceed confidently and optimize exposure as required while avoiding unnecessary risks. After utilizing a curet to enlarge the bur hole and stripping the skull from the underlying dura, the B1 tool with the footplate is used to extend the craniotomy to the desired limit. Finally, four additional shallow partial-thickness holes are made in the cranium outside the craniotomy. The coordinates of these points, which serve as internal fiducials, are then entered into the stereotactic database as reference points that can be used later to detect any displacement of the system and allow for reregistration.

After homeostasis of the bone and dura is achieved using small amounts of bone wax, Surgicel, and Gelfoam, ultrasound is used to localize the lesion in real time. This serves to double check the stereotaxis and is a reference for echogenicity of the metastatic lesions, should there be a need to rely on this tool due to significant brain shift or malfunction of the stereotactic device.

The dura is then opened to expose the lesion. In general, we prefer to use a no. 15 blade to incise the dura and complete the opening with dural scissors, taking care to preserve the cortex. A trapdoor or cruciate incision is preferred **(Fig. 14–3).**

Electrophysiological Mapping Technique

When lesions are located on or near eloquent regions of the brain, intraoperative stimulation mapping is used to identify the boundaries of these critical regions. This facilitates optimum resection with maximum safety.

Somatosensory evoked potentials (SSEPs) can be used to accurately map the primary motor cortex in patients with lesions near this region that have good power (4-/5 or greater). This can be done with the patient under general anesthesia, with minimal muscle paralysis. A subdural electrode grid of the

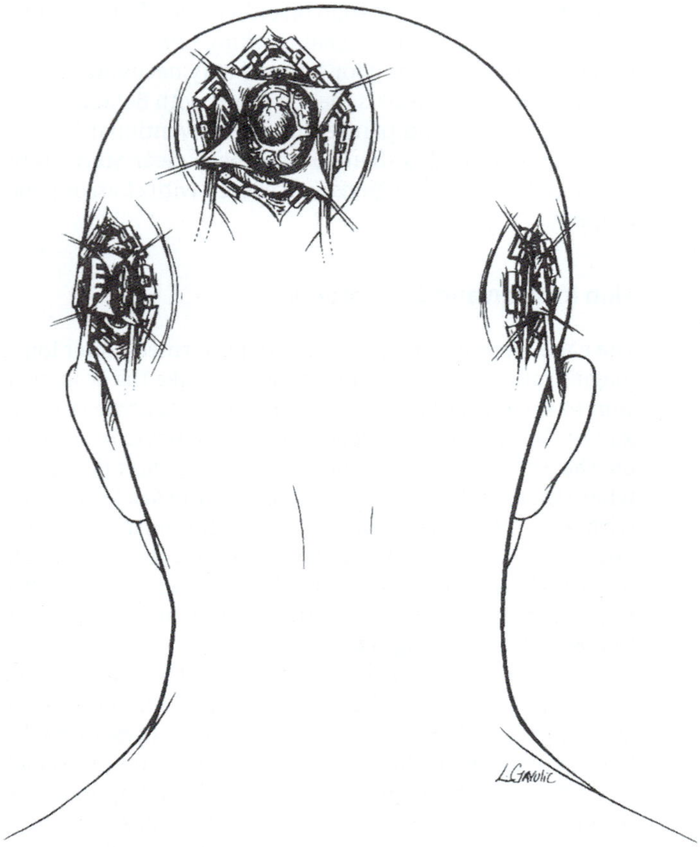

Figure 14–2 Illustrative case. A right temporal and occipital lesion and a left occipital lesion have been localized using stereotactic guidance. Incisions have been made at each site, and small self-retaining retractors placed. (From Sloan AE, Perez-De La Torre R, Diaz FG. Stereotactic Resection of Brain Metastasis, Neurosurgery Operative Atlas (AANS). AANS 2000 with permission.)

appropriate size is placed along the cortex at a right angle to the central sulcus **(Fig. 14–4A,B)**.

Patients with more profound hemiparesis, however, are best mapped using awake mapping techniques. If SSEPs fail to identify the location of the central sulcus, the patient is awakened and the position of the primary motor and sensory cortex is identified by stimulation with a 1.25 msec pulse, with a frequency of 1 to 60 Hz and an amplitude of 1 to 20 mA. The sensory region is identified by transient, localized sensation during stimulation, while the motor strip is localized by transient focal movement during low-voltage stimulation **(Fig. 14 –4C)**.

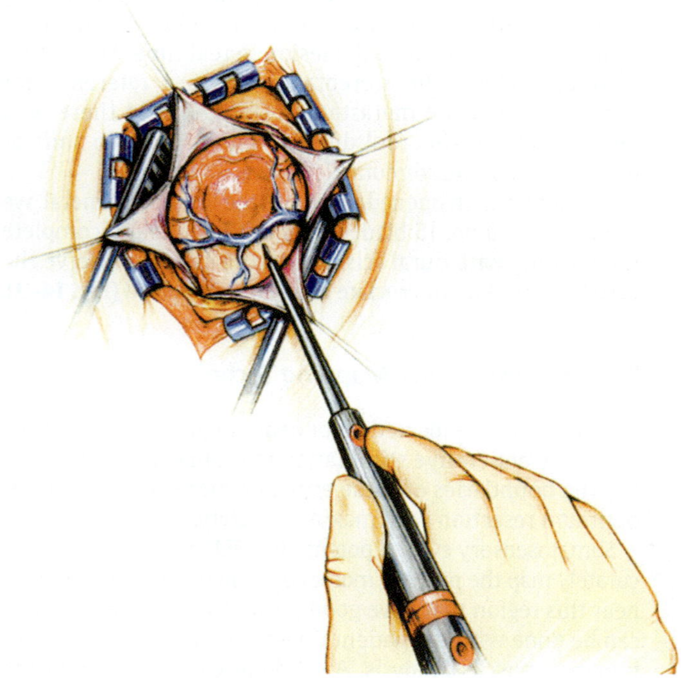

Figure 14–3 A cruciate incision has been made in the dura, and the dural leaves retraced with 4–0 Neurolon suture. The stereotactic probe is then used to precisely localize the lesion. (From Sloan AE, Perez-De La Torre R, Diaz FG. Stereotactic Resection of Brain Metastasis, Neurosurgery Operative Atlas (AANS). AANS 2000 with permission.)

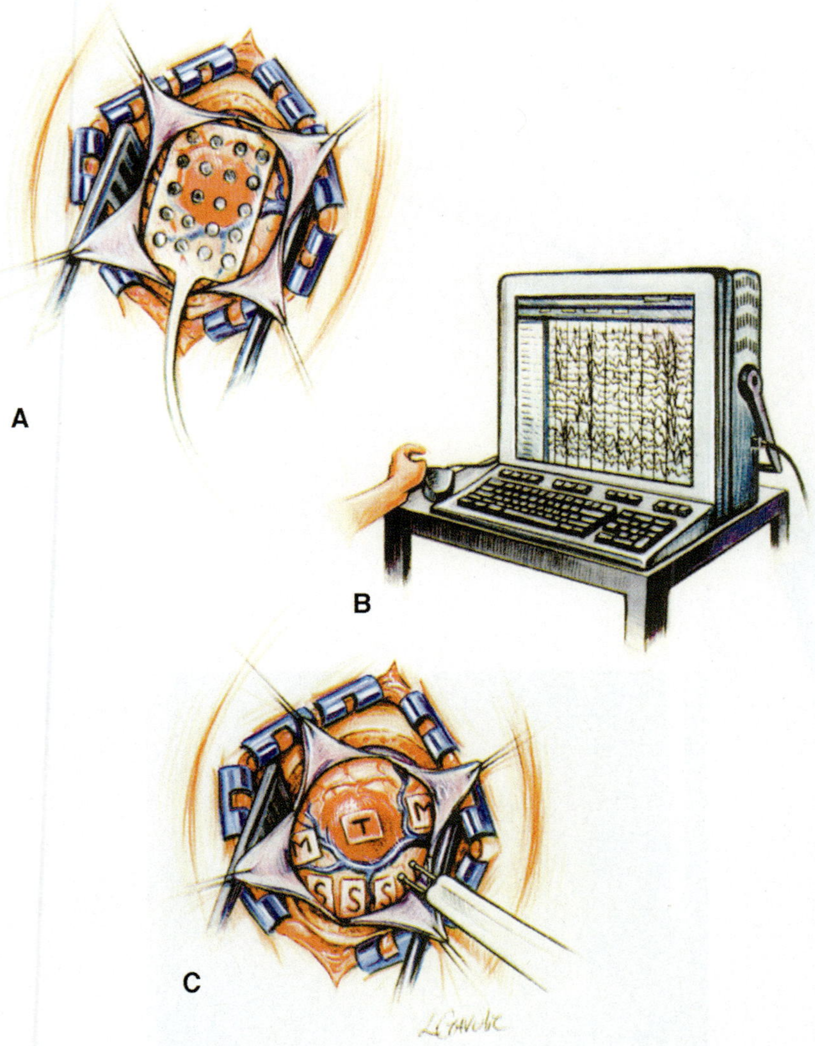

Figure 14–4 Functional mapping of the motor strip. **(A)** A 4 × 5 grid of electrodes is placed on the cortex for somatosensory evoked potentials. **(B)** Each 1 × 5 strip is sequentially activated in an effort to identify a phase reversal that will localize the position of the central sulcus and the primary motor and sensory cortices. **(C)** Stimulation mapping utilizing a bipolar electrode to stimulate the cortical surface. When the motor cortex is stimulated with sufficient current, the involved extremity can be observed to contract. As mapping proceeds, small tabs are placed on the brain to identify primary motor regions (M), primary sensory cortex (S), and tumor (T). (From Sloan AE, Perez-De La Torre R, Diaz FG. Stereotactic Resection of Brain Metastasis, Neurosurgery Operative Atlas (AANS). AANS 2000 with permission.)

Language function can only be mapped on awake patients with relatively good language functions. We stimulate the cortex near the relevant regions at 60 to 100 Hz with pulses 1 msec in duration, while carrying the intensity from 1 to 20 mA. The parameters tested depend on the patient's condition and the location of the lesion, but generally include following simple and complex commands, object naming, comprehension, repetition, and spontaneous speech. The naming tasks are rehearsed preoperatively with the neurophysiologist. Any anomia, lack of comprehension, dysphasia response, or speech arrest not present preoperatively serves to identify the eloquent region. A spread of epileptiform discharges from nearby regions of the brain, however, can confound the identification of regions of primary language cortex. Subdural grids are used to monitor afterdischarge potentials to exclude this possibility. Intraoperative seizures are managed by irrigating the brain with ice-cold Ringer's lactate solution, which stops the seizure activity immediately.

Intraoperative ultrasound facilitates the real-time identification of tumor limits. It is also somewhat helpful in identifying the consistency of these lesions as well as any brain shift due to CSF leakage, and as such is a useful adjunct to stereotactic resection. Metastases are usually hyperechoic, whereas lesions characteristic of radiation necrosis are usually hypoechoic **(Fig. 14–5)**.

Resection

Brain metastases typically seed the subcortical white matter. Most can be approached using a transsulcal approach with minimum to no resection of surrounding brain, and we prefer to use this approach whenever possible. In contrast, gliomas may occur in any part of the brain. Nonetheless, because most resectable gliomas are well circumscribed and appear to infiltrate successive gyri, the transsulcal approach is also preferred.

Under loupe magnification, the arachnoidal adhesions between the sulci are gently stretched apart and then sharply divided with microscissors. The approach proceeds along the pial banks, taking care to avoid damaging vessels running along it. Once the depth of the sulcus is reached, a small corticectomy is made at the point nearest the lesion guided by stereotaxis and ultrasound. When working in

A

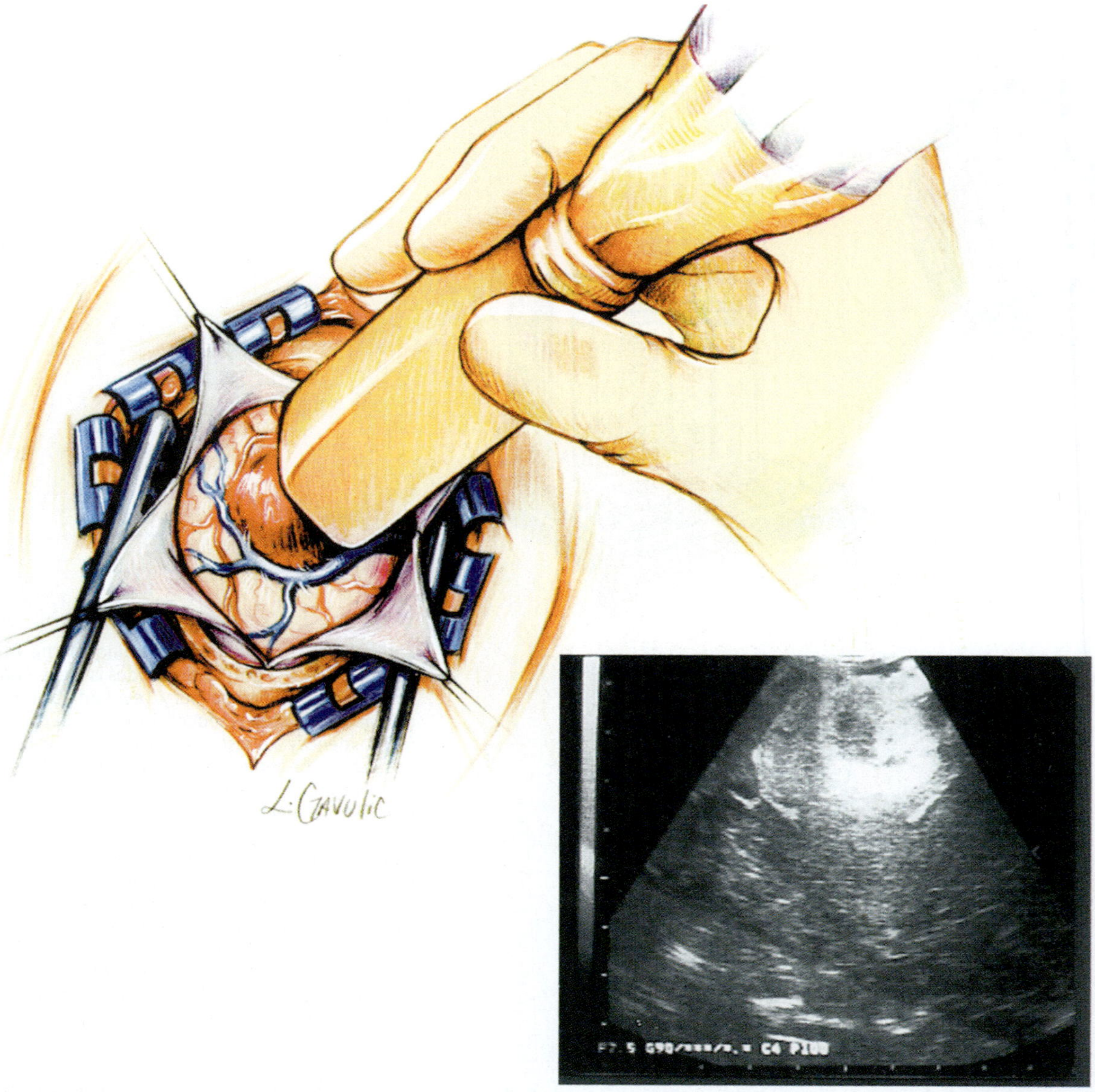

B

Figure 14–5 **(A)** Intraoperative ultrasound probe allows real-time localization of the lesion and is a useful adjunct to stereotactic resection. **(B)** Brain metastases are often hyperechoic to brain on ultrasound as illustrated here. Edema is also visualized here as a diffuse hyperechoic region around the lesion and is bounded by the pial banks, which are seen as curvilinear hyperechoic structures. (From Sloan AE, Perez-De La Torre R, Diaz FG. Stereotactic Resection of Brain Metastasis, Neurosurgery Operative Atlas (AANS). AANS 2000 with permission.)

eloquent regions or in areas more than 1-cm deep into the brain parenchyma, this step, and those that follow, are usually done under microscopic magnification.

Subtleties of the technique employed vary according to the pathology of the lesion being resected. For example, a generous lobotomy may be indicated in patients with high-grade gliomas of the nondominant frontal or temporal pole. In contrast, when resecting firm, well-circumscribed lesions such as renal cell carcinoma, the goal is to be as precise as possible, resecting the tumor while leaving surrounding brain, which may be gliotic but functional, as intact as possible. In such cases, the lesion is dissected circumferentially, taking care to retract the lesion rather than the surrounding brain. The management of cystic lesions varies depending on the pathology. In resecting a cystic or friable brain tumor, particularly melanoma or adenocarcinoma of the lung, great care is taken not to enter the tumor cyst to avoid spilling the contents, potentially seeding the resection cavity unless absolutely necessitated by the size or location of the lesion. This is especially true of intraventricular tumors. In contrast, because gliomas have already infiltrated the surrounding brain, decompression of intratumoral cysts is often indicated to facilitate resection and minimize retraction. Resection of 1 to 2 mm of grossly infiltrated white matter may also be indicated during resection of gliomas or infiltrative metastatic lesions such as melanoma brain metastasis where this can be tolerated without inducing a neurological deficit. Care should be exercised to distinguish vessels feeding or draining the tumor, which should be sacrificed, from those lining the pial banks, which should be spared. Particular care must be used in the insular region because critical Middle cerebral artery (MCA) branches supply-

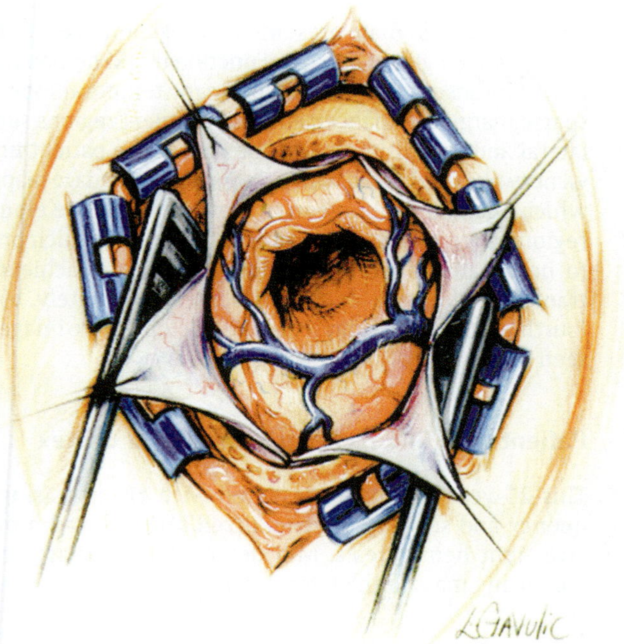

Figure 14–6 The resection bed is inspected after resecting a lesion to identify any residual disease. Hemostasis has been achieved, and the vessels at the perimeter of the lesion, as well as the vessel along the deep wall of the resection cavity, have been preserved. (From Sloan AE, Perez-De La Torre R, Diaz FG. Stereotactic Resection of Brain Metastasis, Neurosurgery Operative Atlas (AANS). AANS 2000 with permission.)

ing critical structures deep to the tumor often traverse the tumor margins and must be identified and preserved.

For deep lesions, a small corticectomy is occasionally required. In these cases, intraoperative mapping should be employed to identify eloquent cortex and avoid it. The cortical incision is planned perpendicular to the long axis of the gyrus, and the cortex and white matter is gently spread (not resected) with the bayoneted bipolar. We prefer to excise a small gyrus between transversing vessels rather than partially excising a larger region and inducing significant stretch injury. Typically, we use the Budde self-retaining retractor to facilitate the exposure, and the lesion is resected under the microscope.

After the lesion has been resected and hemostasis achieved, the resection bed is inspected for any residual tumor **(Fig. 14–6)**. Discoloration or vascular oozing usually signifies infiltrating disease. Vasospasm is occasionally observed during this step as well and is treated with local application of papaverine-soaked Gelfoam. We do not routinely line the resection bed with hemostatic material, although others may do so. However, when inserting Gliadel wafers, Surgicel is used to fix wafers to the wall of the resection cavity. Some have also employed fibrin glue for this purpose.

Closure Techniques

A watertight dural closure is completed using 5–0 Neurolon suture in a continuous running fashion. This is particularly important for posterior fossa lesions, or when Gliadel wafers have been implanted. Duraplasty is performed, if required, to achieve adequate closure. Two or three dural tackup sutures are placed in the dural and tied to the bone to avoid epidural fluid collections. A layer of Gelfoam may also be used to minimize CSF leakage, particularly in the setting of reoperation or if Gliadel is used. The craniotomy flap is secured with titanium miniplates. Hemostasis of the galea and the scalp is accomplished with judicious use of the bipolar cautery and with closely spaced 3–0 Vicryl sutures. This minimizes the tension on the skin and helps avoid the need for subgaleal drain except following pterional approaches. Finally, the skin is closed with staples or 3–0 nylon sutures. This should be done with care because many patients will be receiving either or both whole brain radio-therapy (WBRT) and chemotherapy shortly after their surgery, which impedes skin healing. A compressive dressing is rarely required if the aforementioned steps have been done meticulously, and a small cotton dressing secured with tape or op-cite is usually all that is needed. The dressing is left in place for 1 day and then removed.

◆ Postoperative Management

Postoperative care is critical to the success of the surgery. Control of intravascular volume, blood pressure, sodium and anticonvulsant levels, and nutrition is essential to preventing medical complications and promoting recovery in the postoperative period. Steroids are typically maintained at high levels for the first few postoperative days, then rapidly tapered. Patients implanted with Gliadel wafers and those undergoing brachytherapy continue moderate steroids for 30 days postoperatively prior to a more gradual taper. Prophylaxis of deep venous thrombosis with thigh-high stockings and pulsatile boots is also crucial. These are placed in the operating room and remain in place until the patient is ambulatory. Early ambulation is encouraged, and nonambulatory patients are started on subcutaneous heparin on the fifth postoperative day. Physical and occupational therapy consults as well as consults for rehabilitation are ordered for the first postoperative day, when indicated. Postoperative MRI is routinely obtained within the first 3 postoperative days to facilitate differentiation of residual tumor versus postoperative inflammatory response.

◆ Illustrative Cases

Patient with Multiple Brain Metastasis

This 42-year-old female with a history of metastatic carcinoma of the breast with well-controlled primary disease presented with increased headaches and seizures after radiotherapy of temporal and occipital lesions on the right. MRI demonstrated that both lesions had increased in size and a new left occipital lesion was also identified. She was symptomatic, had a Karnotsky Performance Scale score of 90, was in recursive partitioning analysis class I, and had failed previous treatment. She underwent resection of all three lesions in a single operation. Parts of the procedure are illustrated sequentially in **Figs. 14–2 through 14–6.** Pre- and postoperative MRI are seen in **Fig. 14–7.**

Patient with Glioma in Wernicke's Area

This 27-year-old male presented with generalized seizures with postictal global aphasia. Functional MRI demonstrated a hypointense lesion in the dominant temporal lobe with sparse marginal enhancement, and eloquent regions superolateral and anterosuperior to the lesion. The patient underwent awake craniotomy with intraoperative language mapping, which enabled the surgeon to identify and spare eloquent regions. A gross-total resection of the lesion, which proved to be an anaplastic oligodendroglioma, was achieved. A transient receptive aphasia resolved completely by the fourth postoperative day. Pre- and postoperative images are seen in **Fig. 14–8.**

Patient with Glioma Deep in the Motor Cortex

This 21-year-old male presented with an increasing frequency and severity of generalized seizures and progressive right hemiparesis. MRI demonstrated a large cystic enhancing mass in the left primary motor cortex extending

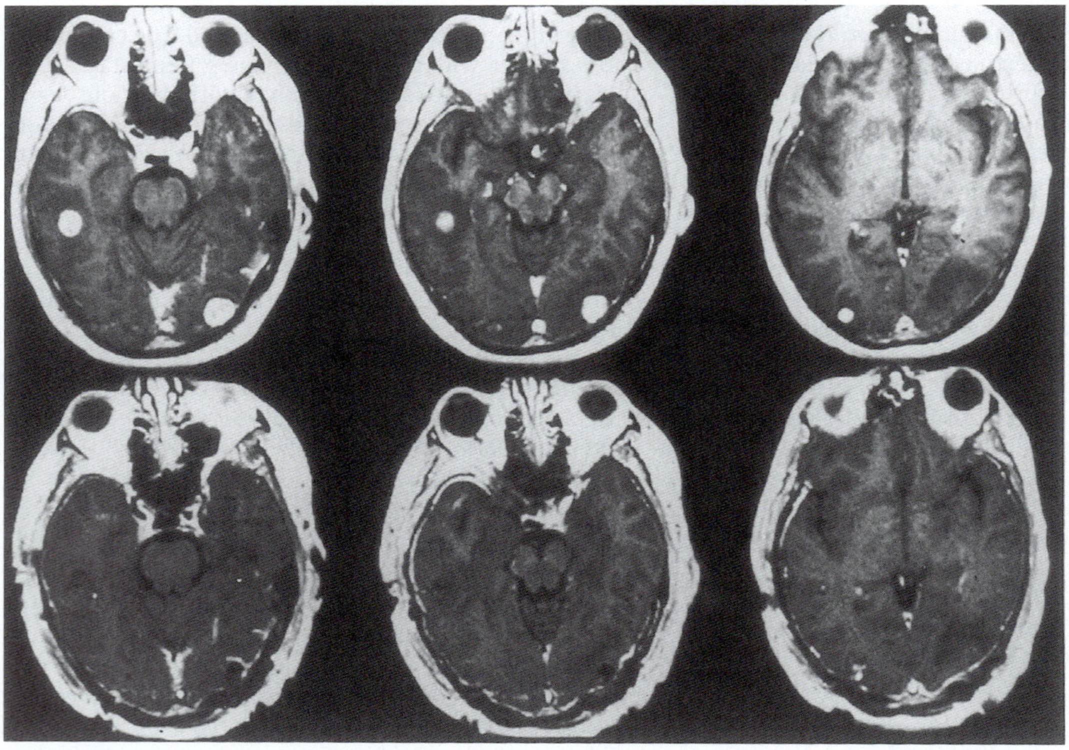

Figure 14–7 Preoperative (upper) and postoperative (lower) magnetic resonance imaging of illustrative case. Note minimal postoperative edema as early as the third postoperative day. (From Sloan AE, Perez-De La Torre R, Diaz FG. Stereotactic Resection of Brain Metastasis, Neurosurgery Operative Atlas (AANS). AANS 2000 with permission.)

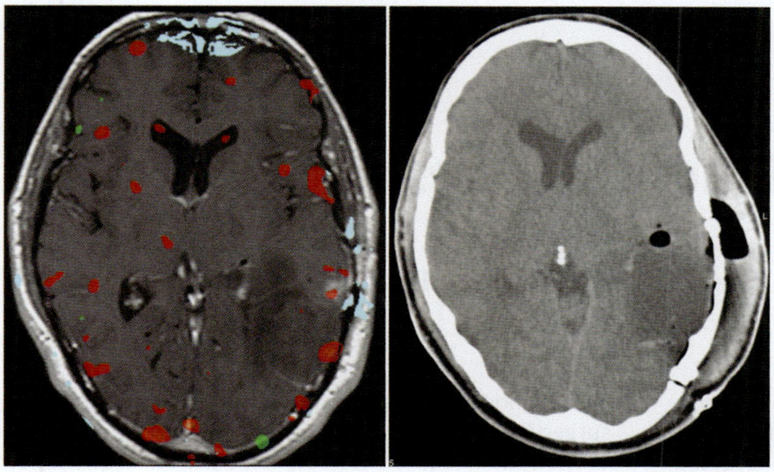

A B

Figure 14–8 Glioma in Wernicke's area. **(A)** Preoperative MRI. **(B)** Postoperative CT.

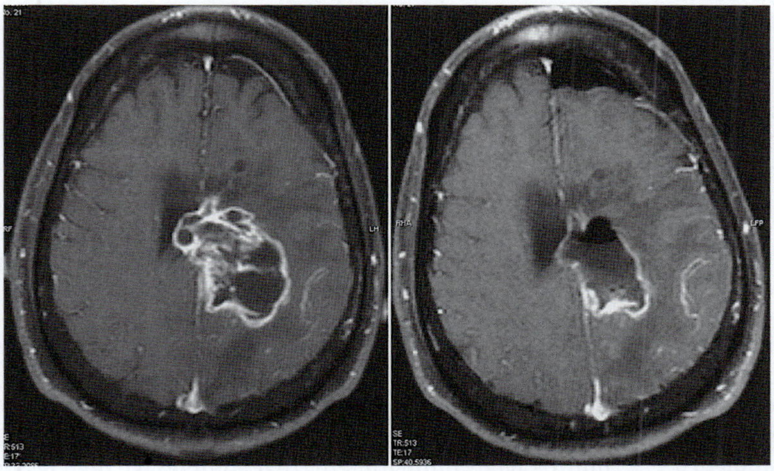

A B

Figure 14–9 Glioma deep in the motor cortex. **(A)** Preoperative MRI. **(B)** Postoperative MRI.

into the ventricle. The patient underwent craniotomy with motor mapping. The posteroinferior margin of the tumor infiltrated the primary motor cortex and consistently induced focal motor movement in the right lower extremity when stimulated and thus was spared. A near-complete resection was achieved, and the patient's hemiparesis markedly improved. Pre- and postoperative MRIs are seen in **Fig. 14–9.**

15

Radiosurgery of Intracranial Lesions

John S. Yu, Anne Luptrawan, Robert E. Wallace, and Behrooz Hakimian

In 1951 Swedish neurosurgeon Lars Leksell coined the term *radiosurgery* to denote a noninvasive technique that precisely delivers a single high dose of radiation to a targeted area of brain through an intact skull. The desired biological effect of radiosurgery is the destruction of a targeted area in the brain while avoiding nearby normal tissue and critical structures. Leksell, along with biophysicist Dr. Borje Larsson, introduced the first gamma knife in Europe in 1968. Radiosurgery can be performed using two devices: gamma knife and linear accelerator. Photon and proton beam radiation are two forms of radiation sources used to perform stereotactic radiosurgery.

◆ Gamma Knife Radiosurgery

Gamma knife is a multisource photon-based device that houses 201 fixed cobalt-60 sources. Cobalt-60 emits gamma ray photons. These photons travel as high-energy beams and are delivered at a predictable and easily quantifiable rate. The gamma knife device allows precise delivery of radiation to a target. The cobalt-60 sources deliver 201 separate beams of radiation, which converge onto a predetermined central target. Only at the point where these beams cross is radiation delivered high enough to effectively destroy the cells of the abnormal brain lesion. The amplitude of radiation at this point of convergence is so high that it allows for "scalpel-like" precision. The targeted tissue absorbs the radiation, leading to cell death. This process of cell death occurs over time, usually weeks to months. The end result of treatment is typically shrinkage of the lesion, halting further growth of the lesion or causing total obliteration of the lesion. When used with a stereotactic head frame, the precision of radiation delivery is 0.3 mm.

The radiobiological effect of gamma knife radiosurgery is different from that of conventional fractionated radiotherapy. Conventional radiotherapy usually involves the delivery of large volumes of irradiation, which may deliver radiation to normal brain tissue. Conventional radiotherapy also includes fractionated radiotherapy, which involves fractionation or dividing radiation treatment into multiple smaller daily doses. Normal brain tissue can tolerate fractionated radiation but it is not tolerated by the brain tumor, which results in the control of tumor growth. Gamma knife radiosurgery, on the other hand, delivers the entire dose of radiation in a single sitting. In fact, a single given dose with the gamma knife produces three times the biological effectiveness as the same dose in fractionated radiation. Inhomogeneity of the radiation dose is another inherent characteristic of gamma knife radiosurgery. This results in the delivery of radiation at the center of the tumor that is twice the dose delivered at the tumor periphery.

◆ Modified Linear Accelerator Radiosurgery

The linear accelerator (linac) is another radiosurgery tool used to effectively treat brain lesions. Unlike a natural emission of gamma ray photons produced by the gamma knife cobalt-60 sources, photons are created via the linac by accelerating electrons along a linear path and colliding with a metal target. The single stream of photon radiation simulates multiple stationary beams by using multiple noncoplanar arcs around the patient's head while the patient rotates on a turntable (couch) in each of four positions. Multiple beams of radiation can also be shaped with multileaved collimators to treat complex-shaped lesions.

Linac delivers very precise and uniform irradiation, but unlike the gamma knife device, it also allows for fractionation of treatment. Fractionation of treatment divides treatments into multiple sessions using smaller doses, or fractions, of radiation. This treatment strategy is referred to as stereotactic radiotherapy. Fractionation allows for treatment of larger lesions and lesions that are intrinsically part of a critical structure while minimizing effects on surrounding normal brain as compared with the gamma knife. Radiosurgery using the linac device can be more cost-effective as compared with gamma knife, particularly if institutions already use linacs for other applications.

◆ Patient Selection

Radiosurgery is considered an effective alternative treatment to conventional surgery and radiation therapy. It is an effective treatment option for patients who are considered high-risk candidates for conventional surgery. High-risk patients are those who are at high general anesthesia risk, too ill to undergo conventional surgery, or have lesions that are considered inoperable due to inaccessibility. Radiosurgery has been shown to safely and effectively treat patients with intracranial lesions that are considered inoperable using conventional surgery techniques. It is also an effective option for patients who have failed other forms of treatment, including conventional open surgery, conventional radiotherapy, and chemotherapy. At the same time, radiosurgery may also be utilized in conjunction with conventional surgery and radiotherapy, especially for patients with aggressive conditions. Radiosurgery is increasingly used as a first-line therapy for benign tumors, such as acoustic neuromas and meningiomas due to the efficacy in tumor control.

Radiosurgery treatment of intracranial lesions is limited primarily by size. Patients with lesions measuring greater than 3.5 to 4.0 cm are not appropriate candidates for radiosurgery because treatment of such lesions runs the risk of delivering an excessive amount of radiation to surrounding normal brain tissue.

The goals of stereotactic radiosurgery are to prevent tumor recurrence in the long term, maintain patient function, and prevent occurrence of new neurological deficits or adverse radiation effects. Another aim of radiosurgery is to deliver a more localized sphere of high-dose irradiation than would be achieved with conventional radiotherapy. Utilizing radiosurgery reduces the risk of damage to nearby healthy brain tissue and cranial nerves, allows for irradiation treatment near critical areas such as the brain stem and optic chiasm, and allows for safe treatment of large lesions up to 4.0 cm.

The most common clinical indications for the use of stereotactic radiosurgery include management of benign brain tumors such as meningiomas, acoustic neuromas, craniopharyngiomas, and pituitary tumors; malignant tumors such as primary and recurrent gliomas, metastatic tumors, arteriovenous malformations (AVMs); functional disorders such as trigeminal neuralgia; and movement disorders.

Meningiomas

Radiosurgery is an effective alternative to surgical resection for the treatment of well-circumscribed, small, benign, intracranial meningiomas. After treatment with gamma knife, 53 to 74% of meningiomas decreased in volume, 17 to 40% had no enlargement, and only 7 to 9% had increased in volume.

Vestibular Schwannomas (Acoustic Neuromas)

Radiosurgery has been shown to effectively control the growth of acoustic neuromas. After gamma knife radiosurgery, tumor regression was 32 to 73%, no growth in tumor size was 25.5 to 59%, and only 1.9 to 3% of patients had increase in growth and underwent conventional surgery after radiosurgery. Overall tumor control rate after gamma knife radiosurgery was 92%.

Pituitary Tumors

Radiosurgery is safe and effective therapy for patients with pituitary tumors. After radiosurgery, 29 to 50% showed a decrease in tumor volume, 36 to 67% showed no change in tumor size, and 14% showed an increase in tumor size.

Craniopharyngiomas

Radiosurgery is being used increasingly as an adjunct to other therapies to treat craniopharyngiomas. In one series, volume reduction of residual tumor after treatment with bleomycin was noted in 74% of patients. In another series, tumor control was achieved in 87%, and 84% had fair to excellent clinical outcome in an average follow-up period of 36 months, when cysts were treated with adjuvant stereotactic aspiration and/or Ommaya reservoir implantation prior to radiosurgery. In a study of eight patients who underwent stereotactic neuroendoscopy and subsequent treatment with intracavitary bleomycin and radiosurgery, a reduction of the entire tumor volume of greater than 90% was observed in three of eight cases and reduction greater than 50% in four of eight cases.

Trigeminal Neuralgia

Radiosurgery is a safe and effective way to treat the pain associated with trigeminal neuralgia. After treatment with radiosurgery for medically refractory trigeminal neuralgia, 40 [14] to 51.2% of patients reported excellent pain control, 17.1 to 30% reported good control. A decrease in pain medication usage was noted in 66% of patients. Recurrence of pain/treatment failure was reported in 23.9 [13] to 30% of patients.

Arteriovenous Malformations

The treatment of AVMs using radiosurgery is both effective and well tolerated. Several series showed obliteration rates of AVMs to be between 77 and 81.3% on follow-up angiography. In a retrospective study of 118 patients treated with radiosurgery, hemorrhage occurred in 6% of patients.

Malignant Primary Brain Tumors

Radiosurgery is typically adjunctive therapy for malignant primary brain tumors and has been shown to be clinically effective and safe in improving patient outcomes. Some publications have demonstrated increasing likelihood of local tumor control and prolongation in overall survival. Standard management of malignant primary brain tumors such as glioblastomas and grade 3 anaplastic astrocytomas is open surgical resection, with the goal of resecting as much tumor as safely possible, and subsequent postoperative external beam radiotherapy (EBRT). However, because of the aggressive nature of malignant gliomas (overall survival is 1 year for glioblastomas, and 2 to 3 years for anaplastic astrocytomas), patients continue to experience tumor recurrence even after high doses of EBRT. Brachytherapy and stereotactic radiosurgery are two approaches currently utilized to deliver higher doses of radiation to the tumor bed; controlling and slowing tumor growth in malignant gliomas. However, radiation boost via brachytherapy (temporary implants that deliver radiation to the tumor bed) is associated with prolonged hospital stay and higher rates of radiation necrosis. Because of increasing availability and less invasive means, radiosurgery is progressively replacing brachytherapy, with promising results.

Presently, the most common role of the gamma knife in the treatment of malignant gliomas is to provide a radiation boost in addition to conventional radiation therapy. In a series of 31 glioblastoma patients treated with EBRT plus gamma knife radiosurgery boost, an overall survival of 25 months was produced, compared with an overall survival of 13 months when patients received EBRT alone.

Metastatic Tumors

Radiosurgery is effective in controlling metastatic brain tumors and is considered a safe and effective treatment option. Brain metastases are excellent targets for radiosurgery because these tumors are usually spherical, small, and well demarcated from the surrounding normal brain tissue, unlike primary brain tumors. Forty percent of patients treated with radiosurgery demonstrated no further growth, 30% of patients demonstrated a decrease in tumor size, and 20% of patients demonstrated virtual disappearance of the tumor. Treatment of multiple brain metastases with gamma knife radiosurgery produces median survival rates similar to patients treated for a single metastasis.

◆ Contraindications to Gamma Knife Radiosurgery

Tumor or lesion size greater than 4.0 cm in maximum diameter; tumor or lesion edge less than 3 mm from the optic chiasm.

◆ Alternatives to Radiosurgery

Alternatives to radiosurgery should be discussed with each patient. Taking into consideration the patient's neurological problem, these include conventional open brain surgery, conventional radiation therapy, and fractionated stereotactic radiotherapy using a linac or gamma knife. The option not to undergo any treatment should also be presented to the patient. These treatment options along with their risks and benefits should be discussed with each patient considering radiosurgery.

◆ Preoperative Management and Operative Procedure

Gamma Knife Radiosurgery

The procedure for gamma knife radiosurgery is typically performed on an outpatient basis. The procedure involves ~3 to 4 hours. However, the age of cobalt-60 sources (decay with a half-life of ~5 years), dose of radiation to be delivered, size of the patient's head, and tumor location play a role in the total actual treatment time. Duration of treatment usually ranges from ~10 to 60 minutes. Large or irregularly shaped lesions usually require more than one gamma knife exposure. These "multiple isocenters" are delivered sequentially during a single sitting.

Linear Accelerator–Based Radiosurgery

Placement of Stereotactic Head Frame

If the patient is anxious, a mild sedative with Ativan or Valium 30 minutes prior to application of the stereotactic head frame may be helpful. Placement of the stereotactic head frame is performed by a neurosurgeon. The neurosurgeon fits the patient for the appropriate-sized Cosman-Roberts-Wells (CRW) stereotactic head frame. The head frame provides regional immobilization, holding the head still during the procedure and creating a fixed target. The stereotactic head frame also functions to provide the team with a set of exact coordinates on imaging equipment to precisely target the lesion to be irradiated. The head frame is made of aluminum alloy and is relatively light in weight.

The head frame has four sites where the frame is attached to the skull with mounting pins. Before attaching the head frame, two frontal and two occipital sites are prepped with Betadine and injected intradermally with a local anesthetic such as lidocaine. The patient will feel pressure as the pins are secured; however, if the patient complains of sharp pain, more local anesthetic should be administered. The neurosurgeon places two frontal and two occipital pins to immobilize the frame. Skull fractures have been known to occur if pins are secured too tightly.

Image Acquisition and Computerized Dose Planning

After the head frame is secured, image acquisition computed tomographic (CT) scan or angiography is performed. The type of study obtained is determined by the type of lesion: CT scan is indicated for tumors, angiography is indicated for AVMs or other vascular lesions. Image acquisition is necessary at this stage to identify the exact location and size of the intracranial lesion to be treated. These images are then fused with magnetic resonance (MR) images that were obtained previously. The following describes the process for stereotactic radiosurgery (SRS) in which high-energy x-ray treatment is delivered in one session. The course of events for multiple-session (on sequential days) stereotactic radiotherapy (SRT) follows the same steps over several days. On the treatment day, the surgeon affixes to the patient's head a rigid stereotactic frame (i.e., Brown-Roberts-Wells [BRW]/CRW for SRS) **(Fig. 15–1).** For SRT, this device is a relocatable frame (i.e., Gill-Thomas-Cosman frame [Integra Radionics Inc., Burlington, MA]) allowing reproducible positioning for each of the sequential treatment sessions. The frame establishes the absolute coordinate system for treatment, to which all radiation beam orientations and motions are related. CT scans are taken in the position fixed by the connection of the rigid frame to the imaging couch, and prior MR (or other) images are fused to the CT using mutual information technologies. The three-dimensional (3-D) CT image set provides an accurate spatial description of the patient as well as the spatial distribution of electrons with which the high-energy x-rays interact to deliver the dose. MR images (and other image types) are used

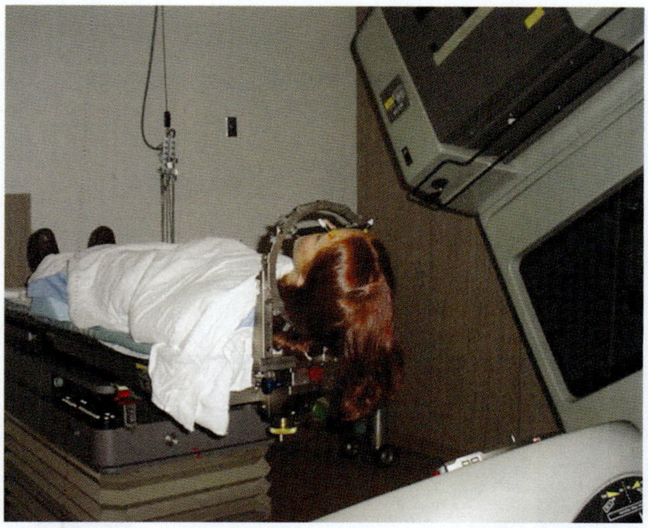

Figure 15–1 Patient after placement of stereotactic head frame and undergoing stereotactic radiosurgery treatment with linear accelerator.

to discriminate radiation targets (benign and malignant tumors or other structures) from normal and eloquent anatomy. Fusion maps this MR information onto the spatially accurate CT images. To image tumors, typical MR specifications are 2 to 3 mm thick slices with no gaps, T1 weighting, and postcontrast image acquisition, and follow specifications particular to the neurosurgical interest. The CT image axial planes are imaged using a fiducial system that allows direct mapping of the location of CT (and MR) pixels into the stereotactic coordinate system of the rigid head frame. An attachment system, symmetrical to that on the CT, connects the rigid head frame to the therapy radiation machine and thereby establishes the mapping between the stereotactic coordinate system and the orientation and motion of the radiation beams used in treatment. So the use of rigid attachment of the patient's head to a frame, a CT scanner, and a treatment machine allows the development of a plan for therapy that will be as precise as these connections allow. Using specialized equipment, the mechanical stability of the frame attachment to the patient's head is evaluated upon its placement and just prior to treatment to establish that there had been no movement of the frame while the patient waited for treatment. The mechanical accuracy of the fiducial device is subpixel size for a modern CT scanner. The mechanical accuracy of the aim of the treatment machine is verified prior to treatment and has magnitude depending on the radiation system in use. Typically, this is on the order of one fourth to one third of a millimeter. This is done using a system of film and a precise mechanical apparatus. Similarly, the accuracy of the image fusion is important in defining the radiation targets. Modern mutual information algorithms can reduce the imprecision to submillimeter pixel dimensions. The net uncertainty in the position, or more important, the border of a target or an important normal tissue structure, is then on the order of 1 mm with attention paid to technique. Mechanical alignment and its quality assurance are integral to maintaining the integrity of the stereotaxy. Other sources of uncertainty in target position derive from the ambiguity in target definition in the images, particularly with regard to different image interpretation among a group of observers/ readers.

The CT and MR images, and identified targets and normal anatomy (to "miss"), having been established in the stereotactic space, a computer-aided radiation therapy design system is used to plan the treatment. The orientation and possible motions of radiation beams to treat the target(s) are evaluated interactively. The 3-D distribution of the radiation dose is predicted for a given proposed beam arrangement and the doses to identified structures can be evaluated in 3-D detail. To do this, a radiation and mechanical model of the treatment machine and adjunct stereotactic accessories are maintained in the treatment planning program. The relationships among the head frame stereotactic coordinates, those of CT and MR images, and those of the treatment machine are captured in the planning program via the CT fiducial device. The accuracy of the treatment planning software in predicting dose is maintained through standardized and legally mandated quality assurance of the radiation-producing machines. Furthermore, an independent method is used to certify the calculations for each particular treatment.

Once the planning is completed, the information that describes the steps to administer the radiation is transferred to a database/control system to ensure that treatment occurs as planned. Prior to treatment, the patient is attached to the treatment machine couch using the rigid frame attachment, reproducing that of the CT and planning. During treatment, a radiation therapist downloads the parameters stored for the patient under treatment, checks that these are for the correct patient, makes adjustments for the direction and motion of the machine, and engages radiation for the radiation fields dictated by the plan. After treatment, the patient is detached from the treatment couch, and the rigid head frame is removed.

The use of modern linacs in radiosurgery allows the treatment of odd-shaped tumors using shaped fields. More traditional spheroidal targets, common in gamma knife therapies, are also possible using circular field "cones" that move about the target at a fixed distance, along an arc of a circle. An example of shaped fields is shown in **Fig. 15–2A–C**, where a meningioma is shown treated with 10 conformal radiation fields. **Fig. 15–2A** shows the 3-D volume of the prescription dose in the upper left panel, and the 3-D dose distributions in each of three principal planes through a central point in the tumor. **Fig. 15–2B** depicts the planned shape of one of the 10 fields and **Fig. 15–2C** is a predicted transmission x-ray with the target and field indicated. Each of these figures is used in planning, either to shape the field or to evaluate the planned distribution of radiation dose. In particular, aside from the directions and relative intensity ("weight") of planned treatment fields, the display in **Fig. 15–2B** allows the manipulation of the beam-shaping leaves of the treatment machine (shown as the yellow and blue bars in the figure). By moving these, a planner can evaluate the effects of leaf position on desired/desirable dose to the target. Noncoplanar arcs or radiation using circular beams of radiation are used for smaller and more spherical targets such as metastatic brain tumors **(Fig. 15–3).**

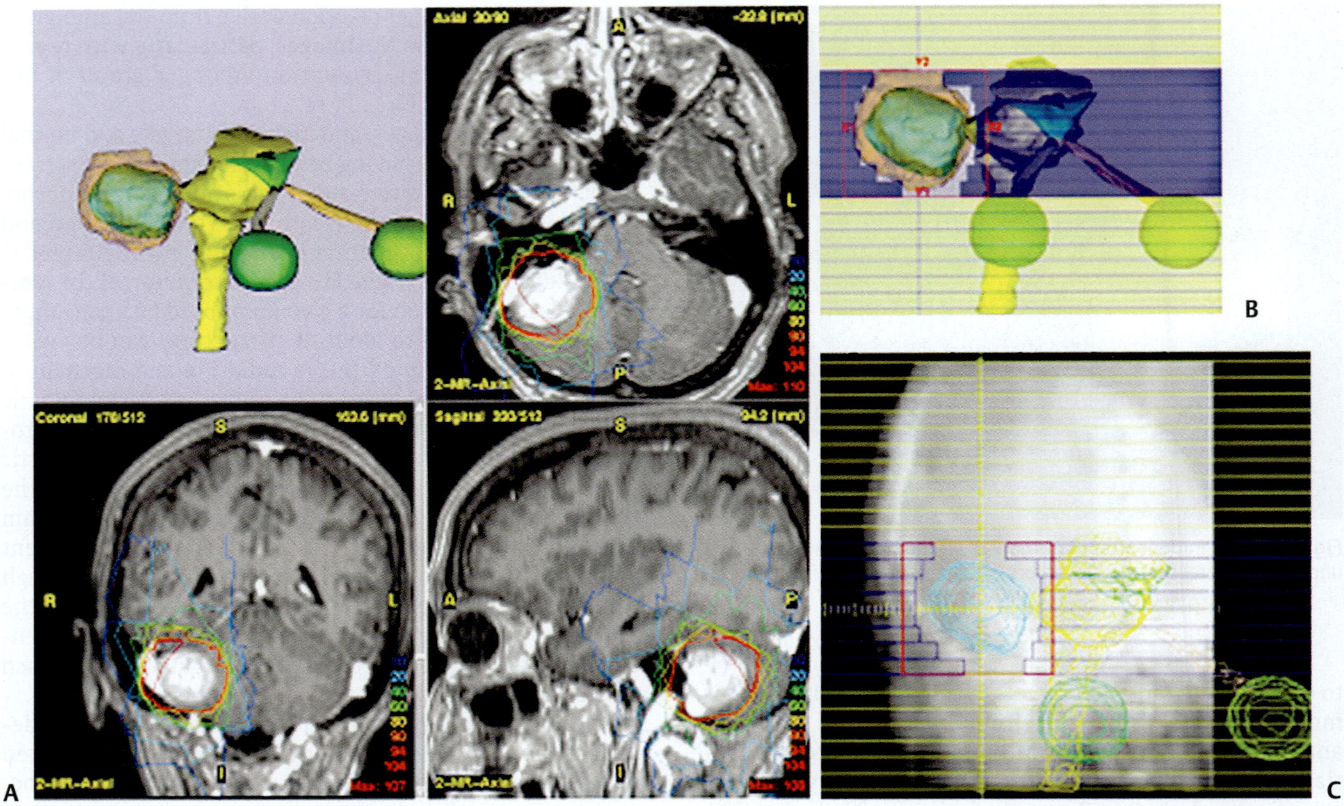

Figure 15–2 An example of shaped fields where a meningioma is shown treated with 10 conformal radiation fields. **(A)** The three-dimensional (3-D) volume of the prescription dose in the upper left panel, and the 3-D dose distributions in each of three principal planes through a central point in the tumor. **(B)** The planned shape of one of the 10 fields. **(C)** Predicted transmission x-ray with the target and field indicated.

◆ Postoperative Management

After the treatment is complete, the head frame is removed. Bleeding from the pin sites is common. Applying gauze and pressure should halt the bleeding. Occasionally, patients may experience headaches or nausea. Analgesics such as acetaminophen and antiemetics may be given before the patient is discharged home. The use of steroids is case- and physician-specific.

◆ Complications

Radiosurgery is designed to deliver a high dose of radiation to a small area in the brain. It has been successfully used in the past 40 years, treating many benign and malignant brain tumors successfully. The use of linac- and gamma knife–based radiosurgery has made this modality more popular and the utility has significantly increased. With this in mind, one should use radiosurgery judiciously because many patients with benign tumors will live a normal life, and complications can be devastating if they happen. Delivery of excessive amounts of radiation to normal brain tissue is a potential complication of radiosurgery. Radiation reactions and radiation necrosis are two primary types of complications that may occur after treatment with radiosurgery. Radiation reactions appear as hyperintense signal areas surrounding the originally treated lesion (perilesional) on T2-weighted MR images and are more suggestive of a glial inflammatory response rather than true edema. Clinical symptoms of perilesional radiation reactions usually occur with reactions in eloquent areas of the brain such as in speech areas and the internal capsule. Treatment for symptomatic radiation reactions is corticosteroids such as dexamethasone. Radiation reactions rarely produce neurological deficits because most subside over time. The occurrence of radiation reactions is largely dose dependent, with an increased likelihood of complications occurring with higher doses of radiation.

A more serious reaction to radiosurgery is radiation necrosis. Radiation necrosis is a result of either death of tumor cells and associated reaction in surrounding normal brain tissue, or necrosis of normal brain tissue surrounding previously treated metastatic brain tumor. Twenty to 25% of patients with primary malignant brain tumors treated with gamma knife radiosurgery experienced radiation necrosis. If significant clinical symptoms persist despite treatment with corticosteroids, surgical resection of the area of severe radiation reaction or necrosis would be indicated to improve the patient's quality of life.

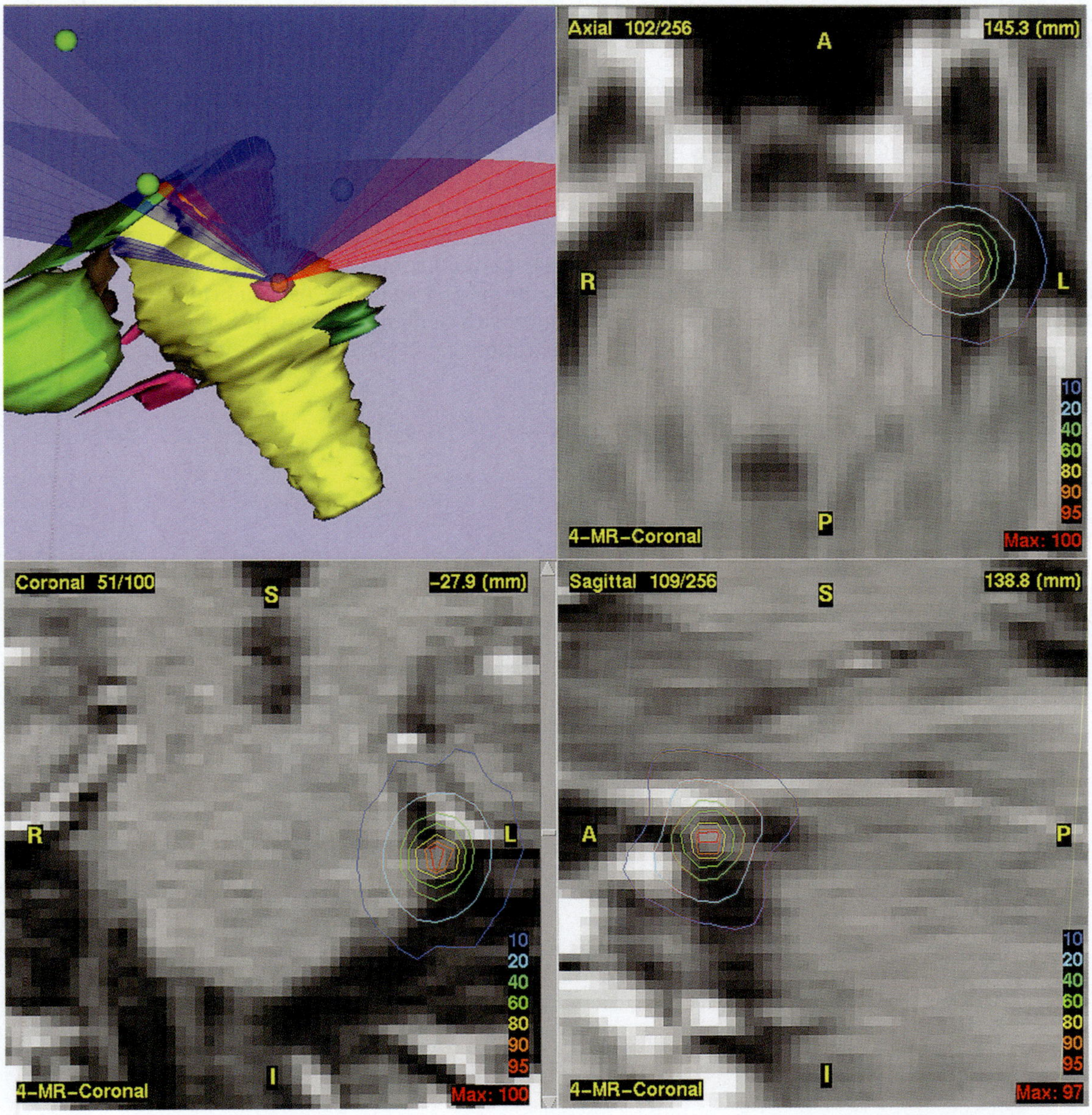

Figure 15–3 Moving fields are using a 5-mm "cone" aperture to describe the radiation distribution shown in the axial, coronal, and sagittal slices through the rotation center. Paths of the arcs are shown in the upper left panel. The treatment couch can rotate relative to the fixed plane in which the radiation beam moves in arcs. Oblique arc paths occur when the couch is rotated from perpendicular to the plane of radiation beam motion.

In general, one should decrease the total dose delivered in a single fraction as the irradiated volume increases. The dose-volume histogram should be looked at to decide whether the dose intended to an area is safe or even warranted. The reported data indicate that the risk of necrosis is anywhere from 1 to 7% in the patients treated for brain metastasis. Most studies indicated a range of 3 to 4%. Of course not everyone with radiological abnormality of necrosis requires treatment. Gerosa et al reported a necrosis rate of 7% for treatment variably sized and histological metastatic disease. They also reported some of the longer median survivals for patients with metastatic diseases. In addition, many of these patients may require whole brain radiation therapy, and with no doubt this could explain the risk of this magnitude. As indicated, this risk is dose and volume dependent. With the aggressive nature of metastatic tumors, even this high risk should be acceptable.

Although the risk of necrosis for malignant tumors may be acceptable, it would be difficult to justify this risk in patients with benign diseases. Fortunately, benign diseases, in general, require a lower dose of radiation for optimal control. Although acoustic neuromas were being treated with doses of 15 Gy in the past with gamma knife, the doses used are now on the order of 12.5 to 13 Gy. It is invariably noted that meningiomas close to the optic nerve or skull base may require doses that will exceed the tolerance doses of the cranial nerves. Single-fraction radiosurgery often limits the dose to these structures and could potentially underdose these most critical areas. Fractionated stereotactic radiotherapy is being used to treat these regions with excellent control and minimal risk to these structures. More conventional dose regimens of 1.8 to 2 Gy/fraction for a total of 50 to 54 Gy have shown excellent control of the tumor without any significant morbidity. Selch et al, in a review of 45 patients treated with fractionated stereotactic radiotherapy, reported minimal acute side effects. They also reported one patient with cerebrovascular accident 6 months after completion of the treatment. None of the patients in this publication reported long-term neuropathy, tumor edema, cognitive dysfunction, endocrine dysfunction, or secondary malignancy.

◆ Conclusion

As described here, radiosurgery can be utilized successfully to treat numerous neurosurgical conditions. Its induction into the neurosurgical armamentarium has largely replaced conventional microsurgery and radiotherapy with documented clinical efficacy. The utilization of radiosurgery for the treatment of intracranial lesions as we have discussed is effective, safe, and cost-effective and has been shown to improve patient outcomes and prolong overall survival. However, radiosurgery should be used judiciously because many patients with benign tumors will live a normal life, and complications can be devastating if they occur.

Section V

Surgical Management of Meningiomas

16

Surgical Management of Meningiomas of the Sphenoid Wing Region: Operative Approaches to Medial and Lateral Sphenoid Wing, Spheno-orbital, and Cavernous Sinus Meningiomas

Michael R. Chicoine and Sarah C. Jost

Meningiomas of the sphenoid wing have classically been categorized as arising from either the medial or the lateral sphenoid wing **(Fig. 16–1A,B)**. Often, distinction between tumors in this location can be made based on anatomical considerations, but meningioma growth does not always respect these arbitrary anatomical boundaries. Sphenoid wing meningiomas may extend into the orbit, in which case the term *spheno-orbital meningioma* may be more appropriate **(Fig. 16–2)**. Medial sphenoid wing meningiomas may also extend into the cavernous sinus **(Fig. 16–3)**. A meningioma may involve one of these regions, or any possible combination of these regions. We adopt a "building block" approach to tumors of the skull base, in this case removing portions of bone from the frontal, temporal, orbital, and anterior clinoid regions as necessary to optimize exposure and minimize disturbance of brain, cranial nerves, and other critical structures.

This chapter discusses neurosurgical approaches to meningiomas that involve regions of the sphenoid wing. The tumors discussed will be medial and lateral sphenoid wing meningiomas, spheno-orbital meningiomas, and cavernous sinus meningiomas. The general surgical approach to these tumors is similar, typically involving a frontotemporal or pterional craniotomy with additions or modifications as dictated by the unique anatomical and physiological challenges posed by the particular tumor of interest. We describe how various modifications of these approaches are used for the most common meningiomas involving the sphenoid wing. The reader should bear in mind that larger meningiomas of the sphenoid wing

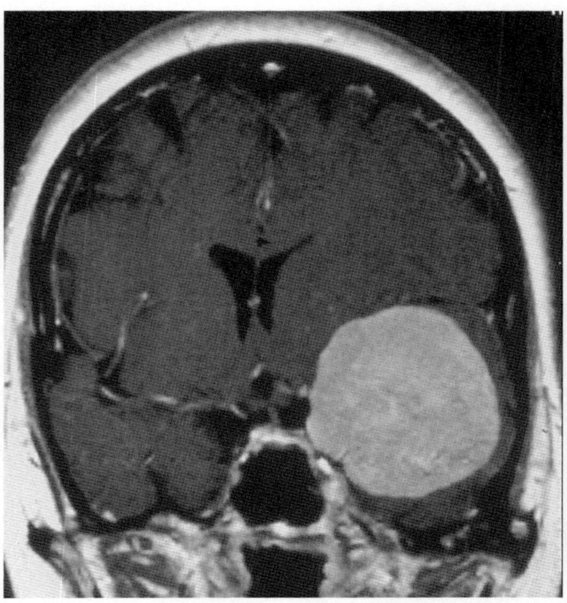

A

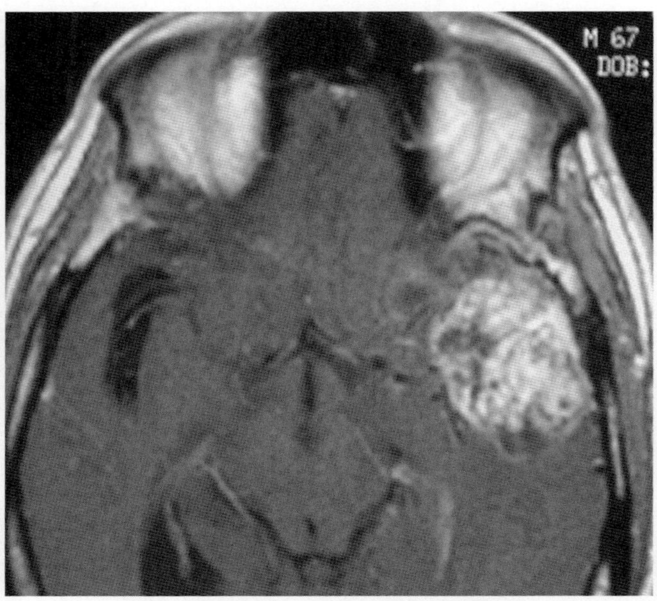

B

Figure 16–1 (A) Medial sphenoid wing meningioma as seen on T1-weighted magnetic resonance imaging (MRI) with gadolinium. **(B)** Lateral sphenoid wing meningioma as seen on T1 MRI with gadolinium.

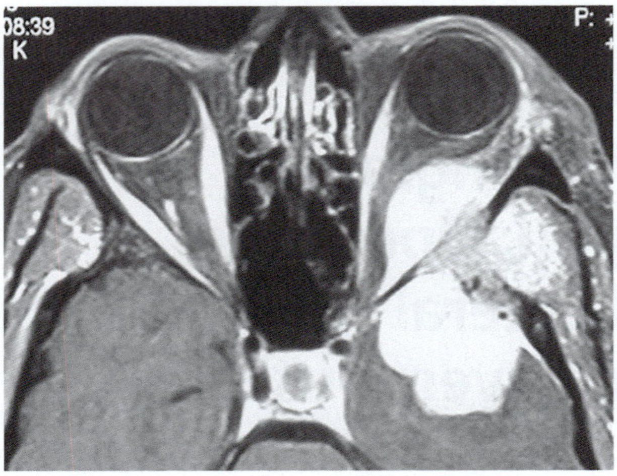

Figure 16–2 Magnetic resonance imaging of a spheno-orbital meningioma.

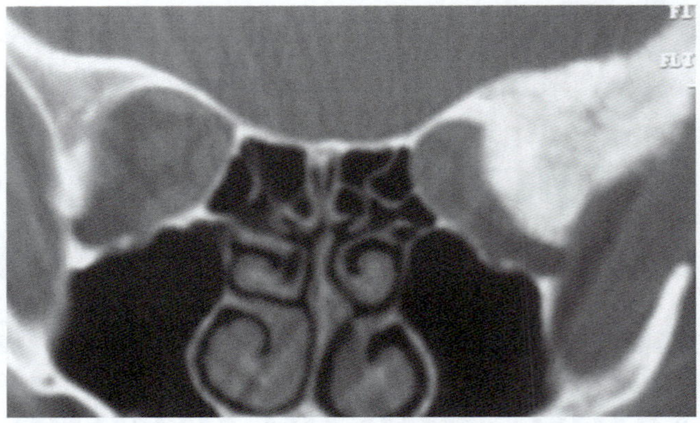

Figure 16–4 Coronal computed tomographic scan of a hyperostotic spheno-orbital meningioma.

may also involve adjacent anatomical regions, such as the sella turcica, the planum sphenoidale, the petroclival region, or the infratemporal fossa. More complex lesions such as these may require combinations of approaches described in this chapter with approaches described in other chapters of this text.

◆ Anatomy

Meningiomas that arise in the anterior skull base account for up to 30% of all intracranial meningiomas. Of these, approximately half originate in the region of the sphenoid wing. Tumors of the sphenoid ridge typically arise from the lesser wing of the sphenoid bone. Sphenoid wing meningiomas are the most common of the basal meningiomas. These meningiomas may be associated with hyperostosis of the sphenoid ridge **(Figs. 16–4 and 16–5)** and may extend to the dura of the frontal, temporal, orbital, and sphenoidal regions. Less commonly than hyperostosis these meningiomas may cause bony destruction **(Fig. 16–6).** Medial sphenoid wing meningiomas may extend medially through the wall of the cavernous sinus, anteriorly into the orbit, laterally into the temporal lobe, and superiorly into the frontal lobe.

Meningiomas are believed to arise from the arachnoid cap cells that line the inner dura and typically grow at the border between these cells and the dura. As a meningioma grows, the pia and arachnoid stretch over the surface of the tumor, forming the tumor capsule. In regions where there is a continuous flow of cerebrospinal fluid (CSF), a cleavage plane is maintained that allows the surgeon to dissect the meningioma from adjacent neurovascular structures. This may permit more complete resection of extensive or complex tumors. These tissue planes are most evident at the time of initial surgery, and may no longer be apparent if there have been prior surgeries or radiation treatments.

Local adhesions or anatomical complexity may limit the surgeon's ability to achieve a complete resection. In addition, meningiomas have been reported to escape their arachnoid planes and invade into adjacent cranial nerves or cerebral arteries. In these cases, more specialized approaches may be of benefit. Additionally, the surgeon may decide to leave residual tumor to minimize damage to crucial arteries, venous structures, or nerves.

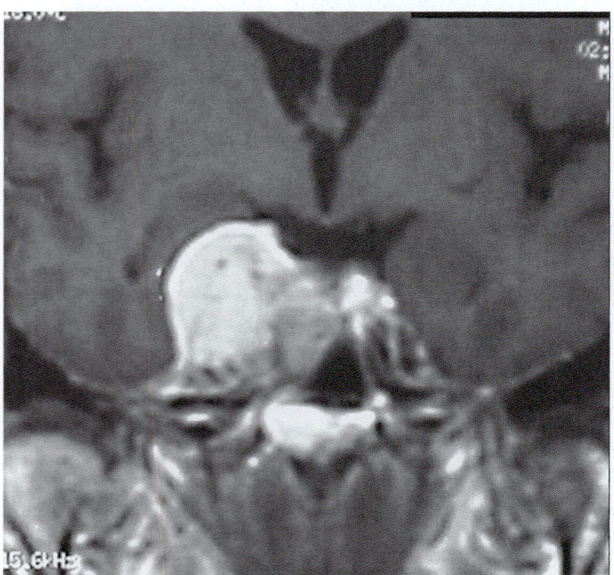

Figure 16–3 Magnetic resonance imaging of a sphenocavernous meningioma.

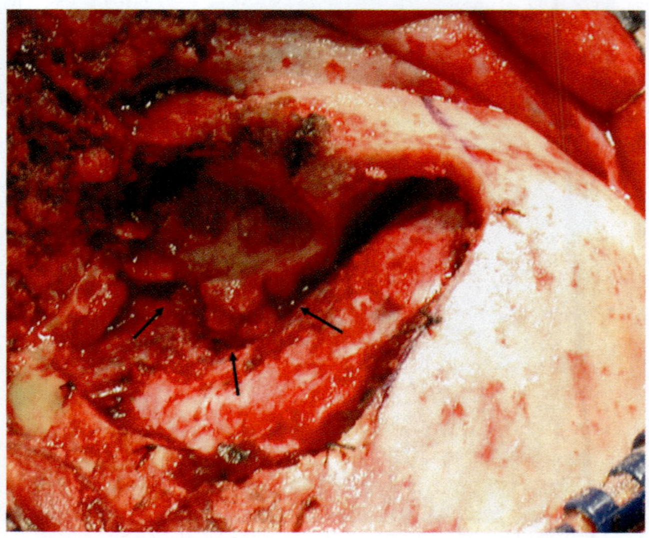

Figure 16–5 Intraoperative photograph after left frontotemporal craniotomy demonstrating hyperostosis. Areas of hyperostosis are demarcated with arrows.

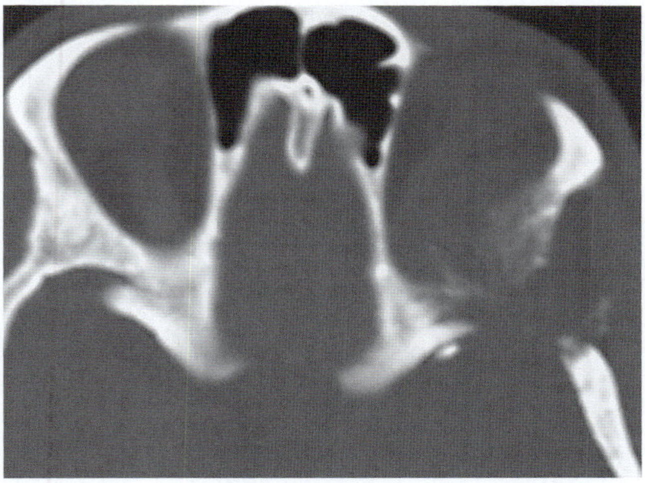

Figure 16–6 Computed tomography of an osteolytic spheno-orbital meningioma.

Lateral sphenoid wing meningiomas typically grow from the sphenoid ridge and extend laterally (**Fig. 16–1B**). Tumor growth can extend into the anterior or middle cranial fossae, displacing adjacent cortex medially. Lateral sphenoid wing meningiomas rarely encase the middle cerebral artery (MCA) and can grow to a large size before causing neurological symptoms.

Medial sphenoid wing meningiomas can present more of a challenge to the surgeon. The tumors are typically adjacent to or encase arteries of the anterior circulation, including the internal carotid artery (ICA), MCA, or anterior cerebral artery (ACA) (**Fig. 16–7**). The optic nerves, chiasm, and tracts can be involved, as can the third cranial nerve. Additionally, given the deeper location of these tumors, significant brain retraction may be required for adequate visualization of these structures. For medial sphenoid wing meningiomas, particularly those that are larger in size, we often utilize the addition of the orbitozygomatic osteotomy to the standard frontotemporal craniotomy to optimize exposure and minimize brain retraction.

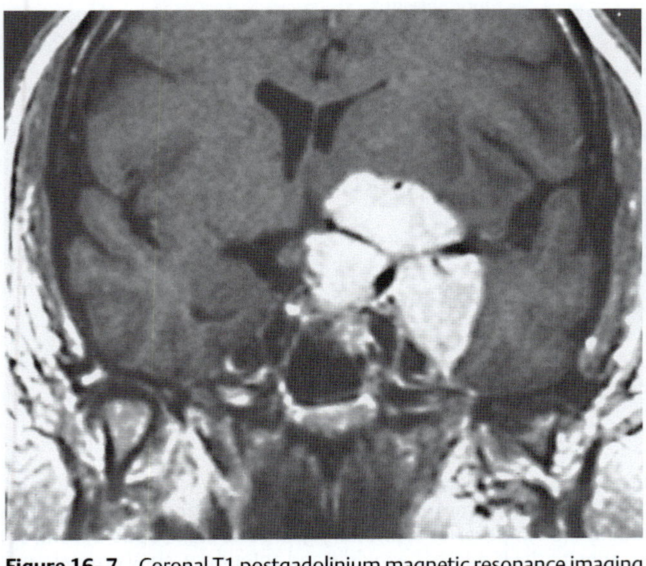

Figure 16–7 Coronal T1 postgadolinium magnetic resonance imaging of a medial sphenoid wing meningioma with encasement of the internal carotid artery, middle cerebral artery, and anterior cerebral artery.

Spheno-orbital meningiomas arise along the sphenoid ridge but extend anteriorly and medially to involve the orbit (**Figs. 16–2, 16–4, and 16–5**). These tumors can be associated with extensive hyperostosis of the adjacent bone, and dissection with subsequent reconstruction of the orbit is an additional challenge to the surgeon. Presentation of these tumors is often related to involvement of the optic apparatus, either through a change in vision or through proptosis.

Cavernous sinus meningiomas are reported to arise from the arachnoid cap cells of the cavernous sinus, or they may grow into the sinus as part of a larger tumor involving the medial sphenoid wing, orbit, or other areas of the middle fossa (**Fig. 16–3**). The anatomy of the cavernous sinus must be understood to treat these tumors. The neurovascular structures within the cavernous sinus as well as structures encountered during an approach to the lesion include cranial nerves II, III, IV, V, and VI, deep venous structures, and the ICA and its branches.

An understanding of the triangles between the cranial nerves and a knowledge of what critical structures will be encountered in each of these triangles facilitates surgical management of tumors within the cavernous sinus. Organization of the cavernous sinus region into a series of anatomical triangles was first described by Dolenc, and later was refined and expanded by other authors. The triangles of the cavernous sinus described by Dolenc were divided into three regions: (1) parasellar region—anteromedial triangle, paramedical triangle, and Parkinson's triangle; (2) middle fossa region—anterolateral (Mullan's) triangle, lateral triangle, posterolateral (Glasscock's) triangle, and posteromedial (Kawase's) triangle; (3) paraclival region—inferomedial triangle and inferolateral (trigeminal) triangle. The boundaries of these triangles are described in **Fig. 16–8A,B.**

Essential to understanding the various approaches to the cavernous sinus is the basic knowledge that the lateral wall is composed of two layers of dura and that the outer layer is the anteromedial continuation of the temporal lobe dura (**Fig. 16–9**). Understanding this concept, one recognizes that the outer layer of the lateral wall of the cavernous sinus can be stripped from the inner layer via an extradural subtemporal approach, thereby exposing cranial nerves III, IV, and VI enmeshed in the inner membranous layer without opening the dura.

More medially located sphenoid wing meningiomas carry a greater risk for surgical morbidity. The potential risks may sway the surgeon to a more conservative approach in treating meningiomas of the medial sphenoid wing region. The surgeon may decide that adequate resection is not possible and may manage these tumors without surgical intervention, sometimes using fractionated radiation or radiosurgery. In other situations, a partial resection is performed and radiosurgery or external beam radiation is used to treat residual tumor mass. However, partially resected medial sphenoid wing tumors have one of the highest recurrence rates of all meningiomas. Through an adequate understanding of microsurgical anatomy and application of appropriate neurosurgical techniques, the goal is to minimize surgical morbidity and maximize cytoreduction. This approach decreases the chance of tumor recurrence and potentially

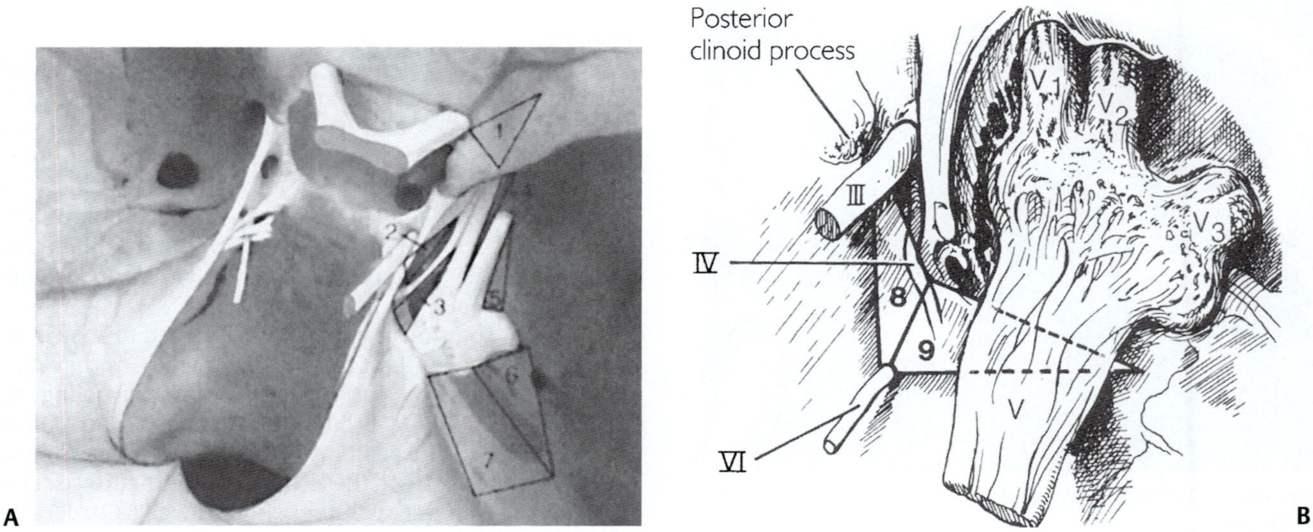

Figure 16–8 Triangles of the cavernous sinus and their borders: **(A)** (1) Anteromedial triangle: medial, optic nerve; lateral, oculomotor nerve; base, dural edge. (2) Paramedial triangle: medial, oculomotor nerve; lateral, trochlear nerve; base, dural edge of tentorium. (3) Parkinson's triangle: medial, trochlear nerve; lateral, V1 trigeminal nerve; base, dural edge of tentorium. (4) Anterolateral triangle: medial, V1 trigeminal nerve lateral, V2 trigeminal nerve; base, line between V1 in the superior orbital fissure and foramen rotundum. (5) Lateral triangle: medial, V2 trigeminal nerve; lateral, V3 trigeminal nerve; base, line between foramen rotundum and foramen ovale. (6) Posterolateral (Glasscock's) triangle: medial, greater superficial petrosal nerve; lateral, line between foramen spinosum and the arcuate eminence; base, V3 trigeminal nerve. (7) Posteromedial (Kawase's) triangle: medial, superior petrosal sinus; lateral, greater superficial petrosal nerve; base, V3 trigeminal nerve. **(B)** (8) Inferomedial triangle: medial, line between posterior clinoid and abducens nerve at Dorello's canal; lateral, line between Dorello's canal and trochlear nerve at edge of tentorium; base, petrous apex. (9) Inferolateral (trigeminal) triangle: medial, line between Dorello's canal and trochlear nerve at edge of tentorium; lateral, line between Dorello's canal and petrosal vein at the petrosal sinus; base, petrous apex. (With permission from Robertson JT, Coakham HB, Robertson JH. Cranial Base Surgery, P. 180 Churchill Livingstone, 2000; London)

increases the effectiveness of postoperative radiation while possibly decreasing deleterious effects of radiation.

◆ Patient Selection

The presentation of a patient with a meningioma of the sphenoid wing region will depend on the anatomical location of the tumor. Patients with lateral sphenoid wing tumors may not present until the tumor is quite large. They may present with a longstanding history of unilateral headaches, or they may experience seizures. Patients with medial sphenoid wing meningiomas may present with headaches or seizures, but they may also present with symptoms related to compression of medial cranial nerves. Especially in the dominant hemisphere, compression of the anterior temporal lobe may cause cognitive changes. This can be overlooked as slowly progressive dementia, especially in an older patient. Patients

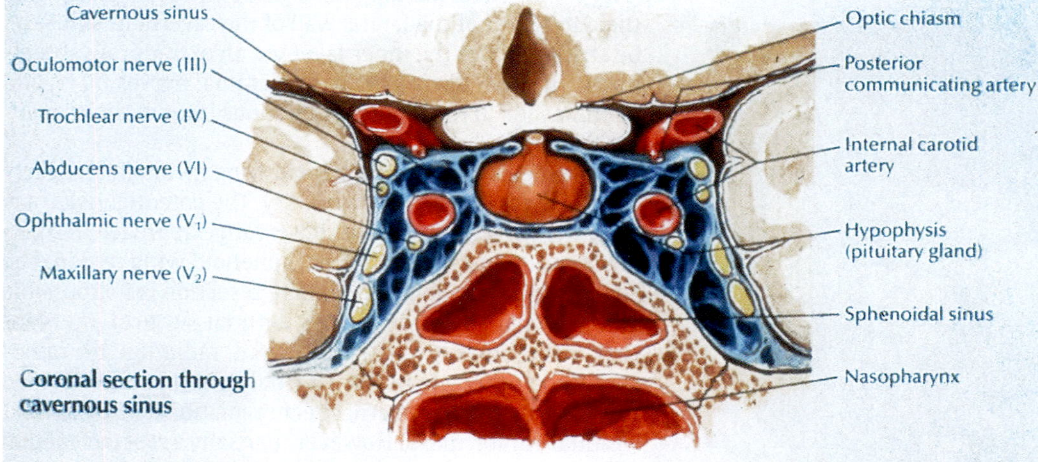

Figure 16–9 Drawing of the cavernous sinus region in coronal section demonstrating that the outer layer of the lateral wall of the cavernous sinus is made up of the dura of the anteromedial temporal lobe. The perineural sheaths of cranial nerve II, IV, and V_1 form the inner membranous layer of the lateral wall of the cavernous sinus. Also illustrated are the neurovascular relationships of CN II, III IV, V_1, V_2, and VI and the internal carotid artery (ICA). Note adjacent structures, including the temporal lobe, pituitary gland and stalk, optic chiasm, bifurcation of the ICA into the middle and anterior cerebral arteries, and the sphenoid sinus.

with tumors of the spheno-orbital region often present with symptoms of visual loss and proptosis along with fronto-orbital headaches. Cavernous sinus tumors will often present with cranial nerve abnormalities, including extraocular motor dysfunction or facial numbness or pain. Patients can also present with retro-orbital headaches.

◆ Preoperative Management

Although meningiomas are often visible on computed tomographic (CT) imaging, magnetic resonance imaging (MRI) is an essential component of the clinical approach to these lesions. Gadolinium-enhanced multiplanar MRI assists with identification of the ICA, MCA, and ACA, as well as important structures like the optic nerve. The extent of dural involvement or extension into the cavernous sinus can also be estimated on MRI. CT is more useful for identifying the extent of bony involvement, especially in cases of hyperostosis.

The utility of angiography has been debated in the preoperative management of meningiomas. For many meningiomas, including smaller or convexity-based lesions, surgical intervention may be undertaken without angiography, but for meningiomas of the sphenoid wing region, we frequently find angiography to be quite useful. Understanding the anatomical variants of the arteries, as well as displacements, stenoses, or occlusions secondary to meningioma mass are important to delineate with preoperative angiography **(Fig. 16–10A)**. At present, we do

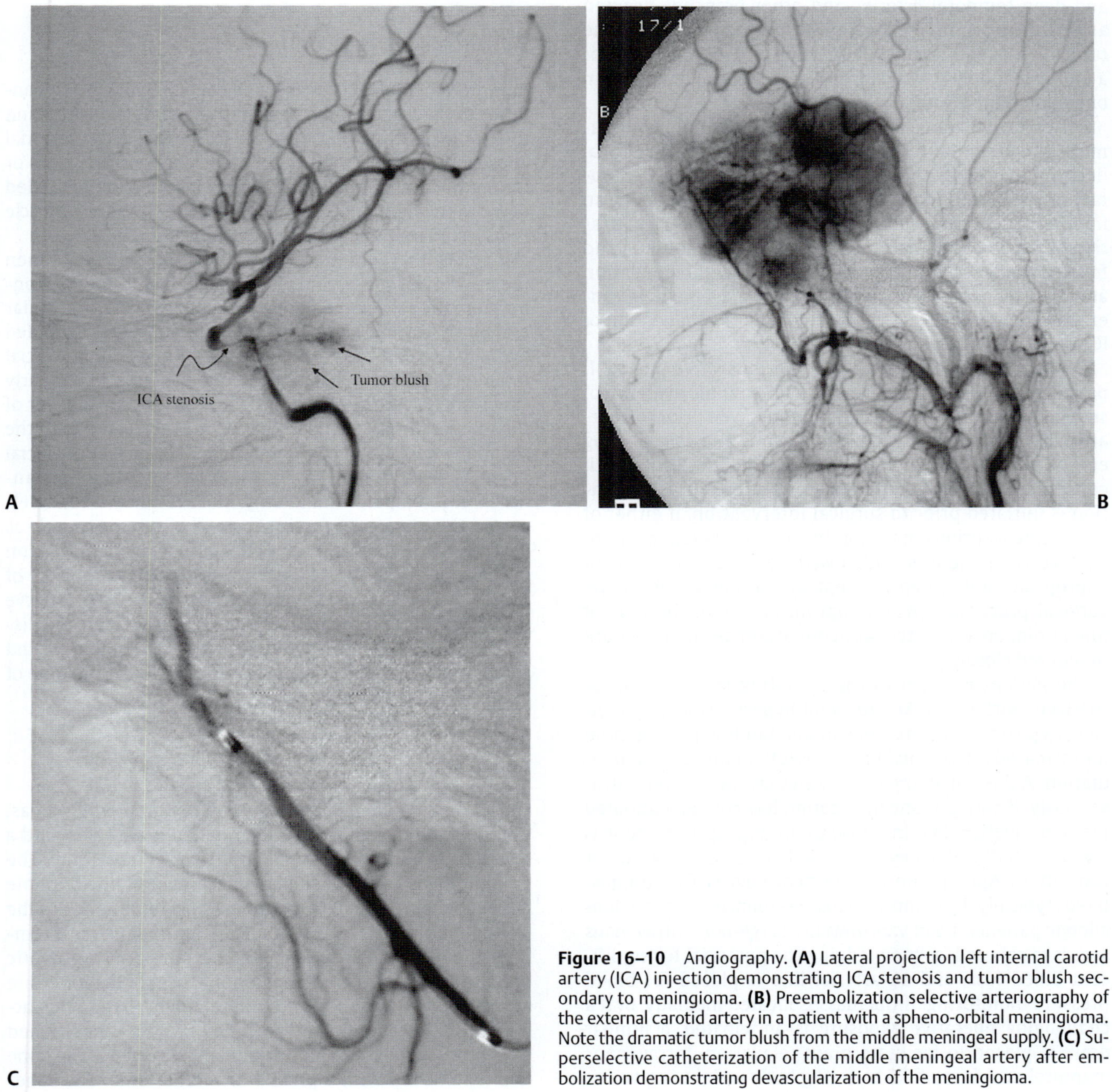

Figure 16–10 Angiography. **(A)** Lateral projection left internal carotid artery (ICA) injection demonstrating ICA stenosis and tumor blush secondary to meningioma. **(B)** Preembolization selective arteriography of the external carotid artery in a patient with a spheno-orbital meningioma. Note the dramatic tumor blush from the middle meningeal supply. **(C)** Superselective catheterization of the middle meningeal artery after embolization demonstrating devascularization of the meningioma.

not feel that many of these variations can be fully assessed with current techniques of magnetic resonance angiography (MRA) or computed tomographic angiography (CTA). In rare instances, temporary balloon occlusion testing may be warranted if the tumor threatens arterial occlusion. Meningioma tumor vascularity shared with the pial blood flow from MCA or ACA branches has been demonstrated to predict a higher incidence of peritumoral edema as well as a greater likelihood of a higher histopathological grade meningioma [World Health Organization (WHO) grade II or III].

For lateral tumors, much of the tumor's blood supply often comes from branches of the external carotid artery. Superselective arterial catheterization with preoperative embolization of the middle meningeal artery, the artery of the foramen rotundum, the accessory meningeal artery, and deep temporal arteries and other branches deemed amenable to sacrifice may minimize blood loss, soften the tumor consistency thereby facilitating resection, provide for a more clear operative field, and decrease the length of an operation **(Fig. 16–10B,C)**.

For cavernous sinus and large medial sphenoid wing tumors, the potential for iatrogenic ICA injury, or a surgical decision to occlude the ICA, must be kept in mind. Temporary balloon occlusion testing of the ICA therefore can be an important preoperative adjunct measure. Good visualization of the vascular anatomy of the ICA, MCA, and ACA and full knowledge as to the adequacy of collateral circulation are important aspects of preoperative management. In general, we do not feel that the added risk of embolization of ICA feeders is advisable.

Corticosteroids are used in the perioperative period. If patients have signs, symptoms, or radiographic evidence of significant cerebral edema, steroids are given prior to operative intervention, using dexamethasone at a dose of 4 mg every 6 hours. If patients have presented with seizures or if concern is high for seizure activity, antiepileptic medication is initiated prior to surgical intervention. If either of these interventions has not been undertaken prior to surgery, the patient is loaded with corticosteroids and an appropriate antiepileptic agent at the beginning of the surgical procedure. When appropriate, as in the case of phenytoin, postoperative anticonvulsant serum levels are monitored closely.

The patient is taken to the operating room and anesthetized, with care taken to avoid hypertension, hypotension, hypoxia, or hypercarbia, understanding the potential for increased intracranial pressure (ICP) in this patient population. A dose of 10 mg of dexamethasone is given intravenously. If antiepileptic medication has not been initiated preoperatively, a loading dose of an appropriate agent is given (18 mg/kg of phenytoin is used most commonly at our institution). Appropriate antibiotic coverage is also administered (typically 2 g of intravenous cefazolin, or for penicillin-allergic patients, 1 g of vancomycin). Large-bore intravenous access is ensured, acknowledging the potential for significant blood loss, and an arterial line is placed for blood pressure monitoring. If the mass is located medially, or if a challenging operative exposure is anticipated, a lumbar drain is placed to facilitate brain relaxation. Intravenous mannitol at a dose of 0.5 to 1 g/kg body weight is given at the time of the craniotomy.

◆ Operative Procedure

Surgery is performed with the patient supine. The thorax is elevated 15 degrees for unobstructed venous drainage, and the head is extended and rotated 30 degrees to the side contralateral to the lesion **(Fig. 16–11A,B)**. This positioning places the medial sphenoid ridge in a vertical position. The head is secured using the Mayfield three-pin fixation device (Schaerer Mayfield, Cincinnati, Ohio) **(Fig. 16–11B–D)**. When draping, if extensive dural or bony resection is planned, the possible need for fascia lata or fat graft should be anticipated. If a tumor is adjacent to or extensively involves the ICA, the neck in the region of the cervical carotid artery should be prepped in anticipation of a possible need for proximal carotid artery control, or rarely, a bypass procedure.

Skin Incision

A frontotemporal incision is made beginning 0.5 to 1 cm anterior to the tragus and coursing to the midline just behind the frontal hairline **(Fig. 16–11A–C)**. If a standard pterional approach is planned (for small medial sphenoid tumors or for readily accessible lateral tumors), dissection is carried down to the temporalis muscle **(Fig. 16–12)**, and the muscle is dissected from the bone to expose the pterion.

If an orbitozygomatic osteotomy (OBZ) is planned, then the entirety of the zygoma is exposed, including the frontozygomatic process, temporozygomatic process, and malar eminence. The exposure of the malar eminence is extended laterally to a point 2 to 3 mm medial to the zygomatic facial foramen to preserve its neurovascular contents. In our early experience with the OBZ approach, the superficial layer of the temporalis fascia and its fat pad were elevated with the skin flap to preserve the frontotemporal branch of the facial nerve as described by Yasargil as we would do for a standard frontotemporal craniotomy. More recently we have elevated the temporalis fascia separately from the muscle as described by Zabramski and colleagues to avoid dissection of the superficial fat pad and further reduce the chance of injury to the frontotemporal branch of the facial nerve **(Fig. 16–13)**. The temporalis muscle is then incised and dissected off of the bone, leaving a superior cuff of muscle and fascia attached to the bone for approximation at the time of closure **(Fig. 16–14)**.

Bone Flap

For all four types of sphenoid wing region meningiomas, the first step in removing the bone flap is based around a standard frontotemporal (i.e., pterional) craniotomy. The craniotomy is accomplished by placement of one bur hole at the keyhole (i.e., a few millimeters posteroinferior to the frontal zygomatic process), a second in the squamous temporal bone immediately above the temporal zygomatic process, and a third at the posterior aspect of the exposure at the level of the superior temporal line. When anticipating an OBZ osteotomy, the keyhole bur hole is positioned so it exposes the frontal lobe dura and periorbita. The bone flap is removed with a pneumatic craniotome. The sphenoid wing between the anterior two bur holes is scored

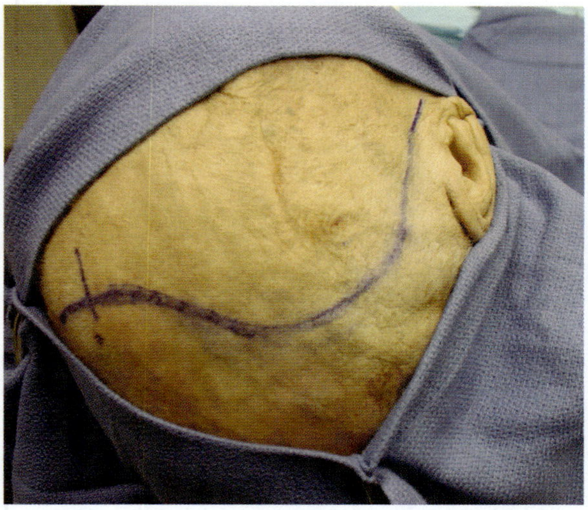

A

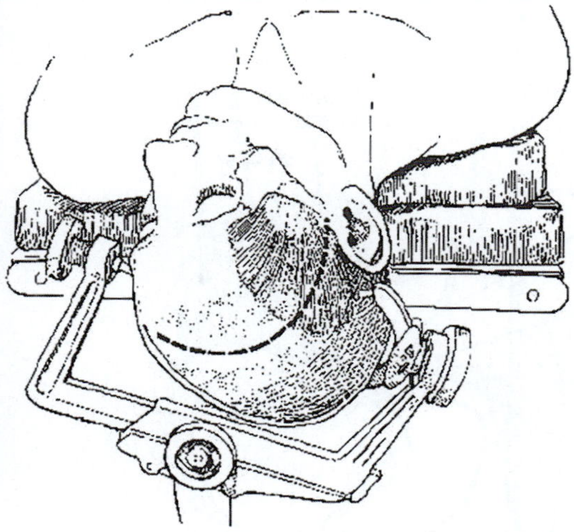

B

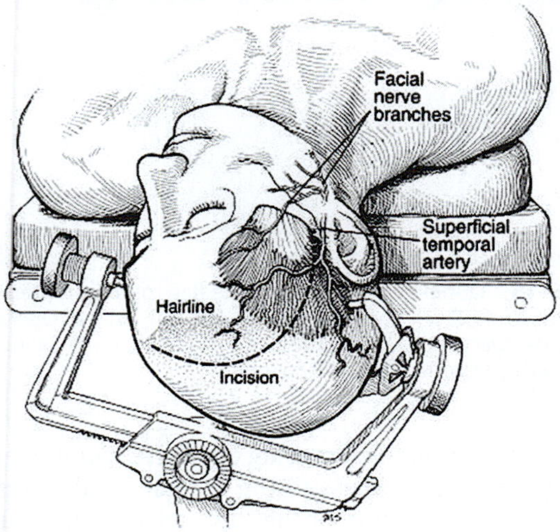

C

Figure 16–11 **(A)** Patient position and incision. **(B)** Diagram of patient position in head holder and incision. (From LeMole GM, Henn JS, Zabramski JM. J Neurosurg 99:924–930, with permission.) **(C)** Patient position, incision, and locations of critical arterial and nervous structures. (From Zabramski JM, Kiris T, Sankhla SK, et al. J Neurosurg 1998:337.)

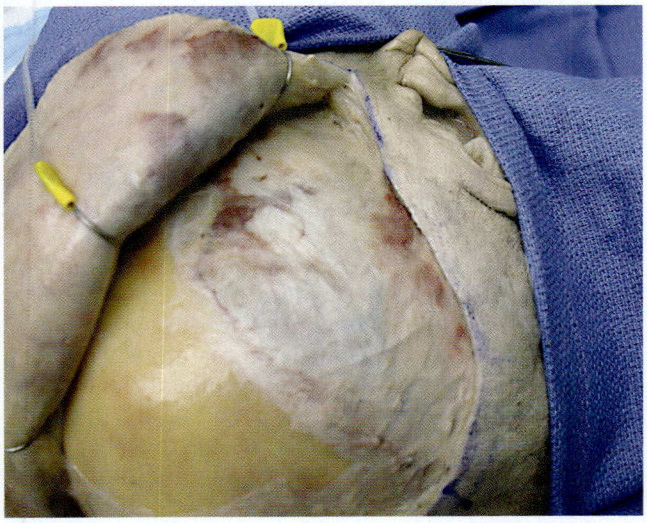

Figure 16–12 Temporalis dissection for standard frontotemporal craniotomy.

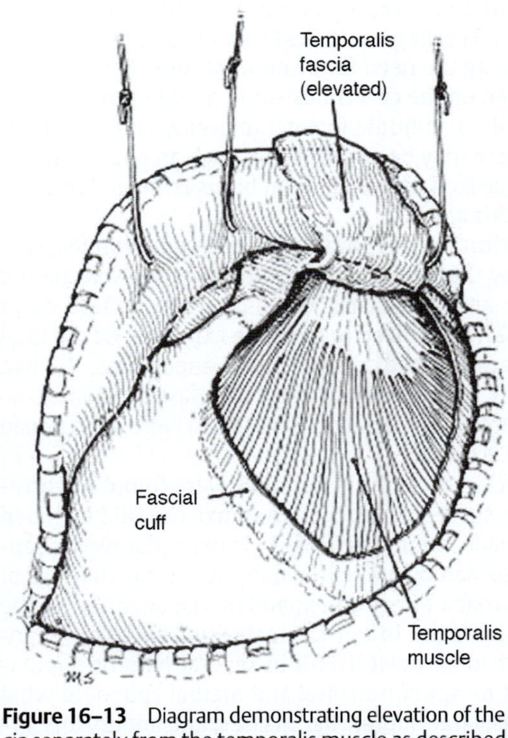

Figure 16–13 Diagram demonstrating elevation of the temporalis fascia separately from the temporalis muscle as described by Zabramski. (From Zabramski JM, Kiris T, Sankhala SK, et al. Orbitozygomatic craniotomy: technical note. Journal of Neurosurgery 1998;89:336–41, figure from 337, with permission.)

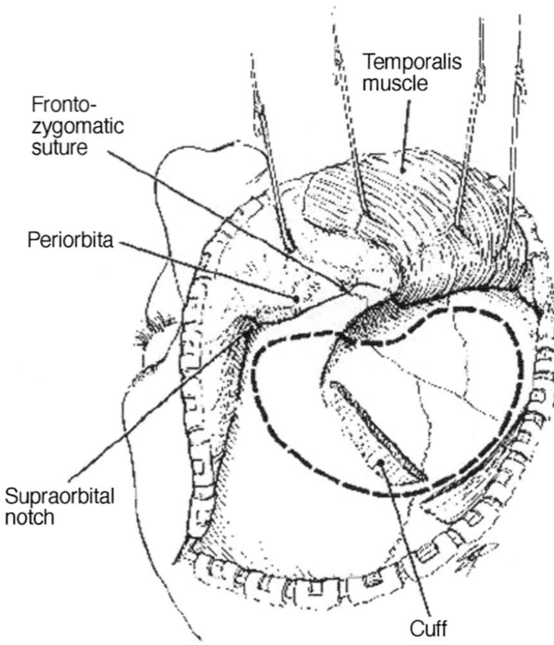

Figure 16–14 Diagram of the temporalis dissection for a frontotemporal craniotomy with orbitozygomatic osteotomy. (From Lemole GM, Henn JR, Zabramski JM. Modifications to the orbitozygomatic approach. Journal of Neurosurgery 2003;99:925, with permission.)

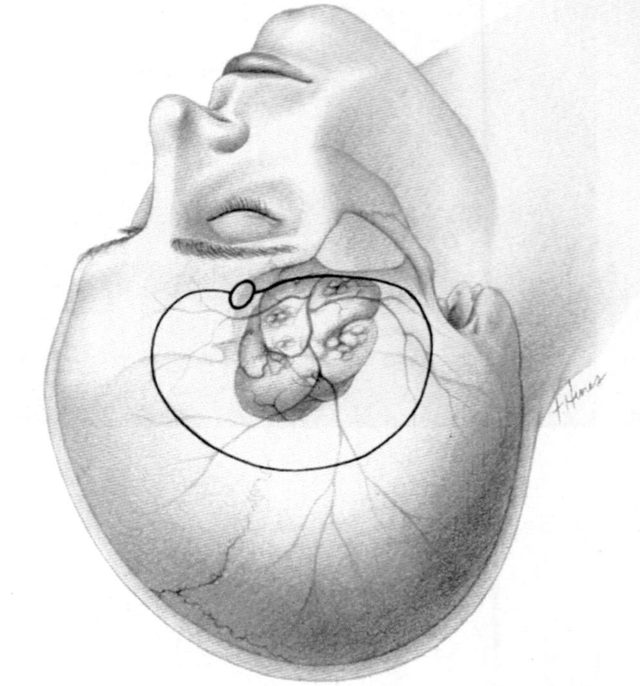

Figure 16–15 Outline of a standard bone flap for a right pterional craniotomy. (From Tew JM, van Loveren HR, Keller JT. Atlas of Operative Microneurosurgery. Vol 2, Brain Tumors. Philadelphia: WB Saunders; 2001:52, with permission from WB Saunders.)

with the drill to be fractured as the bone flap is removed **(Fig. 16–15).**

The standard frontotemporal craniotomy will be sufficient for many small medial sphenoid wing tumors and for lateral sphenoid wing tumors. For larger medial sphenoid wing tumors, spheno-orbital meningiomas, and tumors extending into the cavernous sinus, the addition of an OBZ approach is often helpful in widening the operative field and minimizing the need for brain retraction. For some tumors centered on the cavernous sinus, a more posterior approach based on a middle fossa craniotomy and a subtemporal exposure may be appropriate. Such an approach will not be emphasized in this chapter, but is reviewed in other chapters of this atlas.

At our institution, 140 frontotemporal craniotomies were performed by the senior author (MRC) over a 4-year period for vascular and neoplastic lesions. In 33 of these cases (23%), an OBZ was utilized to facilitate exposure. Of the total cases, 11 patients had a total of 16 aneurysms, 15 had meningiomas, and seven had other neoplastic lesions. Seventy-nine percent of meningiomas (15/19) were approached using an OBZ exposure.

The characteristics of a lesion that were found to correlate with the surgeon's decision to utilize the OBZ included large size, and location (particularly lesions that were deep-seated and/or had orbital extension). It is clear that use of the OBZ approach offers an expanded visualization of the middle cranial fossa. In our clinical experience this exposure was felt to be most useful in several patient populations, including spheno-orbital and medial sphenoid wing meningiomas, large suprasellar masses, and aneurysms, especially those involving the terminal segment of the ICA and the vertebrobasilar junction. Based on our experience, clinical variations on the foregoing operative requirements, including a need for access to the medial middle cranial fossa, the cavernous sinus, or the suprasellar region, ought to lead a surgeon to consider expansion of the operative exposure through the use of the OBZ technique.

Once the decision is made to add the OBZ approach, the bone flap can be removed either as two separate pieces or as one single piece. First we describe the two-piece technique. In this case, the bone flap described for a pterional craniotomy is removed, and the temporalis muscle is moved back into an anatomical position so that four bone cuts can be made to achieve the OBZ. These cuts are performed with a small-diameter side-cutting bit to optimize fit when the flap is reconstructed. Prefitting cranial fixation plates and drilling the screw holes prior to elevation of the OBZ flap facilitates correct anatomical reconstruction at the time of closure. Prior to performing the OBZ the periorbita is dissected from the superior and lateral orbital walls, avoiding exposure of periorbital fat **(Fig. 16–16A).**

After removing the frontotemporal bone flap and thinning the lateral sphenoid wing with a cutting bit, the first cut is made across the supraorbital ridge extending into the frontal craniotomy. The second cut is made across the temporal-zygomatic process. The third cut is across the malar eminence of the zygoma proximal to the zygomaticofacial foramen. The depth of the malar cut is protected with a dural elevator placed in the inferior orbital fissure (IOF) from within the orbit between the periorbita and the lateral wall of the orbit. The fourth cut is made in the roof and lateral wall of the orbit (i.e., floor of the anterior cranial fossa) from the first cut across laterally to the IOF protecting the intraorbital contents and the frontal lobe dura. This fourth

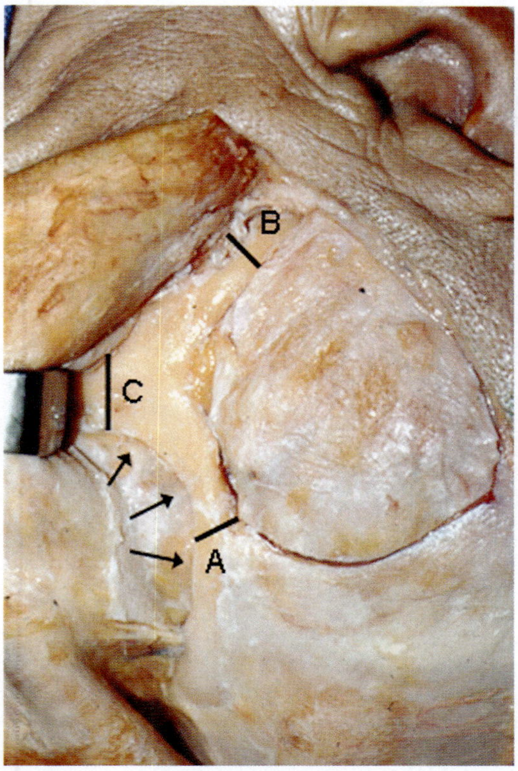

A

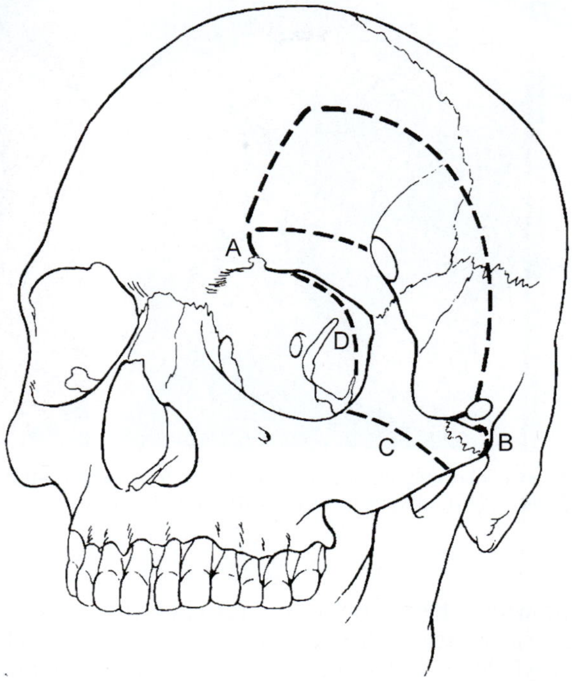

B

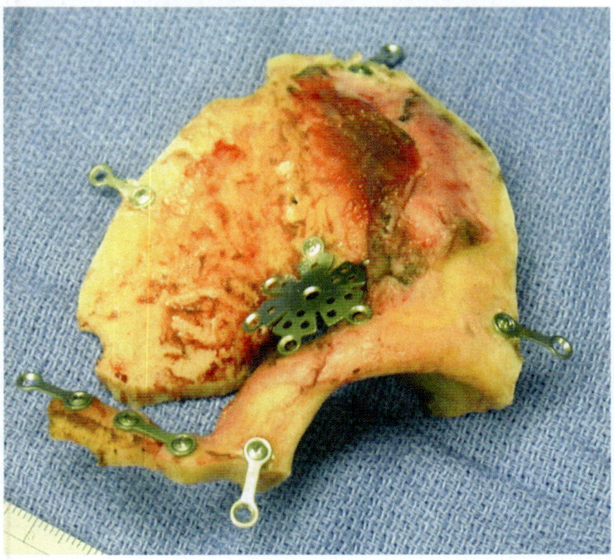

C

Figure 16–16 **(A)** Dissection of periorbita prior to orbitozygomatic (OBZ) osteotomy and bony cuts for the OBZ osteotomy indicated on dissection and on the bone flap following removal. A, supra-orbital ridge; B, temporal zygomatic process; C, malar eminence of the zygoma. Arrows indicate periorbital dissection. **(B)** Bony cuts for the OBZ osteotomy. Dashed lines indicate the cuts for a right-sided pterional craniotomy and OBZ osteotomy. Letters A through D are the cuts for the osteotomy, and cuts A, B, and C correspond to the cuts shown in **(A)**. **(C)** Single-piece, right-sided, frontotemporal OBZ bone flap.

cut can also be made with a small curved osteotome. The remaining bony connections of the lesser and greater wings of the sphenoid are fractured as the OBZ flap is reflected inferiorly as an osteoplastic flap based on the masseter. The locations of these cuts and their corresponding locations on the bone flap are indicated in **Fig. 16–16A-C.**

Alternatively, the OBZ can be taken as a single piece with the frontotemporal craniotomy. With this approach the frontotemporal craniotomy and OBZ are removed in a single piece. As already described, three bur holes are placed. The craniotomy is performed as for the two-piece technique except that the cut from the superior temporal bur hole to the frontal bone medial to the supraorbital nerve is modified. Rather than extending this cut laterally to join with the keyhole bur hole, the cut ends at the orbital rim **(Fig. 16–16B,C).** The sphenoid bone between the keyhole and inferior squamotemporal bur hole is scored with the drill.

Next the four cuts for the OBZ are made in the same fashion as for the two-piece technique. The first cut meets the anterior extent of the frontal cut of the craniotomy. Typically this cut is made lateral to the supraorbital nerve, but if necessary for exposure can be made medially in which case the bone around the supraorbital foramen is cut to mobilize the nerve. The second and third cuts are made in the temporal zygomatic process and in the malar eminence as already described. The fourth is again made from the first cut across laterally to the IOF. In making the fourth cut in the one-piece technique, the surgeon does not have the advantage of

A 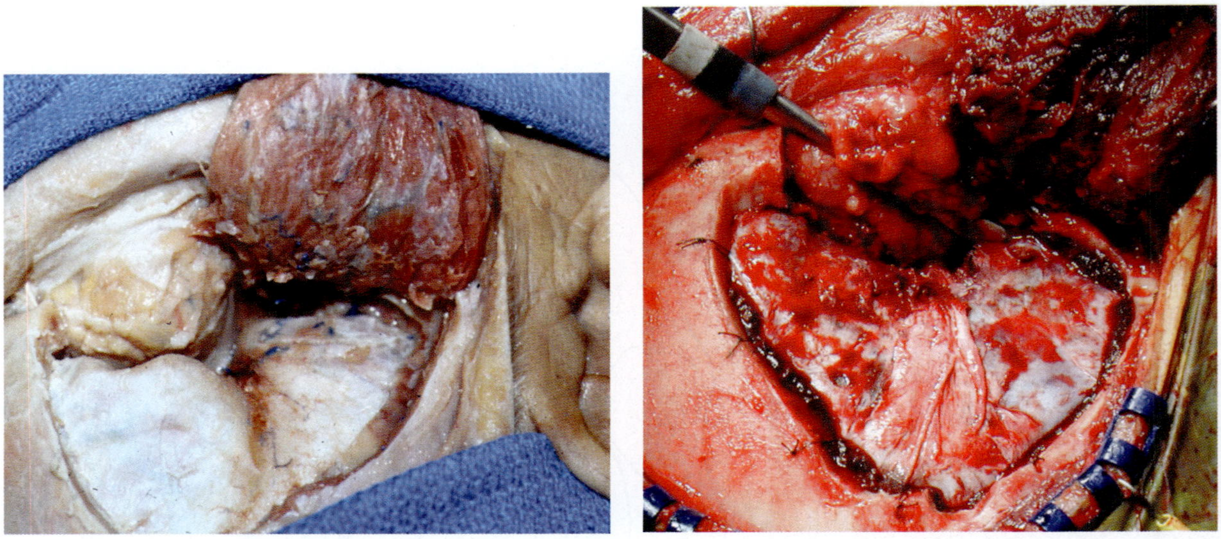 B

Figure 16–17 Appearance following removal of the bone flap for a right frontotemporal craniotomy orbitozygomatic osteotomy with the bone flap removed in a single piece. **(A)** Cadaveric dissection. **(B)** Surgical dissection.

viewing the cut from within the anterior fossa. Protection of the frontal lobe dura can be accomplished with a dural elevator through the keyhole while the cut is made from the orbital side. After all cuts have been completed, the frontotemporal craniotomy and OBZ are fractured from the sphenoid bone in a single piece **(Figs. 16–16C and 16–17).**

For spheno-orbital meningiomas, the orbital bone may be extremely hyperostotic. Removing this hyperostotic bone is a part of the frontotemporal flap, but it may require more attention if the bone is extensively thickened. Craniectomy of the hyperostotic bone may be necessary prior to elevation of the frontotemporal and OBZ flaps. Once the orbital roof has been removed, the orbit, superior orbital fissure, optic canal, and in some cases the foramen spinosum, rotundum, and second division of the fifth nerve can be unroofed in an extradural fashion. We prefer to do this with the aid of the operating microscope using small cutting and diamond burs. Following completion of bone removal, bone edges are sealed with bone wax for hemostasis, Surgicel Fibrillar (Ethicon, Summerville, New Jersey) is placed in the epidural plane at the edge of the cranial opening, and peripheral tackup sutures are placed in the dura and secured to twist holes. Attention to hemostasis is important prior to dural opening because epidural and bony bleeding is commonly encountered.

Dural Opening

When the bone flap has been removed, the dura is visible. For lateral tumors, the lesion may be visible through the dura. For more medial tumors, the brain may be under some tension, and CSF can be removed using the lumbar drain. For the standard frontotemporal craniotomy the dura is opened over the anterior and middle cranial fossae in a semicircular fashion using Metzenbaum scissors, and the dural flap is temporarily sutured to the temporalis muscle. In cases utilizing an OBZ approach, we typically open the dura using a Y-shaped incision with the main limb of the Y extending over the sylvian fissure, and the two shorter limbs extending overt the anterior aspect of the frontal and temporal dural exposures, respectively. Additional modifications of the dural opening are often necessary because large portions of dura may be resected with the meningioma itself. For laterally located and spheno-orbital tumors, some degree of tumor resection may begin at this point. For more medially located tumors and cavernous sinus meningiomas, a dissection of the sylvian fissure is required prior to resection.

Opening the Sylvian Fissure

At this point, the operating microscope is brought into the field. The arachnoid of the sylvian fissure is opened widely, beginning distally. Attention is focused on identifying distal branches of the MCA, acknowledging that more proximal vessels may be encased by tumor. The exposed brain is covered with Bicol (Codman Division of Johnson & Johnson, Raynham, Massachusetts), which we find to be less adherent to the brain than cottonoids. Brain retraction is minimized. The fissure opening is extended proximally toward the sphenoid wing. Anterior and lateral bridging veins are identified, and only if necessary, coagulated, and divided. Exposing and widely opening the basal cisterns provides additional brain relaxation and further expands the field of view. Once the sylvian fissure has been opened, self-retaining retractors are used intermittently over the frontal and temporal lobes as needed, affording visualization of the anterior and basal aspects of the meningioma but minimizing undue pressure on the brain.

Tumor Resection

The blood supply to meningiomas arises largely from branches of the external carotid artery (and in some cases from parasitization from ICA, MCA, or ACA branches). Some meningiomas contain extensive vascular networks, and therefore cutting into a heavily vascularized meningioma can result in brisk arterial bleeding. Typically, for sphenoid wing region meningiomas, extradural identification, coagulation, and sectioning of the middle meningeal artery at the foramen spinosum significantly reduce tumor vascularity.

For laterally located tumors, tumor removal begins with attention to the medial and basal aspect of the tumor, where there may be less readily accessible feeding vessels. These should be addressed and coagulated in an attempt to devascularize the tumor capsule. If the tumor is large, it may be useful to debulk prior to medial resection. If the tumor has been embolized, a large portion of the mass may be necrotic, soft, and readily removed. An ultrasonic aspirator, monopolar cutting loops, Metzenbaum scissors, or a no. 15 blade scalpel can be used at this point to assist in debulking the tumor. During medial and superior resection, close attention should be paid to vessels adjacent to the tumor capsule. The MCA is often displaced superiorly and medially by lateral sphenoid wing meningiomas. Use of cottonoids within the dissection plane can help the surgeon to separate the tumor from the brain and critical adjacent vascular structures. When the tumor adheres densely to the vessel, it is preferable to leave a small portion attached to the MCA rather than damage or sacrifice the vessel. Through repeated debulking of the tumor, with tension on and resection of the tumor capsule, an aggressive removal of the tumor can usually be achieved.

For more medially located tumors, attention is initially paid to the inferior and anterolateral aspect of the tumor. Debulking the lateral tumor mass provides improved exposure for the more delicate dissection of tumor from the involved ICA branches and the cranial nerves. Again, by identifying the plane between the tumor capsule and the brain parenchyma, dissection and subsequent resection proceed. As the resection proceeds medially into the middle fossa, the posterior communicating artery is identified and traced toward the incisura. The ICA and, at its bifurcation, the ACA and MCA vessels are identified. Tumor, wherever possible, is dissected from these vascular structures. Attention must also be paid to the small perforating vessels arising from the A_1 and M_1 segments, as damage to these vessels can cause significant morbidity.

When a sphenoid wing tumor extends anteriorly to involve the orbit and optic canal, attention must also be paid to the fragility of the optic nerve. The optic nerve is often displaced medially and superiorly by sphenoid wing tumors, and vision has often been compromised by tumor growth prior to operative intervention. The dissection must be undertaken to balance the goal of achieving a complete resection with minimization of vision loss. The tumor surrounding the proximal optic nerve is exposed and resected by elevating the frontal lobe. Prior to any significant dissection in the region of the optic nerve, the anterior clinoid process and the bone over the superior aspect of the optic canal are removed using a high-speed drill **(Fig. 16–18).** Often this is performed early in the operation, prior to the dural opening. The dura overlying the optic nerve including the falciform ligament can be opened using microscissors. These maneuvers untether the optic nerve from the optic canal, facilitating gentle mobilization for dissection and resection of the tumor.

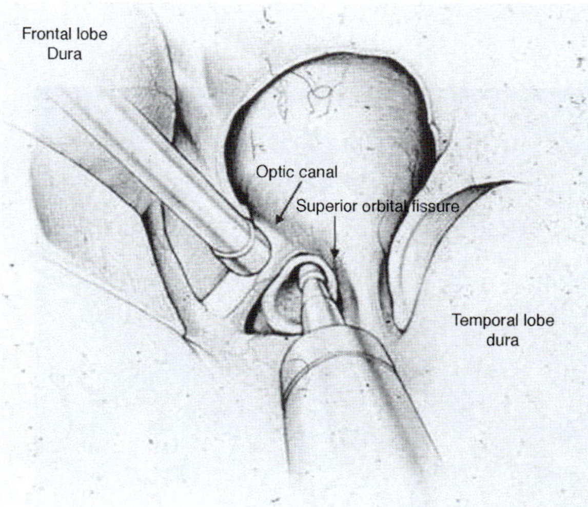

Figure 16–18 Diagram demonstrating extradural removal of the right anterior clinoid process and unroofing of the right optic canal and superior orbital fissure. (From Tew JW, van Loveren HR. Atlas of Operative Microneurosurgery.Vol. 1: Aneurysms and Arteriovenous Malformations. Philadelphia: WB Saunders; 1994:87, with permission from WB Saunders.)

Extension of a medial sphenoid wing tumor into the cavernous sinus poses a challenge to the neurosurgeon. A decision is made whether to open the cavernous sinus and attempt further resection, or as is most commonly done, to knowingly leave residual tumor in the sinus, with a potential for adjunctive postoperative radiation. The balance here lies between the potential for morbidity involving the carotid artery, venous structures, and cranial nerves III through VI with the known increased likelihood of recurrence given a subtotal resection. If tumor growth has affected the function of the intracavernous cranial nerves, resection can be undertaken with less fear of surgical morbidity. If the nerves are functioning normally preoperatively, typically the tumor is left to prevent significant postoperative morbidity. If intracavernous resection is undertaken, a preoperative temporary balloon occlusion test may be appropriate in conjunction with preoperative angiography with consideration for carotid occlusion or sacrifice with tumor resection, but rarely would we advocate such an approach.

Following resection of the bulk of the tumor, the surgeon will have good visualization of the sphenoid ridge. All dural attachments should be removed. Any bone that appears involved should also, when feasible, be removed.

Closure

The dura should be approximated primarily wherever possible. When tumor location has necessitated extensive dural resection, fascia lata autograft or dural replacement graft can be used to reconstruct and close the dura. We typically prefer bovine pericardium. In cases of deep dural resection, approximation may not be possible. In these cases an autologous adipose graft may be utilized to augment dural closure. When resection requires removal of hyperostotic or tumor infiltrated bone, reconstruction of the orbit or adjacent bony

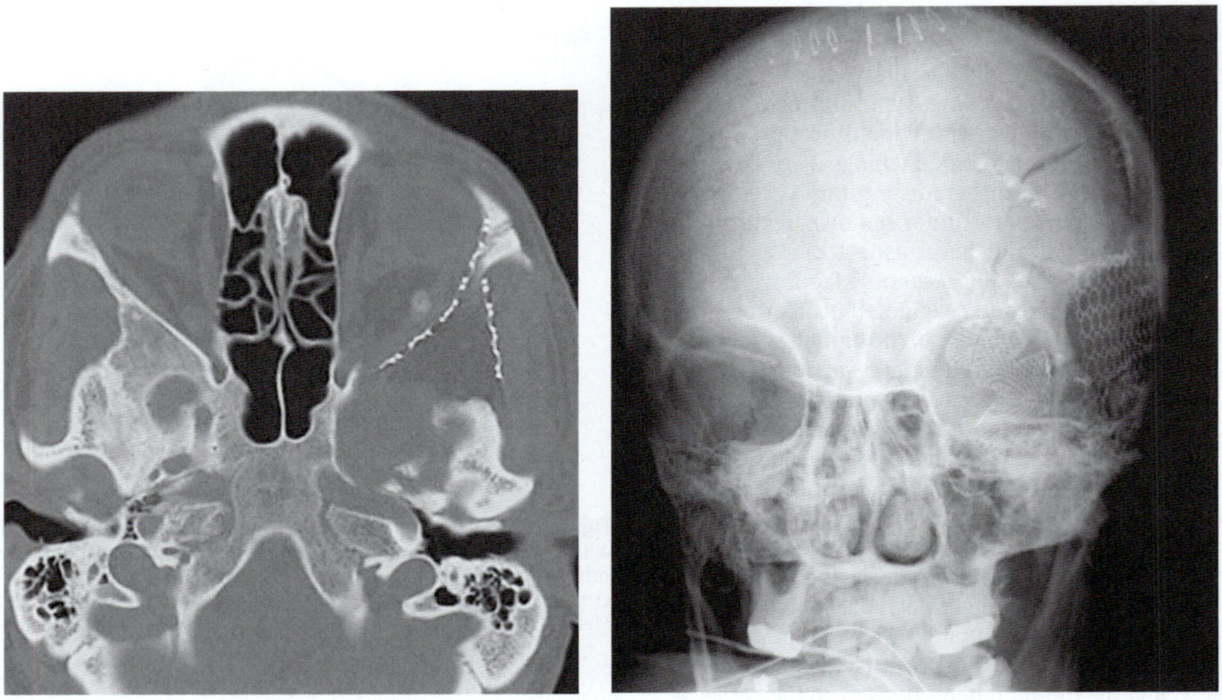

A B

Figure 16–19 Reconstruction of the orbit using titanium mesh. **(A)** Axial bone-window CT of head. **(B)** AP Skull x-ray.

structures is performed using titanium mesh **(Fig. 16–19).** This is often done with the assistance of an ophthalmological surgeon. "Dead space" from resection of large areas of hyperostotic bone or extracranial tumor is also obliterated using autologous adipose tissue from the thigh or abdominal region. Once reconstruction of dura and the orbital walls is complete, the bone flap is replaced, or if largely removed with the tumor, the squamous temporal bone is reconstructed with titanium mesh, acrylic cranioplasty, or other bone substitutes **(Fig. 16–20).** The flap is secured with cranial fixation plates and screws. The temporalis muscle is reapproximated, and the galea is closed with absorbable sutures. The skin is closed with staples or interrupted nonabsorbable suture.

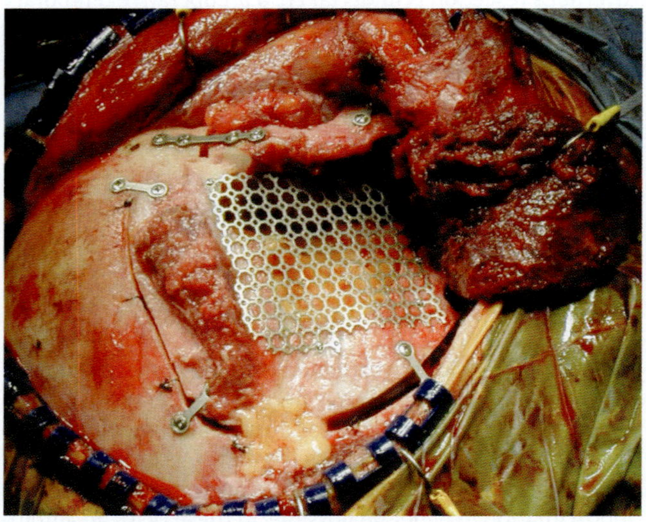

Figure 16–20 Replacement of a bone and soft tissue defect following removal of a hyperostotic right spheno-orbital meningioma using titanium mesh and autologous adipose.

◆ Postoperative Management

Patients are typically extubated immediately postoperatively, continued on corticosteroids, and admitted to the intensive care unit. Antiepileptic medications are continued for at least 1 week postoperatively, at the discretion of the treating surgeon. Postoperative cerebral edema can be problematic, particularly for larger medial sphenoid wing tumors, and patients may require osmotic therapy with mannitol in addition to corticosteroids. If there is significant concern for residual tumor, higher histopathological grade (WHO grade II or III), or other features that increase the potential for recurrence, the patient may undergo fractionated radiation or radiosurgery after full recovery.

◆ Conclusions

Tumors arising from the sphenoid wing region are varied in their extent, location, and complexity. Considering them as a functional unit, however, gives the surgeon the ability to understand how variations on and modifications of the standard frontotemporal craniotomy can give the surgeon more control over tumor resection and the ability to minimize postoperative surgical morbidity.

17

Surgical Management of Convexity Meningiomas

Michael P. Steinmetz, Ajit Krishnaney, and Joung H. Lee

◆ Patient Selection

Convexity meningiomas (CMs) are meningiomas arising from the meninges overlying the frontal, temporal, parietal, and occipital cortex, and not involving any of the major dural venous sinuses, the tentorium, or the falx cerebri. Clinical presentation may vary depending on the tumor's particular location. Seizures, headaches, and focal neurological deficit(s) are common presentations. With wide use of computed tomography (CT) and magnetic resonance imaging (MRI) done today as part of routine evaluations for headaches, minor head trauma, and various neurological complaints such as dizziness and visual changes, incidental meningiomas are being detected with an increasing frequency. Surgical removal of CMs is one of the most rewarding procedures performed by neurosurgeons because the surgery is often straightforward and the outcome excellent, with complete resection providing a cure for most patients.

MRI provides accurate diagnosis. On T1-weighted MRI, the majority of meningiomas are isointense, whereas the remainder are slightly hyperintense to the gray matter. Gadolinium-enhanced T1-weighted images reveal dramatic and usually homogeneous enhancement in meningiomas and, often, their associated "dural-tail." **(Fig. 17–1A,B)**. On T2-weighted sequences, nearly 50% of all meningiomas are hyperintense, whereas the other half are isointense to the gray matter. T2-weighted sequence is also highly sensitive in delineating the extent of peritumoral edema. However, dural-based metastasis, lymphoma, sarcoid, hemangiopericytoma, sarcoma, and pleomorphic xanthoastrocytoma have been found in patients who were thought to have a CM based on their preoperative MRI scans. These lesions, therefore, should be included in the differential diagnosis for patients presenting with an extra-axial lesion overlying the cerebral convexity. Cerebral angiography is rarely needed for most patients with CMs. In our practice, a preoperative embolization is considered only for patients with large CMs (>6 to 7 cm) **(Fig. 17–1C-F)**.

Surgery is the treatment of choice for most patients with CMs. Primary goals of surgery include (1) total resection of the tumor and the involved surrounding bone and dura when possible, and (2) reversal or improvement in neurological deficits/symptoms caused by the tumor. Given the benign nature of meningiomas and the established efficacy of adjuvant radiation, the goal of total removal must be balanced by the physician's basic credo to "do no harm." When total removal carries a significant risk of morbidity, a small piece of tumor may be left, with further plans of observation followed by reoperation or radiation when the tumor is noted to be growing or causing new symptoms. However, observation alone, with periodic (usually yearly) follow-up neurological and MR evaluations, is reasonable for elderly patients, especially if they have minimal or no symptoms caused by the tumor. Because people are living healthier and longer lives today, the age at which a person is considered "elderly" is debatable. The patient's absolute age is no longer important in the decision-making process in the management of convexity meningiomas; however, it may be reasonable to consider those with less than 10 to 15 years remaining in their life expectancy as elderly. In addition, observation may be an appropriate option for the following people regardless of their age: (1) patients with incidental small tumors with no surrounding edema, and (2) patients who insist on nonintervention after a thorough discussion of all treatment options. However, these patients must be compliant with the necessary radiographic and neurological follow-up evaluations.

◆ Preoperative Management

Symptomatic patients with a significant amount of peritumoral edema seen on T2-weighted MRI may be started on dexamethasone as an outpatient with surgery planned within 1 to 2 weeks. Anticonvulsants are started preoperatively only for patients who present with seizures. Otherwise, a loading dose of phenytoin is given at induction of anesthesia and then therapeutic levels are maintained postoperatively for up to several weeks, depending on the tumor size, brain manipulation required during surgery, and extent of perioperative swelling. For tumors large enough to cause visual symptoms/deficits or located in the occipital region, a detailed preoperative ophthalmologic evaluation, including a formal visual field testing, is obtained. Preoperative embolization is reserved for patients with large CMs (>6 to 7 cm).

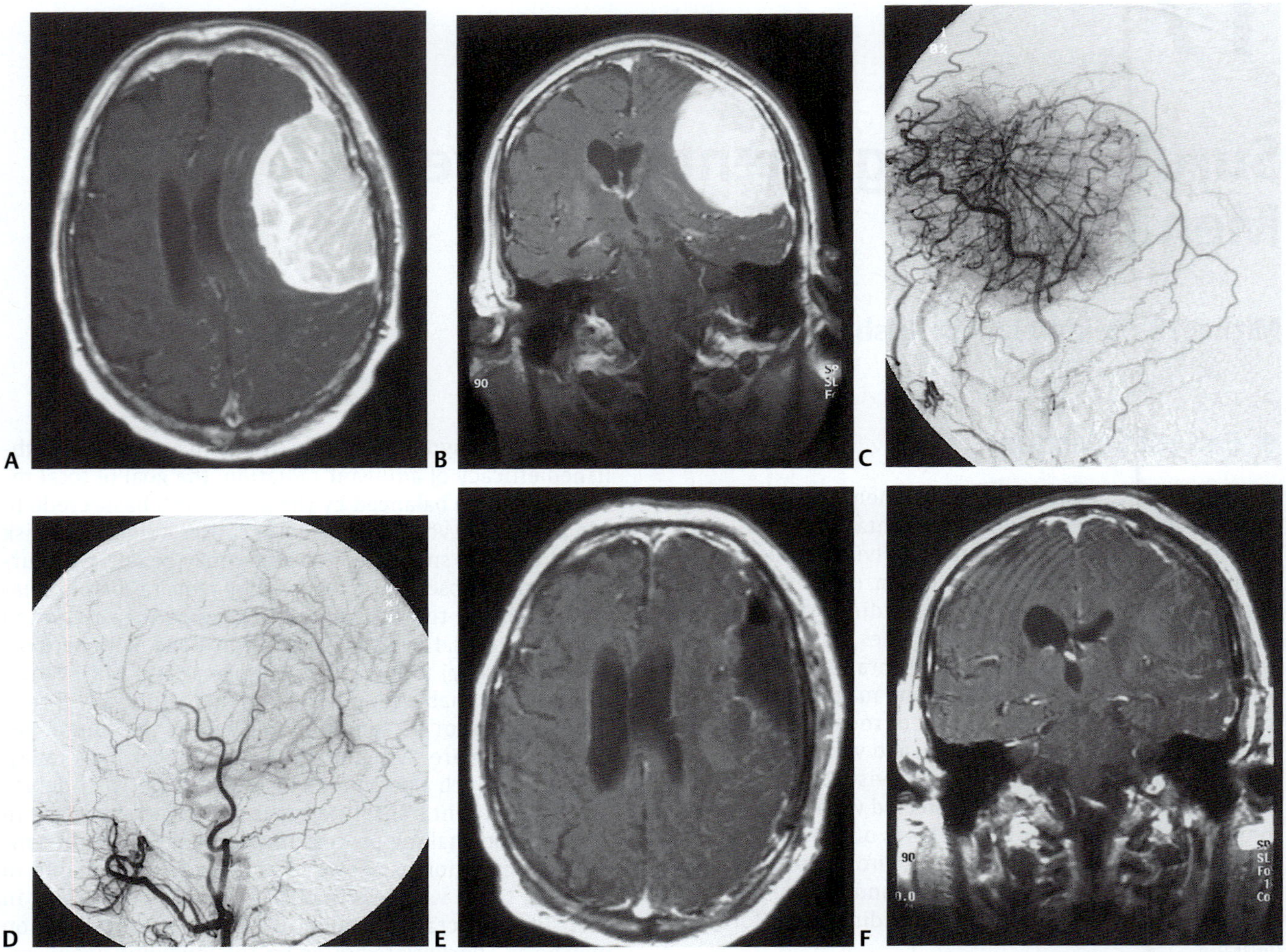

Figure 17–1 **(A,B)** A large left frontal convexity meningioma is demonstrated. There is mass effect involving the frontal and temporal lobes. **(C)** Angiography demonstrates a significant tumor blush, **(D)** which has resolved following embolization. **(E,F)** Using the techniques outlined in the chapter, the tumor was removed successfully and there is significant resolution of the mass effect.

◆ Operative Procedure

Convexity meningiomas require surgical approaches that are primarily dictated by their locations. The following, which are general principles for meningiomas of most locations, hold true for CMs as well:

1. Optimal patient positioning, incision, craniotomy, and tumor exposure
2. Early tumor devascularization
3. Internal decompression/extracapsular dissection
4. Preservation of adherent or adjacent neurovasculature
5. Removal of involved dura and bone
6. Closure

Patient Positioning, Skin Incision, Craniotomy

The patient positioning, appropriate incision placement, and selection of the optimal approach for tumor exposure are the critical elements of successful meningioma surgery. The patient is positioned in such a way that safety is maximized. Moreover, the ideal position must allow for an approach that provides complete exposure of the tumor and the involved surrounding bone and dura. At the same time, maximal brain relaxation must be achieved by use of gravity and uncompromised venous drainage. The head should be no lower than the level of the heart, regardless of the position selected, and undue severe neck rotation or flexion must be avoided. In addition, the surgeon's comfort for the duration of surgery must be maintained.

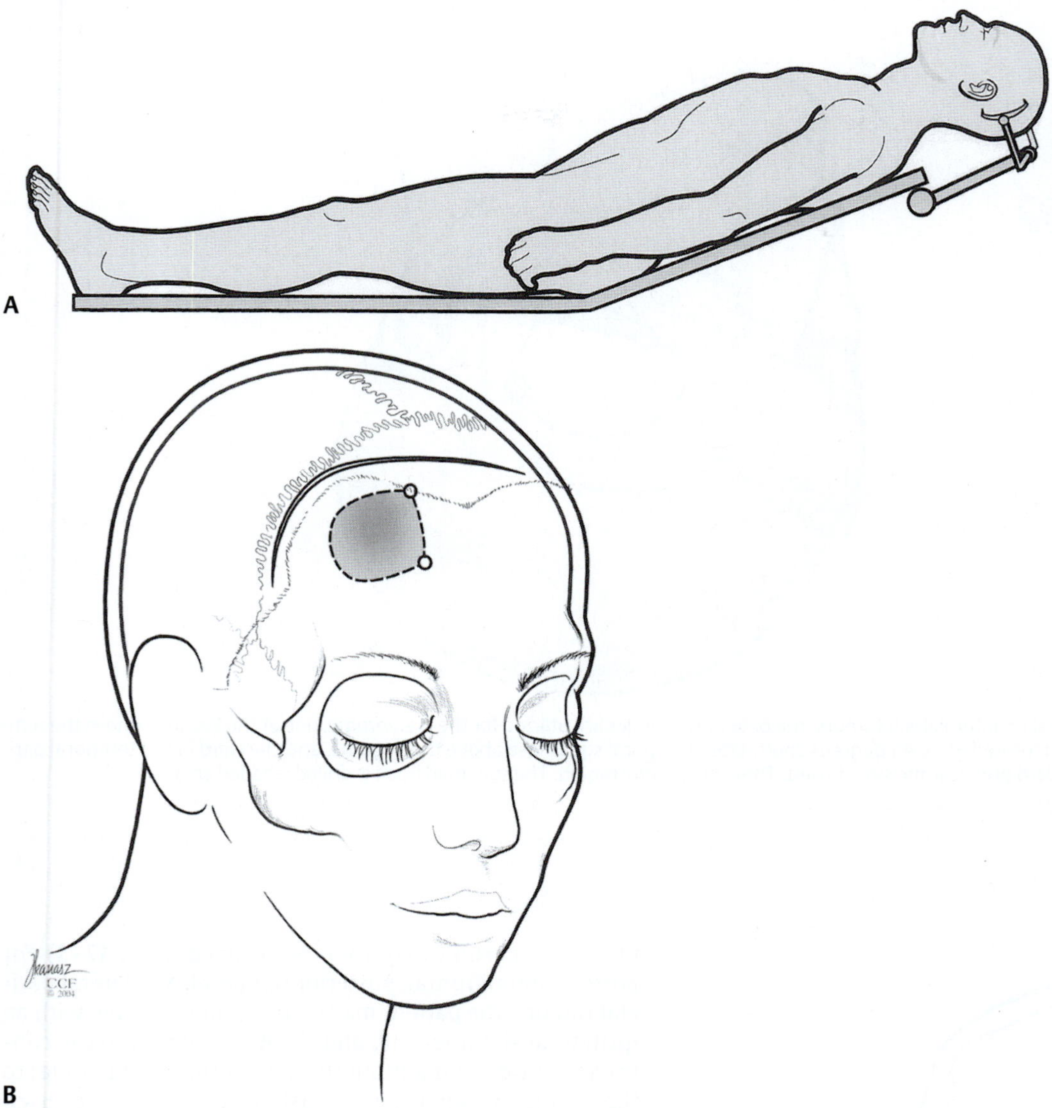

Figure 17–2 **(A)** For anterior frontal tumors, the patient is positioned supine with the nose straight up. **(B)** The incision extends from the side of the tumor above the zygoma and across the midline immediately behind the hairline. The length of the incision depends on the size of the planned craniotomy. The authors prefer to place two bur holes in the midline or immediately off the midline. The lower bur hole is placed immediately above the frontal sinus.

Depending on the tumor location, the patient may be positioned supine or prone. The planned scalp flap should contain the tumor in the center. Of important note, the incision must be planned to avoid any visible cosmetic defect or significant compromise to the scalp vascular supply. If a horseshoe-shaped incision is planned, the depth must not exceed the width of the flap. The size of the scalp and bone flaps must be large enough to allow for maximal exposure of the tumor, the involved bone and dura, as well as the limits of the dural tail, as noted on preoperative MRI scans. With the availability of frameless computer-assisted navigation systems, the exact extent of the tumor and the dural tail may be fully delineated during surgery. Computer-assisted navigation may also aid in accurate and optimal placement of the incision and craniotomy, especially in patients with a small CM.

For anterior frontal tumors, the patient is positioned supine with the nose straight. A bicoronal incision placed within the hairline is utilized **(Fig. 17–2),** For frontotemporal or anterolateral tumors, the patient is positioned supine with the head turned to the side contralateral to the tumor by 30 to 45 degrees. A standard curvilinear

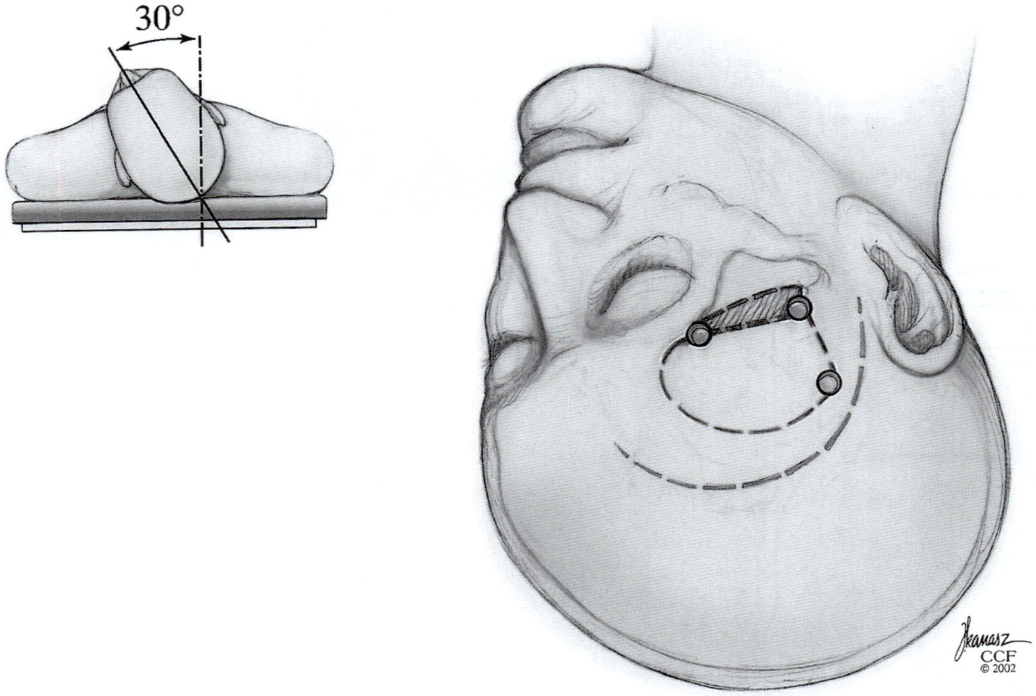

Figure 17–3 For frontotemporal or anterolateral tumors, the patient is positioned supine with the head rotated 30 to 45 degrees contralateral to the side of the tumor. A standard pterional incision is used. Three bur holes are utilized for the craniotomy, one at the keyhole, one in the temporal squamosa above the zygoma, and the third in the temporal parietal region. The sphenoid bone is drilled (shaded area).

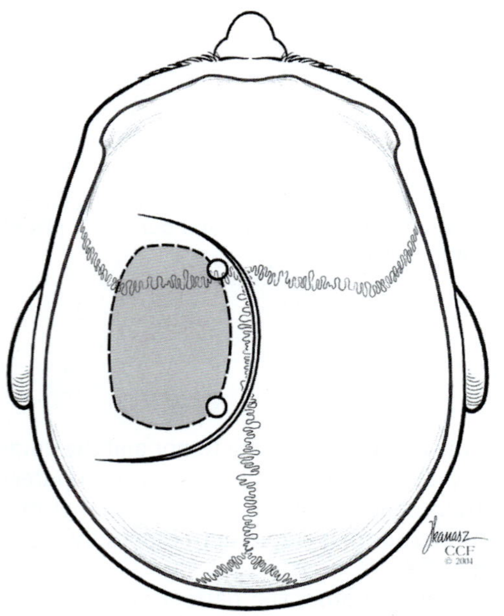

Figure 17–4 For posterior frontal and parietal tumors, the patient is positioned supine. The head is rotated until the side of the head is parallel to the floor. A horseshoe incision is utilized. Two bur holes are used based on the midline or immediately off the midline.

pterional incision may then be utilized. **(Fig. 17–3)** For posterolateral frontal, posterior temporal, and lateral parietal tumors, the patient may be positioned supine, with an ipsilateral shoulder roll, and the head rotated to the contralateral side to maintain the side of the head parallel to the floor. A horseshoe incision may then be used **(Fig. 17–4).** Lastly, for tumors located in the medial parietal or occipital regions, the authors prefer the prone position **(Fig. 17–5).**

A craniotomy is planned large enough to completely expose the tumor and the surrounding involved dura, as delineated by gadolinium-enhanced T1 MRI, with a 1- to 2-cm circumferential margin. After making one or two bur holes, craniotomy is performed. The free bone flap is dissected off of the underlying dura with the aid of Penfield dissectors. In patients with severe calvarial involvement by the tumor, performing a craniotomy around the tumor, followed by lifting off of the free bone flap as previously described, may be difficult or harmful to the underlying brain. Instead, the tumor eroding through the calvarium is removed with a rongeur, and the margin of skull defect through which the tumor eroded is removed either with a rongeur or with a high-speed 6-mm cutting bur until normal dura is exposed circumferentially around the tumor.

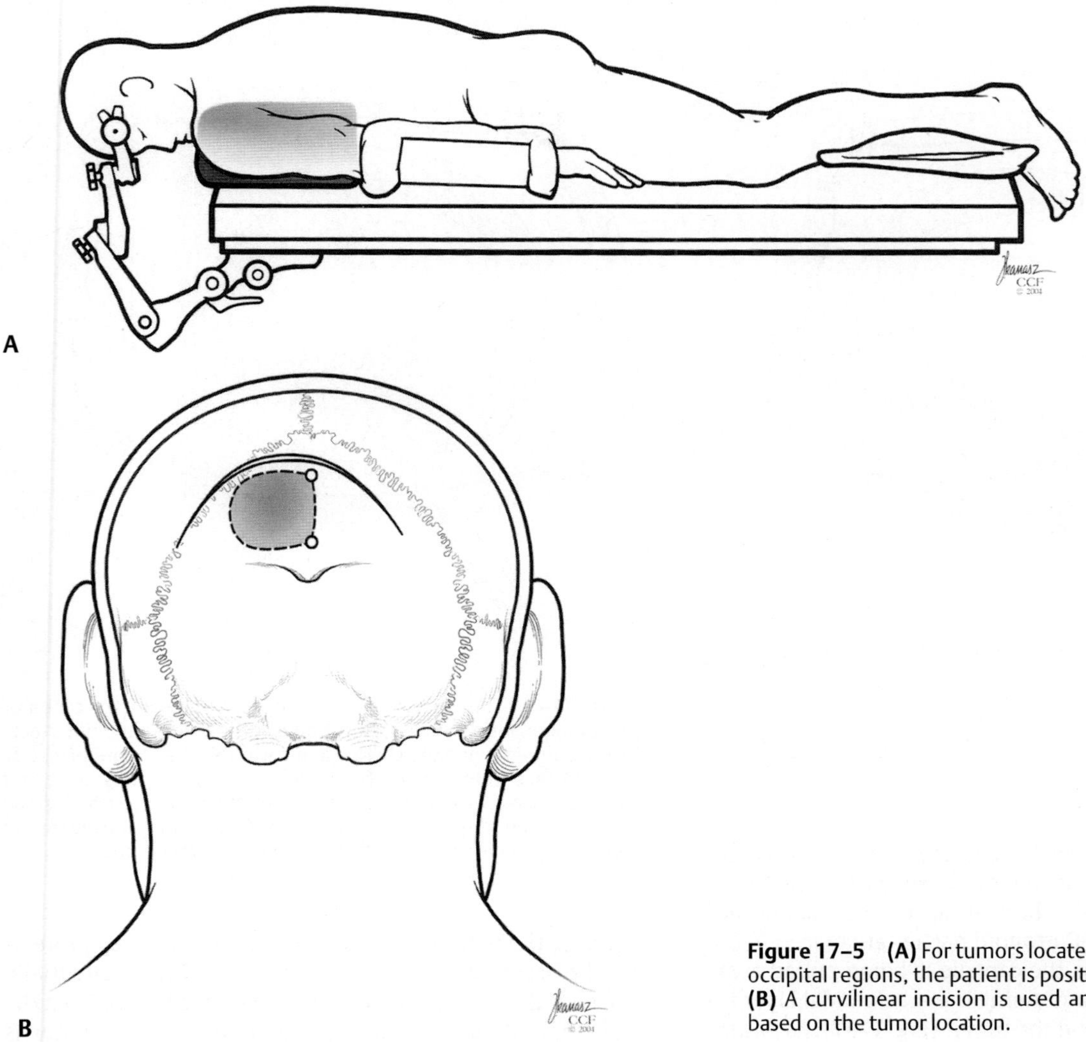

Figure 17–5 **(A)** For tumors located in the posterior parietal or occipital regions, the patient is positioned in the prone position. **(B)** A curvilinear incision is used and a craniotomy is planned based on the tumor location.

In most situations, several options exist in selecting the patient's position, incision, surgical approach, and exposure. The final selection must be based on what is best for the patient and the surgeon, based on the surgeon's knowledge, past experience, and preference.

Tumor Devascularization

Meningiomas may be quite vascular, and therefore, early tumor devascularization is paramount. Preoperative embolization may be utilized for large CMs. In CMs not embolized, upon dural exposure prior to opening the dura, extra time should be expended to coagulate all of the tumor-feeding vessels—most commonly the branches or the main trunk of the middle meningeal artery.

Internal Decompression and Extracapsular Dissection

The dura is next opened sharply with a 1-cm border beyond the tumor or the dura involved by tumor **(Fig. 17–6).**

Although small meningiomas may be removed en bloc, internal decompression is a key initial step in actual tumor removal for most sizeable meningiomas, including those of the convexity locations, following adequate exposure and initial devascularization. Internal debulking is performed until a thin rim of exposed portion of the tumor is remaining. This internal debulking minimizes brain retraction and facilitates extracapsular dissection. Following initial internal decompression, extracapsular dissection is initiated by identifying a layer of arachnoid (maintained in most meningiomas) at

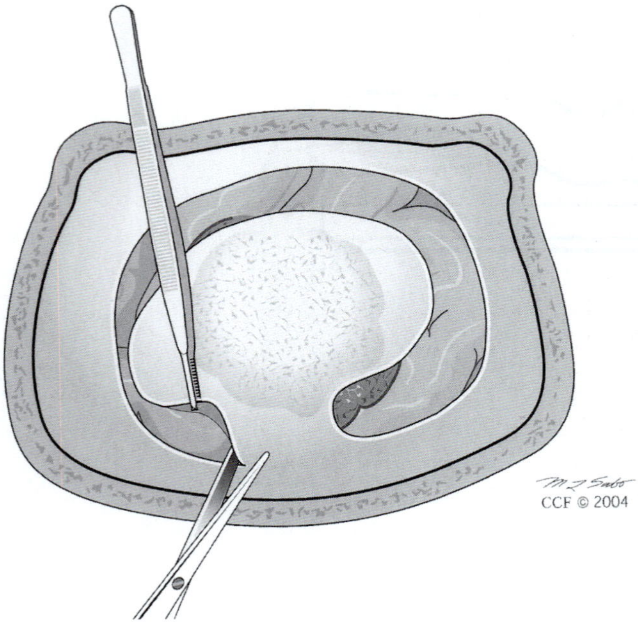

Figure 17–6 The dura is incised surrounding the tumor, ideally with a 1-cm margin.

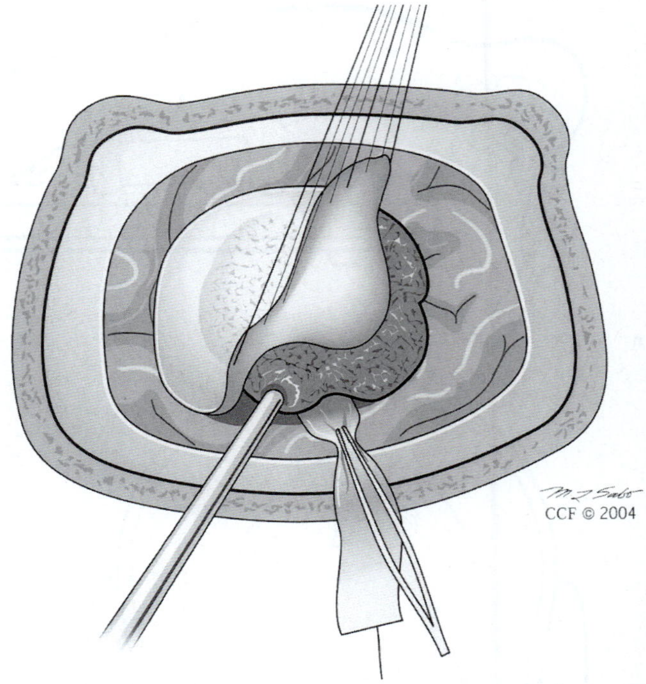

Figure 17–7 The capsule of the tumor is pulled toward the center of the tumor exposing a layer of arachnoid at the brain–tumor interface. This arachnoid is opened sharply and cottonoid patties are placed at this interface between the brain and tumor. As patties are being placed sequentially around the tumor, they are used to gently strip the arachnoid from the tumor capsule, covering the brain and arachnoid together, thereby protecting the brain from surgical trauma.

the brain–tumor interface. As surgery progresses, rather than increasing brain retraction to expose more of the tumor hidden under the brain, the thinned capsule is pulled toward the center of the tumor. Cottonoid patties are placed in the brain–tumor interface as the capsule is being pulled away from the brain, while maintaining the arachnoidal layer intact between the brain and the tumor **(Fig. 17–7).** As patties are being placed sequentially around the tumor, they are used to gently strip the arachnoid from the tumor capsule, covering the brain and arachnoid together, thereby protecting the brain from surgical trauma. Patties are sequentially placed until the tumor is completely dissected free from the brain **(Fig. 17–8).** After complete dissection, the tumor is completely removed from the brain, thus exposing the tumor bed and the patties **(Fig. 17–9).**

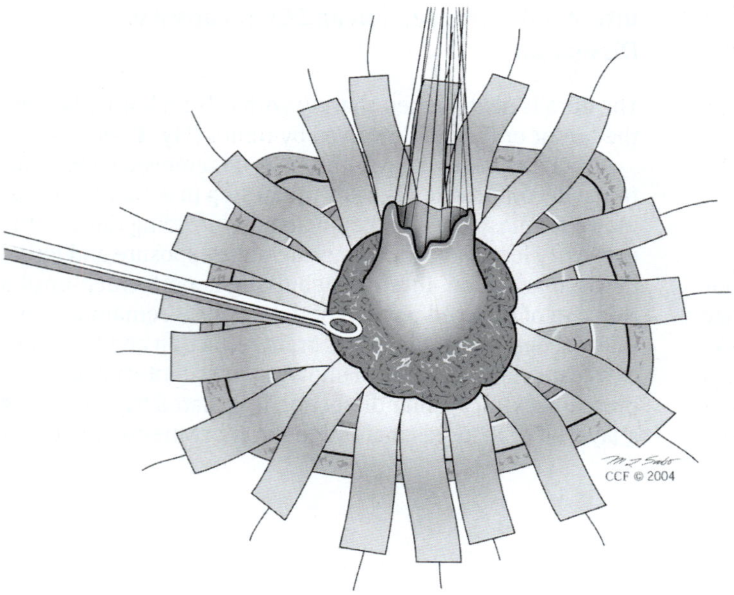

Figure 17–8 Patties are sequentially placed between the brain and tumor until it is completely dissected free from the brain.

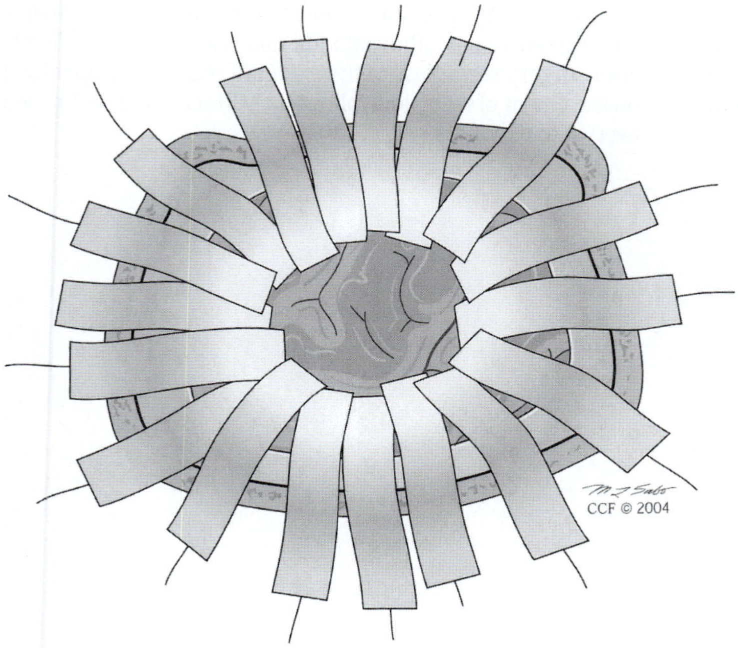

Figure 17–9 After the tumor is completely dissected free, it is removed from the brain thus exposing the tumor bed and the patties that have been placed.

Preservation of the Adherent or Adjacent Neurovasculature

During extracapsular dissection, any adherent sizeable cortical veins are carefully dissected and preserved to prevent any risk of postoperative venous infarction. Small arteries attached to the tumor surface are thoroughly inspected. As a rule, no artery or arterial branch is sacrificed except when the vessel is definitely confirmed to be a tumor feeder. Commonly, loops of vessels may be encased by the tumor or may course onto the capsule surface and become adherent. In these situations, the surgeon may initially misinterpret these vessels as tumor feeders. Before concluding that a vessel is a tumor feeder and therefore amenable to coagulation, the afferent and efferent course of the vessel must be fully appreciated. It is very rare for meningiomas to have feeders directly from major intracranial arterial trunks or their main branches. Therefore, no vessels coming directly off the MCA or its main branches in a large CM overlying the sylvian fissure should be coagulated. If any appreciable vasospasm occurs while dissecting tumor off arteries, small pieces of Gelfoam soaked in papaverine applied directly onto the vessel readily reverse the spasm.

Portions of tumor capsule are sequentially devascularized and completely dissected from the surrounding cortical surface, and blood vessels are further removed in segments until the entire tumor is removed.

Removal of the Involved Dura and Bone and Closure

After tumor removal, the undersurface of the remaining dural margin is carefully inspected circumferentially. The bone flap is also carefully examined, and any bone involvement is removed. This may easily be performed with a high-speed cutting bur.

The dural defect may be repaired with a commercially available dural substitute. Currently, the authors prefer to use synthetic collagen-based dural substitutes. A synthetic graft may simply be laid over the dural defect without the need for suture. The bone flap is then replaced and secured with titanium miniplates. When there is a cranial defect following removal of the involved calvarium, cranioplasty is performed using methylmethacrylate.

◆ Postoperative Management

Follow-up evaluations consist of careful neurological examination and MRI scans with and without gadolinium. Steroids, started preoperatively on patients with CMs causing neurological symptoms or those with radiographic peritumoral edema, are gradually weaned over several days. An antiepileptic, usually phenytoin, is administered for 1 to 6 weeks, depending on the tumor size, brain manipulation required during surgery, and extent of perioperative swelling. For patients with preoperative visual field defect due to occipital CMs, detailed neuro-ophthalmologic evaluations are an important part of follow-up management. Following resection of all meningiomas, a postoperative baseline MRI scan is obtained on day 1 or 2 after surgery. For benign tumors, following confirmation of total removal on postoperative MRI, further follow-up evaluation with imaging studies is performed every 1 to 5 years, depending on whether a Simpson grade I or II removal was achieved. Following a rare instance of subtotal CM removal, subsequent follow-up with MRI is done every year, with plans of either repeat surgery or adjuvant radiation if and when there is clinical or radiographic progression of the residual tumor. If the tumor is noted to be clinically and radiographically stable for a few years after initial surgery, the frequency of follow-up may be decreased to every 2 to 3 years.

For atypical meningiomas, after initial postoperative MRI following either subtotal or total removal, subsequent evaluations with MRI are performed every 6 months for the first 2 years. As with benign tumors, radiation or a repeat surgery is considered in the presence of documented clinical or radiographic progression of the residual tumor. With malignant meningiomas, adjuvant radiation is administered shortly after surgery regardless of the extent of resection. Depending on the extent of resection, follow-up MRI scans are performed every 3 to 6 months.

18

Surgical Technique for Removal of Clinoidal Meningiomas

Joung H. Lee, James J. Evans, Michael P. Steinmetz, and Jeong-Taik Kwon

Clinoidal meningiomas (CMs) are meningiomas arising from the meningeal covering of the anterior clinoid process (ACP). These tumors have been referred to by various other terms, such as medial or inner sphenoid wing meningiomas. In the literature predating the wide use of magnetic resonance imaging (MRI), which aids in correctly identifying the site of origin in most meningiomas, CM was often reported under the loose category of "suprasellar" meningiomas. In large meningiomas encompassing both the cavernous sinus (CS) and the clinoidal region, the exact site of origin, based on preoperative imaging studies, or at times even after an intraoperative inspection, is often difficult to determine. In these large tumors, the clinoidal origin is assumed in our practice if greater than two thirds of the tumor is extracavernous in location. Those tumors extending to the clinoidal region, but originating from the tuberculum sella, optic canal, orbital roof, planum sphenoidale, or middle or lateral aspects of the sphenoid wing, are not considered as CMs.

◆ General Considerations for Removal of Clinoidal Meningiomas

In 1983, Dolenc introduced an extradural technique of complete removal of the ACP. This technique, described as a component of a more extensive approach, was originally advocated as a critical step necessary to gain safe entry into the CS for direct surgical management of intracavernous vascular lesions. Later, the "Dolenc approach" was utilized for CS tumors, clinoidal segment internal carotid artery (ICA) and upper basilar aneurysms, and giant pituitary adenomas. Subsequently, a few others presented their experience with this technique, with some modifications, applied to surgery of a small number of parasellar/periclinoid region tumors such as craniopharyngiomas and suprasellar meningiomas.

Removal of the ACP provides improved exposure of the optic nerve (ON) and the ICA, enhancing access to the pathology around these structures as well as within the optic canal. Additionally, by opening the optic nerve sheath (ONS) as an extension of the dural incision following anterior clinoidectomy, the ON can be decompressed and visualized early and mobilized safely during surgery, thereby reducing the risk of intraoperative injury to the ON. In cases of large tumors encasing the ON and the ICA, the traditionally recommended surgical technique for removal has been to first identify the distal middle cerebral artery (MCA) branches and follow these vessels proximally toward the ICA with further tumor removal and dissection. However, until the ICA and eventually the intradural ON are located, surgery progresses very slowly. More importantly, the risk of intraoperative neurovascular injury persists during surgery because the exact location of the ON and ICA remains unknown to the surgeon, and the ON remains compressed. During this time, any minor surgical retraction, dissection, or tumor manipulation may add further compression to the ON, especially against the falciform ligament. To circumvent these critical problems, the ON can be exposed and simultaneously decompressed early in the surgery by unroofing the optic canal, followed by anterior clinoidectomy and then opening the ONS. The location of the optic canal, and therefore, the intracanalicular segment of the ON, is fairly constant; only the intradural cisternal segment of the ON varies in location depending on how the tumor causes nerve displacement during its growth. The exposed ON can then be followed from the optic canal proximally, toward the tumor in the intradural location. As tumor resection progresses further, the ICA can be readily found adjacent to the exposed distal intradural segment of the ON. Complete ONS opening, along the length of the nerve within the optic canal to the anulus of Zinn, relieves any focal circumferential pressure on the ON contributed by the falciform ligament. ON decompression, thus achieved, leads to reduced intraoperative injury to the nerve because the force of retraction is then dispersed over a much larger surface area. Moreover, if the tumor recurs, because the ON is already decompressed from the surrounding falciform ligament and optic canal, the patient's impending visual deterioration may be delayed.

In this chapter, we describe a skull base technique, modified from the original Dolenc approach, consisting of extradural clinoidectomy coupled with optic canal unroofing and ONS opening. We also outline several key advantages provided by the skull base technique, and our current indications for its use. The advantages provided by the skull base technique include (1) early localization and exposure of the ON and the adjacent ICA, (2) complete decompression and mobilization of the ON, (3) expansion of various operative windows, (4) facilitation of access to difficult locations, and (5) facilitation of aggressive removal of tumor, as well as the involved bone and dura.

◆ Patient Selection

Indications for the use of the skull base technique for CMs (and other tumors in the periclinoid region) in our practice include those lesions (1) causing ON or chiasmatic compression based on preoperative ophthalmologic evaluations, (2) encircling or covering the ON and ICA on preoperative MRI studies, (3) extending into the optic canal, subchiasmatic/infraoptic regions, or CS, (4) in patients with limited operative windows (e.g., patients with prefixed chiasm), and (5) causing extensive involvement of the surrounding bone and dura. When tumors are relatively small (3 cm or less) and not causing any significant preoperative visual deficits, surgical resection can be done utilizing standard pterional craniotomy without the added skull base exposure.

For relatively young patients, those with at least 15 years remaining in their life expectancy, we recommend surgery at the time of tumor detection regardless of the size, even in incidental tumors. This immediate intervention is a conscious attempt to provide these patients with total resection and the best possible outcome before these tumors become larger and pose increased surgical risks.

Alternatives to Surgery

Treatment options other than surgery include observation and radiation therapy. Final treatment plans must be individualized for each patient based on age, overall condition, and the patient's personal wish after a thorough discussion of all options. Because people are living longer and healthier lives, there is no specific age limit above which no surgery is recommended. However, given the fact that many meningiomas are slowly progressive, nonoperative options may be considered for patients with less than 10 to 15 years remaining in their life expectancy. Observation alone is reasonable for patients in this group if they have minimal or no symptoms; for those in this age group with significant neurological deficits or with documented radiographic progression, radiation therapy or radiosurgery may be a good option. Radiosurgery can be utilized for lesions less than 2.5 to 3 cm in diameter. However, the tumor's proximity to the optic apparatus must be carefully analyzed to avoid any radiation injury to the optic nerve/chiasm. For those patients with residual tumors following initial resection, adjuvant radiation, either in the form of radiosurgery or radiation therapy (conventional or conformal) depending on the size and proximity to the optic apparatus, may be considered.

◆ Preoperative Management

Symptomatic patients with a significant amount of peritumoral edema seen on preoperative T2-weighted MRI may be started on dexamethasone as an outpatient for 1 to 2 weeks. Anticonvulsants are started preoperatively for patients who present with seizures. Otherwise, a loading dose of phenytoin is given at induction of anesthesia, and then therapeutic levels are maintained postoperatively for 1 to 6 weeks, depending on the tumor size, brain manipulation required during surgery, and extent of pre- and postoperative swelling. All patients undergo detailed neuro-ophthalmologic evaluations pre- and postoperatively.

Routine preoperative angiogram is no longer performed in these patients in our practice. In the past, patients with large clinoidal tumors completely circumscribing the ICA and its branches underwent a test balloon occlusion (TBO) of the ICA. Such information may be helpful because it allows the surgeon to plan the extent of resection around the ICA. For patients passing the TBO, an aggressive tumor resection may be pursued, and in the rare event of intraoperative ICA injury, the surgeon has the options of direct ICA repair, bypass, or ICA sacrifice. However, if the patient does not pass the TBO, tumor resection around the ICA may be more limited to prevent a devastating stroke. Another option is to perform an arterial bypass in preparation for an aggressive tumor resection. Embolization is not possible in these tumors because their main vascular supply is from branches of the ophthalmic artery, ICA, and surrounding small pial vessels.

◆ Operative Procedure

The same basic principles of meningioma surgery apply to CM removal as well, with minor modifications dictated primarily by the unique anatomical considerations inherent to the clinoidal region. These basic surgical principles, applicable to CM, include (1) optimal patient positioning, incision, bone removal; (2) when possible, tumor devascularization; (3) early localization, exposure, and decompression of the ON and ICA; (4) following the ON and ICA into the tumor; (5) internal tumor debulking; (6) extracapsular devascularization and dissection; (7) preservation of the adherent/surrounding neurovasculature; (8) removal of the involved bone and dura; (9) dural reconstruction and closure.

The surgical steps involved in the skull base technique utilized in removal of CMs can be summarized as follows: (1) frontotemporal craniotomy, (2) sphenoid ridge drilling, (3) limited posterior orbitotomy, (4) posterolateral orbital wall removal (to completely decompress the superior orbital fissure), (5) optic canal un-roofing, (6) complete extradural anterior clinoidectomy, and (7) dural opening, with dural incision extending into the falciform ligament and the ONS.

Positioning

After induction of general anesthesia, the patient is placed in the supine position, with the head fixed in a Mayfield three-pin head holder. The head is then rotated 30 degrees to the side contralateral to the tumor. The head of the bed is elevated ~20 degrees.

Incision

A standard curvilinear frontotemporal incision is made following injection of 15 mL of 0.5 % Xylocaine/1:200,000 epinephrine. The incision is initiated just above the palpated zygoma, 1 cm anterior to the tragus, extending superiorly, then curving anteriorly from the superior temporal line to the midline, just to the limit of the hairline. The skin flap and the underlying temporalis fascia/muscle are elevated and reflected anteriorly as separate layers.

Craniotomy

A standard frontotemporal craniotomy is performed. The craniotomy is extended into the anterior frontal region by 1.5 to 2 cm from the "key hole," made parallel to the superior orbital rim to allow for subsequent extradural exposure of the orbital roof and optic canal. The size and shape of the frontal sinus are carefully appreciated from the preoperative MRI, so that if possible, entry into the lateral margin of the frontal sinus is avoided during the frontal extension of the craniotomy. If the frontal sinus is entered, it is repaired with a temporalis muscle graft followed by reinforcement with a pericranial flap.

Skull Base Technique

The lateral sphenoid ridge is drilled, followed by performing a limited posterior orbitotomy. The sphenoid bone drilling is achieved by using a 6-mm round cutting bur. Orbitotomy and subsequent skull base drilling are then performed using a 4-mm coarse diamond bur. The posterolateral orbital wall is then removed to completely decompress the superior orbital fissure. The roof of the optic canal is then drilled with a diamond bur. During this stage, copious irrigation is critical to prevent potential ON damage by the heat generated from drilling. The bone overlying the optic canal is made paper-thin with the drill, and the remaining bone is then easily removed using a microdissector or a microcuret. While the medial aspect of the optic canal roof is being drilled, entry into the ethmoid or sphenoid sinus must be avoided. If an entry is made, a small temporalis muscle graft is used to cover the opening at the time of closure, further reinforced using a piece of blood-soaked Gelfoam. This extradural dissection and exposure requires some degree of frontal lobe retraction. Rather than using a fixed retraction system, we prefer dynamic retraction utilizing the suction tip held in one hand of the surgeon to gently retract the brain. Although many neurosurgeons advocate using lumbar cerebrospinal fluid (CSF) drainage, in our practice the lumbar drain is not used. We believe that the CSF in the subarachnoid space (including within the ONS) protects the brain and ON from intraoperative injury.

After exposure of the ON within the optic canal is completed, the dura is then circumferentially dissected off the ACP. The ACP is now ready to be removed. In situations of significant hypertrophy of the ACP, the center of the ACP and hypertrophied optic strut is drilled, followed by removal of the remaining ACP by using a small straight-tipped Lempert rongeur. With nonhypertrophic ACP removal can be done by gently manipulating the ACP to fracture the optic strut. During this maneuver, one must be careful not to cause any damage to the adjacent ON, ophthalmic artery, or anterior loop of the ICA. If the fracture technique cannot be performed using minimal force, then the remainder of the ACP can be drilled intradurally under direct visualization. Often, brisk venous bleeding is encountered from the triangular space occupied by the removed ACP. This can be readily controlled by gently packing the extradural triangular space with a small piece of Gelfoam. Aggressive packing should be avoided to minimize compressive injury to the ON or the oculomotor nerve. A brief summary of these extradural steps is as follows: (1) a standard frontotemporal craniotomy, (2) lateral sphenoid wing removal, (3) posterior orbitotomy, (4) complete bone removal surrounding the superior orbital fissure, (5) optic canal unroofing, and (6) anterior clinoidectomy **(Figs. 18–1 through 18–4).**

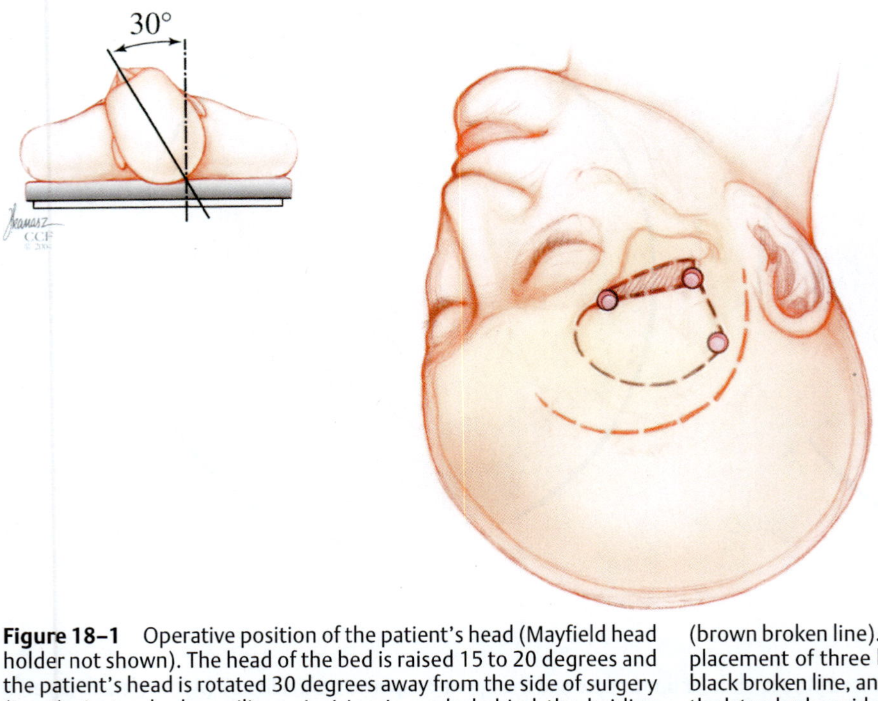

Figure 18–1 Operative position of the patient's head (Mayfield head holder not shown). The head of the bed is raised 15 to 20 degrees and the patient's head is rotated 30 degrees away from the side of surgery (inset). A standard curvilinear incision is made behind the hairline (brown broken line). A frontotemporal craniotomy is turned following placement of three bur holes. The craniotomy flap is depicted by the black broken line, and the shaded area represents the bone drilled from the lateral sphenoid wing after performing the craniotomy.

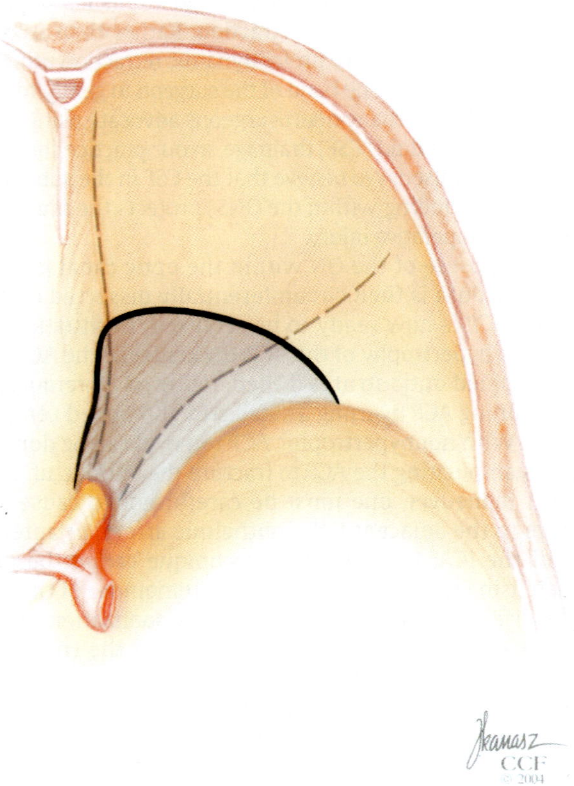

Figure 18–2 The shaded area depicts the bone removed during the skull base technique, including the lateral sphenoid wing, posterolateral orbital wall, posterior orbital roof, optic canal roof, and anterior clinoid process.

Dural Opening

The dura is opened in two steps. First, a frontotemporal curvilinear opening is made centered over the sylvian fissure, followed by a second incision bisecting the dural flap directed toward the falciform ligament. An operating microscope is brought in at this point, and the dural incision is continued from the falciform ligament along the length of the exposed ONS within the optic canal, extending to the anulus of Zinn. Cutting of the falciform ligament, and subsequently the ONS, is best performed by using a right-angle arachnoid knife or a "beaver blade." This completes the full exposure and decompression of the extradural ON, which can then be followed easily toward the tumor with exact knowledge of the ON's location (**Figs. 18–5 through 18–7**). The intradural ICA, located immediately lateral to the prechiasmatic ON, is easily identified by dissecting and removing tumor around the already exposed ON. In comparison, **Fig. 18–7** upper left depicts the conventional intradural exposure, not utilizing the skull base technique and opening of the ONS, in which the tumor is noted to be covering all the critical neurovascular structures.

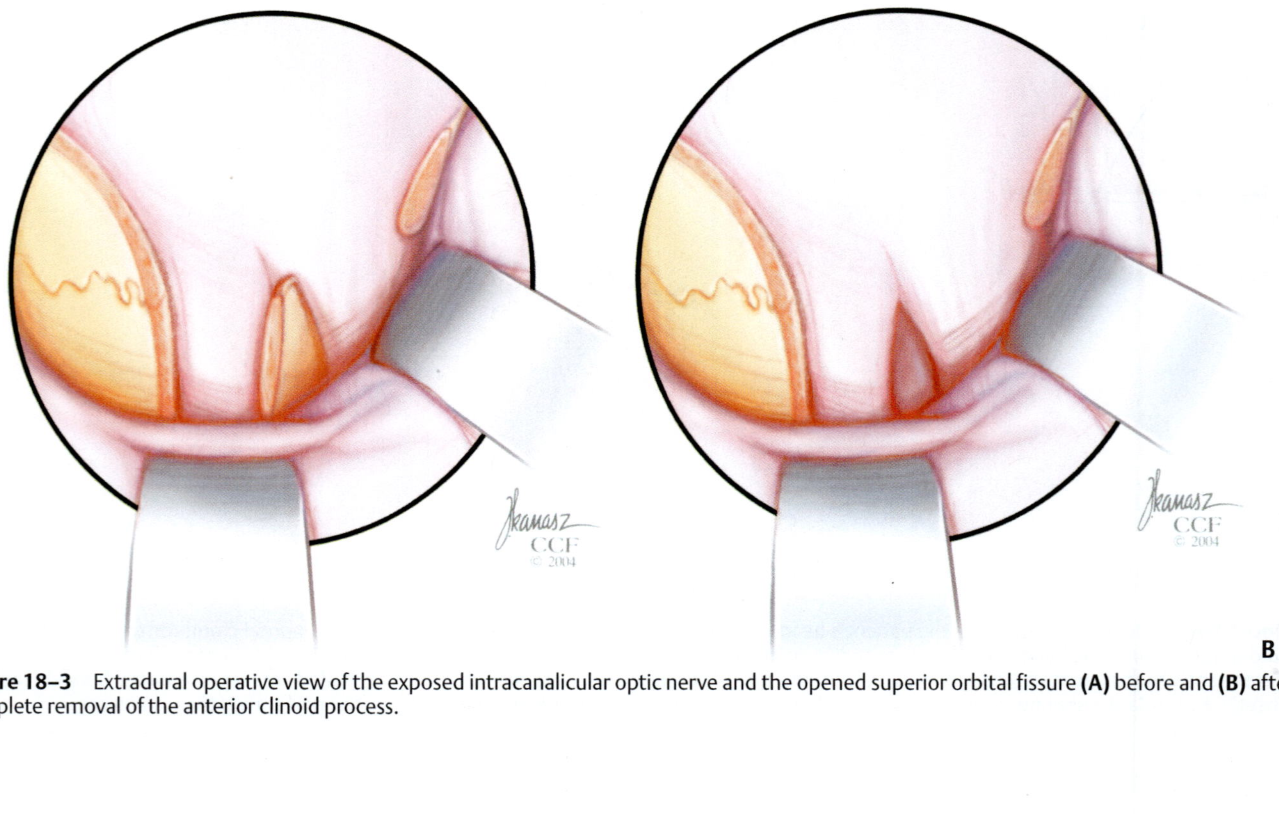

A B

Figure 18–3 Extradural operative view of the exposed intracanalicular optic nerve and the opened superior orbital fissure **(A)** before and **(B)** after complete removal of the anterior clinoid process.

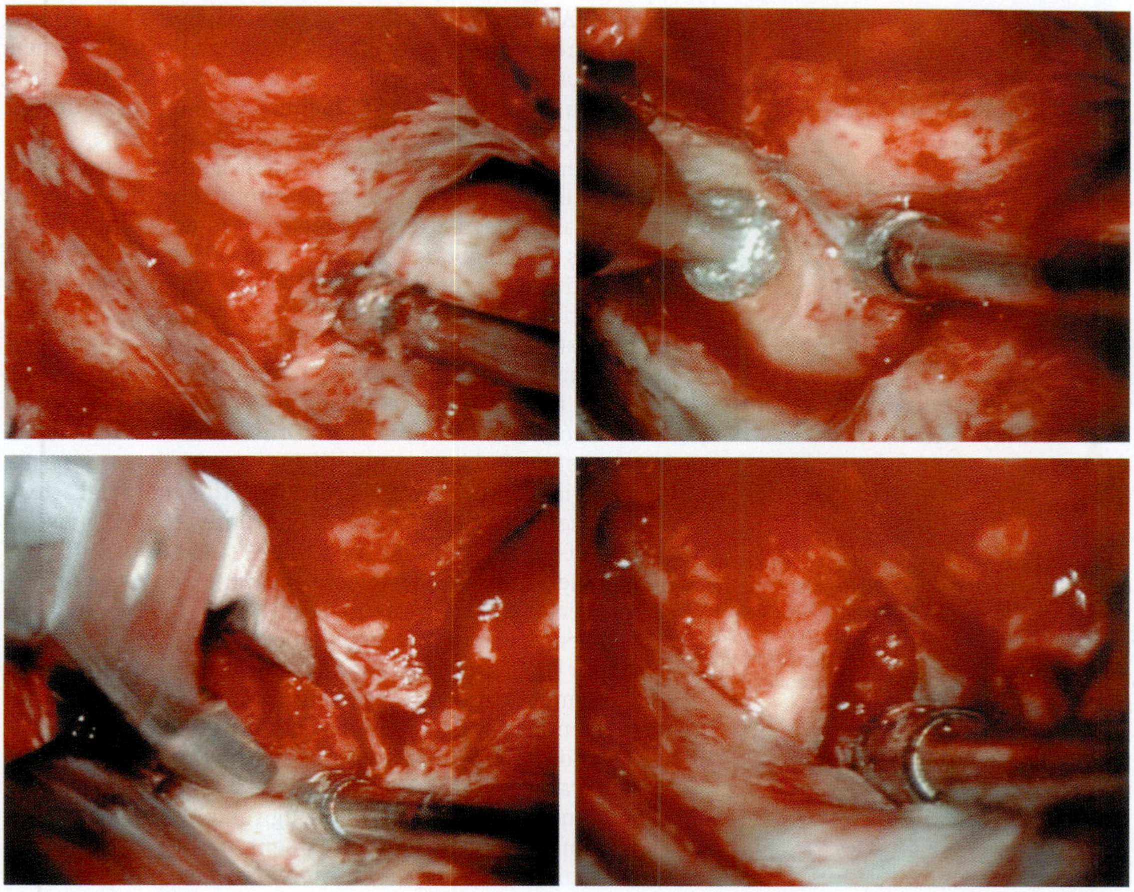

Figure 18–4 Intraoperative photographs of the right-sided extradural skull base technique. Upper left: Posterior orbitotomy is completed, and the superior orbital fissure is completely opened. Upper right: Unroofing of the optic canal is being performed with a 4-mm diamond bur. Lower left: The anterior clinoid process (ACP) is being manipulated to fracture off of the remaining attachment at the optic strut. Lower right: Extradural view of the exposed intracanalicular optic nerve after completion of the skull base technique including extradural removal of the ACP.

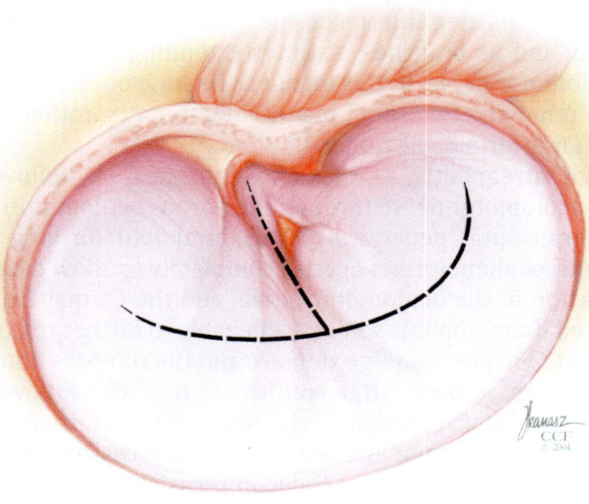

Figure 18–5 Extradural view after completion of the skull base technique, including (1) frontotemporal craniotomy, (2) lateral sphenoid wing removal, (3) posterior orbitotomy, (4) superior orbital fissure decompression, (5) optic canal unroofing, and (6) extradural anterior clinoidectomy. The dural incision (broken line) is made in two steps: First, a frontotemporal curvilinear opening is created, centered on the sylvian fissure, followed by bisection of the dural flap toward the optic sheath and extending across the falciform ligament and to the anulus of Zinn.

Tumor Removal

Although the tumor may completely cover, circumscribe, and/or displace the intradural ON and the ICA, with the ON now exposed and decompressed, and with the intradural ICA localized, subsequent tumor removal can progress with ease. Moreover, because the ON is no longer compressed by the falciform ligament following complete opening of the ONS, the ON can now be safely manipulated and gently retracted to enlarge the interoptic and opticocarotid spaces during subsequent tumor removal. The undersurface of the ON and chiasm is also readily and safely explored. In most cases, as the arachnoid around the ON and ICA is maintained, careful dissection of the tumor off of these critical neurovascular structures is possible. Tumor extension into the optic canal is also removed, with care exercised to prevent any damage to the ophthalmic artery. The tumor is removed, in large part, using suction and bipolar coagulation. In firm tumors, an ultrasonic aspirator or careful use of microscissors facilitates piecemeal removal. Central tumor debulking facilitates dissection of the tumor off of the surrounding critical neurovascular structures.

After initial debulking of the anterior aspect of the tumor, having established the exact intradural locations of the ON

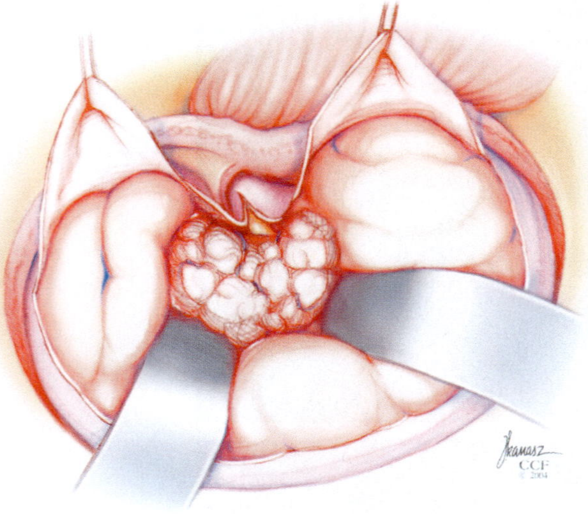

Figure 18–6 View of a clinoidal meningioma following completion of the skull base technique and extending the dural incision into the optic sheath. The optic nerve is readily identified in the exposed optic canal and completely decompressed at the onset of tumor removal. Tumor resection progressed by following the optic nerve proximally. The combination of early identification and decompression leads to prevention of intraoperative optic nerve injury.

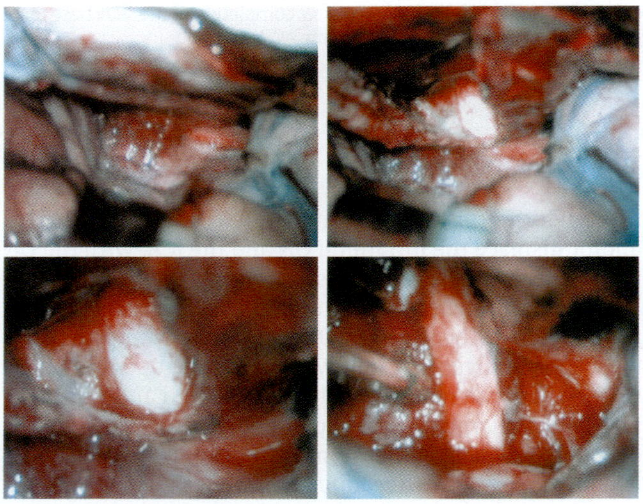

Figure 18–7 Intraoperative photographs of tumor and optic nerve exposure. Upper left: View of the clinoidal meningioma following a conventional technique of tumor exposure, not utilizing the skull base technique. Note that the tumor covers the optic nerve and internal carotid artery (ICA). Upper right: Following completion of the skull base technique, the optic nerve within the canal is readily localized. The initial dural flap has been bisected with microscissors. The optic sheath has not been opened. Lower left: The same view as the Upper right under higher magnification. Lower right: The optic nerve is completely exposed and decompressed by opening the optic sheath. A linear contusion is seen where the falciform ligament was compressing on the nerve. The optic nerve is further exposed proximally as tumor removal progresses. The ICA (not shown) can be readily located just lateral to the exposed intradural optic nerve.

and ICA, attention may be directed at exposure and removal of the remainder of the tumor. The sylvian fissure is opened, and both the frontal and temporal lobes gently retracted. Particular attention is paid to preserve branches of the ICA and MCA. In large tumors, several arterial branches are often seen coursing into the tumor or around the capsule. Until their final course can be determined, confirming that these are indeed arterial branches feeding the tumor, the vessels should not be sacrificed. When dissecting the tumor off of the ON or the chiasm, fine vessels coursing on the undersurface (which provide main blood supply) to the optic apparatus must be preserved. In dissecting the tumor extending into the suprasellar region, the pituitary stalk, which is usually displaced posteriorly and medially, must be recognized and preserved. Other neurovascular structures of critical importance include the oculomotor nerve, posterior communicating artery, anterior choroidal artery, and their branches, which are encountered during dissection of the inferior pole, and the A1 and M1 main trunks and their branches, which are encountered during dissection/removal of the posterior segment.

When dealing with a large tumor (>5 or 6 cm), the senior author (JHL) prefers to approach the tumor by subdividing the tumor into several segments or poles: (1) the anterior segment, located directly above the anterior prechiasmatic ON and the proximal ICA (proximal to the posterior communicating artery). This is the anterior pole of the tumor first encountered upon following the intracanalicular ON proximally; (2) the lateral segment, located lateral to the ICA main trunk, dorsal to the ICA branches (posterior communicating and anterior choroidal arteries) and the oculomotor nerve, and includes the portion of the tumor extending into the middle fossa floor; (3) the medial segment, located medial to the ICA main trunk, surrounding or displacing the posterior prechiasmatic ON and optic chiasm; (4) the posterior segment, located posterior to the ICA bifurcation, sometimes circumscribing the MCA, anterior cerebral artery (ACA), and their branches; (5) the inferior segment, located inferior to the optic chiasm and the ICA trunk and its branches, at times extending ventral to the oculomotor nerve. In this manner, the surgeon is, in principle, removing five small manageable tumors, rather than one large formidable tumor.

Not infrequently, a CM extends into the CS by following the oculomotor nerve through the porous oculomotoris or via transdural penetration. The dural fold forming the porous oculomotoris is opened completely to allow decompression of the oculomotor nerve, and the CS may be explored if the tumor is soft and amenable to further removal. If the CS involvement is extensive and the tumor is fibrous, surgery is stopped after confirmation of the following: (1) gross-total resection of the intradural extracavernous portion of the tumor and removal of any accessible tumor-involved dura and bone, (2) decompression of the ON, and (3) decompression of the oculomotor nerve. Any involved dura not possible to remove is aggressively coagulated. Occasionally, the distal carotid dural ring may be involved by the tumor, which should also be removed down to the base. Any further bony hyperostosis is drilled using a 2- or 4-mm diamond bur, with care taken not to enter the surrounding sphenoid or ethmoid sinuses.

Closure

The dura is reapproximated with multiple interrupted sutures. The dural defect along the skull base is covered with commercially available collagen dural substitute. No attempt is made for a watertight closure because this is neither necessary nor possible following extensive resection of the dura involved by tumor at the skull base. The bone flap is replaced and secured with titanium miniplates and screws. Closure of the temporalis muscle/fascia and the scalp is then performed in a routine fashion.

◆ Postoperative Management

Because of the proximity of the ON to the ACP, patients with CM most commonly present with monocular visual deterioration, which is often unrecognized by patients until visual loss is severe and the tumor has reached a significant size. These tumors are often formidable to resect completely and safely, especially when their size becomes large enough to encircle, compress, and/or displace the adjacent ON, the ICA and its branches, and the oculomotor nerve. In the past, common morbidity associated with CM surgery included injury to the optic and oculomotor nerves, the ICA, and its branches. Total resection was possible in only a minority of cases, leading to early tumor recurrence and further deterioration of the patient. Many neurosurgeons, even today, recognizing the relatively high incidence of poor postoperative outcome for patients with these tumors, recommend conservative subtotal resection with or without postoperative radiation therapy. Others advocate an even more conservative approach, using radiation as the sole treatment. Additionally, most asymptomatic patients with CM are often observed with serial MRI scans.

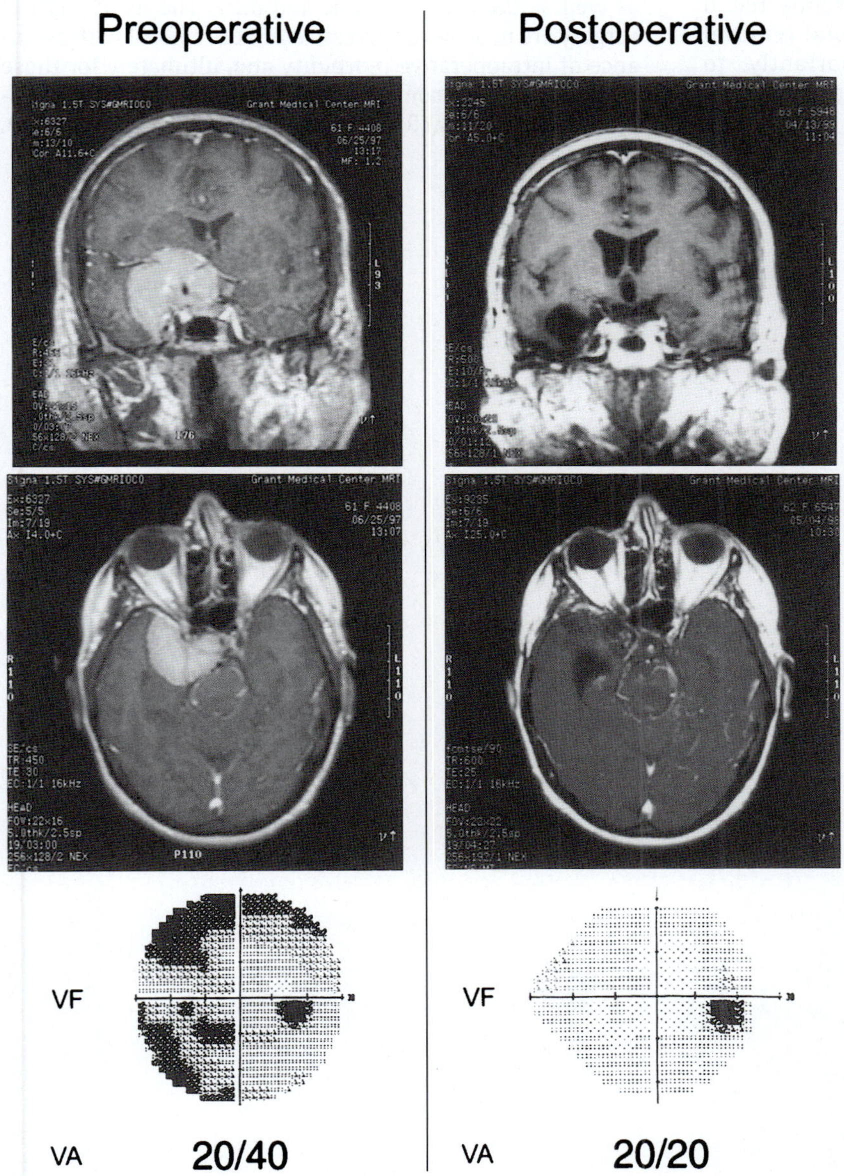

Figure 18–8 Upper and Middle Left: Preoperative coronal (upper) and axial (middle) contrast-enhanced T1-weighted magnetic resonance imaging (MRI) obtained in a 61-year-old woman. A 5-cm right clinoidal meningioma is present, encasing both the right internal carotid artery and optic nerve. Lower Left: She presented with decreased visual acuity (20/40) and visual field deficit as depicted on her Humphrey's perimetry. Upper and Middle Right: Postoperative contrast-enhanced MRI reveals complete resection of the tumor. Lower Right: Her visual acuity returned to 20/20 and her preoperative visual field deficit completely resolved.

During the past few decades, the primary goal of surgical management for patients with CM focused on maximizing the extent of resection and reducing the operative morbidity/mortality without any particular attention paid to enhancing visual outcome. In fact, reporting has been very limited regarding the patients' visual status. Moreover, the past views regarding postoperative visual recovery in patients with CM have been quite pessimistic. Poor visual outcome was previously attributed to an ischemic mechanism of preoperative visual loss, and visual deficits were considered mostly irreversible. At best, only a fraction of the patients with preoperative visual deterioration experienced visual improvement after removal of their CM (up to 30 to 40%), and many even noted visual worsening. There is a clear need for further efforts directed at improving the overall, and particularly, the visual outcome in patients with CM. Today, with advances in neuroimaging, which allows the detection of small tumors at the onset of symptoms, in addition to improved microsurgical techniques, skull base exposures, and neuroanesthesia, CM surgery can be far less risky. We propose that by utilizing the surgical technique delineated in this chapter, it is possible to attain gross total removal with minimal morbidity, and more importantly, to achieve postoperative visual improvement in the majority of patients with CM.

◆ Summary

The surgical steps involved in the skull base technique utilized in removal of CMs can be summarized as follows: (1) frontotemporal craniotomy, (2) sphenoid ridge drilling, (3) limited posterior orbitotomy, (4) posterolateral orbital wall removal (to decompress the superior orbital fissure), (5) optic canal unroofing, (6) complete extradural anterior clinoidectomy, and (7) dural opening, with dural incision extending into the falciform ligament and the ONS.

The described skull base technique provides several critical advantages, which result in improved extent of resection and outcome. These include (1) early localization and exposure of the ON and ICA; (2) complete mobilization and decompression of the ON and ICA, which prevent or minimize intraoperative neurovascular injury; (3) expansion of various operative windows, particularly the opticocarotid triangle; (4) facilitation of access to difficult locations, especially in dealing with tumor extension into the orbit, sella, optic canal, CS, orbital apex, or the infraoptic and subchiasmatic regions; and (5) facilitation of aggressive removal of tumor as well as the involved bone and dura. The main goals of surgery are to achieve aggressive tumor removal with avoidance of intraoperative morbidity and, ultimately for those with preoperative compromised vision, to provide improvement in their visual function following surgery **(Fig. 18–8).**

19

Surgical Management of Olfactory Groove Meningiomas

Michael W. McDermott and Andrew T. Parsa

Olfactory groove meningiomas arise most commonly at the posterior aspect of the cribriform plate at the junction of the suture line separating the sphenoid bone from the orbital part of the frontal bone. Frequently a small depression can be found, with the smaller tumors in the region of the ethmoid spine at the posterior edge of the crista galli, or laterally in and around the region of the posterior ethmoid foramen. As pointed out by Cushing, for the largest tumors it is impossible to determine the exact point of origin, but early on he observed several pathological specimens that suggested the exact location as just described.

◆ Patient Selection

In the past, these tumors tended to grow to very large sizes before diagnosis, whereas now, tumors are more frequently discovered at a small size. Not all meningiomas in this region require surgery, and frequently interval observation with imaging studies to document growth may be all that is required. This is particularly true for calcified tumors seen in older patients. Documented tumor growth of more than 2 mm per year on magnetic resonance imaging (MRI) may be used in a younger patient to recommend surgical intervention. For patients who are symptomatic from their olfactory groove meningioma, the decision to operate involves consideration of many factors related to the patient, the tumor, and definable surgical risk:benefit ratios. Patient factors such as age, expected survival, performance status, general neurological condition, and associated medical conditions should be considered. Sense of smell should be documented by history and exam. The surgeon also needs to decide whether the tumor is responsible for symptoms and signs. Tumor factors such as size and associated edema in the surrounding brain will help determine the surgical approach to be selected and the difficulty to be encountered defining the arachnoid plane between tumor and brain.

Olfactory groove meningiomas account for ~10 to 18% of meningiomas in a surgical series. They arise in the midline in the region of the crista galli and olfactory groove, and displace the olfactory tracts laterally. Larger, giant meningiomas from this region displace the optic chiasm posteriorly. The A2 segment of the anterior cerebral artery is typically pushed posteriorly and superiorly, whereas the medial orbital frontal and frontal polar arteries are displaced to the lateral side of the tumor. Blood supply to these tumors is predominantly from anterior and posterior ethmoid arteries off the ophthalmic artery, as well as sphenoidal branches from the middle meningeal artery and pial supply from branches of the anterior cerebral artery.

Clinical Presentation

The most common clinical presentation is that of slow onset of change in mental status; insight, judgment, motivation, and mood. Frequently, this is not so much noted by the patient, but rather by family members. Late in the clinical course for large tumors, patients may complain of headache and of reduced vision. Seizures are also not uncommon with large tumors. Rarely do patients complain of loss of sense of smell or taste. The Foster Kennedy syndrome of anosmia, unilateral optic atrophy, and contralateral papilledema was attributed to about one third of the patients described by Cushing for this tumor location.

◆ Preoperative Evaluation

Physical Examination and Medical History

The history and physical examination, as in all cases, is important to establish the baseline of neurological function or deficit. This is particularly true for small tumors in this region that are operated on and to document the presence or absence of olfaction. The status of optic nerve heads, visual acuity, and Humphrey visual field testing should be done for the larger tumors, where there is concern regarding optic pathway compression.

Medication use should also be documented, and aspirin and antiplatelet agents discontinued at a minimum of 7 to 10 days prior to elective procedures. For those with concomitant cardiac conditions, consultations with the attending cardiologist should be made before discontinuation of these antiplatelet agents.

Elderly patients in the seventh, eighth, and ninth decades of life should be evaluated for comorbid medical conditions and referred for appropriate consultations prior to consideration of surgery. All patients over the age of 70 are evaluated 2 weeks ahead of time in our anesthesia preoperative clinic.

Radiographic Evaluation

Psammomatous meningiomas are particularly common in the olfactory groove region, and therefore many of these tumors will have some degree of calcification, particularly at their base. Thin-cut computed tomographic (CT) scans with or without contrast can be done, but mainly the without-contrast scans in the coronal plane are done to evaluate for the presence or absence of bony hyperostosis and the need for basal skull base bone resection to complete the tumor removal. MRI in the axial and coronal planes is also valuable to determine whether there is any extension into the ethmoid sinuses, and also to evaluate the degree of surrounding vasogenic edema. The amount of edema is usually correlated with the amount of pial blood supply. The greater the edema, the greater the pial blood supply, and the more difficult the dissection will be to separate tumor capsule from surrounding brain. Cerebral angiography is only required for the largest tumors, to document blood supply and the position of the anterior cerebrals on the posterior aspect of these large tumors. Angiography will confirm supply from the ethmoid arteries, which can be divided during the initial orbital dissection for the largest tumors. Knowing that medial orbital frontal or frontal polar arteries are an important source of pial blood supply assists the surgeon with planning the surgical steps for devascularizing the tumor early on in the procedure.

◆ Preoperative Preparation

In preparation for the surgery, the surgeon should again review the anatomy of important bony, arterial, venous, and brain parenchymal structures. A list of equipment needed to carry out the procedure expeditiously should be made and requested when booking the surgery, such as the preoperative imaging, use of intraoperative image-guided systems, surgical microscope, ultrasonic aspirator, and cutting loops.

Preoperative preparation of the patient should include the use of steroids several days to weeks before surgery for those tumors with abundant associated vasogenic edema. Although there is no good information about the use of prophylactic anticonvulsants for patients with large tumors or associated vasogenic edema, we use anticonvulsants for 1 week around the time of surgery, following guidelines set down for their use in severely head injured patients.

◆ Operative Procedure

Intraoperative Monitoring

Intraoperatively, patient positioning and padding of extremities to avoid compression neuropathy are important considerations. For the larger tumors, lumbar subarachnoid drains are routinely used, or for those tumors where a transbasal approach will be necessary with entry into the ethmoid sinuses to accomplish complete tumor removal.

Table 19–1 Selection of Surgical Approaches

Tumor	Size	Surgical Approach
Small, medium	<3 cm	Unilateral Pterional Subfrontal Cranio-orbital
Large, giant	>3 cm	Bifrontal, extended

Small to Medium Tumors (< 3 cm)

Patient position: supine, with ipsilateral shoulder elevation

Head rotation: 20 to 30 degrees

Approaches: unilateral subfrontal, pterional, or supraorbital

For small to medium-size tumors less than 3 cm, we prefer a unilateral frontotemporal cranio-orbital approach with supraorbital osteotomy to limit the frontal lobe retraction (**Table 19–1**). A lumbar subarachnoid drain is generally not used for these smaller tumors.

The operation begins with the patient positioning as already noted. To get the scalp flap down low enough, we prefer a bicoronal scalp incision **(Fig. 19–1)**. The patient's head is placed in a Mayfield pin headrest with a single pin a fingerbreadth above the pinna and the two-pin arc on the opposite side with one pin on the mastoid process and the second pin in the temporo-occipital region. Placing the Mayfield in this position prevents the patient from sliding back through the pin set during the procedure. The ipsilateral shoulder on the nondominant side is elevated with a 1 L IV bag covered in foam, and the head is gently rotated 20 to 30 degrees to the opposite side. The neck is flexed on the chest, and the head gently extended on the neck such that the supraorbital margin is parallel to the floor and uppermost in the surgical field. The scalp is routinely shaved back 1.5 cm from the hairline, and a bicoronal skin incision is marked out. Importantly, no draping should be placed over the frontal scalp or supraorbital margin because this may increase the pressure on the skin and orbit once the scalp flap is turned down over the orbital region for the low bony exposure. During long procedures this excessive pressure may compromise blood supply to the scalp flap. Therefore, ophthalmic ointment is placed into the eyes, and the eyes are covered with small waterproof dressings. Then the upper face and scalp are prepped as one in the usual manner. Disposable towels are stapled a centimeter behind the incision line, down at the level of the zygomatic arch, and then across the zygoma just below the orbit, across the nose to the opposite side.

The incision line is injected with a combination of Xylocaine and Marcaine with 1:100,000 of epinephrine, and the skin incision fashioned in the usual way. For longer procedures, Michel clips are placed on skin edges for hemostasis to avoid prolonged potentially ischemic occlusive forces that may occur with the plastic scalp clips. The loose areolar

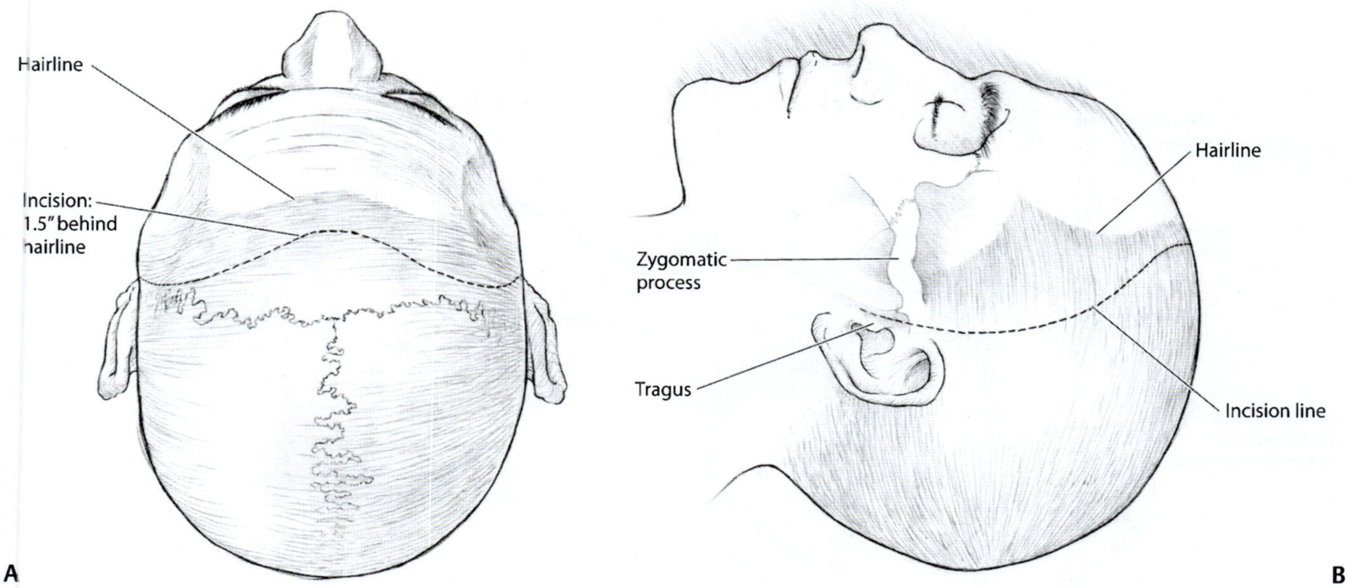

Figure 19–1 **(A)** Vertex and **(B)** lateral view of incision for both approaches.

tissue below the galea is dissected, and the subgaleal space and the scalp flap turned down forward over a single rolled gauze. The pericranium is then elevated from the superior temporal lines bilaterally, and then posteriorly just behind the coronal suture from one side to another. The pericranium is then rolled forward off the frontal bone to the supraorbital margin, and then following the course of the front zygomatic process down past the suture on the operating side. The temporalis muscle is then disinserted from the superior temporal line, leaving a small cuff of muscle. The main part of the temporalis muscle is then dissected from the temporalis fossa, and the superficial and deep fascia are taken down off the posterior aspect of the frontozygomatic process. One is always careful to dissect the superficial and deep temporal fascia, reflecting the fat between these two layers up forward with the scalp flap, to avoid injury to the frontalis branch of the facial nerve.

Once the temporalis is reflected posteriorly and retracted, this allows for the placement of a bur hole at the key point and a second hole just below the muscle cuff posteriorly. The dura is then dissected with a right-angle Penfield no. 4, and the pneumatic powered drill with the foot pedal attachment is then used to fashion a free frontotemporal bone flap. The anterior cut is along the supraorbital margin to the midline and then falls away from the midline a short course back ~2 cm, before curving gently toward the lateral frontal bone at the posterior aspect of the muscle cuff. The bone flap is then gently elevated by dissecting the dura with a Penfield no. 3 and Penfield no. 1, and the dura is then reflected off the roof of the orbit.

At this point, with the aid of operating loups and the headlight, the pericranium is reflected over the supraorbital margin on the nondominant side. The supraorbital nerve is dissected from the notch, and if a foramen is present, a small channel can be made on either side of the foramen with the drill, and the remaining bone can be fractured with a small periosteal elevator. The surgeon then approaches from the orbital side, looking up toward the roof of the orbit to dissect the periorbita and try to maintain its integrity. Any small holes in the periorbita can eventually be repaired with figure-of-eight 4–0 sutures or covered with a collagen sponge.

Once the periorbita is dissected off the roof and lateral wall of the zygoma, supraorbital osteotomy can be performed with an oscillating saw or with the pneumatic air drill using the footplate attachment **(Fig. 19–2)**. It is important to make the medial cut close enough to the midline to remove that portion of the orbital roof that rises up from the region of the crista galli and protects the valley of the olfactory groove. With the supraorbital osteotomy completed, attention should be paid to the frontal sinus, and if opened, the mucosa does not need to be stripped, but the frontal sinus simply packed with bacitracin-soaked Gelfoam. Mucosa on the supraorbital osteotomy bone piece does need to be removed; this portion of the sinus cavity should be drilled out to insure complete sinus mucosa removal.

With the bone work now complete, the dura is opened in a curvilinear fashion based on the floor of the anterior cranial fossa and then sutured forward, retracting the orbital contents forward. A rubber dam is placed over the inferior surface of the frontal lobe and then a self-retaining retractor blade is placed to gently elevate the frontal lobe. The frontal lobe is gently elevated, taking care to divide the arachnoid separating the gyrus rectus and the olfactory bulb and tract, thus allowing the tract to remain on the floor of the anterior cranial fossa. Tumor should come into view just about this time. The surgeon should work from anterior to posterior, dissecting the arachnoid plane and preserving the olfactory tract, and try to identify the posterior aspect of the tumor

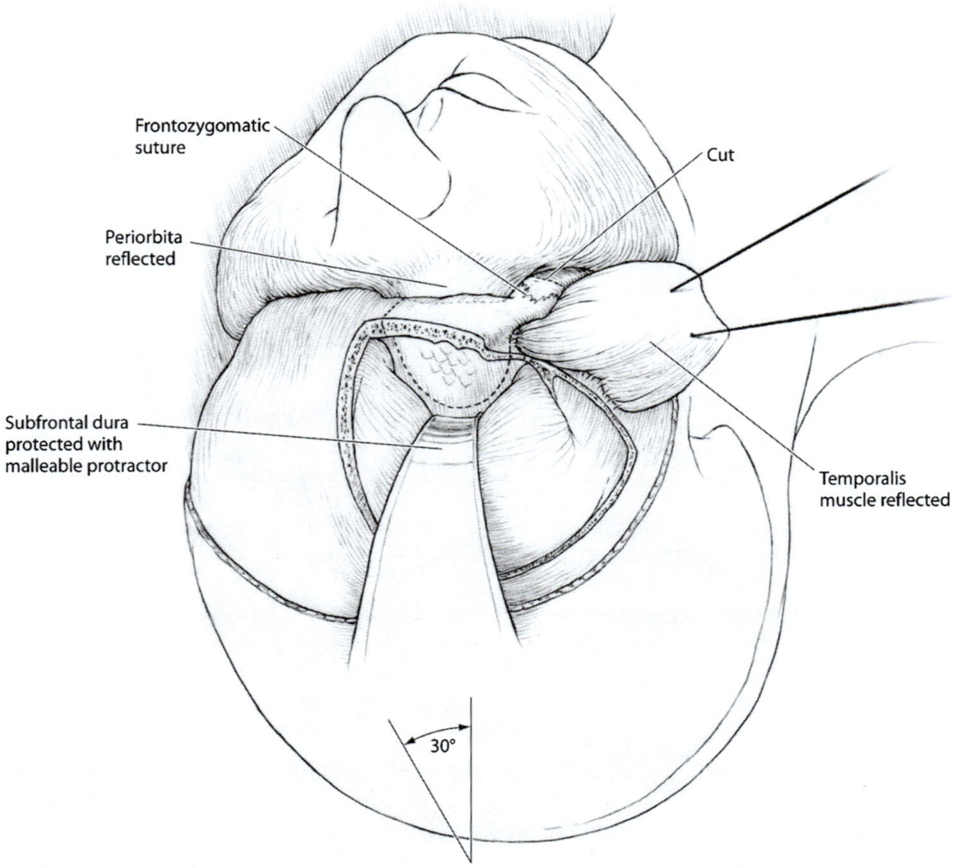

Figure 19–2 After extradural dissection for unilateral approach, dotted lines mark the path for orbital osteotomy through the lateral and supraorbital margin and roof of the orbit.

for these small to medium-size tumors just in front of the planum. Once this is done, coagulation of the basal attachments should be done first, before internally debulking the tumor. Dura in the region of the posterior aspect of the crista galli and ethmoid spine should be excised if possible, and any hyperostotic bone drilled down, using a small rough diamond or smooth diamond bur. It is unusual for small/medium-size tumors to gain access to the ethmoid cavities.

Following removal of the tumor and dural attachments the dura is closed and any openings into the frontal sinus are dealt with by reflecting pericranium over the frontal sinus opening and tacking this pericranium down to the inferior frontal dura with stay sutures. The supraorbital osteotomy bone pieces are positioned and secured with titanium plates and screws. If no frontal sinus opening is present, screws and plates can either be recessed on the anterior aspect of the bone, or the plates can be positioned on the superior aspect of the cut edge of the frontal bone so as not to be evident at all on the convexity side of the skull. The frontotemporal bone flap is repositioned and secured with titanium plates and screws, one at each of the two bur holes, at the key point and just above the pterion, and then a second recessed plate on the posterior medial aspect of the bone flap. It is useful to place the bone plate into compression on the supraorbital bar and to fill any gaps posteriorly with methylmethacrylate or hydroxyapatite crystal to prevent scar adhering to the fibrous tissue, which will fill this gap and create a visible depression in the patient's scalp postoperatively.

Scalp closure is done routinely, with one or two interrupted 3–0 absorbable sutures to align the scalp, and then a running 2–0 absorbable suture for the galea and staples for the skin. One-eighth inch Hemovac drains are placed in the subgaleal space and withdrawn on the morning following the surgical procedure. We have avoided the use of head-wrap dressings because of the potential for pressure necrosis along the skin above the supraorbital region. Ointment is placed along the incision line so that dressings do not stick when removed postoperatively. A loose Flexinet dressing is placed over the scalp and face, and then a window cut in the dressing for the eyes, nose, and mouth so that a small portion remains under the chin, preventing the dressing from becoming dislodged.

Large Tumors (>3 cm)

Position: supine

Head rotation: 0 degrees

Approach: bifrontal, extended frontal craniotomy **(Fig. 19–3)**

The bifrontal, extended frontal approach is preferred for large and giant tumors of the olfactory groove. For these

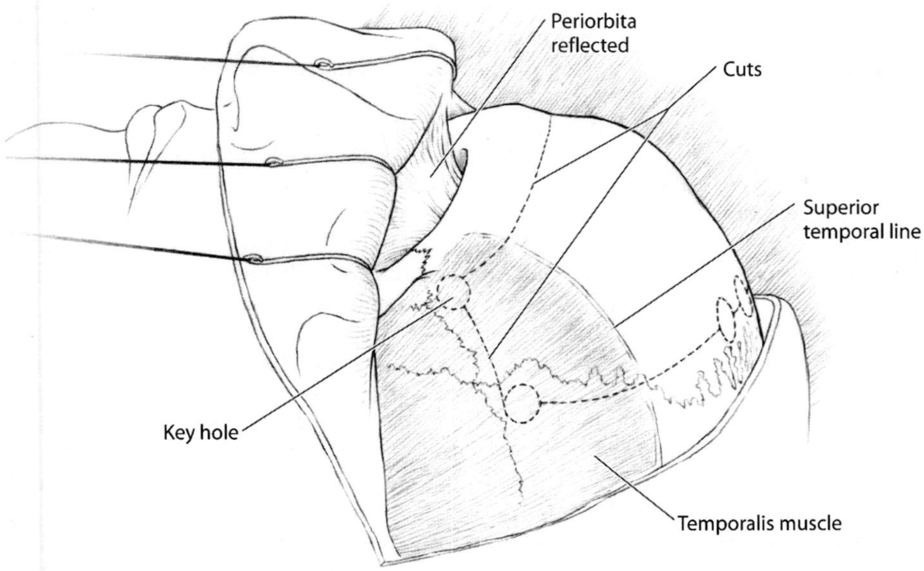

Figure 19–3 Lateral view of lines for a craniotomy for a bifrontal, extended frontal approach. Bur holes for access to the anterior fossa are below the muscle cuff.

large tumors, or when the nasal sinuses must be entered for complete tumor removal, a lumbar subarachnoid drain is inserted and 20 mL allowed to drain by gravity at the beginning of the case. More cerebrospinal fluid can be removed during the case as necessary. The patient is again positioned supine, with care and attention to padding extremities, and the neck is flexed on the chest, the head extended on the neck to bring the supraorbital region uppermost in the surgical field. Skin and scalp preparation is as for the small to medium-size tumors as already described. In some cases of giant tumors, there may be extension of the tumor through the bone of the anterior cranial base through to the ethmoid sinuses; the surgeon should be prepared for this and consult with otolaryngology colleagues for their assistance during this portion of the dissection and repair.

For these large tumors predominant blood supply is from the anterior and posterior ethmoidal arteries, which are found in the frontal-ethmoid suture in the medial wall of the orbit **(Fig. 19–4).** The anterior ethmoid foramen is ~24 mm behind the nasolacrimal crest, the posterior foramen another 12 mm posterior, and the optic canal another 6 mm back. A useful sequence to remember these distances is "24, 12, 6." Dissection of periosteum off both frontal bones proceeds on both sides as described earlier. The periorbita is continuous with the periosteum and dissected on both sides. On approaching the medial aspect of the supraorbital margin, medial to the supratrochlear nerves, the ligamentous insertion of the trochlea is taken down with a periosteal dissector. Releasing the trochlea allows dissection of the medial periorbita so that the frontoethmoid suture can be found. Using a Rhoton microdissector the periorbital sleeve extending into the foremen is dissected front, top, and bottom, then coagulated and cut.

In most cases we leave the posterior ethmoid artery intact because of its proximity to the optic canal and potential for either retraction or thermal injury to the optic nerve during its exposure.

Once the ethmoid arteries on both sides and the orbits have been dissected, then the bifrontal craniotomy can proceed. The temporalis muscle is disinserted from the superior temporal line bilaterally and reflected inferiorly to expose the temporal fossa and key point. A bur hole is made at the key point at the junction of the superior temporal line and frontozygomatic process and then a second hole again below the muscle cuff in the region of the pterion. One hole is placed on either side of the midline posteriorly just in front of the coronal suture and the underlying dura is dissected with a right-angled Penfield no. 4. The bur holes on either side of the midline are made in an ovoid shape, with the long axis of the bur hole parallel to the coronal suture. This allows easier access for the Penfield no. 3 dissector to dissect the dura across the midline. The footplate attachment for a pneumatic drill is then used to connect the bur holes, but no bur holes are placed low on the supraorbital region. The cut across the midline low and anteriorly is made with straight collar attachment on the drill. The bone flap is elevated and if difficulties are encountered then the flap can be converted into a bipartite or tripartite flap. With patients over 70 we routinely begin with removing the right frontal flap first, then dissect under direct vision across the midline to the left. Pieces can be connected one to another using titanium plates and screws with countersinking or recessing the screws and plates along the midline to prevent any cosmetic difficulties.

Once the bone flap is elevated the dura is reflected off the roof of the orbit bilaterally. With one operator protecting the intracranial dura and using the pneumatic drill, the second protects the orbital contents, and the footplate attachment for the pneumatic drill is then used to begin the supraorbital osteotomy out laterally at the frontozygomatic suture extending back a short distance into the lateral wall of the orbit and then across the roof of the orbit toward the midline. The anterior cut from the intracranial side is limited by the medial wall of the orbit and so the drill is

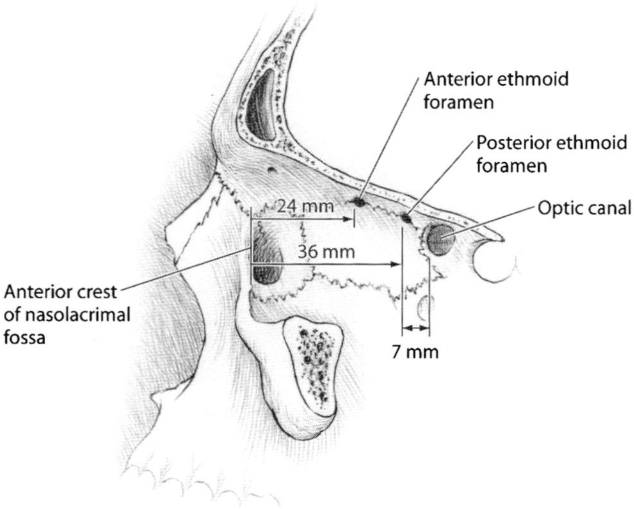

Figure 19–4 Medial wall of the orbit with positions of the ethmoid foramina and optic canal.

switched out again to a straight collar. This can then be used to extend the cut on the intracranial side across just in front of the crista galli into the ethmoid air cells. Next, a horizontal cut is made just above the nasofrontal suture. This is connected with the cuts along the medial aspect of the orbit. Then the supraorbital osteotomy bone piece can be elevated, usually with little resistance. The frontal sinus mucosa need not be excised or removed from the remaining frontal sinus but simply covered with antibiotic-soaked Gelfoam and then covered with a small $^1/_2 \times 3$ in. cottonoid pledget. Any mucosa in the supraorbital osteotomy bar must be removed with a drill to prevent development of a mucocele later on.

Drill holes are placed in the margins of the craniotomy posteriorly and laterally, but not anteriorly, and the dura tacked up. Bleeding along the midline superior sagittal sinus is controlled with the bipolar, and usually three 1×3 in. pieces of Gelfoam. Methods such as head elevation and irrigation and digital compression will assist with hemostasis along the midline.

Once the hemostasis has been secured, the dura is opened a fingerbreadth above the supraorbital region and sutured forward over the orbital contents. The superior sagittal sinus is divided using a suture ligation technique with 2–0 braided nylon. With this approach, for large olfactory groove meningiomas, the tumor usually presents right up against the dura, and dissection can begin along the base. Taking the ethmoidal arteries will reduce the blood supply, but many other small branches may persist, and these can be taken with the bipolar. Once the base has been dissected, internal debulking can be accomplished. Interactive image-guided surgical systems improve the efficiency of resection in allowing the surgeon to more accurately predict positioning within the debulked cavity. Dissection of the margins of the tumor from surrounding brain is usually somewhat difficult for these larger tumors, which rarely have a preserved arachnoid plane and frequently have a component of pial blood supply, which must be identified, dissected, coagulated, and divided.

On the posterior aspect of the tumor, the optic apparatus will be pushed back and down by olfactory groove meningiomas. The arachnoid in this region is almost always intact but the surgeon must not get fooled by compressed, edematous gyrus rectus on the posterior edge, mistaking this for the optic chiasm. Care must be taken to work out toward the lateral margins of the tumor posteriorly, out toward the medial aspect of the sylvian fissure, which is afforded easily by this bifrontal extended frontal approach **(Fig. 19–5)**, to identify the optic nerves. Remember that the posterior aspect of the olfactory tract always runs lateral and superior to the optic nerve.

Once the tumor is excised, any hyperostosis in the region of the anterior cranial base must also be removed. This is usually done with a small cutting or diamond bur. If the ethmoid or sphenoid sinuses are entered, then the dural defect must be repaired, and we have chosen to do this extradurally, after tumor removal and repair of the dura incision just above the orbits. The dura is then reflected off the roof of the orbit, bilaterally, and the dural defect is then exposed. A bovine pericardial graft is then sutured onto this inferior basal dura, with nonabsorbable braided nylon suture. The ethmoid sinuses are filled with gelatin sponge from above and below by an assisting head and neck surgeon. This nasal packing is removed 10 to 14 days postoperatively with endoscopic assistance under monitored anesthesia care. The inferior basal closure is augmented with a collagen sponge, and then the pericranial flap harvested during the opening is reflected down over the frontal and ethmoid sinus opening posteriorly to the remaining ledge of the tuberculum. Usually, lateral tack-up sutures are placed in the posterior lateral dura to maintain the flap position.

For closure the supraorbital osteotomy bone piece is repositioned and secured with a small gap at the nasofrontal suture line to avoid constriction of the pericranial flap used for reconstruction. If the sphenoid and ethmoid sinuses were not entered during tumor removal and extradural resection was not required, then the pericranial flap is reflected over the frontal sinus, the supraorbital bar is replaced, and the additional pericranium beyond the frontal dural repair suture line is excised **(Fig. 19–6)**. Pericranial tissue that becomes congested postoperatively has been reported to act as a mass lesion, and therefore any additional tissue should be excised if not needed. The bifrontal bone flap is repositioned and secured with titanium plates, and two tack-up sutures are placed on each side. The bifrontal bone flap is placed in close contact with the supraorbital bar to limit postoperative cosmetic problems **(Fig. 19–7)**. A gap along the posterior aspect of the craniotomy can be filled with hydroxyapatite paste. After skin closure and dressings the lumbar subarachnoid drain is removed.

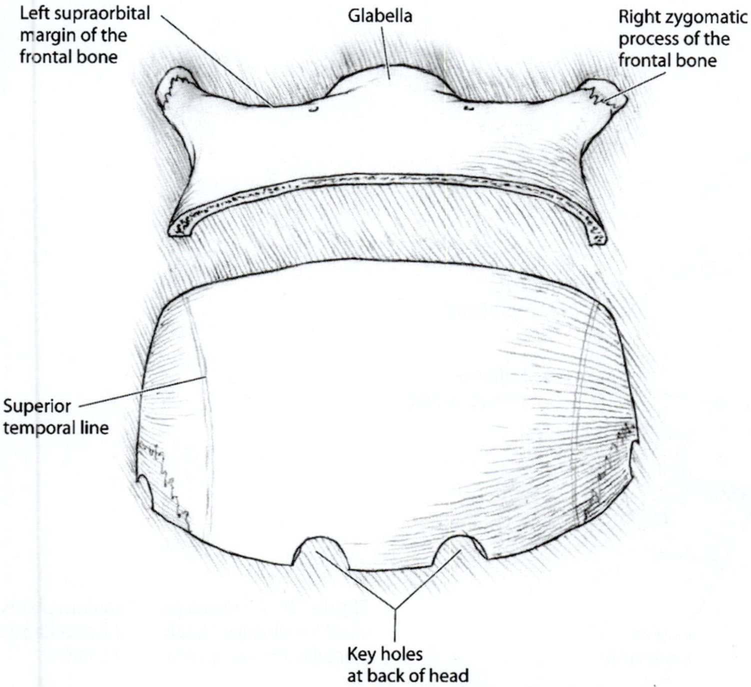

Figure 19–5 Exploded view of bone flaps for a bifrontal, extended frontal approach.

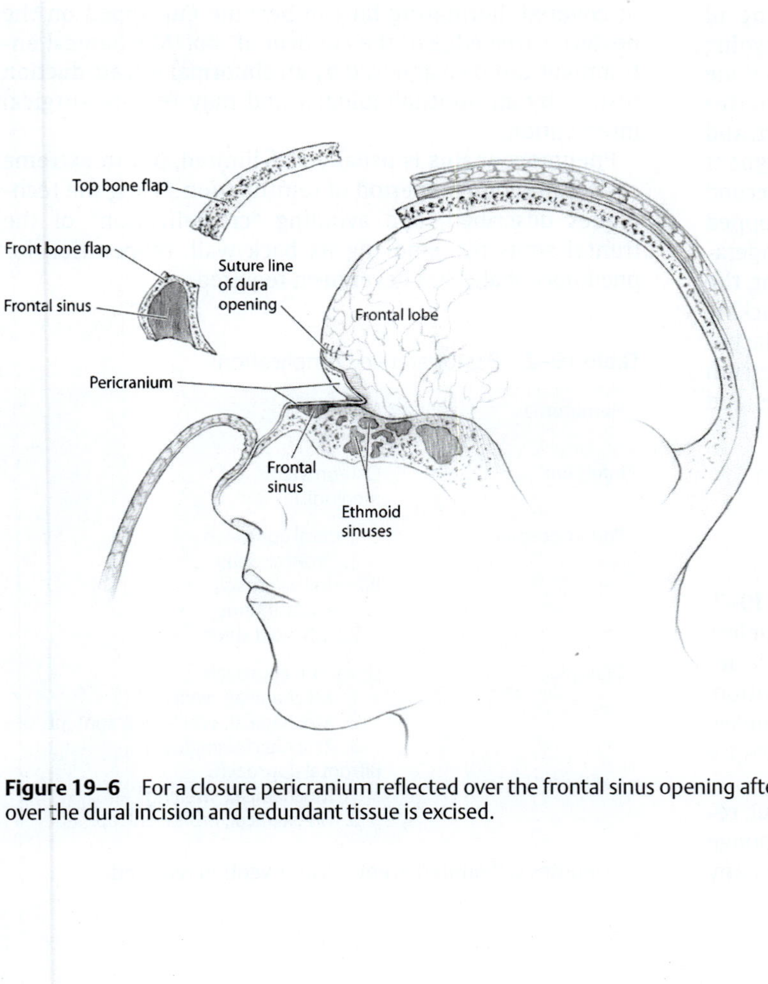

Figure 19–6 For a closure pericranium reflected over the frontal sinus opening after which a supraorbital bar is attached. The pericranium runs up over the dural incision and redundant tissue is excised.

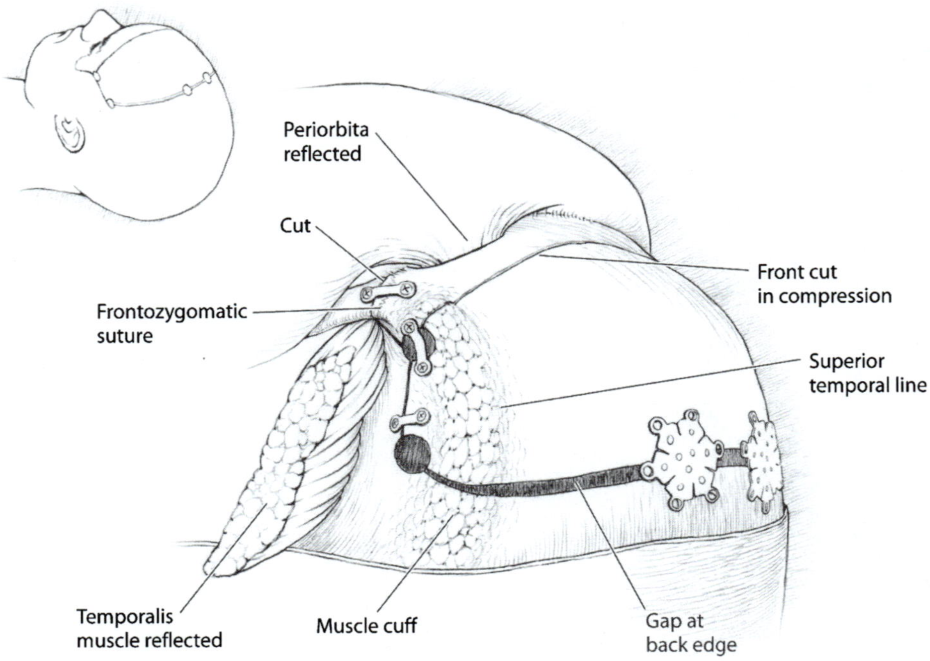

Figure 19–7 Positions of titanium plates used for closure. A bifrontal bone flap is placed in the compression anteriorly.

◆ Postoperative Management

Standard postoperative measures are instituted and the patient observed overnight in the neurosurgical intensive care unit. Hemovac drains are removed at the end of the first postoperative day and low-molecular-weight heparin begun for venous thrombosis prophylaxis on the morning of the second day postoperatively. For patients undergoing bifrontal, transbasal operations a baseline CT scan is done the morning of the first day postoperatively. Postoperative MRI scans are delayed until the patient is awake, alert, and cooperative, and unlike baseline scanning for malignant glioma, there is no need to get the scan on the first or second day. Anticonvulsants are continued for 7 days then stopped without tapering. Patients recovering from unilateral operations are discharged at 3 to 5 days, and those having the more extensive procedures at 5 to 7 days. Any nasal packing is removed 10 to 14 days postoperatively by the otolaryngologist and they usually like to maintain broad spectrum antibiotic coverage until the packing is out. Sutures and staples are left in for 10 to 14 days.

◆ Complications

Possible surgical complications are listed in **Table 19–2.** Postoperative epidural blood collections are observed unless associated with an alerted level of consciousness. These are rare but when symptomatic require immediate attention. Cerebrospinal fluid leaks are managed with lumbar drainage for 3 to 5 days, after allowing a period of 12 hours to elapse for those already on low-molecular-weight heparin.

Periorbital swelling is common on days 2 to 3 but resolves over time. Covering with absorbable collagen sponge or repairing any openings in the periorbita will avoid any orbital entrapment syndromes. With orbital osteotomy a minor amount of ptosis can be seen and is usually transient. Double vision is not a problem with bifrontal approaches when the trochlea is taken down on both sides, and after unilateral procedures it is mechanical and self-limited. However if the periorbital defects are not repaired or covered, herniating fat can become entrapped on the posterior free edge of the cut orbital roof. Mechanical entrapment can be diagnosed by an abnormal forced-duction testing by an ophthalmologist and may require surgical intervention.

Pneumocephalus is usually self-limited, but in extreme cases can require a period of reintubation. Using the techniques described, and avoiding "cranialization" of the frontal sinus by removing its back wall, reoperation for pneumocephalus has never been required.

Table 19–2 Postoperative Complications

Hematomas	Epidural Subdural
Infection	Osteomyelitis Meningitis
Pneumocephalus	Unilateral approach 1. Frontal sinus Bifrontal approach 1. Frontal sinus 2. Ethmoid sinus
Diplopia	Unilateral approach 1. Mechanical, swelling* 2. Mechanical, orbital entrapment 3. Trochlea taken down* Bifrontal approach 1. Mechanical, swelling* 2. Mechanical, orbital entrapment

* Denotes self-limited event; no intervention required.

Development of signs suggesting a bone flap infection are managed early and aggressively with reoperation, debridement, placement of an antibiotic irrigation and drainage system, replacement of bone, and intravenous antibiotics for 6 weeks. Meningitis is rare, despite entrance into the frontal sinuses on a routine basis.

◆ Follow-Up

The risk of recurrence is related to the grade of surgical resection, including tumor, dural attachments, and bone. For all cases MRI is done on an annual basis until 10 years postoperatively and then every 2 years. Options for documented recurrence include reoperation, external irradiation, and radiosurgery.

◆ Conclusion

Overall the outcome of surgery for patients with olfactory groove meningiomas, large or small, can be gratifying. With proper patient selection and use of appropriate surgical techniques, surgeons should be confident that they can provide an excellent quality of life and superior surgical outcomes.

20

Petrosal Approach for Resection of Petroclival Meningiomas

James K. Liu and William T. Couldwell

Although petroclival meningiomas represent a small percentage of meningiomas that reside in the posterior fossa, their treacherous location in proximity to the cranial nerves, the basilar artery and its perforating branches, and the brain stem makes them one of the most formidable lesions encountered in skull base surgery. These tumors may grow to a surprisingly large size with minimal symptoms. If left untreated, however, persistent tumor enlargement in this location will ultimately result in fatality. Prior to 1970, the risk of mortality from resection of petroclival meningiomas exceeded 50%, and some deemed these tumors "inoperable." The development of microsurgical techniques and modern skull base approaches, however, has made safe removal of these tumors feasible; improved surgical results now achieve less than 5% mortality. Nevertheless, these tumors remain a surgical challenge because of the relatively high incidence of permanent complications associated with their removal, primarily cranial neuropathies and vascular injury to the brain stem perforating vessels.

Although there is some variation in the definition of petroclival meningiomas in the literature, we believe that petroclival meningiomas should be strictly defined as those meningiomas involving the upper two thirds of the clivus with dural attachments at or medial to the cranial nerve foramina (fifth to eleventh cranial nerves, **Fig. 20–1**). Also considered in this group of meningiomas are those that arise directly from Meckel's cave and extend directly into the posterior fossa, which Cushing described as "gasseropetrosal" meningiomas. With continued growth, such tumors invariably become both supra- and infratentorial and occupy both medial and lateral positions to the fifth cranial nerve.

Precise classification of petroclival meningiomas is important from an anatomical and surgical standpoint because the origin of dural attachment can predict the direction of cranial nerve displacement, which can significantly determine surgically induced morbidity. Because petroclival meningiomas arise medial to the cranial nerve foramina, these tumors tend to displace the cranial nerves posteriorly in that the cranial nerves are interposed between the surgeon and the tumor. These tumors often displace the brain stem contralaterally and engulf the basilar artery or its

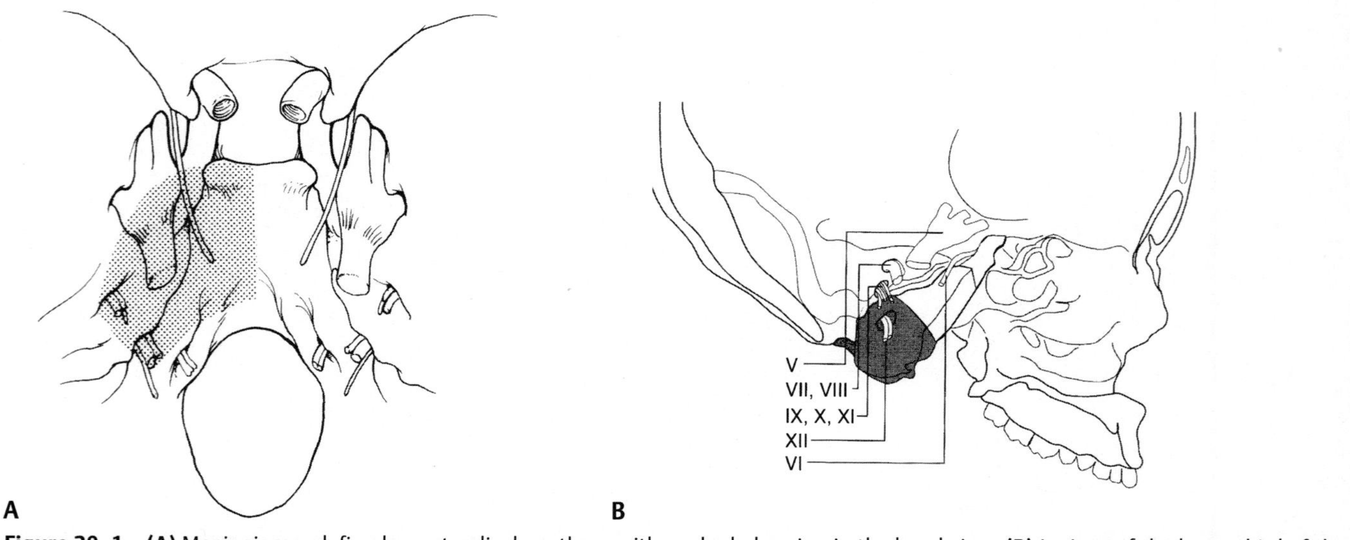

Figure 20–1 **(A)** Meningiomas defined as petroclival are those with basal attachments at or medial to the skull base foramina of the fifth through eleventh cranial nerves. This area is demonstrated by the shaded region in the basal view. **(B)** Lesions of the lower third of the clivus (shaded area) are best considered as foramen magnum meningiomas when planning surgical strategies.

perforating vessels supplying the brain stem, making surgical removal very challenging. In contrast, posterior petrous meningiomas arise lateral to the cranial nerve foramina and tend to displace the fifth through eighth cranial nerves anteriorly. The surgical morbidity of removing such tumors is significantly lower than that of petroclival meningiomas. Meningiomas that arise from the lower third of the clivus at or medial to the hypoglossal canal are best considered as foramen magnum meningiomas **(Fig. 20–1)**.

The petrosal approach (also referred to as the combined petrosal approach or transpetrosal approach) is useful for extensive lesions that involve both supratentorial and infratentorial compartments located at the petroclival and posterior cavernous sinus regions. Although many variations of this approach have been described in the literature, the basic petrosal approach involves a mastoidectomy and an L-shaped temporo-parieto-occipital craniotomy. Various degrees of temporal bone can be removed (retrolabyrinthine, translabyrinthine, or transcochlear), depending on the extent of the lesion and the preoperative hearing status of the patient. In the retrolabyrinthine approach, the presigmoid dura is exposed while the integrity of the otologic structures is maintained to preserve hearing. The translabyrinthine approach involves removal of the semicircular canals, allowing for more medial exposure at the expense of hearing. The transcochlear approach involves additional skeletonization and transposition of the facial nerve posteriorly to allow further drilling of the cochlea and the remainder of the petrous bone. These latter two approaches are usually reserved for those who do not have serviceable preoperative hearing. A combined petrosal approach incorporates an anterior petrosectomy (extended middle fossa approach), with the posterior petrosectomy allowing for maximal exposure from multidirectional viewing angles.

◆ Patient Selection

The goals of surgery should be tailored to the individual patient, considering the age of the patient, the location of the tumor, and the presenting symptomatology. For asymptomatic lesions in elderly patients, a period of observation may be warranted until symptomatic brain stem compression is evident because most tumors in this location are slow growing. The size of the lesion is a significant factor in determining the surgical morbidity and mortality. The goal should be total removal of tumor whenever possible while preserving or improving neurological function. Total removal provides the best chance for a surgical cure or long-term tumor control. The first attempt at resection offers the best chance at complete removal when the arachnoidal membranes are intact because these facilitate dissection of neurovascular structures.

Some situations, such as tumor involvement of the cranial nerves or tumor adherent to the brain stem and its vasculature, may preclude total removal without increasing significant morbidity and incurring new neurological deficits. In these instances, a subtotal removal with resection of the symptomatic portion of the mass may be chosen. If, for example, a patient has a compressive petroclival tumor that extends into the cavernous sinus but has no significant cranial neuropathies (diplopia), a subtotal resection (removing the compressive posterior fossa mass) and subsequent stereotactic radiosurgery to the residual cavernous sinus tumor may minimize postoperative morbidity while maximizing tumor control. This strategy may be considered in the elderly patient with associated medical problems. If, on the other hand, symptomatic cranial neuropathies are present because of tumor in the cavernous sinus, especially in a young patient, a more aggressive radical resection of the tumor should be considered. If tumor is encasing the cavernous carotid artery and an oncological resection is planned with sacrifice of the carotid artery, a cerebrovascular bypass may be necessary. In instances where the tumor encases the basilar artery, adheres to the brain stem or vasculature, or parasitizes the brain stem perforators, a more conservative approach that leaves a small remnant of tumor may be considered if radical removal might result in potential devastating neurological morbidity. Many of these decisions regarding the justification of radical removal must be made intraoperatively based on the surgeon's judgment of the risk involved with resection.

◆ Preoperative Preparation

Radiographic Evaluation

Preoperative high-field thin-section magnetic resonance (MR) imaging with and without gadolinium enhancement is performed to delineate the size, location, and extent of the tumor. The relationship of the tumor to the brain stem, cranial nerves, cavernous sinus, temporal bone, and neighboring vasculature is carefully examined. The degree of supratentorial extension should be assessed because it will be critical in determining the appropriate surgical approach (see later discussion). Evidence of tumor encasing the basilar artery and its respective branches and any potential adherence of the tumor to the brain stem can be determined on these images. Specifically, loss of the arachnoidal plane on T1- and T2-weighted images as well as edema of the brain stem on T2-weighted images may be indications of pial invasion. A computed tomographic (CT) scan of the skull base is useful to evaluate for hyperostosis in the temporal bone.

MR angiography and MR venography are particularly useful for assessing cerebrovascular anatomy and the blood supply of the tumor and for confirming patency and connection between the two transverse sinuses. In patients who have tumor involving the cavernous sinus and cavernous carotid artery, a conventional angiogram is performed with a balloon occlusion test to assess the risk involved with performing a carotid artery sacrifice and subsequent reconstruction of the carotid artery with a high-flow bypass. Angiography is also useful for visualizing the vertebrobasilar circulation and its relationship to the tumor. If there is unilateral encasement of the vertebral artery by the tumor, a specific balloon occlusion test is performed on the artery to assess the risk of resection. Preoperative embolization of these tumors is generally not necessary because their blood supply can be interrupted early in the operation during extradural bone removal.

Preoperative Hearing Status

The status of the patient's preoperative hearing influences what type of surgical approach or degree of temporal bone resection is most appropriate. Hearing is often already diminished because the cochlear nerve is prone to early injury from tumor growth. In patients with suspected hearing loss or with tumor in the region of the seventh–eighth nerve complex, a preoperative formal audiogram is performed. If functional hearing is significantly impaired (>50 dB hearing loss or <50% speech discrimination score), a translabyrinthine or transcochlear exposure that sacrifices hearing may be considered; these approaches provide increased exposure of the petroclival region and allow early interruption of the tumor's blood supply through removal of the temporal bone and the tumor attachment. If, however, functional hearing is intact (<50 dB hearing loss or >50% speech discrimination score), a retrolabyrinthine exposure is performed to preserve hearing.

Intraoperative Monitoring

Intraoperative monitoring, including brain stem auditory evoked responses (BAERs), somatosensory evoked potentials (SSEPs), electroencephalography (EEG), motor evoked potentials (MEPs), and facial nerve monitoring, is performed in all cases. It is important to obtain baseline BAER and SSEP prior to surgery in cases of large tumors with brain stem compression because subclinical impairment may be detected in some patients. Preoperative knowledge of any impairment is important because suboptimal recordings have been noted following the induction of anesthesia in some cases. In patients whose tumor involves the lower cranial nerves, an electromyographic endotracheal tube can be used for tenth nerve monitoring, and electrodes directly placed into the sternocleidomastoid muscle can be used for eleventh nerve monitoring.

Anesthetic Techniques

A Foley catheter and an arterial line for continuous blood pressure monitoring are placed in all cases. We reserve placing a central line for patients with significant medical and cardiac histories. At the start of surgery, the patient is administered high-dose intravenous corticosteroids, which are continued throughout the duration of surgery (20 mg of dexamethasone every 2 hours). Intravenous antibiotic prophylaxis (1 g cefazolin) is administered prior to the skin incision and is continued every 6 hours during the procedure and for 24 hours postoperatively; if a lumbar drain is placed, antibiotic prophylaxis is continued until the drain is removed.

The anesthesiologist must strive to minimize intracranial hypertension while maximizing cerebral perfusion during the operation, especially during bone and tumor removal. Normotensive anesthesia is the goal. We generally use a balanced combination of intravenous narcotics, low-dosage inhalational agents, and propofol. The use of muscle relaxants is avoided except during opening and closing to enable MEP and cranial nerve recording. Because propofol is a rapid-acting agent with a short half-life, it allows for a smooth induction and rapid emergence from anesthesia following prolonged skull base operations. It is also ideal for immediate production of burst-suppression EEG for cerebral protection during temporary vascular occlusion.

Choosing the Appropriate Surgical Approach

The main purpose for selecting a skull base approach is to provide access to otherwise inaccessible tumors by removing bone at the skull base to reduce brain retraction. Choosing the appropriate skull base approach depends primarily on the location of the lesion and the extent of skull base attachment revealed by careful examination of preoperative imaging studies. The approach must provide exposure that creates the shortest distance to the lesion, adequate visualization of the lesion, control of critical neurovascular structures, and minimized brain retraction. Ideally, an approach is chosen to expose and enable immediate interruption of the tumor blood supply at the base of the skull; this may be accomplished intra- or extradurally, depending on the location of the attachment. It is also important to determine whether the lesion lies intradural or extradural because an approach that traverses a contaminated cavity (such as the transoral approach) may pose a relatively higher risk of meningitis for intradural lesions, especially when obtaining an adequate dural closure is difficult. Concepts of keyhole microneurosurgery should be applied to all cases of skull base surgery. A "minimally invasive approach" should translate as an approach that provides adequate exposure associated with minimal disruption of normal anatomy. In some cases, the use of endoscopy, image-guided stereotaxy, or intraoperative MR imaging may serve as an adjunct in facilitating the skull base approach. The surgeon's experience and familiarity with the surgical approach should also be considered.

The potential skull base approaches to access petroclival meningiomas include anterior petrosal (extended middle fossa), posterior petrosal (presigmoid retrolabyrinthine transtentorial), combined petrosal, retromastoid/retrosigmoid, and primary transtemporal approaches **(Fig. 20–2)**. Generally, the more medial the dural attachment, the more lateral the bone removal that will be necessary for exposure. The most common approach used for smaller petroclival meningiomas confined primarily in the infratentorial space is a retromastoid/retrosigmoid approach. However, for larger tumors with a broad base of attachment or those tumors with supra- and infratentorial extension, the combined petrosal (or simply "petrosal") approach is used. This approach is ideal for large tumors centered about the petrous apex

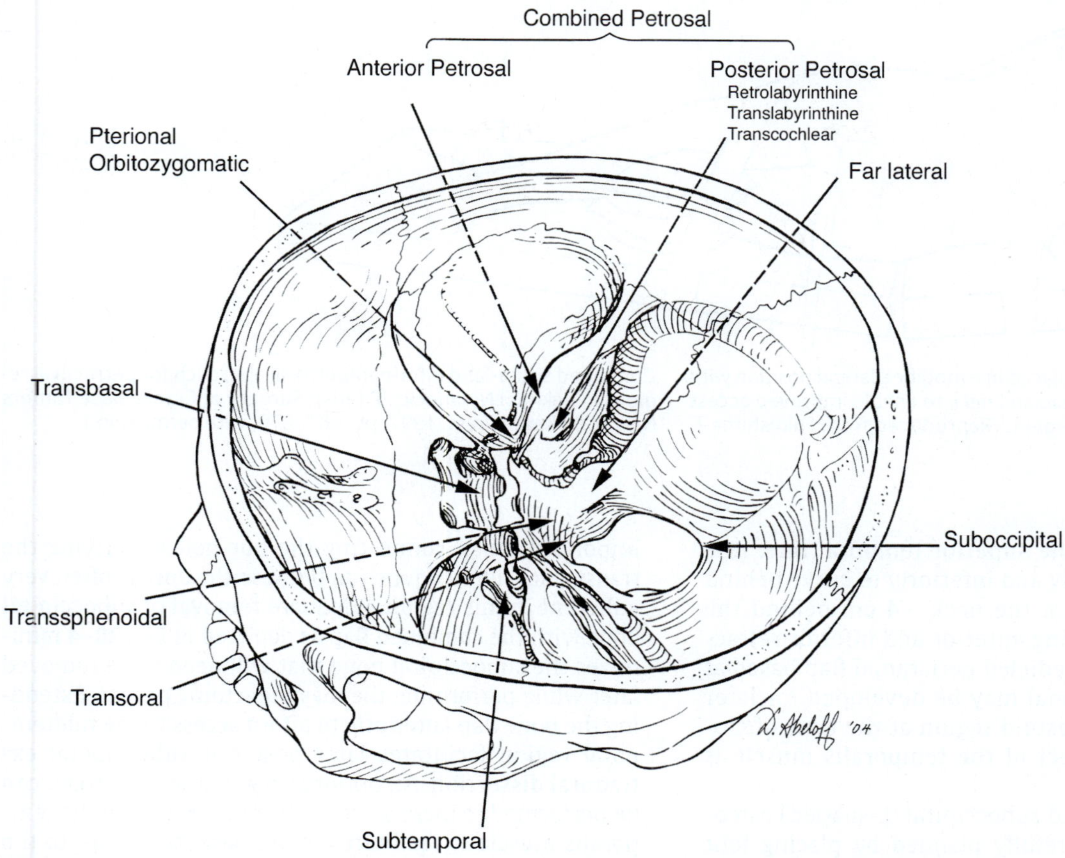

Figure 20–2 Diagram illustrates various skull base approaches to the clivus and petroclival regions. Note that combined petrosal approach allows multiple surgical trajectories to the petroclival region with variable degrees of petrous bone removal (with permission from William T. Couldwell and James K. Liu).

with a large basal attachment that necessitates extensive basal exposure of the petroclival region. It offers several advantages, including direct surgical trajectory and shorter operative distance to the anterior brain stem and petroclival regions, preservation of the transverse and sigmoid sinuses (including the drainage of the vein of Labbé), early interruption of the tumor's vascular supply, and minimal retraction of the temporal lobe and cerebellum. Temporal bone removal can be tailored depending on the patient's preoperative hearing status using the retrolabyrinthine, translabyrinthine, and transcochlear approaches. The simultaneous exposure of both supra- and infratentorial compartments eliminates the need for staged approaches that might be caused by anatomical limits (i.e., retromastoid/retrosigmoid combined with a subtemporal approach).

◆ Operative Procedure for Petrosal Approach

Patient Positioning

The patient is placed in the lateral position and the head is held in three-point pin fixation with the sagittal suture parallel to the floor; the head should be laterally flexed ~10 to 15 degrees to increase the access to the suboccipital and lateral neck region **(Fig. 20–3).** Although the head of the table is elevated slightly to facilitate venous drainage, raising the head significantly should be avoided to minimize the risk of venous air embolism when dissecting around major venous sinuses. An axillary roll is placed, and the contralateral arm rests on a Krauss armrest. The elevated arm is distracted inferiorly toward the foot of the table to provide more room for the surgeon above the shoulder. All pressure points are carefully padded with foam or gel pads. Pillows are placed between the legs, and pneumatic compression stockings are used during the procedure and continued postoperatively in the intensive care unit. The patient is secured to the operating table with wide adhesive tape to allow safe rotation of the table during the operation to improve the surgeon's line of sight. In all cases, either the abdomen or lateral thigh should be prepped and draped for later harvesting of autologous fat and fascia for wound closure. Intravenous corticosteroids, antibiotics, and mannitol are administered at the time of the skin incision, as discussed previously.

Skin Incision and Craniotomy

A pre- and postauricular incision is made that begins at the zygoma anterior to the tragus and extends upward

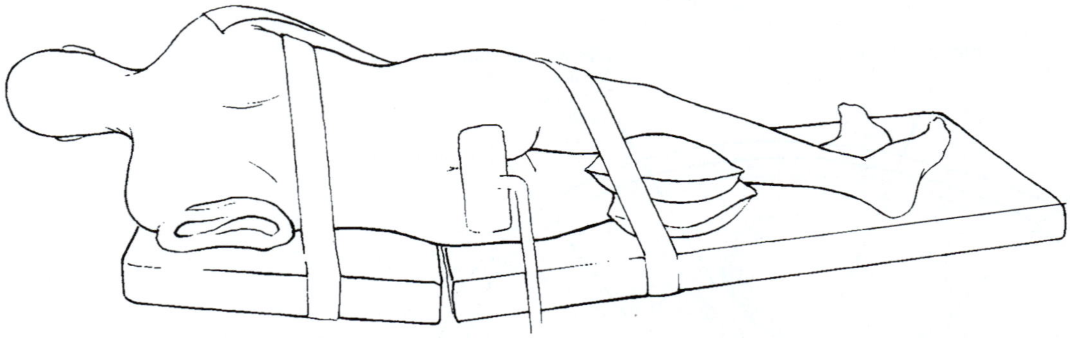

Figure 20–3 The patient is placed in a modified lateral position with slight lateral flexion of the head and neck to enable improved access to the inferior suboccipital region. (Reproduced from Fukushima T. Combined supra- and infra-parapetrosal approach for petroclival regions in Sekhar LN, Janecka IP (eds): Surgery of Cranial Base Tumors New York: Raven Press, 1992, pp. 661–670, with permission.)

behind the hairline to the superior temporal line. It is then extended posteriorly and inferiorly to curve behind the ear and down toward the neck ~4 cm behind the mastoid process. Following anterior and inferior retraction of the scalp flap, a pedicled pericranial flap based at the external auditory canal may be developed for later reconstruction of the mastoid region at the time of closure. The posterior aspect of the temporalis muscle is then reflected forward.

A temporo-occipital and suboccipital (L-shaped) osteoplastic craniotomy is carefully planned by placing four bur holes that straddle the transverse sinus and transverse–sigmoid junction **(Fig. 20–4).** This bone flap will eventually provide exposure of both supra- and infratentorial compartments as well as the transverse and sigmoid sinuses. Precise planning of the bur holes and margins of the bone flap is critical because improper positioning of this flap will limit surgical exposure and increase the likelihood of injury to the major venous sinuses. The width of the sinus is ~10 mm, so the distance between the bur holes used to straddle the sinus should be planned accordingly. In most cases, the right sinus is larger than the left, but this should be verified on the preoperative MR venogram. The lateral pair of holes should be planned to straddle the transverse–sigmoid junction. Stereotactic image guidance may be used to place the holes precisely to avoid sinus injury. One hole should be placed with its posterior margin at the squamosal–parietomastoid junction; the other should be placed below the superior nuchal line along the posterior body of the mastoid bone (just anterior to the "trigeminal keyhole"). The second, more posterior pair of holes should straddle the sinus ~3 cm posterior (just behind the asterion) on either side of the nuchal line. Satisfactory placement of the bur holes will allow separation of the bone overlying the sinus to be performed under direct vision to avoid violation of the sinus. The wall of the sinus is a dome that forms an impression in the bone; it must be separated completely using a thin dural separator. If the dura is completely separated from the bone, the assistant may depress the sinus while performing the craniotome cuts; if there is any question regarding the separation of the sinus from the overlying bone, the cuts directly over the sinus should be made with a diamond bur. This is especially important when connecting the bur holes overlying the transverse–sigmoid junction because the dura is often very adherent in this region. Adequate removal of suboccipital bone with the combined flap as depicted in **Fig. 20–4** minimizes the suboccipital bone that will need to be removed later while performing the mastoidectomy proper. Extending the bone flap anteriorly to afford access to the midtemporal region facilitates later posterior subtemporal extradural dissection. An optional zygomatic osteotomy can be performed to increase inferior mobilization of the temporalis muscle to facilitate a more basal trajectory to the

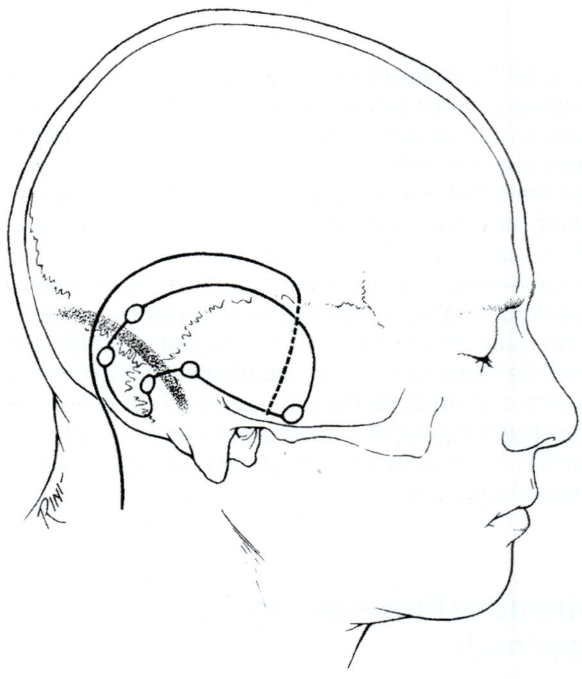

Figure 20–4 The combined supra- and infratentorial petrosal approach scalp incision is planned to enable elevation of a combined temporo-occipital and suboccipital craniotomy flap. The dotted line indicates an optional extension of the incision to facilitate retraction of the scalp flap. Bur holes are placed straddling the transverse sinus, extending laterally to its junction with the sigmoid sinus.

middle fossa. Following elevation of the bone flap using a high-speed craniotome, the surgeon is left with only the remaining triangular-shaped mastoid region, from the supramastoid crest to just posterior to the sigmoid sinus.

Mastoidectomy and Posterior Petrosal Bone Removal

After elevating the temporo-occipital bone flap, a mastoidectomy is performed. As an alternative to standard mastoid drilling, we prefer to perform a cosmetic mastoidectomy, which involves the elevation of the outer table of mastoid bone prior to mastoid drilling. This technique preserves the outer table as a separate bone flap for later mastoid reconstruction at the time of closure. The margins of the outer table of mastoid to be removed are defined by the root of the zygoma, the external auditory canal, and the outer contour of the mastoid to the tip of the mastoid process. Using an oscillating saw or a fine high-speed cutting drill, the outer cortical table is undercut and gently elevated, carefully leaving the insertion of the sternocleidomastoid muscle intact **(Fig. 20–5)**. It is important not to cut deeply into the mastoid sinus to avoid inadvertent injury to the sigmoid sinus and otologic structures.

After the outer table of the mastoid is removed, the remainder of the traditional mastoidectomy is performed with a high-speed drill. If the patient has serviceable preoperative hearing, a retrolabyrinthine exposure is performed. In this approach, the mastoid air cells are sequentially removed to expose the mastoid antrum, which is ~1.5 cm deeper than the intersection of the root of the zygoma and spine of Henle. Within the mastoid antrum, the lateral

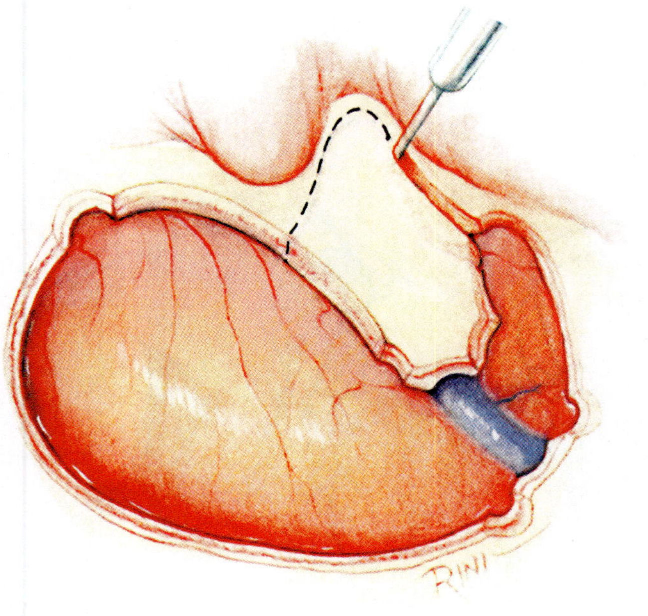

Figure 20–5 Following the elevation of the combined supra- and infratentorial bone flap, a cosmetic mastoidectomy is performed by undercutting the outer table of the mastoid bone using an oscillating saw or a fine high-speed cutting bur as depicted. This split-thickness bone flap is used for later cosmetic reapproximation. The remainder of the mastoid is drilled in the standard fashion, with labyrinth or cochlear removal as deemed necessary for tumor removal.

semicircular canal can be identified. The sigmoid sinus is skeletonized to the jugular bulb, and the middle fossa and presigmoid dura are exposed. The sinodural angle, which marks the entrance of the superior petrosal sinus into the transverse–sigmoid junction, is identified. The remaining semicircular canals and fallopian canal containing the facial nerve are skeletonized with a high-speed diamond drill and copious irrigation. Bone removal should be limited to this extent to prevent damage to the patient's hearing. If, however, the patient has nonserviceable preoperative hearing, additional temporal bone removal with a translabyrinthine or a transcochlear exposure can be performed at this juncture. The translabyrinthine approach, which involves complete removal of the semicircular canals, provides more medial exposure of the petroclival junction. We rarely perform the transcochlear approach, which involves facial nerve transposition, because gain of exposure is minimal at the expense of invariable transient facial nerve palsy. If needed, a total petrosectomy can be performed for lesions that are more extensive.

Anterior Petrosal Bone Removal (Extended Middle Fossa)

Additional removal of the anterior petrous apex through the extradural middle fossa exposure may be considered in patients with larger tumors that require enhanced petroclival exposure. This maneuver is suitable for tumors that involve the petrous apex and upper clivus and extend into Meckel's cave, Dorello's canal, or the posterior cavernous sinus. The anterior petrosectomy also provides a supratentorial to infratentorial trajectory to the anterolateral aspect of the brain stem between the fifth and seventh cranial nerves. Combining both anterior and posterior petrosal approaches (combined petrosal approach) increases the exposure of the petroclival junction and provides multiple surgical trajectories of visualization; limited exposure of the petroclival region from the presigmoid window can be complemented by viewing from the subtemporal window, and vice versa.

The subtemporal dura is elevated extradurally to expose the floor of the middle fossa. The middle meningeal artery at the foramen spinosum is cauterized and cut to allow more medial dissection. The outer layer of the lateral wall of the cavernous sinus (dura propria) is elevated extradurally to identify the gasserian ganglion and the inferior aspect of V3 as it exits through the foramen ovale. The petrous apex (Kawase's triangle), which is bordered by V3 anteriorly, the greater superficial petrosal nerve (GSPN) and petrous internal carotid artery laterally, the internal acoustic canal (IAC) posteriorly, and the petrous edge medially, is carefully removed with a high-speed diamond drill. Caution should be taken not to violate the cochlea, which is located anteromedial to the geniculate ganglion (intersection of the GSPN and IAC).

Dural Incision

The dura is opened along the anterior border of the sigmoid sinus and along the temporal lobe base, while the venous

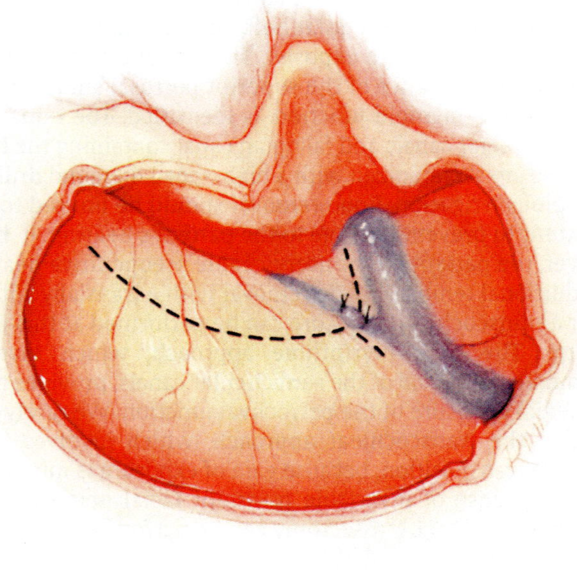

Figure 20–6 The dural opening (dotted line) is performed low and parallel to the base of the skull so the superior petrosal sinus can be ligated well clear and below the junction of the vein of Labbé with the transverse–sigmoid sinus junction. Care must be taken to avoid injury to the vein of Labbé with dural opening. This will enable the cerebellum, the temporal lobe, and the sinuses to be retracted as a unit following division of the tentorium to provide clear access to more medial structures.

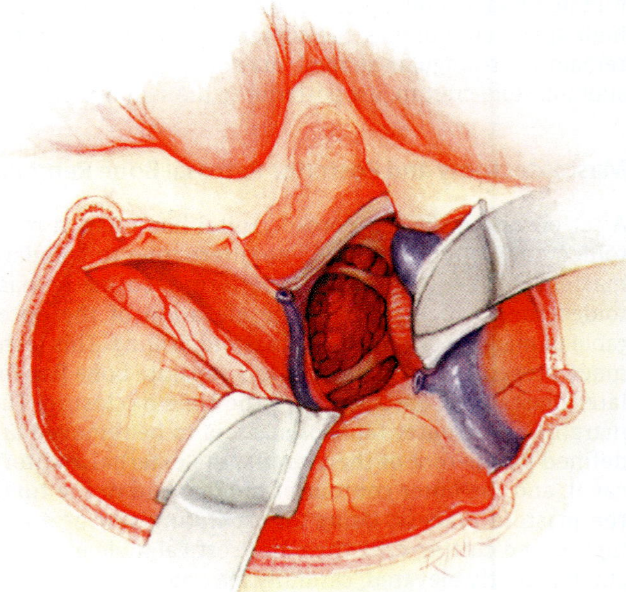

Figure 20–7 Placement of self-retaining retractors on the posterior temporal lobe and cerebellum is followed by aspiration of cerebrospinal fluid and gentle traction. The tumor will soon be visualized, and the surgeon should attempt to identify the lower cranial nerves (IX to XI), the trigeminal and trochlear nerves, and the VII/VIII complex and their respective relationships to the tumor.

drainage of the temporal lobe is carefully inspected **(Fig. 20–6).** The superior petrosal sinus is then ligated with a silk suture and divided just anterior to the transverse–sigmoid junction. This maneuver should be performed with extreme caution not to violate the vein of Labbé, which sometimes may have a variable course in this region. In many cases, the vein of Labbé courses inferior to the temporal lobe for some distance and may also adhere to the dura prior to entering the sinus. In some instances, the vein may duplicate or bifurcate prior to its junction with the sinus. The vein of Labbé may be dissected off the cortical surface with care to enable subsequent retraction of the temporal lobe without traction on the vein.

After the dura is opened, the tentorium is divided just posterior and adjacent to the petrosal sinus, parallel to the petrous pyramid. Depending on the size of the tumor to be removed, variable amounts of tentorium will be exposed. Care must be taken to identify and avoid injuring the trochlear nerve along the inferior border of the tentorium near the incisura. In addition, the trigeminal nerve may be displaced by tumor and be adjacent to the tentorial edge. Self-retaining retractors are then placed to retract the posterior temporal lobe and the transverse and sigmoid sinus complex together with the cut edge of the tentorium and cerebellum **(Fig. 20–7).**

Tumor Removal

After the dura is opened, the basilar cisterns are opened and cerebrospinal fluid (CSF) is gently aspirated to facilitate further brain relaxation. Once the tumor has been exposed, the relationship of the tumor to the cranial nerves and major vasculature must be elucidated **(Figs. 20–7 and 20–8).** It is useful to consider the tumor in the context of four major orientations (superior, inferior, medial, and lateral), and dissection should proceed systematically. Inferiorly, attention must be

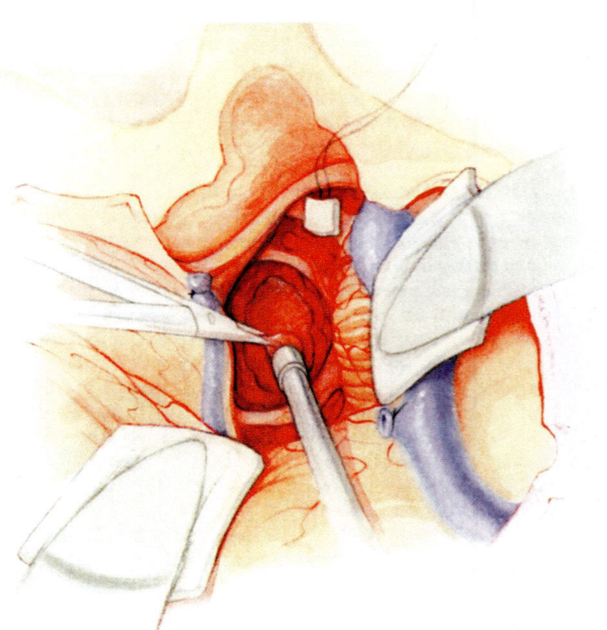

Figure 20–8 Resection of the tumor proceeds in an organized fashion with dissection in a "four-quadrant" pattern. Inferiorly, the tumor is isolated from the lower cranial nerves, which are protected using small pledgets of wet Gelfoam followed by small cottonoid patties. Through a series of extracapsular dissections and debulking of the center of the tumor with microscissors or the ultrasonic aspirator, the tumor is removed.

paid to the location of the vertebral artery, the posterior inferior cerebellar artery, and the ninth–eleventh nerve complex. Effort must be made early during the course of the dissection to identify the fourth and fifth nerves superiorly. The sixth cranial nerve is usually displaced medially, anteriorly, and often inferiorly. It is the most difficult to identify until late in the dissection when most of the tumor has been removed. The seventh and eighth cranial nerves are frequently stretched laterally by the tumor; however, in much larger tumors, these nerves may be embedded within the tumor. By carefully studying the relationship of the major neurovascular structures on the preoperative images, these important landmarks can be anticipated and safely protected during the dissection.

If the lesion is highly vascular, the blood supply to the tumor must be interrupted early in the procedure. The majority of the tumor devascularization is achieved by the petrous bone resection prior to the dural opening; however, tumors located very medially may still receive vascular input from the remaining clival attachment. Larger tumors will likely require intracapsular debulking to allow infolding of the capsule followed by extracapsular dissection. Tumor removal is readily accomplished with the use of bipolar coagulation and microscissors. If space permits, an ultrasonic aspirator may be utilized, although the senior author (WTC) has found this device unwieldy for use in this critical location in many cases. Care must be exercised not to injure intervening cranial nerves and arteries that may be coursing through the tumor or displaced along the margins of the tumor.

With careful piecemeal removal of the tumor, each nerve may be identified and preserved accordingly. In most cases, an adequate plane of dissection between the nerves and the tumor can be established to allow safe removal of the tumor. Careful electromyographic recording and stimulation will aid in locating and preserving the facial nerve. Excessive manipulation of the tenth cranial nerve may result in bradycardia and hypotension. Placing wet pledgets of Gelfoam and thin paddies over the respective nerves protects them from trauma and desiccation during the procedure. The arachnoid planes over uninvolved regions of the cerebellum, cranial nerves, and brain stem are left intact, if possible. In a distinct minority of cases, the tumor may truly invade the nerve, and establishment of adequate dissection planes may not be possible. If oncological removal is to be attempted and nerve function is already impaired, consideration may be given to sacrificing the intervening nerve with the tumor and performing a primary repair or cable grafting (usually with the sural nerve).

As the dissection and tumor removal proceed, the medial aspect of the tumor will invariably be adjacent to and often significantly deforming the brain stem and the basilar artery and its perforating branches. The basilar artery is often displaced to the contralateral side if it is not encased by the tumor. If the arachnoid planes have been preserved adjacent to these structures, dissection will proceed in a straightforward manner. However, in some cases the tumor may be adherent to these structures, making continued dissection hazardous. Some large tumors may parasitize the blood supply from the paramedian perforating branches of the basilar artery. Manipulation or interruption of these branches may risk brain stem infarction as a result of thrombosis or vasospasm. In these cases, it may be more prudent to leave a thin remnant of tumor capsule adherent to the brain stem or important perforating branches to reduce the risk of brain stem infarction.

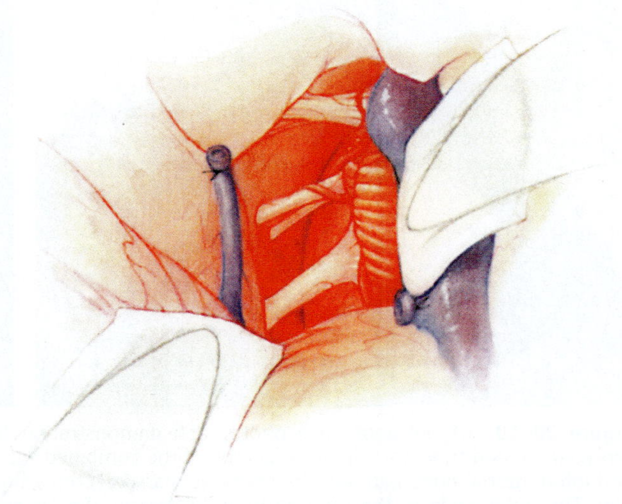

Figure 20–9 Following removal of the tumor, hemostasis is meticulously secured and the tumor bed is covered with a single layer of Surgicel. The self-retaining retractors are removed and the wound is copiously irrigated. Dural closure is performed, and a fascial graft is harvested to enable complete closure of the dura. The mastoidectomy defect is then filled with harvested fat, and the outer table of the mastoid is replaced with titanium miniplate fixation (see **Fig. 20–10**).

Once tumor removal has been accomplished **(Fig. 20–9)**, meticulous hemostasis is performed with a bipolar cautery. The wound is irrigated and the tumor bed is lined with a single layer of Surgicel. The anesthetist performs a Valsalva maneuver or jugular compression to ensure adequate venous hemostasis prior to closure.

Wound Closure

The dural leaflets are reapproximated with interrupted 4–0 Nurolon sutures. In cases in which a primary watertight closure of the dura is not possible, an autologous fat fascia graft is harvested for subsequent repair. After the dura is closed with the fascial graft, the previously developed pericranial graft can be used to supplement the dural closure. Fibrin glue can also be used to reinforce against a CSF leak. The mastoidectomy and petrosectomy defects are obliterated with autologous fat to tamponade the dural patch, with care not to produce unnecessary mass effect against the dura. The residual mastoid air cells are obliterated with wax, and the eustachian tube, if violated, is plugged with muscle to prevent formation of a CSF fistula.

The temporo-occipital bone flap and the outer table of mastoid bone are replaced over the craniotomy defect and fastened with titanium miniplates and screws **(Fig. 20–10)**. The outer table of the mastoid bone tamponades the fat graft against the dural closure to minimize CSF leaks. The soft tissues are reapproximated in multiple layers. A lumbar drain is employed for prophylaxis against development of a CSF fistula in all cases that require fat and fascial grafting.

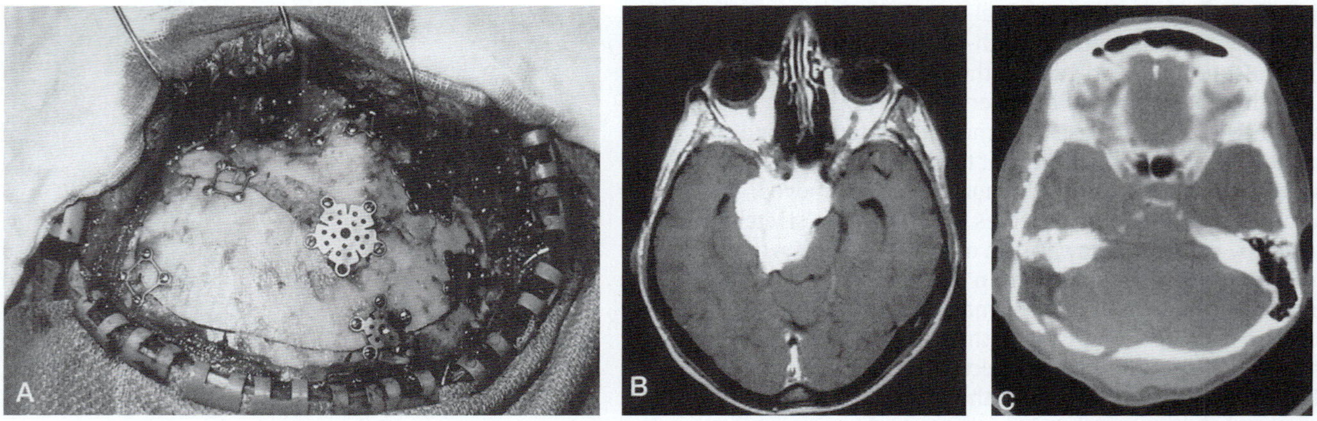

Figure 20–10 **(A)** Intraoperative photograph demonstrating the replacement and titanium miniplate fixation of the combined supra- and infratentorial bone flap and the cosmetic mastoidectomy bone flap. The outer table of the mastoid bone buttresses the fat graft placed in the drilled mastoid cavity below. The bur holes are covered with titanium bur hole covers. (From Couldwell WT, Fukushima T. Cosmetic mastoidectomy for the combined supra- and infratentorial transtemporal approach. J Neurosurg 1993;79:460–461, with permission). **(B)** Gadolinium-enhanced magnetic resonance imaging of a 56-year-old woman who presented with a 6-month history of progressive gait ataxia demonstrates a large right petroclival meningioma displacing the brain stem and basilar artery. The patient underwent a petrosal approach for resection of the tumor. **(C)** Postoperative computed tomographic scan shows resection of the tumor with a fat graft placed in the mastoid defect. Note the smooth contour and lack of bony defect following reconstruction using a cosmetic mastoidectomy.

◆ Postoperative Management

If the operative procedure was extensive, as often is the case with removal of these tumors, the patient may remain intubated until stable in the intensive care unit. Careful postoperative management includes monitoring of blood pressure, arterial blood gases, and urine output. Significant elevations of systolic blood pressure (>20 mm Hg over preoperative blood pressure) are treated aggressively with intravenous antihypertensive agents to minimize the risk of a postoperative hemorrhage; some patients with marked brain stem compression from the tumor may exhibit significant fluctuations in blood pressure in the early postoperative period. Corticosteroids are continued postoperatively and tapered slowly over the following 3 to 5 days. H2 blockers are continued until the patient completes the steroid taper and resumes adequate oral intake.

Following extubation, the patient's swallowing function is carefully evaluated, especially if the ninth–tenth nerve complex was dissected free from the tumor. If there is a suspected risk for aspiration, a thin, flexible nasoenteric feeding tube (Dobhoff tube) can be placed to provide early nutrition. True vocal cord paralysis may be a potentially lethal complication, and every effort must be made to avoid the risk of aspiration in the presence of this complication. An early evaluation by flexible endoscopy by an otolaryngologist is performed to assess mobility of the vocal cord and protection of the airway. A percutaneous feeding tube may be required if the patient is at significant risk for aspiration.

Temporary CSF diversion with a lumbar drain is continued postoperatively for another 3 days if there is no evidence of a CSF leak. Caution is taken to avoid overdrainage, which may result in significant pneumocephalus, cranial nerve palsies, and possibly intracranial hemorrhage. Usually, 5 to 10 mL per hour are drained only under close supervision. The head of the bed is maintained at a maximum of 20 degrees to avoid pneumocephalus.

Measures to reduce the risk of deep venous thrombosis include administration of subcutaneous heparin (5000 U every 12 hours) beginning on postoperative day 1 and mechanical prophylaxis with continuous pneumatic compression devices. Aggressive ambulation, physical therapy, incentive spirometry, and pulmonary toilet cannot be overemphasized to prevent postoperative pulmonary complications.

◆ Complications

Despite a significant reduction in the mortality rate from surgical removal of petroclival meningiomas, postoperative morbidity in these patients is still considerable, largely from associated permanent cranial nerve palsies. The size of the lesion is related to the risks of surgical morbidity and mortality, with removal of larger tumors associated with a greater percentage of complications. Cranial nerve palsies are the most frequent complication encountered, especially when tumor within the cavernous sinus is removed. As noted previously, the decision to completely remove tumor in this region surgically must be made based on individual circumstances.

Additional difficulty arises when tumor either encases the basilar artery or lies between the artery and brain stem. In such instances, extreme care must be exercised during tumor removal because interruption of perforating vessels may result in brain stem infarction. In cases in which the tumor is adherent to the vascular structures or the tumor has parasitized the pial blood supply, a more conservative approach that leaves a thin remnant of adherent tumor is advocated.

In elderly patients, especially those with associated medical problems, the goals of surgery must be limited. In a patient who has a tumor that is causing symptomatic brain stem compression but minimal or no cranial nerve palsies, a subtotal resection (removal of the compressive mass while leaving the tumor invading the cavernous sinus or adherent to the brain stem) may be a more appropriate strategy. Because many of the tumors in this location are slow growing, asymptomatic lesions in elderly patients clearly warrant an observation period before attempting surgical removal.

21

Surgical Management of Tentorial Meningiomas

Daniel R. Pieper

Less than 3% of all intracranial meningiomas arise from the tentorium. The site of origin along the tentorium determines the appropriate surgical approach. Multiple classification systems have been introduced over the years; however, the system described by Yasargil appears to be the most surgically applicable **(Fig. 21–1)**. Yasargil describes the tumor as arising from (1) the inner ring, or free edge, of the tentorium (T1–T3); (2) the outer ring, which runs along the transverse sinus (T5–T7); or (3) the intermediate ring, the area of the tentorium between the inner and outer rings (T4). The site of origin is then further categorized by their location along their respective ring, anterior, lateral, or posterior. Finally, the tumors can be described as primarily supratentorial, infratentorial, or both.

Preoperatively identifying the relationship of the tumor to structures of the deep venous system, dural venous sinuses, brain stem, and cranial nerves allows the surgeon to better plan for the surgical endeavor. Unfortunately it is not always possible to differentiate between petroclival and tentorial meningiomas preoperatively; however, differentiating between these origins at the time of surgery, prior to the resection, has significant implications regarding the method of dissection. Tentorial meningiomas, unlike petroclival meningiomas, arise lateral to cranial nerve V and, therefore, have an origin outside the arachnoidal layers of the basilar cisterns, which provides a plane of dissection between the tumor, the brain stem, blood vessels, and cranial nerves. Identifying dural venous sinus invasion preoperatively and intraoperatively is essential in determining the limits of resection in tentorial meningiomas.

◆ Patient Selection

As with all intracranial meningiomas, tentorial meningiomas are more common in middle-aged females. Tentorial meningiomas typically present with nonspecific signs and symptoms including headache, visual changes, and papilledema. Tumors located along the inner ring have a higher incidence of cranial nerve or brain stem disturbances, particularly (1) ocular dysmotility due to extraocular cranial nerve (III, IV, and VI) compression or brain stem compression as in Parinaud's syndrome, and (2) disturbances of the trigeminal nerve presenting as trigeminal neuralgia, atypical facial pain syndrome, or facial hypesthesia. Tumors involving the supratentorial compartment may have associated visual field disturbances when there is compression of the calcarine cortex, or dysphasias or seizure disorders or both with compression of the temporal lobe. Infratentorial extension may typically be associated with signs and symptoms of cerebellar compression. Elevated intracranial pressure may be present when there is significant involvement of a major dural venous sinus major, especially the torcula, or secondary to obstructive hydrocephalus due to aqueductal compression.

Since the introduction of nonsurgical modalities for the treatment for meningiomas there has been ongoing debate as to the management of meningiomas. These modalities have included radiosurgery, hormonal manipulation, and chemotherapy; however, to date, these interventions remain an adjunct to surgical resection. Personal experience has suggested that the patient's best, and sometimes only, chance of cure occurs at the first operation. Therefore, the surgeon's objective should be one of surgical removal of the tumor while preserving, if not improving, the patient's function. In situations where vital structures are involved in tumor, which in the case of tentorial meningiomas are typically the venous sinuses, a gross total resection may not be possible; however, this is a decision to be made intraoperatively. In these cases, depending on the amount and location of residual tumor, adjunctive modalities may be considered.

◆ Preoperative Preparation

Preoperative evaluation by magnetic resonance imaging (MRI) with gadolinium enhancement in all three planes is necessary to evaluate the tumor and its relationship to the intracranial structures. Additionally, radiographic examination of the cerebrovascular anatomy, either by conventional angiography or magnetic resonance angiography (MRA) and venography (MRV) will provide further details necessary for surgical planning. In differentiating severe versus total vascular occlusion, especially of a venous sinus, cerebral angiography is more sensitive when compared with MRV. Therefore, it is my practice to obtain a venous phase angiogram prior to the sacrifice of a major venous sinus.

The necessity of other preoperative examinations is determined by the location of tumor. These additional tests

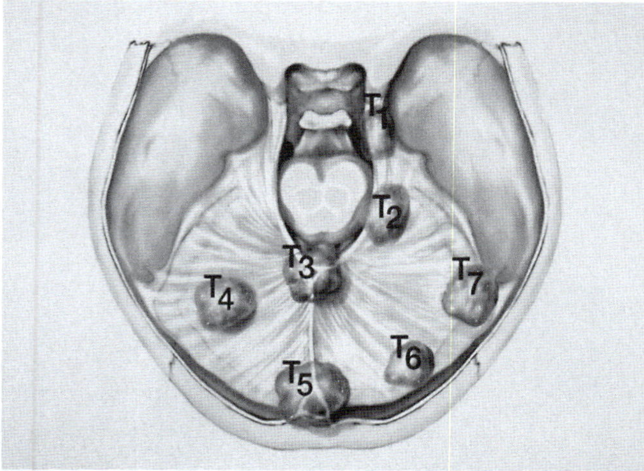

Figure 21–1 The classification of tentorial meningiomas as described by Yasargil. Under this classification system tumors are described as involving the inner ring (T1–T3), the intermediate ring (T and T8), or the outer ring (T5–T7). (Reproduced with permission from Yasargil MG. Microneurosurgery. Vol 4B, p. 37. Stuttgart: Thieme; 1996.)

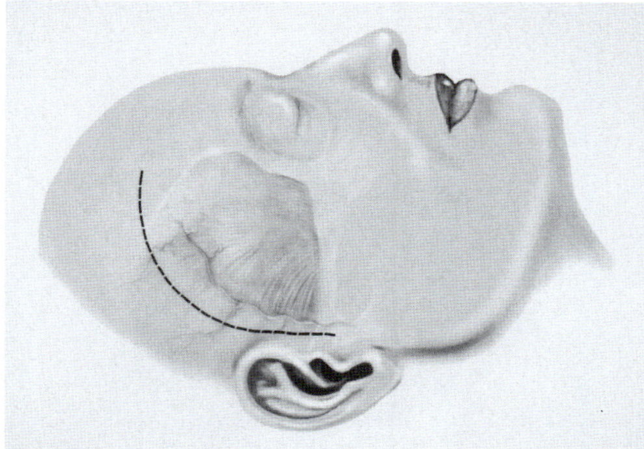

Figure 21–2 Incision used in the extended middle fossa approach. (Reproduced with permission from Kaye AH, Black PM. Operative Neurosurgery. London: Churchill Livingstone; 2000.)

may include neuro-ophthalmologic evaluation, formal visual field testing, audiometry, facial nerve electromyography (EMG), electronystagmography (ENG), vocal cord motility examination, or swallowing.

◆ Operative Procedure

When approaching tentorial meningiomas, the choice of approach must be specifically tailored in each case. Two major anatomical variables are evaluated when determining the best route of approach to the tumor. The first variable is dependent on the location of the tumor along the tentorium: anterior, lateral, or posterior **(Fig. 21–1)**. The second identifies whether the tumor is supratentorial, infratentorial, or both. In the majority of cases an approach that provides access to both the supra- and infratentorial compartments is preferable because this allows better visualization during the resection of the tumor's tentorial origin as well as control of the dural venous sinuses.

T1 Lesions

For tumors arising anteriorly along the inner ring (T1) the extended middle fossa approach including petrous apicectomy is utilized. This approach provides access to Meckel's cave as well as the posterior fossa. In cases where there is a significant supratentorial component this can be converted to a cranio-orbitozygomatic approach.

Extended Middle Fossa Approach

A preauricular incision is made avoiding injury to the superficial temporal artery (STA) and frontalis branch of the facial nerve as it crosses over the zygomatic arch. The incision is carried superiorly to the superior temporal line and extended anteriorly to the edge of the hairline. The skin flap is then reflected anteriorly **(Fig. 21–2)**.

An incision is made through the superficial and deep layers of the temporalis fascia 1 cm posterior to the lateral orbital. The temporalis fascia is then dissected along the zygomatic arch in a subperiosteal fashion and reflected with the skin flap. This maneuver preserves the frontalis branch of the facial nerve, which courses between the layers of the temporalis fascia at this point. A zygomatic osteotomy is performed by making oblique cuts through the zygoma flush with the malar eminence and at the root of the zygoma **(Fig. 21–3)**. The temporalis muscle and fascia are dissected along the superior temporal line and reflected inferiorly with the zygoma.

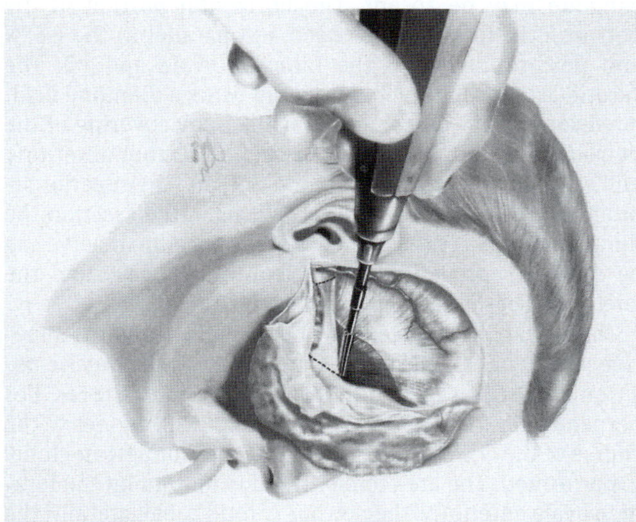

Figure 21–3 Oblique cuts are made in the zygomatic arch flush with the malar eminence and root of the zygoma. (Reproduced with permission from Kaye AH, Black PM. Operative Neurosurgery. London: Churchill Livingstone; 2000.)

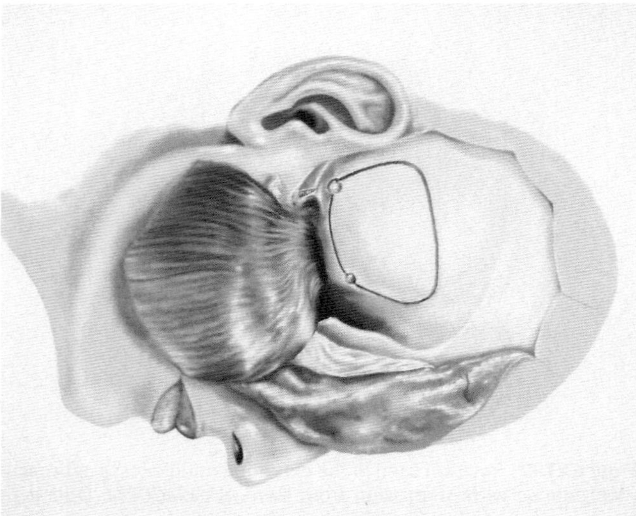

Figure 21–4 Inferior displacement of the temporalis muscle and zygoma providing exposure of the floor of the middle fossa. Bur holes are placed along the floor of the middle fossa. A temporal craniotomy is then performed as shown. (Reproduced with permission from Kaye AH, Black PM. Operative Neurosurgery. London: Churchill Livingstone; 2000.)

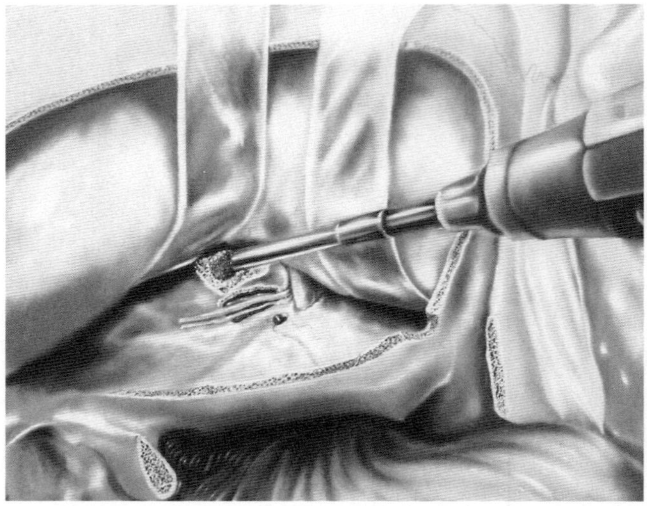

Figure 21–5 After identifying and transecting the middle meningeal artery at the foramen spinosum, the V3 is identified anteromedially exiting via the foramen ovale. The greater and lesser superficial petrosal nerves are identified exiting via the facial hiatus. The horizontal portion of the petrous internal carotid artery is identified posterior to the foramen ovale and paralleling the greater superficial petrosal nerve. Drilling of the petrous apex is performed. (Reproduced with permission from Kaye AH, Black PM. Operative Neurosurgery. London: Churchill Livingstone; 2000.)

Bur holes are placed along the floor of the middle fossa just above the residual zygomatic root and more anteriorly along the floor of the middle fossa. A temporal craniotomy is made flush with the floor of the middle fossa extending posteriorly along the petrous bone **(Fig. 21–4).**

Starting posteriorly and working anteriorly the dura along the floor of the middle fossa is elevated. The middle meningeal artery at the foramen spinosum is identified and transected. Medially to the foramen spinosum, the foramen ovale and V3 are identified. Posteromedially the greater and lesser superficial petrosal nerves are identified (GSPN, LSPN) as they exit from the geniculate ganglion via the facial hiatus and run anteriorly within the sphenopetrosal groove. In some cases the bony covering over the geniculate ganglion may be absent. The horizontal portion of the petrous carotid artery lies deep and parallel to the GSPN and posteriomedial to the foramen ovale and V3. The carotid artery can then be unroofed using a diamond drill; however, it is not uncommon for the bony covering of the petrous carotid to be absent. Dissection further anteriorly will expose the foramen rotundum (V2) and the superior orbital fissure (III, IV, V1, and VI). With sharp dissection the dural covering over the branches of the trigeminal nerve can be removed, providing access to Meckel's cave and the lateral wall of the cavernous sinus **(Fig. 21–5).**

The arcuate eminence is the bony landmark of the superior semicircular canal (SSC). Unfortunately, the precise position of the SSC can be difficult to appreciate. The SSC lies perpendicular to the petrous bone and ~120 degrees to the course of the GSPN. At this point the anterior petrosectomy is performed. The area to be drilled is limited by the foramen ovale anteriorly, the petrous carotid canal laterally, the cochlea posteriorly, and the internal auditory canal inferiorly. The cochlea is surrounded by hard compact bone, unlike the bone of the petrous apex, and therefore can be differentiated during drilling of this area **(Fig. 21–5).**

The dura is opened along the floor of the middle fossa. The posterior fossa is entered through Meckel's cave **(Fig. 21–6).** The superior petrosal sinus is identified and either ligated or coagulated and transected sharply. The tentorium can then be divided, with care taken to identify the trochlear nerve along the free edge of the dura and staying posterior to its entrance into the dural fold **(Fig. 21–7).**

T2 and T7 Lesions

For tumors located laterally, either along the inner ring at the incisura (T2) or outer ring (T7), the petrosal approach is

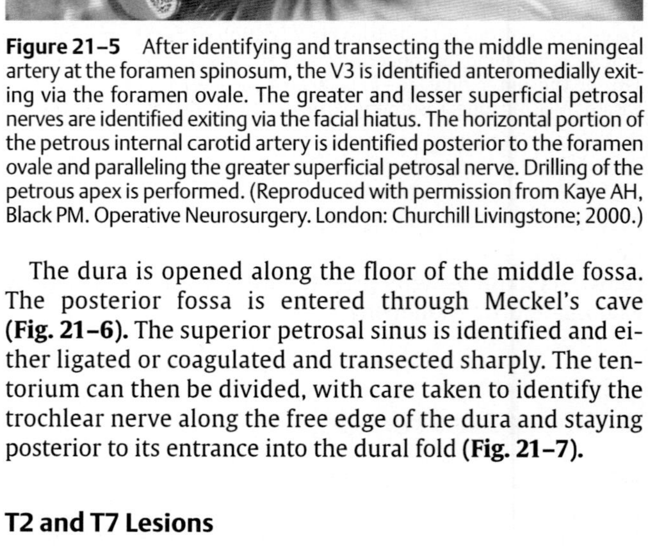

Figure 21–6 The petrous apex has been removed and the horizontal petrous internal carotid artery skeletonized. The dura is opened along the floor of the middle fossa. (Reproduced with permission from Al-Mefty O. Operative Atlas of Meningiomas. Philadelphia: Lippincott-Raven; 1998.)

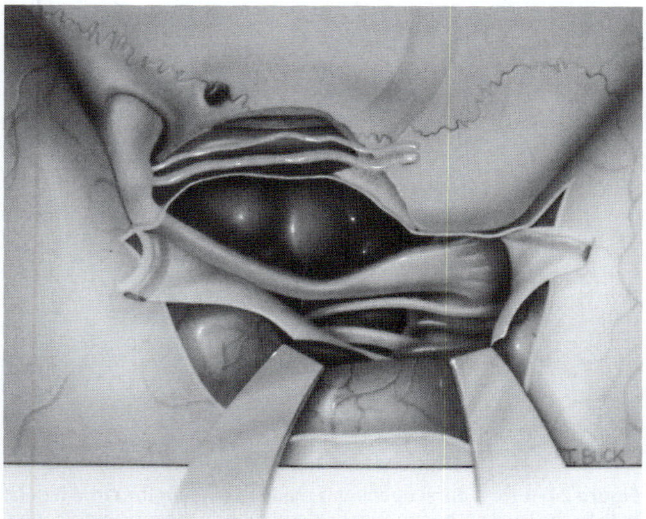

Figure 21–7 The superior petrosal sinus and tentorium have been transected to the level of the incisura. The tumor, arising from the inner ring, is appreciated. The gasserian ganglion and V3, CN III and IV, basilar artery with superior cerebellar artery and anterior inferior cerebellar artery are identified in the posterior fossa. (Reproduced with permission from Al-Mefty O. Operative Atlas of Meningiomas. Philadelphia: Lippincott-Raven; 1998.)

preferred. The petrosal approach affords surgical access to the brain stem laterally and ventrally above and below the incisura, inferiorly to the level of the jugular foramen, and supratentorially to the posterior portion of the cavernous sinus. Additionally, the petrosal approach provides excellent access to the transverse, sigmoid, and superior petrosal sinuses, as well as the tentorial artery.

Petrosal Approach

The patient is placed supine on the operating room table with the ipsilateral shoulder slightly elevated using a shoulder roll, the head rotated 40 to 60 degrees away from the side of the tumor, and the vertex lowered slightly toward the floor. This will place the base of the petrous pyramid at the highest point in the surgical field. A reverse question mark incision is started at the zygoma 1 to 1.5 cm anterior to the tragus to avoid injury to the frontalis branch of the facial nerve as it crosses over the zygoma. The incision is carried 2 to 3 cm above the pinna of the ear and descends 1 to 2 cm medial to (behind) the mastoid process inferiorly to the tip of the mastoid process **(Fig. 21–8).** The skin flap is sharply dissected from the underlying pericranium, temporalis fascia and muscle, and sternocleidomastoid muscle and reflected anteriorly and inferiorly **(Fig. 21–9).** The temporalis fascia is then sharply cut, maintaining its continuity with the periosteum over the temporal and suboccipital areas, and dissected from the temporalis muscle. At this point the sternocleidomastoid is detached along its insertion at the skull base. The temporalis fascia, periosteum, and sternocleidomastoid muscle are then reflected inferiorly as a single unit to be used in the reconstruction at the conclusion of the case. The temporalis muscle is then detached along its insertion at the superior temporal line and reflected anteriorly.

Four bur holes, two on either side of the transverse sinus, are made. The first bur hole is placed just inferior and medial to the asterion, which opens into the posterior fossa below the transverse–sigmoid sinus junction. The second bur hole is placed at the squamosal mastoid junction of the temporal bone along the projection of the superior temporal line. This opens into the supratentorial compartment. The remaining two holes are placed slightly more medial and closer together, flanking the transverse sinus. A temporoparietal craniotomy is performed between the superior two bur holes, and a lateral suboccipital craniotomy is performed between the inferior bur holes. Finally the bridge of bone across the supra- and infratentorial bur holes is cut and the craniotomy flap is elevated. Care must be taken during this maneuver because the dura may be adherent to the bone, especially at the transverse–sigmoid sinus junction **(Fig. 21–10).**

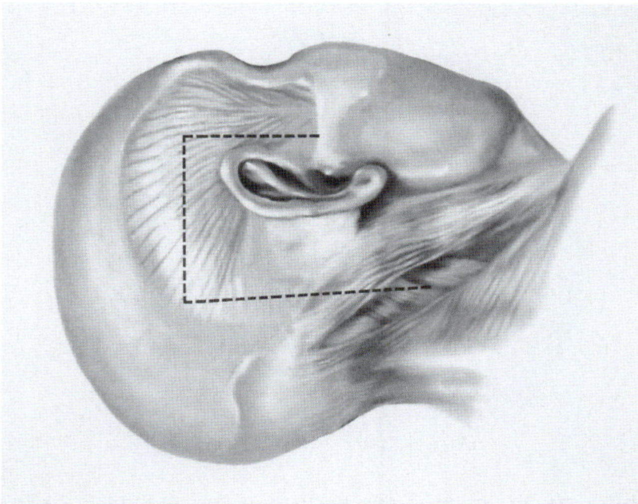

Figure 21–8 Incision used in the petrosal approach. (Reproduced with permission from Kaye AH, Black PM. Operative Neurosurgery. London: Churchill Livingstone; 2000.)

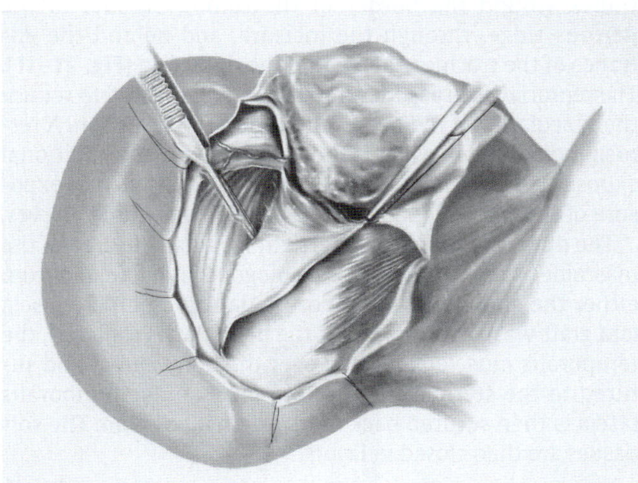

Figure 21–9 Sharp dissection of the temporalis fascia from the underlying muscle. The main trunk of the superficial temporal artery is preserved anterior to the fascial incision to maintain the vascular supply to the temporalis muscle. (Reproduced with permission from Kaye AH, Black PM. Operative Neurosurgery. London: Churchill Livingstone; 2000.)

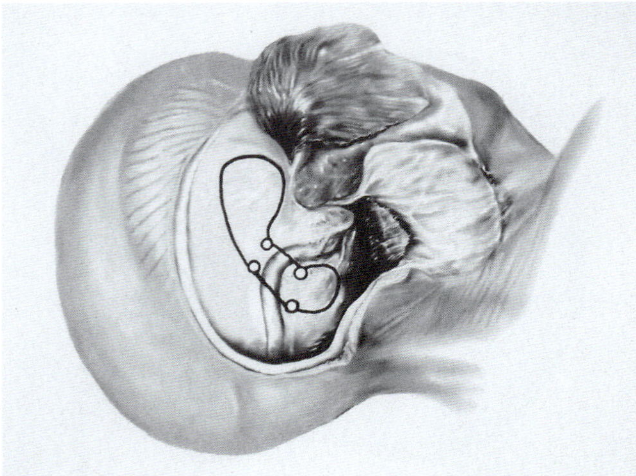

Figure 21–10 Position of the bur holes and the craniotomy used for the petrosal approach. (Reproduced with permission from Kaye AH and Black PM: Operative Neurosurgery. London, Churchill Livingstone, 2000)

The sigmoid sinus is skeletonized down to the jugular bulb. A complete mastoidectomy is performed down to the mastoid antrum, which is usually identified at a depth of 1.5 cm. The solid angle of cortical bone along the medial aspect of the antrum is not violated to protect the otologic structures. The sinodural (Citelli's) angle, which identifies the position of the superior petrosal sinus as it enters the transverse–sigmoid junction, is exposed.

A dural opening is made anterior to the sigmoid sinus down to the jugular bulb and up to the superior petrosal sinus at the transverse–sigmoid junction. The supratentorial incision is made along the floor of the middle fossa and extended along the transverse sinus. Dissection along the vein of Labbé may be necessary to avoid excessive traction and subsequent injury to this vessel. At this point the superior petrosal sinus is either ligated or coagulated and transected at the sinodural (Citelli's) angle. The tentorial incision continues around the border of the tumor, parallel to the petrous ridge, through the incisura, and behind the entrance of the trochlear nerve into the dural fold **(Fig. 21–11)**. The tentorial artery is identified early and divided to reduce the vascularity of the neoplasm during the resection. A retrosigmoid dural incision is then made to provide additional exposure of the tumor along the tentorium, as well as exposure of the cerebellopontine angle and lower cranial nerves.

The dura is closed in a watertight fashion. The area of the mastoidectomy is filled with autologous fat harvested from either the abdominal region or the lateral thigh if a fascia lata graft was necessary. After the bone flap is replaced, the temporalis muscle is rotated over the bony defect and sutured to the sternocleidomastoid muscle. The temporalis fascia is then sutured back to its original position. The soft tissues are then closed in layers.

T3–T6 Lesions

The remaining tumor locations, those involving the posterior inner ring (T3), the intermediate ring (T4), and the

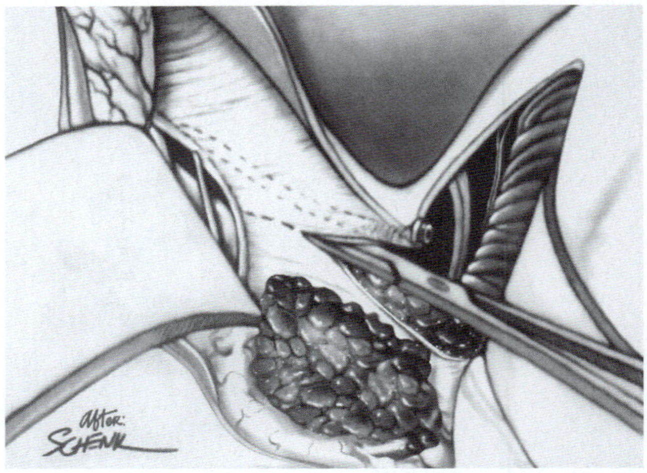

Figure 21–11 A dural opening is made extending from the jugular bulb to the level of the superior petrosal sinus in the presigmoid dura. An additional supratentorial dural incision is made along the floor of the middle fossa extending posteriorly along the distal end of the transverse sinus. The superior petrosal sinus is ligated and transected. The incision continues along the tentorium to the incisura, posterior to the insertion of the trochlear nerve, interrupting the vascular supply to the tumor . (Reprinted with permission from Al-Mefty O, Schenk MP, Smith RR. Petroclival meningiomas. In: Neurosurgical Operative Atlas. Vol 1, no. 5. American Association of Neurological Surgeons; 1991.)

outer ring posteriorly (T5 and 6), are typically approached using a low occipital craniotomy, a suboccipital craniotomy, or a combination of the two depending on the extent of involvement of the supratentorial and infratentorial compartments and the tumor's relationship to the venous sinus.

Combined Occipital-Suboccipital Craniotomy

The patient is positioned on the operating table in a three quarter prone position with the head of the table elevated slightly. The hemisphere ipsilateral to the tumor is placed dependently, which allows the occipital lobe to fall away, minimizing retraction during surgery. The head is placed in the head holder slightly flexed and turned toward the surgeon minimizing any obstruction by the shoulder **(Fig. 21–12)**.

A dorsal midline incision is made extending above and below the external occipital protuberance to allow access to both the supra- and infratentorial compartments. In cases where more lateral access is necessary the superior aspect of the incision can be extended laterally. The incision is carried through the dermal layer only and then sharp subfascial dissection is performed. A curvilinear incision, based inferiorly, is made through the muscle and fascial layers down to the periosteum. This fascial flap is dissected subperiosteally from the occipital bone and reflected inferiorly. By performing the exposure in this way the surgeon is afforded (1) wider exposure laterally; (2) lines of incision that do not overlap, decreasing the risk of cerebrospinal fluid (CSF) leak; and (3) a large tissue flap that can be utilized in the dural closure as necessary.

Bur holes are placed adjacent to the superior sagittal sinus (SSS) and transverse sinus (TS) ipsilaterally **(Fig. 21–13)**. In cases involving both the supra- and infratentorial compartments, we

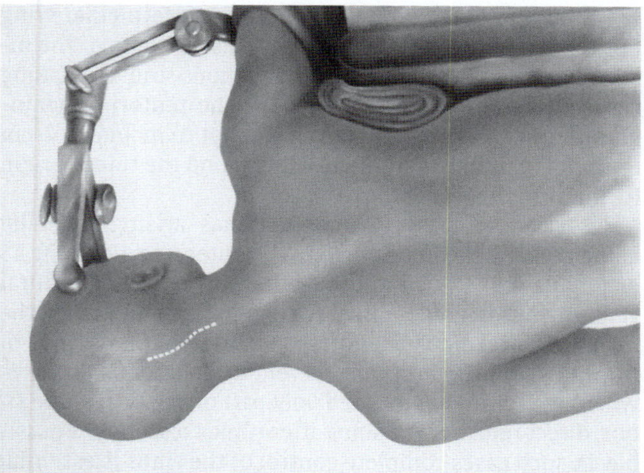

Figure 21–12 The patient is positioned in a three quarter prone position. The side ipsilateral to the tumor is placed dependently and the head is slightly flexed and turned toward the surgeon to minimize any obstruction by the shoulder. A paramedian longitudinal incision is made ipsilateral to the side of the tumor extending both above and below the external occipital protuberance. (Reproduced with permission from Al-Mefty O. Operative Atlas of Meningiomas. Philadelphia: Lippincott-Raven; 1998.)

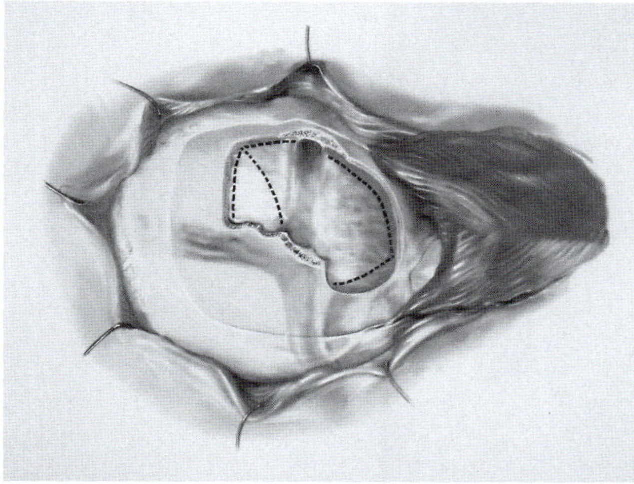

Figure 21–14 The occipital-suboccipital craniotomy is elevated as a single flap, carefully avoiding injury to the underlying transverse sinus, which may be adherent. The dura is then opened as depicted by the dotted lines, allowing access to the supratentorial and infratentorial compartments. The supratentorial dural opening is confined to the ipsilateral side of the tumor; however, the posterior fossa exposure extends across the midline. The dural openings are shown here depicted by the dotted lines (Reproduced with permission from Kaye AH, Black PM. Operative Neurosurgery. London: Churchill Livingstone; 2000.)

typically expose the distal SSS, torcula, and ipsilateral TS. In tumors involving the torcula (T5) distal access along the TS bilaterally is necessary. The occipital and suboccipital craniotomy flap is removed as a single unit, providing access to both the supra- and infratentorial compartments as well as to the SSS, torcula, and TS. When connecting the bur holes across the sinuses we perform a craniectomy using either a high-speed drill or a rongeur. The dura is then carefully dissected free from the overlying bone, carefully avoiding injury to the underlying dural venous sinuses **(Fig. 21–14)**.

Dural openings are made on both sides of the TS, allowing access to the supra- and infratentorium, with the flaps based along the dural sinuses **(Fig. 21–14).** The tumor is approached along the tentorium both supratentorially and infratentorially. A corridor medially along the falx cerebri, where a lack of bridging veins is present, is utilized during the supratentorial approach **(Fig. 21–15)**. The arterial supply

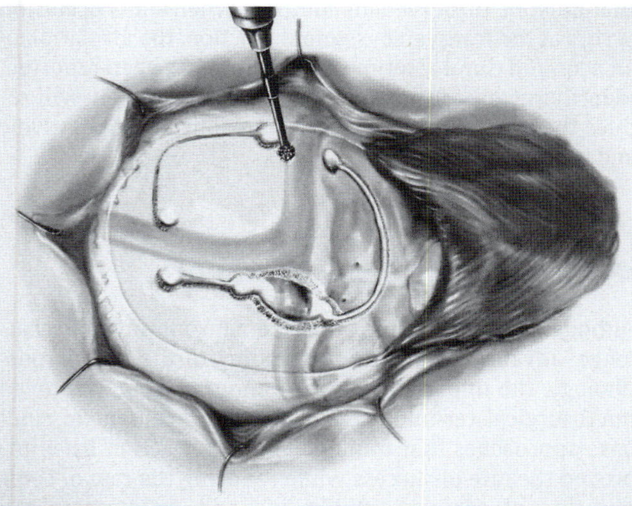

Figure 21–13 Bur holes are placed adjacent to the superior sagittal sinus (SSS) and on either side of the ipsilateral transverse sinus (TS). This exposure is used for those tumors that involve both the supra- and the infratentorial compartments but do not involve the straight sinus. In cases where the tumor crosses the midline, it is necessary to expose the SSS and the contralateral TS. The bur holes are interconnected using a craniotome except across the dural venous sinuses; instead these bur holes are connected by performing a small craniectomy either with a drill (as shown) or a rongeur. (Reproduced with permission from Kaye AH, Black PM. Operative Neurosurgery. London: Churchill Livingstone; 2000.)

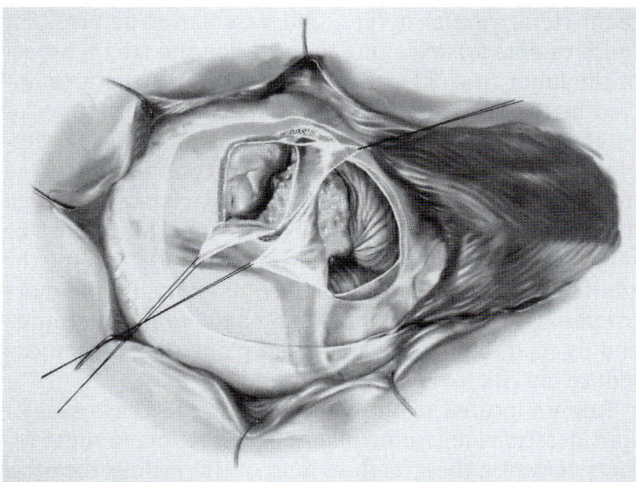

Figure 21–15 The dural flaps are based along the dural venous sinuses providing access both above and below the tentorium. Typically, as represented here, the infratentorial portion of the tumor is larger than the supratentorial component. Tumor resection is performed by interrupting the blood supply along the tentorium, first reducing the amount of blood loss during tumor enucleation. (Reproduced with permission from Kaye AH, Black PM. Operative Neurosurgery. London: Churchill Livingstone; 2000.)

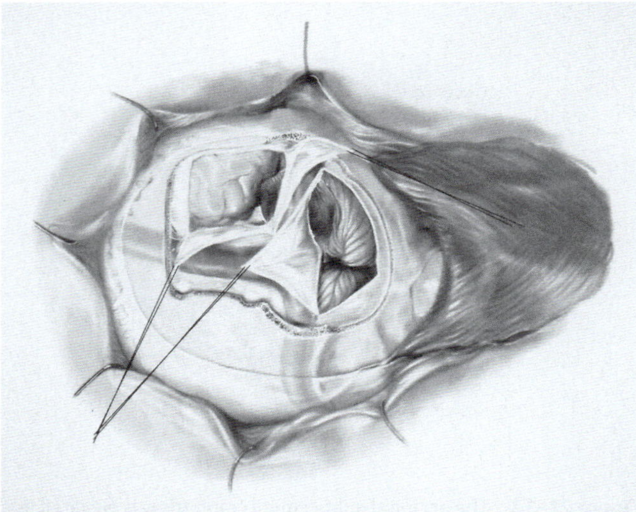

Figure 21–16 The anatomy visualized after tumor removal. A 2-cm tentorial margin is resected circumferentially around the tumor margin, avoiding the dural venous sinuses, to diminish the risk of recurrence. (Reproduced with permission from Kaye AH, Black PM. Operative Neurosurgery. London: Churchill Livingstone; 2000.)

of the tumor is identified along the tentorium and divided prior to the tumor's resection, allowing enucleation of the tumor to be performed with less bleeding. Enucleation of the tumor proceeds while carefully maintaining the arachnoid plane between the tumor and vital structures: brain stem, brain, cranial nerves, arteries, and veins **(Fig. 21–16).**

Tumor Resection

Tentorial meningiomas arising along the inner ring (T1–T3) are invested in multiple layers of arachnoid, unlike those meningiomas that arise from the skull base along the petrous or clivus. These additional arachnoid layers provide a demarcation between the tumor and vital structures: brain stem, cranial nerves, and vascular structures. For those tumors arising along the anterior and lateral aspect of the inner ring (T1 and T2) vital arterial structures, including the anterior choroidal and basilar apex (superior cerebellar, posterior communicating, and posterior cerebral) arteries must be identified and carefully dissected free during the resection. Additionally, cranial nerves III through VI can be displaced by the tumor and must be carefully dissected during the resection. Because of the additional arachnoid plane these vital structures are more commonly displaced rather than engulfed by the tumor, and by maintaining the arachnoid plane the surgeon can reduce the risk to these structures.

Tumors located in the pineal region (T3) have similar considerations regarding planes of dissection. In these tumors, however, the structures most at risk include the basal vein of Rosenthal, precentral cerebellar veins, and the vein of Galen. Cranial nerve IV and the superior cerebellar and posterior cerebral arteries may be displaced and should be identified early during the resection to avoid injury.

Tumors along the lateral aspect of the intermediate ring (T4) typically do not involve the vital structures of the incisura and do not invade the dural venous sinuses, making these tumors one of the easiest of the tentorial meningiomas to resect. If possible we attempt to include a 2-cm tentorial margin circumferentially around the tumor origin to diminish the risk of recurrence.

Resection of tentorial meningiomas arising medially along the straight sinus or along the outer ring along the TS or torcula (T5–T7) is limited by their invasion of the dural venous sinuses. Preoperative angiographic evaluation of the involved dural sinus is necessary to assess the patency of the sinus and the presence of venous collaterals. In cases where the tumor has invaded only part of one wall of the sinus, direct repair of the sinus after tumor resection is possible. In such cases complete control of the sinus is essential proximal and distal to the involved area. When tumor invasion involves more than one wall of the sinus a decision must be made regarding the impact of sacrificing the sinus; such a decision requires a thorough understanding of the venous anatomy preoperatively. Successful repair of a sinus with tumor involving more than one wall either by patch graft or by venous bypass graft has a high incidence of failure. Therefore, in those patients where patency of the sinus is essential for adequate venous drainage of the brain a subtotal tumor resection should be considered.

In cases where the sinus is totally occluded preoperatively, understanding the compensatory hemodynamic changes and their affect on the surgical approach and tumor resection is equally important. Where a major venous sinus is occluded, as in the torcula, venous drainage must use alternative routes, usually in the form of collateral vessels. Formal angiography can provide important information regarding the anomalous venous drainage, identifying vessels that must be preserved. In addition, when sinus occlusion occurs at the transverse–sigmoid junction, the formation of an acquired dural arteriovenous fistula has been reported. Identifying any of these anomalies preoperatively will reduce the risks of untoward complications intraoperatively and postoperatively.

◆ Postoperative Management

Although tentorial meningiomas remain a formidable challenge, advances in the understanding of the tumor morphology, the importance of the venous system, improved microsurgical techniques, and the advancement of skull base approaches that minimize brain retraction have improved the rate of success while reducing the rate of complication of surgery. Establishing and maintaining the arachnoid plane surrounding these tumors significantly reduces the risk to vital structures: brain, brain stem, cranial nerves, arteries, and veins.

Thoroughly understanding the vascular anatomy preoperatively, especially the venous anatomy, dural sinuses, basal veins, and anomalous collaterals, will reduce the risk of unforeseen interruption of the brain's venous drainage.

22

Surgical Management of Tuberculum Sellae Meningiomas

Ossama Al-Mefty and Paulo A. S. Kadri

Meningiomas originating from the tuberculum sellae, chiasmatic sulcus, limbus sphenoidale, and diaphragma sellae are included under the name of *tuberculum sellae meningioma,* representing 5 to 10% of intracranial meningiomas. Although a very short distance separates their origin from the origins of olfactory groove or clinoidal meningiomas, they are distinguished in their clinical, radiological, and surgical considerations. Occupying a subchiasmal position, these tumors usually elevate and displace the optic nerve laterally **(Fig. 22–1A);** thus defects in the visual field due to direct nerve or chiasmal compression, generating the classical "chiasmatic syndrome," which includes primary optic atrophy with bitemporal field defects and an essential normal sellae size. The visual loss is usually asymmetrical and progressive **(Fig. 22–1B).** Pituitary dysfunction is uncommon and late in occurrence, except in patients with diaphragm sellae meningiomas, in which retrochiasmatic growth of the tumor frequently compresses the hypothalamus. In patients with large tumors the third ventricle is displaced upward and hydrocephalus ensues. Cavernous sinus involvement, with ocular motility dysfunction, can also be observed, with the tumor's lateral growth.

The area of attachment of tuberculum sellae meningiomas to the dura is rather small, at least when the tumor is of a small or moderate size, although giant tumors or "en plaque" appearance can also occur. Quite frequently, they invade the bone, causing hyperostosis situated slightly in front of the anterior margin of the sella, and extension of the tumor can be observed inferiorly toward the sellar region and sphenoid sinus. Treatment of tuberculum sellae meningiomas is total surgical removal, including the tumor, dura, bone, and invaded mucosa of the sinus. After tumor removal visual recovery is dramatic, constituting a strong indication for surgery once the diagnosis is made **(Fig. 22–1C).**

Current advances in surgical techniques, and modern anesthesia and neuroimaging, should allow surgical removal in most patients, even of large and complex tumors. A considerable increase in mortality, morbidity, and failure of visual improvement occurs in patients in whom the tumor exceeds 3 cm in diameter. Likewise, the ability to achieve total removal is related to the tumor's size. Hence these tumors should be diagnosed as early as possible and removed totally. A giant size, however, should not temper the surgeon's zeal for total removal of these benign neoplasms. Early devascularization at the base of the tumor provides a bloodless surgical field. Debulking of the central core of the tumor provides the necessary space to dissect the margins of the tumor within the arachnoidal plane. The arachnoid membrane, providing a plane of dissection even when the tumor totally engulfs the cerebral vessels and the optic apparatus, is the best ally of the surgeon. Thus the best chance to achieve total removal is at the first operation when the arachnoid membrane has not been violated.

Tuberculum sella meningioma frequently extend into one or both optic canals, but a plane of dissection separates the tumor from the optic nerves, and this extension should be pursued with the goal of preserving or improving vision. The tumor's involvement of the cavernous sinus no longer deters total removal. Unless serious systemic disease contraindicates major surgery, these tumors are recommended for surgical treatment, and radical removal is the ultimate goal. Either conventional or stereotactic radiation therapy, however, may be an adjuvant in treating recurrence or residual if the tumor is a safe distance of 2 to 3 mm from the optic pathways.

◆ Preoperative Preparation

Modern imaging procedures, such as high-resolution computed tomography (CT), magnetic resonance (MR) imaging, and, in selective cases, angiography, are indispensable in the workup of patients with tuberculum sellae meningiomas. The grade and extension of bone involvement are assessed through axial and coronals cuts of the CT scans, helping to anticipate the extension of surgical bone resection. Contrast-enhanced MR images in multiplanar views is the modality of choice for identifying the lesion and for visualizing tumor extensions into, and encroachment upon, surrounding neurovascular structures, and the extent of dural involvement and cavernous sinus invasion **(Fig. 22–2A–C).** For typical cases, MR angiography (MRA) is adequate in delineating cerebral vasculature and anatomy, identifying arterial encasement and displacement, and revealing associated vascular lesions **(Fig. 22–2D).** Intraoperative neuronavigation has been applied in the last few years and is an important adjunct tool in identifying neurovascular structures at the base of the skull, helping to program the surgery and delineate the extension of bone resection. The very thin stealth MR images provide additional information to the radiological exams. Selective intra-arterial angiography is reserved for

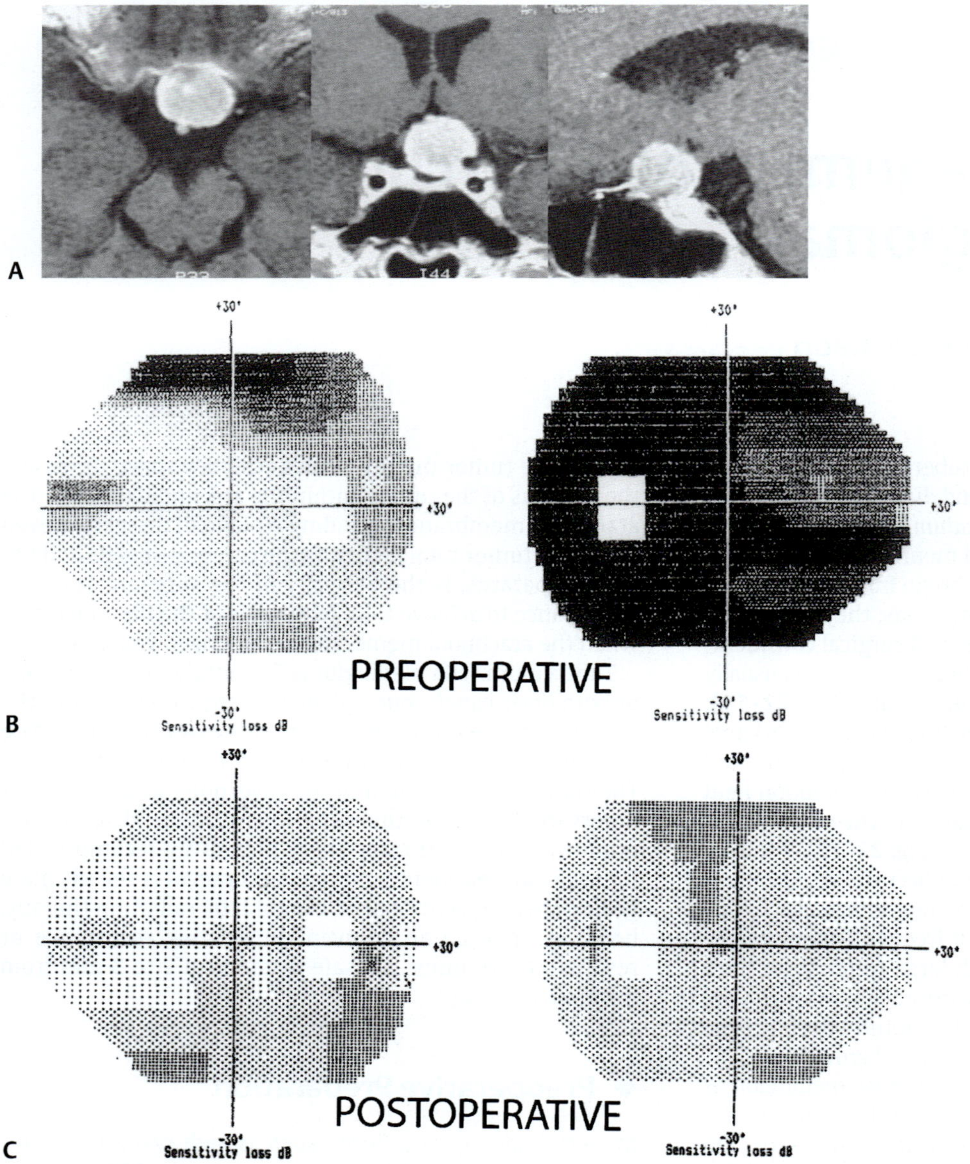

Figure 22–1 **(A)** Contrast-enhanced magnetic resonance images (axial, coronal, and sagittal) demonstrating the typical appearance of a tuberculum sellae meningioma. **(B)** Preoperative visual field of the same patient showing the typical asymmetrical visual loss. **(C)** Postoperative visual field showing the improvement of the visual loss after surgery.

particular situations where associated vascular lesions are suspicious or in prior radiated tumors, and further evaluation is necessary. Because suprasellar meningiomas are fed primarily by the posterior ethmoidal artery (a branch of the ophthalmic artery), preoperative embolization is not usually performed. As for patients with other juxtasellar lesions, a documented visual field and acuity examination and complete endocrinological studies are an integral part of the preoperative evaluation of patients with a tuberculum sellae meningioma.

Dexamethasone is administered to the patient before surgery and antibiotics are given intraoperatively. The author's choice of antibiotics is a combination of vancomycin and a third-generation cephalosporin.

Anesthesia and Monitoring

The successful removal of a tuberculum sellae meningioma depends upon the flawless administration of anesthesia. Premedication is usually withheld; induction is rapid and smooth and should be accomplished with an agent that reduces intracranial pressure. The choice of anesthetic agents should be flexible and tailored to suit the circumstances of each patient. Normotension is the

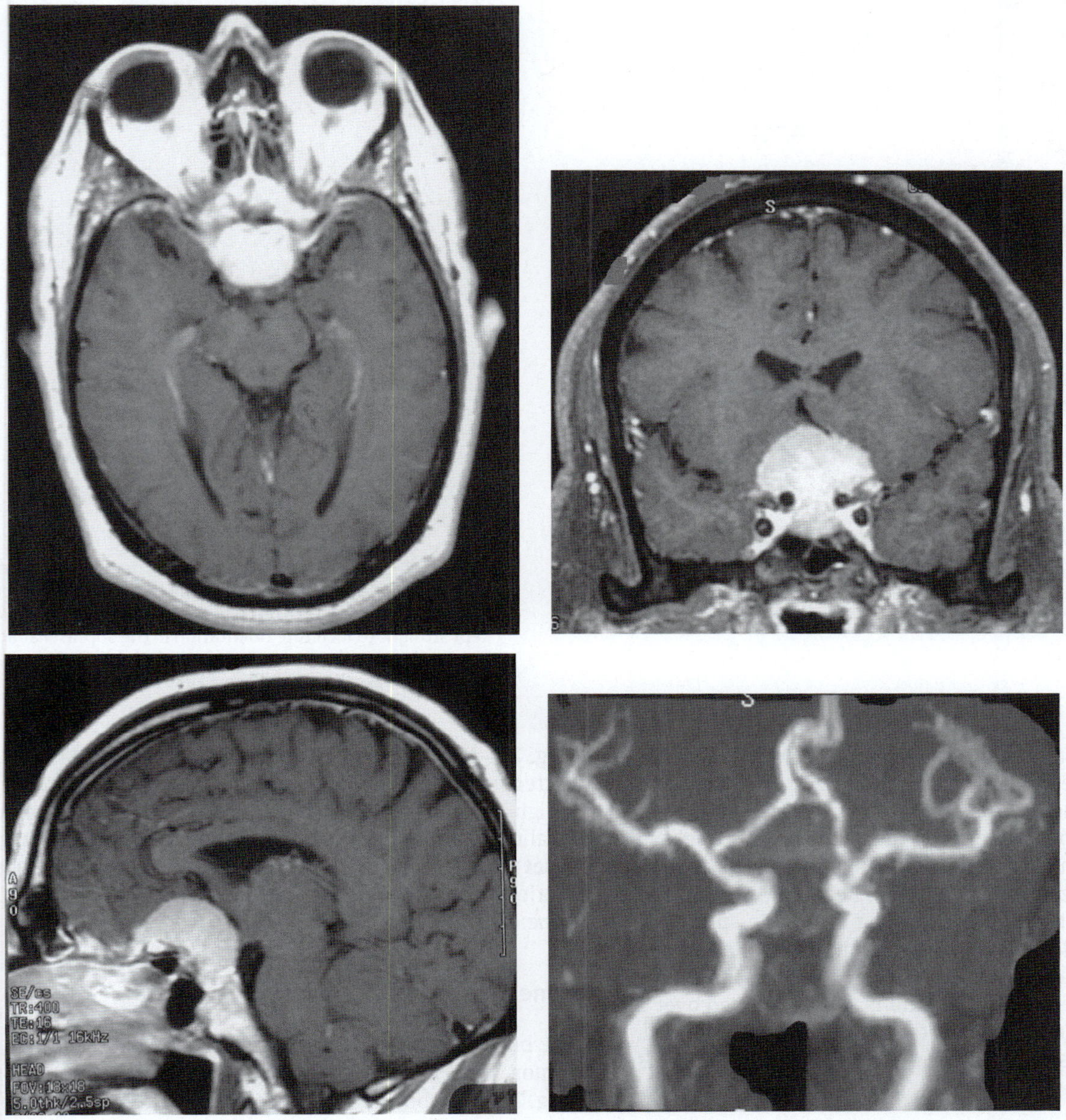

Figure 22–2 Contrast-enhanced magnetic resonance (MR) images—**(A)** axial, **(B)** coronal, and **(C)** sagittal views—of a tuberculum sellae meningioma with invasion of the sphenoid sinus. **(D)** MR angiogram of the same patients showing the upward displacement of the anterior cerebral arteries.

goal, and hypotension should be avoided. Should temporary vascular occlusion be necessary during surgical resection of the tumor, hypertension is induced and a burst suppression by barbiturate is administered for its known cerebral protective effect.

Despite the pressing need for intraoperative monitoring of the visual pathways during surgery of tuberculum sellae meningiomas, visual evoked potential monitoring has been disappointing and is not utilized routinely. Monitoring with brain stem auditory evoked response (BAER) and somatosensory evoked potentials (SSEPs) is used in all surgical cases, and electromyographic monitoring of the ocular muscles is used in cases where the tumor extends into the cavernous sinus.

◆ Operative Procedure

We have used and highly recommend the supraorbital approach to remove tuberculum sellae meningiomas. In this approach, the flap is unilateral or bilateral, depending on the size of the tumor. The highlight of the approach is superb low basal exposure, minimizing frontal lobe retraction.

Patient Position

The patient is placed supine with the head at the foot-end of the table. The table is adjusted so the patient's trunk and head are elevated 20 degrees. The head is then carefully and

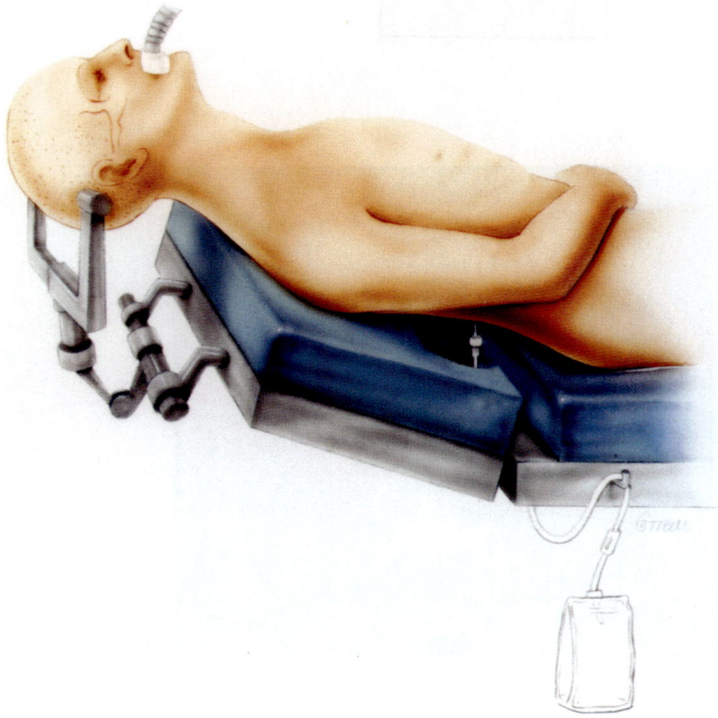

Figure 22–3 The patient's position. The head is elevated ~20 degrees, a lumbar spinal needle is in place. The neck is extended to allow the frontal lobes to fall back. The head is kept straight to facilitate orientation in the suprasellar area. (Reproduced with permission from Al-Mefty O. Surgery of the Cranial Base. Boston: Kluwer; 1989.)

moderately hyperextended and fixed in the Mayfield headrest to allow the frontal lobes to fall backward. To avoid compromising the bicoronal incision, the surgeon must not place the pins too far anteriorly. The head is kept straight to facilitate anatomical orientation. For patients with small and moderate-sized tumors, a spinal needle is inserted and connected to a sterile collection bag through a split mattress (**Fig. 22–3**). A flow control clamp is applied to the draining tube to avoid rapid loss of cerebrospinal fluid. Only 25 to 30 mL of cerebrospinal fluid is slowly drained over a period of 30 minutes just after the craniotomy is completed. If concern of mass effect is present, the spinal drainage is avoided.

Skin Incision and Pericranial Flap

The scalp incision for the supraorbital approach is begun 1 cm anterior to the tragus and proceeds in a curvilinear fashion behind the hairline to the level of the superior temporal line on the opposite side. In this manner, the superficial temporal artery courses posterior to the incision, whereas the branches of the facial nerve are located anteriorly. The scalp is reflected anteriorly with sharp dissection against the galea, leaving thick areolar tissue with pericranial layer attached to the calvarium. Both layers of the temporalis fascia are incised posterior to and along the course of the frontotemporalis branches of the facial nerve until muscle fibers are seen; then the fascia is reflected anteriorly with the fat layer and nerves along with the scalp flap. The temporal muscle is detached from its insertion anteriorly in a subperiosteal fashion and is retracted posteriorly, exposing the junction of the zygomatic, sphenoidal, and frontal bones.

The pericranial flap is then incised as far posteriorly as possible, dissected forward, and reflected over the scalp flap (**Fig. 22–4**). The intact base of this pericranial flap is dissected free from the roof and lateral wall of the orbit. Use of a high-speed air drill may be necessary around the supraorbital notch to free the supraorbital nerve (**Fig. 22–5, right inset**). The periorbita is carefully dissected to avoid fat herniation, from its superior and lateral attachments to the bone.

Bone Flap

The bone flap depends upon the size and extension of the tumor. The flap can be either unilateral supraorbital (**Fig. 22–5**) or bifrontal supraorbital (**Fig. 22–6**) in cases of large or giant tumors. To begin the supraorbital flap, the keyhole is made in the temporal fossa at the frontosphenoidal junction, just behind the zygomatic process of the frontal bone, the McCarthy point (**Fig. 22–5, left inset**). When the hole is drilled, the surgeon will see that its upper half exposes the dura mater of the frontal lobe and its lower half exposes the periorbita, the two membranes being separated by the roof of the orbit. If needed, a second hole is made in the frontal bone above the nasion. To keep it as small as possible, this hole is made with a small bit of the high-speed drill. In adults, this hole will invariably pass through the anterior and posterior walls of the frontal sinus.

The two holes are joined by two bone cuts. The first cut is made with the foot attachment of the drill and passes through the frontal bone ~4 cm above the superior orbital rim, as shown in **Fig. 22–5.** The second cut connects the two holes, crossing the roof of the orbit. This latter bone cut may be performed with a chisel, drill, or Gigli saw.

Using a fine drill, a groove is made from the bur-hole through the medial part of the superior orbital rim. This groove should include both the posterior and anterior walls

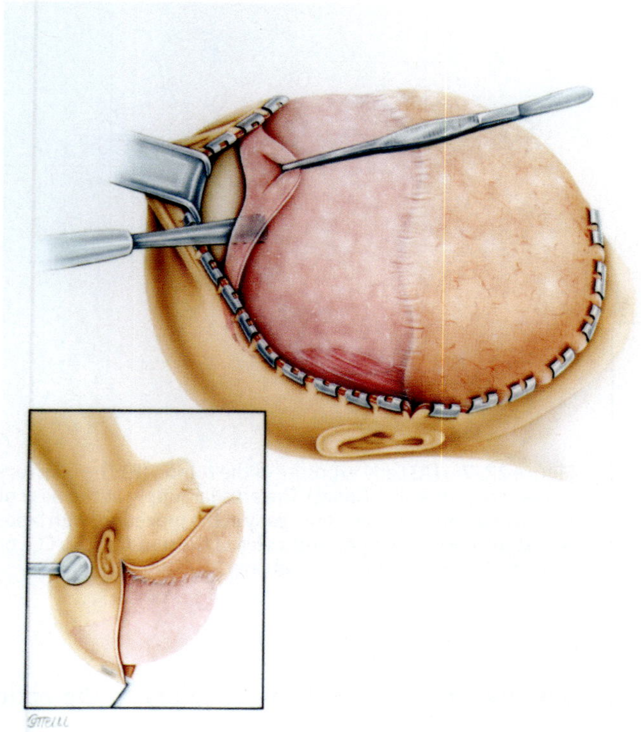

Figure 22–4 Exposure **(inset)** and elevation of a large pericranial flap based anteriorly on the supraorbital and frontal vessels. A large area of the frontal fossa floor can be resurfaced with this flap.

of the frontal sinus and is continued on the medial third of the orbital roof. Using a side-cutting drill, another cut is made across the lateral orbital rim and continued to connect with the keyhole. To avoid the side effects of orbital fat herniation, the surgeon should pay particular attention to keeping the periorbita intact. Injury to the supraorbital nerve and to the trochlear attachment of the superior oblique muscle should be avoided.

The removed and preserved craniotomy flap thus includes the superior portion and the upper half of the lateral portion of the orbital rim, the anterior portion of the orbital roof, and the adjacent frontal bone. After removal of the bone flap the sinus mucosa is exenterated, the posterior wall of the sinus is removed, and the sinus is packed with a small piece of temporalis muscle or Gelfoam, decreasing the risk of infection or potential development of mucocele. All

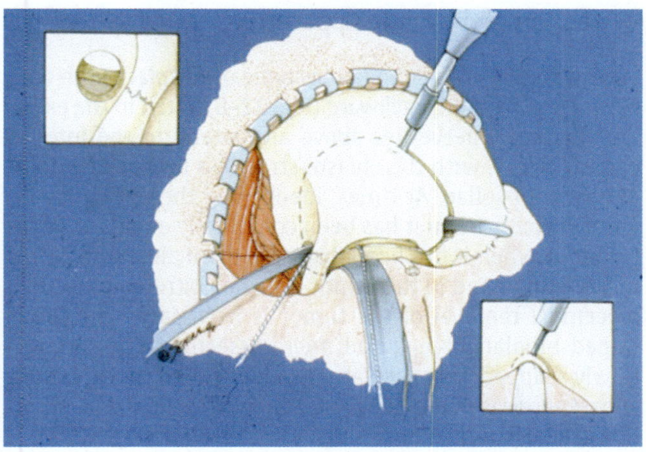

Figure 22–5 The creation of a unilateral supraorbital bone flap is shown. The midline hole and the keyhole are connected by a cut through the frontal bone using a drill with a foot attachment, and through the orbital roof using a Gigli saw. **(Left inset)** The position of the keyhole. **(Right inset)** Freeing the supraorbital nerve from its canal.

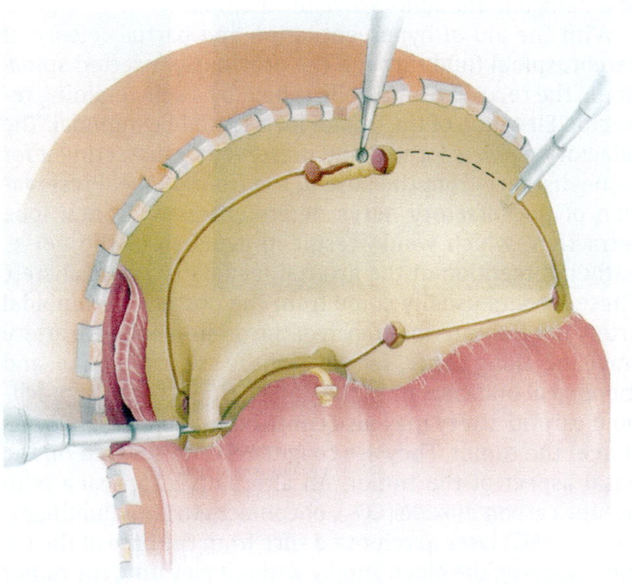

Figure 22–6 A bilateral supraorbital bone flap is shown. Notice the position of the holes and bone cuts.

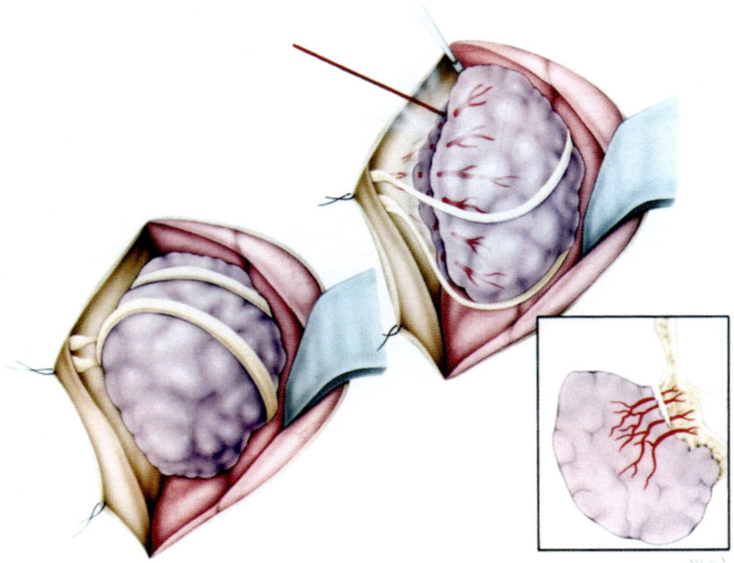

Figure 22–7 **(A)** Early exposure of the tumor. **(B)** The olfactory nerves are preserved. **(Inset)** The arterial supply at the base of the meningiomas is interrupted early in the procedure with bipolar coagulation or by vaporizing a slice of the tumor with a CO_2 or contact yttrium-aluminum-garnet laser.

instruments used in handling the mucosa are disposed of and the surgical team changes gowns and gloves. The dura is tacked up, and the operating microscope is brought into the field before the dura is opened. Opening the dura under the microscope provides a transitional adjustment of the surgeon's dexterity from bone work to fine microsurgical dissection.

Tumor Exposure and Devascularization

When a bifrontal approach is used, the sagittal sinus is divided between two silk sutures and the falx is cut at its lowest limit. Ligating and sectioning the sagittal sinus at the anterior frontal dura should not cause any side effects. Nonetheless, venous drainage in the frontal lobe should be maintained to the sinus above the incision.

With the aid of hyperventilation and partial release of cerebrospinal fluid through the previously inserted spinal drain, the relaxed frontal lobe is held by a self-retaining retractor. Elevation of the frontal lobe should be minimal. The olfactory nerve is located and preserved by dissecting it for some distance from the base of the frontal lobe. Preservation of the olfactory nerve deters excessive frontal lobe retraction, which would result in avulsion of the nerve. Early interception of the arterial feeders is a crucial step. These feeders usually come from the posterior ethmoidal artery but the anterior branch of the orbitomeningeal artery traveling along the lesser wing of the sphenoid bone, and meningeal branches from the dorsal aspect of the supraclinoid carotid artery may also contribute to the vascularization of the tumor. They are coagulated and severed on the basal aspect of the tumor. An alternative approach is to use the carbon dioxide (CO_2), or contact yttrium-aluminum-garnet (YAG) laser to remove a slice from the base of the tumor, reaching the blood supply without elevating the tumor against the frontal lobes **(Fig. 22–7)**. Devascularization is restricted to the midline, which orientation is maintained by observing the falx position to avoid injury to the optic nerves.

Tumor Resection

The tumor is then debulked using the laser or the ultrasonic aspirator. The traditional method of debulking the meningioma using an electrocautery loop is discouraged because it creates a tremendous amount of heat. Once dissection approaches the neurovascular structures, only bipolar cautery end microdissection should be used. By debulking the central core of the tumor, appropriate space is created to proceed with the dissection of the tumor from the optic apparatus, carotid arteries, pituitary stalk, and hypothalamus within the arachnoidal plane, which lessens the need of excessive retraction.

Dissection of the Optic Apparatus

Tuberculum sellae meningiomas typically displace both optic nerves outward and backward **(Fig. 22–8)**, often to the extent that the optic nerve lies above and lateral to the internal carotid artery, with the chiasm stretched far back from the tuberculum sellae. At times, identifying the optic nerve is quite difficult when it has been completely engulfed by the tumor or when it has been distorted to an almost unrecognizable thin band in the tumor capsule. Extremely cautious piecemeal removal of the tumor is necessary, using fine-tipped bipolar forceps and microdissectors. The tumor is slowly stripped from the flattened or engulfed nerve. Despite apparent encasement or severe adherence, a plane of dissection can be obtained under high magnification **(Fig. 22–8)**.

In some instances, the easily identifiable and dissectable optic nerve belongs to the eye with total visual loss, whereas the optic nerve with residual function is encased in the tumor. To preserve the remaining vision, dissection of the nerve and its blood supply must be meticulous. It may be

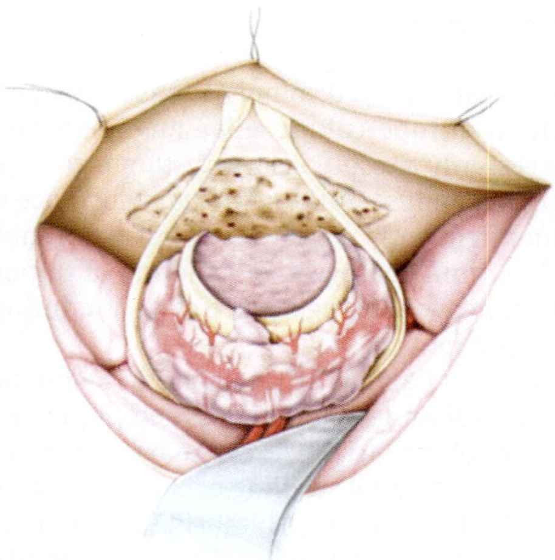

Figure 22–8 The optic nerves are typically displaced laterally and posteriorly. The anterior cerebral artery complex is encased by this tumor. Both vital perforators and tumor feeders originate from the A1 segment, but only the feeders are interrupted. The perforators must be preserved.

necessary to begin dissection at the chiasm to locate and dissect an obscure optic nerve on the other side. Arterial supply to the optic nerves and chiasm should be preserved by the same method of tumor dissection. Sacrificing an optic nerve even in a totally blinded eye is not recommended. Occasionally the patient recovers vision even after total blindness.

Arterial Dissection

As in tumor dissection from the optic nerve, the carotid artery is dissected free from the tumor using an array of microinstruments, including bipolar forceps, microdissectors, and scissors. Adherence and encasement of cerebral vessels should not deter the surgeon from attempting to dissect the tumor free from the involved arteries. Carotid dissection continues to free the ophthalmic artery, the posterior communicating artery, the anterior thalamic perforators, and the choroidal artery. Further dissection of the tumor progresses to the bifurcation of the internal carotid artery and into the sylvian fissure. Dissection continues to free the middle and anterior cerebral arteries. Tumor tissue has either simply displaced these vessels and their perforators or actually engulfed them. The anterior communicating and anterior cerebral arteries are frequently the most difficult to dissect, and commonly supply the tumor. This is the area of vital arterial perforators that may be displaced or encased by the tumor. To facilitate their preservation, the A2 segment should be dissected after the tumor has been thinned out. The Al segments in particular are usually severely stretched or adherent and tend to tear. Should this occur, the surgeon should remain calm, apply a temporary vascular clip (30 g/mm^2) distal, and one proximal, to the bleeding point, and suture the arterial wall with fine 8–0 or 9–0 sutures.

Although the tumor may be supplied by arterial twigs of the anterior cerebral arteries, the surgeon must first be certain that they are tumor feeders and not hypothalamic perforators or optic blood supply. Thus each arterial branch should be dissected and followed to ascertain its eventual course. Particular precision is needed to spare the artery of Heubner and the vital branches to the striatum **(Fig. 22–8)**. As dissection continues, both A1 arteries and the anterior communicating artery are freed from the tumor. The membrane of Liliequist is intact in most cases; consequently, tumor removal from the posteriorly displaced basilar artery is usually easy.

Dissection of the Pituitary Stalk and Hypothalamus

The pituitary stalk can be recognized by its distinctive color and vascular network. A tumor extending backward under the hypothalamus usually displaces the pituitary stalk backward and to one side **(Fig. 22–9)**. Some tumors totally engulf the pituitary stalk, requiring meticulous and tedious dissection. A tumor impinging on the hypothalamus can be removed gently by maintaining a plane of cleavage. Excessive downward retraction of the tumor, however, should be avoided. The arachnoid membrane of Liliequist provides an excellent plane of dissection for tumor removal. Often this membrane comes away with the tumor, leaving the rostral pans, midbrain, oculomotor nerves, and basilar artery and its branches in full view **(Fig. 22–9)**.

Surgical Technique when Tumor Invades the Cavernous Sinus and the Optic Canal

If extensive work in the cavernous sinus is anticipated a cranio-orbital zygomatic approach rather than a supraorbital

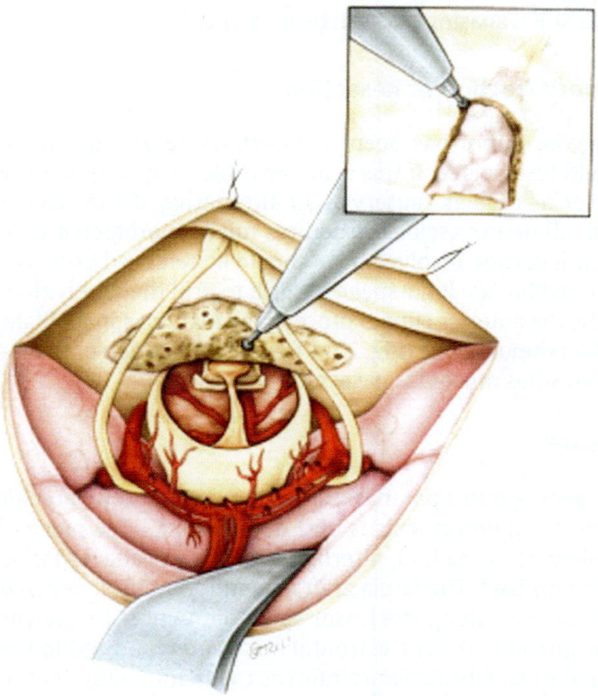

Figure 22–9 The operative field after removal of a tuberculum sellae meningioma. The interpeduncular cistern is seen through the posteriorly displaced optic chiasm. The pituitary stalk is displaced slightly to one side, and branches of basilar artery, which is displaced posteriorly, are seen. The cerebral arteries and perforators are preserved; only feeders to the tumor have been coagulated. At the end of the procedure, the hyperostotic bone is drilled, and the dura at the tuberculum sellae and the plenum sphenoidale is excised. **(Inset)** The optic canal is unroofed to follow a tongue of tumor extending along the optic nerve canal.

approach is preferable because different angles and avenues can be utilized. Through the supraorbital approach, when the tumor extends into the cavernous sinus or the optic canal, the anterior clinoid process, the roof of the optic canal, and the roof of the superior orbital fissure are drilled away with the diamond bit of a high-speed air drill. The dura propria is then opened. Tumor tissue around the optic nerve is removed with bipolar coagulation and microdissectors, and the surgeon must pay particular attention to preserve the ophthalmic and the central retinal arteries. This bony drilling exposes the superior aspect of the cavernous sinus. The internal carotid artery emerges through the superior wall, surrounded and firmly anchored by the dural ring. Beginning with this emergence, an incision is made in the exposed dura and extended posteriorly toward the posterior clinoid process. The internal carotid artery is then followed in retrograde fashion into the cavernous sinus, where it is dissected. In the cavernous sinus space, the tumor is dissected using a bipolar coagulation technique along with microdissectors. Venous hemorrhage is not encountered until the tumor is nearly removed because the venous plexus is compressed. The abducens nerve is the only nerve that courses through the middle of the cavernous sinus space lateral to the carotid artery. Its identification, dissection, and preservation demand particular attention.

If a tear occurs in the arterial wall, the surgeon should be prepared to apply temporary vascular clips of 30 to 40 g/mm^2 pressure and repair the arterial injury with fine microsutures. If the artery is injured beyond repair, it can be reconstructed using a venous graft, or an extracranial-intracranial anastomosis can be performed.

Tumor Attachment Resection

After the tumor has been removed, its dural attachment should be resected. If this is not possible, coagulation using a laser or bipolar cautery is an alternative. If the laser is used, all neurovascular structures must be protected with surgical patties. Involved bone should be removed using the diamond bit of a high-speed air drill to drill the tuberculum sellae, the anterior clinoid process, the planum sphenoidale, or the ethmoid bone **(Fig. 22–9)**. Further resection of the involved sinus mucosa is necessary.

Closure

An opening into a paranasal sinus requires thorough repair of the dural defect; this is best done with a large piece of autologous fascia lata, alternatives such as cadaver fascia can be utilized. The fascia graft, laid intradurally, is secured with sutures along the lesser sphenoid wing. The graft is then spread to cover the frontal fossa and is sutured to the frontal dura. Fibrin glue reinforces the maintenance of the flap in place. The preserved pericranial flap is turned over the frontal sinus and extended over any defect in the floor of the frontal fossa. A titanium microplate is used to reattach the bone flap to the cranial vault. The temporalis muscle is sutured back to the fascia at the lateral orbital rim, and the skin is closed in two layers.

◆ Complications

Myriad potential and reported complications are associated with the removal of tuberculum sellae meningiomas. Although not necessarily a result of surgery, tumor recurrence testifies to surgical failure. Although true recurrence does occur, the tumor frequently regrows as the result of subtotal tumor resection, from conservative handling of tumor attachments, or from overlooking a piece of tumor during intraoperative inspection.

The bicoronal skin flap has an adequate base and blood supply, but acute folding should be avoided. Injury to the superior branches of the facial nerves can be avoided using subfascial dissection. Orbital swelling occurs more often after approaches that excise the orbital rim and roof, but it does not add significant morbidity. Entering the frontal sinus presents a potential source of septic complications and leakage of cerebrospinal fluid. Important precautions to avoid these complications were described earlier.

Injury to cerebral vessels is the most serious intraoperative complication. The complex of anterior cerebral arteries is the most likely to be injured. With microsurgical techniques, however, the cerebral vessels can be dissected freely and safely. Although the small perforators supplying the hypothalamus and brain stem may not produce catastrophic hemorrhage, injury to these vessels produces a devastating neurological deficit. The importance of their preservation cannot be overemphasized, particularly because these vessels are apt to be mistaken for vessels feeding the tumor.

Because of the intimate relationship between the optic apparatus and the tumor, visual impairment may occur as a result of a variety of causes: direct damage from surgical instruments or manipulation or secondary to heating injury from the electrocautery, or interruption of vascular supply to the optic nerve and chiasm, compression by surgically introduced material, development of a suprasellar hematoma, migration of the optic chiasm, or arachnoiditis. The decussating fibers in the central chiasm are supplied solely by the inferior group of arteries arising from the carotid artery. Failure to improve vision because of inadequate tumor removal and optic apparatus decompression should be considered a surgical disappointment at least. A suprasellar hematoma causing visual loss should be removed promptly, although the prognosis for visual recovery is guarded.

Diabetes insipidus is usually transient in patients with this type of meningioma but requires adequate monitoring of electrolyte and serum osmolarity. Partial or complete pituitary deficiency may occur after resection of a tuberculum sellae meningioma. A full endocrinological workup before and after surgery is routine for all of these patients. Hormone replacement therapy is administered as indicated.

The third, fourth, and sixth cranial nerves may suffer temporary or permanent palsy when the tumor is followed into the cavernous sinus. Anosmia frequently occurs after subfrontal exposure and the dissection needed to remove a tuberculum sellae meningioma. A frontal lobe syndrome might be present before, or result from, surgery. Minimal retraction and preservation of the frontal veins should decrease its occurrence.

Section VI

Posterior Fossa Tumors

23

Surgical Management of Jugular Foramen Schwannomas

Madjid Samii

Intracranial schwannomas constitute ~8% of all primary brain tumors. Only 2.9% of all intracranial schwannomas arise from the ninth, tenth, and eleventh cranial nerves. Some series report a higher incidence, due to the inclusion of patients with hypoglossal neurinoma or neurofibromatosis. Schwannomas are more commonly found in females, affecting those aged 14 to 63 years (average 38 years). Younger patients with these tumors should undergo a thorough workup for associated neurofibromatosis type 2. Symptoms are often unilateral and are referable to the deficits of lower cranial nerves, presenting with difficulty in swallowing and phonation. They do not manifest until the tumor attains a large size. Occasionally, these patients present with a cerebellopontine angle tumor such as an acoustic neuroma or a meningioma.

◆ Patient Selection and Evaluation

Because the majority of intracranial schwannomas are benign, slow growing, and do not produce symptoms until they attain a large size, questions arise concerning the benefits of surgery in an asymptomatic patient. Before a decision is made to excise the lesion, it is not unreasonable to establish the growth rate of the tumor by periodic neuroimaging studies. This is particularly important in incidentally discovered lesions confined to the skull bone and upper cervical areas. If the tumors have significant intracranial extension projecting into the posterior fossa, surgical resection is necessary to prevent impending neurological deficits such as cerebellar and brain stem dysfunction. Subtotal resection is an option for symptomatic elderly patients, for patients with significant medical risks, and for patients with neurofibromatosis type 2, in whom bilateral tumors are common. In patients with neurofibromatosis type 2, preservation of the lower cranial nerves, at least unilaterally, should be the goal. With surgical intervention in this area, there is a high probability of producing permanent dysfunction of the lower cranial nerves. Asymptomatic patients with relatively small intracranial tumors discovered during routine examination should be carefully followed and counseled. Relying on the premise that deficits in small tumors are likely to be less severe, some surgeons justify operating on them. We believe that once a clinical and radiological diagnosis has been made, a small asymptomatic tumor needs to be resected after establishing a reasonable growth rate of the tumor. In all other patients, total resection is the goal regardless of size. It is worth noting that compensation of deficits in already paretic lower cranial nerves is better than fully functioning cranial nerves. Prior to surgery, these patients should undergo a thorough medical evaluation to rule out evidence of pheochromocytoma. Accurate radiological and biochemical investigations will differentiate these schwannomas from glomus jugulare tumors, which are the most common type of tumors seen in this area.

Anatomy and Clinical Pathology

The jugular foramen is a canal situated between the lateral portion of the occipital bone and the petrous portion of the temporal bone. The anteromedial compartment (pars nervosa) (which contains the inferior petrosal sinus and the glossopharyngeal nerve) and the posterolateral compartment (pars venosa) (which contains the vagus nerve, accessory nerve, and proximal part of the jugular bulb) are partially separated by a septum. Tumors arising from the accessory nerve are least common when compared with tumors arising from the ninth and tenth nerve complex. Large tumors can traverse the jugular foramen and extend both intra- and extracranially in a dumbbell-shaped fashion. They do not infiltrate the jugular bulb but may occlude it by compression. If the tumor arises proximally in the interior of the jugular foramen, the presentation may resemble a posterior fossa mass, whereas distal lesions appear as a mass in the cervical area of the skull base. However, if the tumor arises in the midregion, it expands the temporal bone and presents as a glomus jugulare tumor without pulsatile tinnitus. Some patients also exhibit signs and symptoms of increased intracranial pressure (ICP), cerebellar and brain stem signs, as well as lower cranial nerve deficit.

Radiological Evaluation

Magnetic resonance imaging (MRI) and computed tomography (CT) are both essential and complementary to each other in diagnosing jugular foramen schwannomas. CT with a bone window delineates the architecture of the jugular foramen and the adjacent skull base. Smooth-edged enlargement of the jugular foramen is a common finding in

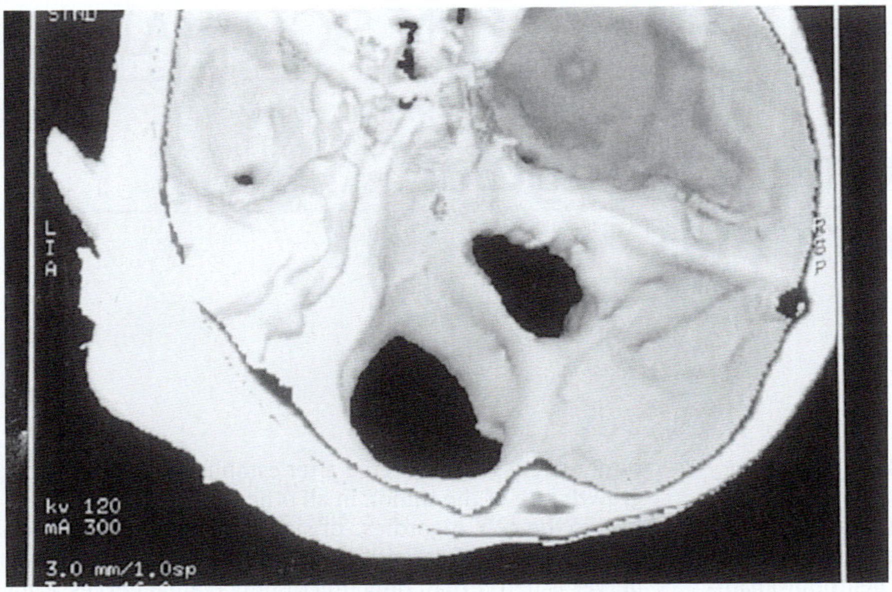

Figure 23–1 Three-dimensional computed tomography demonstrating enlargement of the jugular foramen.

schwannomas **(Fig. 23–1)**, as opposed to irregular bone destruction that is seen in glomus tumors. With contrast, these tumors enhance on CT and MRI; however, the enhancement is less intense than seen in meningiomas and glomus tumors.

The soft tissue details, the vascular supply of these tumors, the relationship of the major vessels, as well as the architecture and patency of the sigmoid sinus and jugular bulb, are well appreciated in MRI and magnetic resonance angiography. Magnetic resonance angiography also provides information regarding the vascularity of the tumor, differentiating it from glomus tumors, where multiple signal voids are a common finding. Cerebral angiography provides information regarding the location and involvement of the carotid artery, as well as the collateral circulation and patency of the sigmoid sinus and jugular bulb. Jugular foramen schwannomas are relatively avascular, and embolization is rarely necessary; angiography is obtained essentially to differentiate these tumors from highly vascular glomus jugulare tumors.

Classification of Tumors

For proper surgical planning, a thorough knowledge of the location of the tumor is mandatory. For this reason, tumor extension is classified into types A to D **(Fig. 23–2** and **Table 23–1)**.

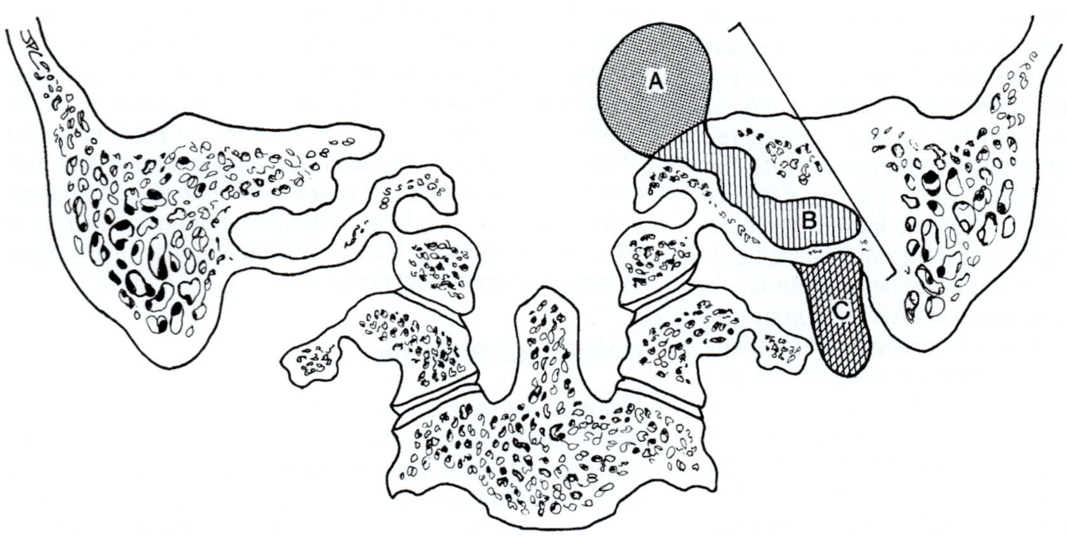

Figure 23–2 Classification of jugular foramen tumors, types A, B, and C. For descriptions, see **Table 23–1**.

Table 23–1 Classification of Extension of Jugular Foramen Schwannomas

Tumor Type	Tumor Extension
Type A	Primarily intracranial with minimal extension into the temporal bone
Type B	Primarily in temporal bone with or without an intracranial component
Type C	Primarily extracranial with minor extension into the temporal bone or into the posterior fossa
Type D	Saddlebag-shaped tumors, traversing the jugular foramen, with intra- and extracranial components

◆ Preoperative Preparation

Starting at midnight before surgery, Solu-Medrol (250 mg every 6 hours) is administered intravenously. The day prior to surgery, a loading dose of Dilantin (1 g) is administered; postoperatively and is continued at 100 mg three times a day. If premedication is used, it may consist of the shorter-acting benzodiazepines such as diazepam or midazolam, which are on call to the operating room. Narcotics should be avoided because they tend to produce respiratory depression and nausea and vomiting, which can result in an increased ICP. Routine monitoring in the operating room consists of pulse oximetry, noninvasive blood pressure measurement, electrocardiography, and capnography. Capnography assesses the level of hyperventilation and is titrated to obtain optimal ICP control. An arterial catheter and one or two large-bore intravenous lines are inserted. A short-acting opioid and an ultrashort-acting intravenous anesthetic (generally thiopental or propofol) are used for induction, followed by a nondepolarizing muscle relaxant for intubation. Intravenous lidocaine (1.0 to 1.5 mg/kg body weight) may be administered prior to laryngoscopy. A combination of these agents permits the smooth induction of anesthesia, thus avoiding hypertension, hypoxia, hypercarbia, and coughing, all of which may increase the ICP.

The hypertensive response to pin fixation of the head may be minimized or eliminated by the prior administration of an intravenous anesthetic. Anesthesia is generally maintained with a narcotic by continuous infusion or intermittent boluses and inhalation of nitrous oxide and isoflurane. The $PaCO_2$ is maintained in the range of 25 to 30 mm Hg. During surgery, it may be necessary to induce hypotension to reduce blood loss and the need for transfusion. A mean arterial pressure of 50 to 60 mm Hg is acceptable in a healthy individual, but may not be tolerated by the patient with cardiovascular disease or hypertension. In highly vascular tumors, deliberate hypotension may be induced by increasing the level of isoflurane or by a direct-acting vasodilator, such as sodium nitroprusside or nitroglycerine.

After intubation, the bladder is catheterized and 20% mannitol is administered intravenously (1 g/kg body weight). Evoked potential monitoring necessitates some modification of the anesthetic technique. If only the sensory modalities are monitored, the level of isoflurane is maintained at $<0.4\%$ and anesthesia is sustained primarily with a narcotic infusion and nitrous oxide. If motor evoked potentials and electromyography are also employed, halogenated anesthetics cannot be used. In this case, propofol and opioid (fentanyl or sufentanil) infusions are substituted and only nitrous oxide is used as an inhalant.

◆ Operative Procedure

Type A Tumors

Type A tumors are primarily intracranial, appearing in the posterior fossa, and are approached via the traditional retromastoid suboccipital route **(Fig. 23–3)**.

The patient is operated on in the semisitting position **(Fig. 23–4)**. Strict precautions are taken to detect and treat air embolism by establishing a central venous line and precordial Doppler. The tip of the central venous catheter should be at the junction of the superior vena cava and the right atrium. The patient's head is fixed in a three-pin Mayfield headholder and is turned 30 degrees to the side of the lesion; it is then flexed and fixed to the bed. Venodyne pneumatic compression boots[DE1] are applied to the lower [[DE1]] extremities, which are elevated to facilitate venous return. To prevent nerve palsies, extreme care is taken to protect all pressure points. A skin incision is made in the retromastoid area 2 to 3 cm behind the mastoid **(Fig. 23–5)**. The incision extends from the top of the external ear, up to 8 to 10 cm toward the neck. The neck muscles are divided vertically and retracted with cerebellar retractors. Using a high-speed drill, a suboccipital craniectomy is performed and should expose the sigmoid–transverse sinus junction; however, a low craniectomy extending to the rim of the foramen magnum is crucial for resection of these tumors **(Fig. 23–6)**. Alternatively, a craniotomy can be done exposing the posterior

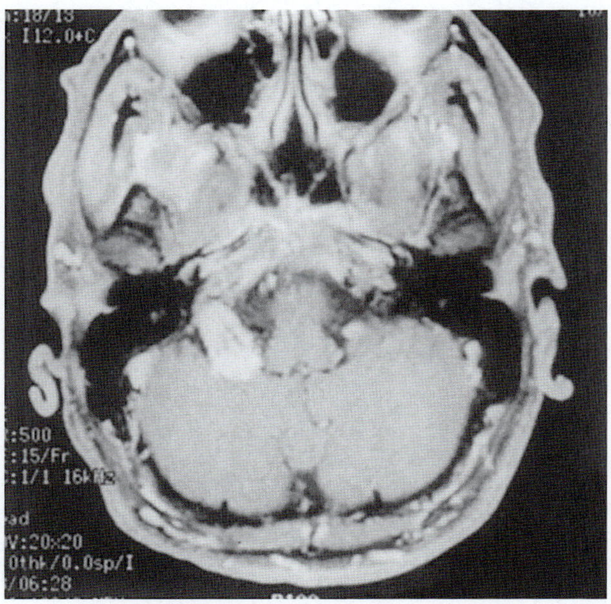

Figure 23–3 Magnetic resonance imaging, axial view, with gadolinium enhancement demonstrating posterior fossa tumor (type A tumor).

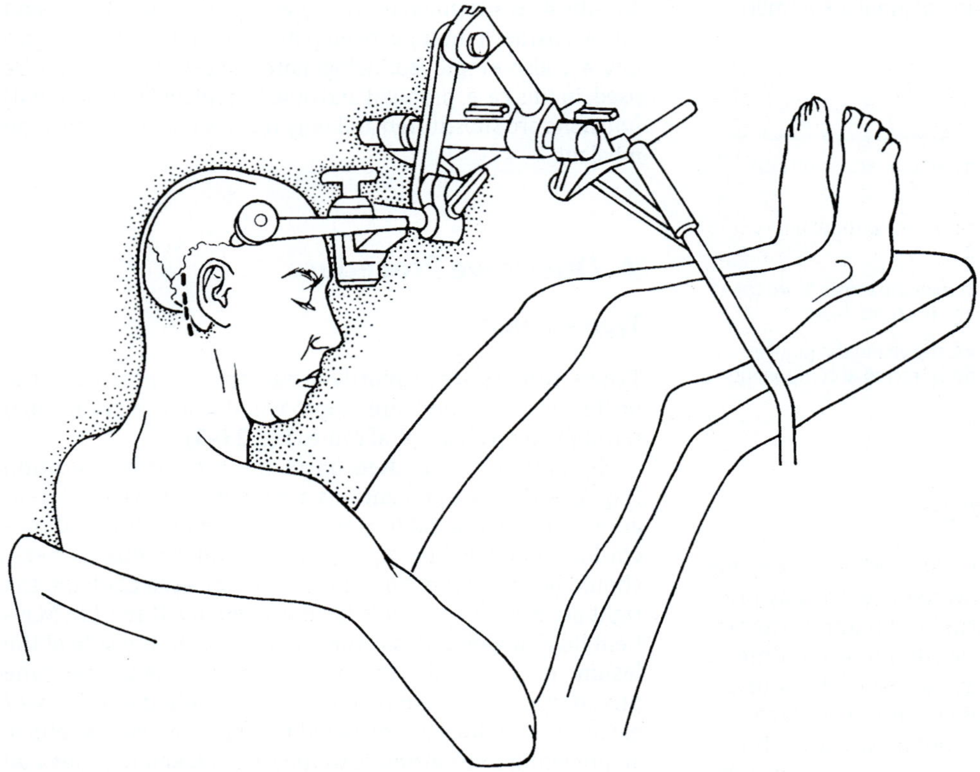

Figure 23–4 Semisitting (lounge) position; used for resection of type A tumors.

fossa with additional drilling. The dura mater is cut several millimeters away from the sigmoid sinus and is reflected medially, exposing the cerebellum. To achieve relaxation of the posterior fossa, cerebrospinal fluid (CSF) is drained from the cisterna magna and the cerebellopontine angle cistern.

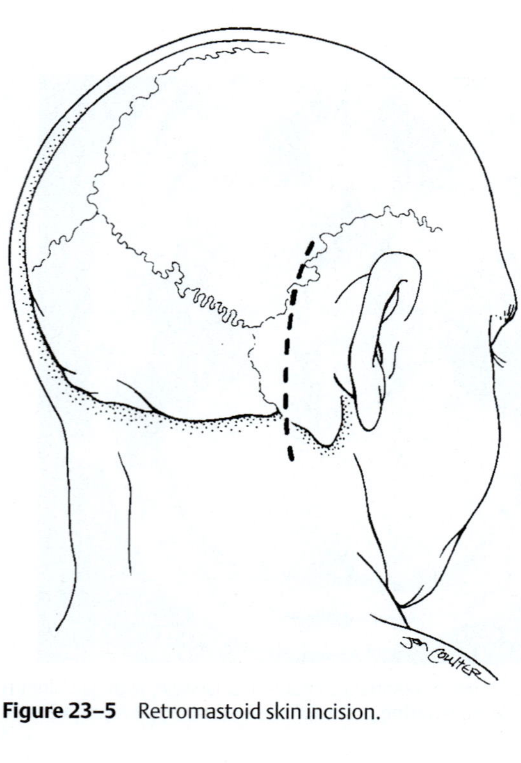

Figure 23–5 Retromastoid skin incision.

At this stage, the cerebellum is covered with cottonoid and the cerebellopontine angle and the floor of the posterior cranial fossa are exposed by retracting the cerebellum medially and upward. This would expose the tumor, the lower cranial nerves, and the adjacent arteries **(Fig. 23–7)**.

It is important to identify the anatomy in this area with particular attention to the relation of the tumor to the sigmoid sinus. Small to medium-sized tumors are situated just anterior to the sigmoid sinus, whereas in larger tumors, the entire distal portion of the sigmoid sinus and jugular bulb are enveloped and may not be obstructed by external compression. Extradural drilling of the jugular foramen may help to better define the tumor margins. Initially, intratumoral debulking is performed so that the tumor shrinks in size and separates itself from the surrounding nerves and sigmoid. In large tumors, it is sometimes difficult to identify the nerves. However, individual nerves can be identified using electromyography. If it is not possible to separate the tumor from the nerves (because lower cranial nerves have multiple rootlets), resection of the tumor is undertaken along with sections of some of the rootlets.

Because the posterior inferior cerebellar artery may be closely associated with tumors in this area, it is essential to identify it during tumor dissection and resection. Intraarachnoidal dissection and debulking using an ultrasonic aspirator with the arachnoid intact is critical to avoid injury to the adjacent structures because they all lie within the arachnoid toward the brain. Once the tumor is resected, the Valsalva maneuver is administered to test for hemostasis, and the dura is closed watertight with 4–0 Nurolon sutures. If necessary, the pericranium is used to patch the dura

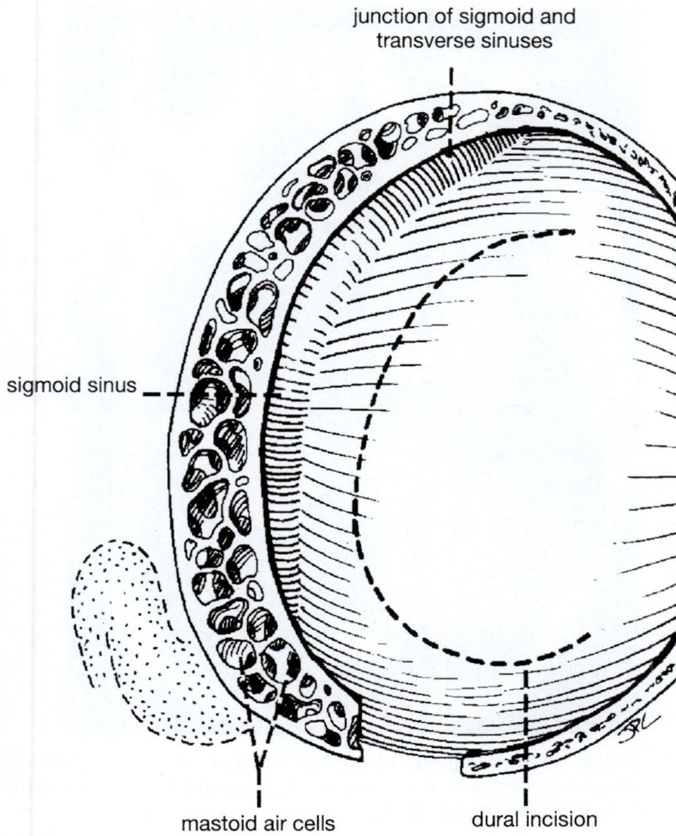

Figure 23–6 A low craniectomy, close to and including the floor of the posterior cranial fossa, with exposure of the lower part of the sigmoid sinus near the jugular bulb. The dural incision can also be seen.

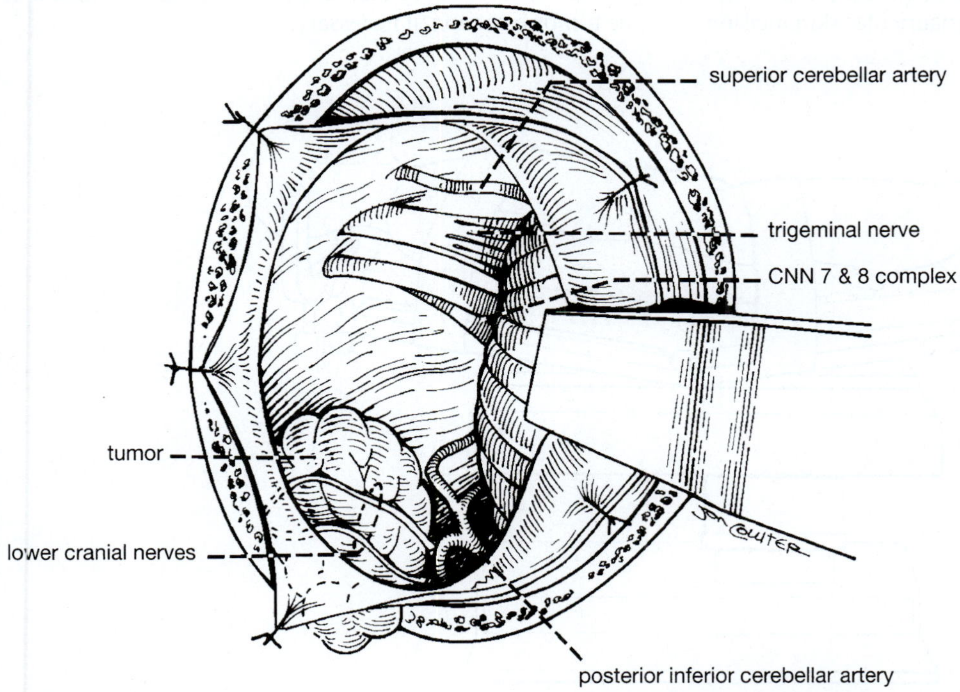

Figure 23–7 Following retraction of the cerebellum, the tumor and the lower cranial nerves are exposed.

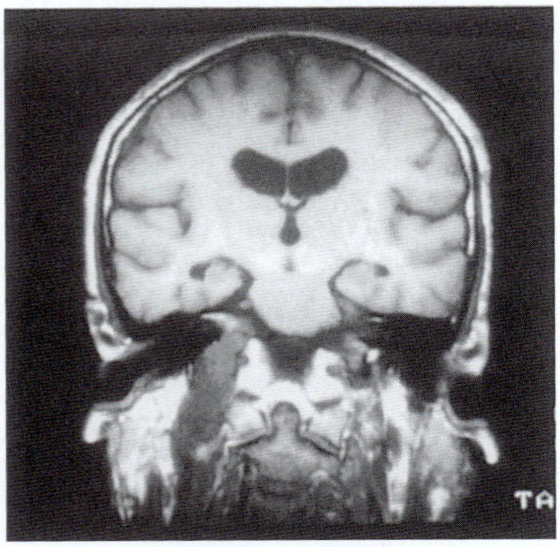

Figure 23–8 Magnetic resonance imaging, coronal view, demonstrating extracranial tumor (type C tumor).

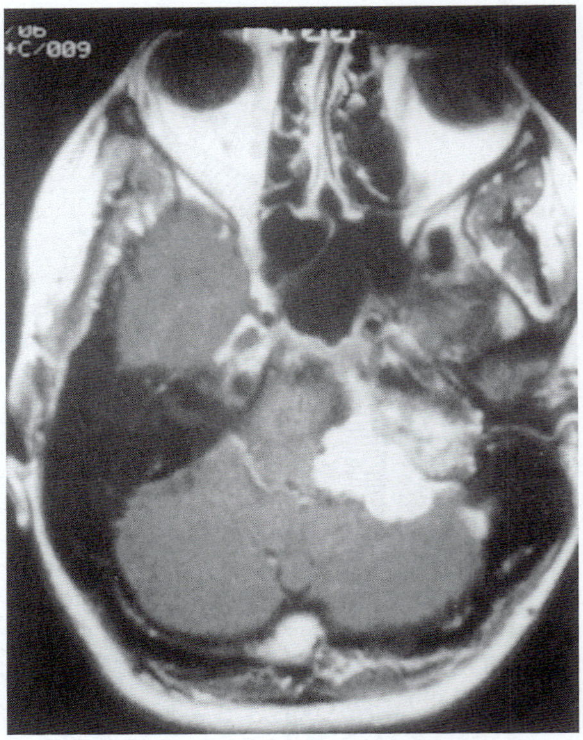

Figure 23–9 Magnetic resonance imaging with gadolinium enhancement demonstrating a saddlebag-shaped tumor traversing the jugular foramen (type D tumor).

and is reinforced with fibrin glue. Mastoid air cells that are opened during the craniectomy are packed with fibrin glue–soaked muscle.

Routine closure of the wound is performed using 0–0 Vicryl sutures for muscle and fascia, 3–0 Vicryl for subcutaneous tissue, and 3–0 nylon or staples for skin.

Types B to D Tumors

Patients harboring tumor types B, C, and D are operated on in the supine position **(Figs. 23–8 and 23–9)**. The head is placed in a three-pin Mayfield headholder and is turned 70 degrees away from the side of the lesion **(Fig. 23–10)** and fixed to the bed. Special care is taken not to compromise the jugular vein. The lower left quadrant of the abdomen and the thigh are prepped to obtain tissue for possible reconstruction during closure. A retroauricular skin incision extending along the anterior border of the sternocleidomastoid muscle to the level of the hyoid bone is marked **(Fig. 23–11)**, and the area of skin incision is infiltrated with 1:100,000 lidocaine to epinephrine. The skin is incised and care is exercised to preserve the greater auricular nerve in the subcutaneous tissue so that it is available as a nerve graft for cranial nerve reconstruction at the conclusion of the tumor resection, if necessary.

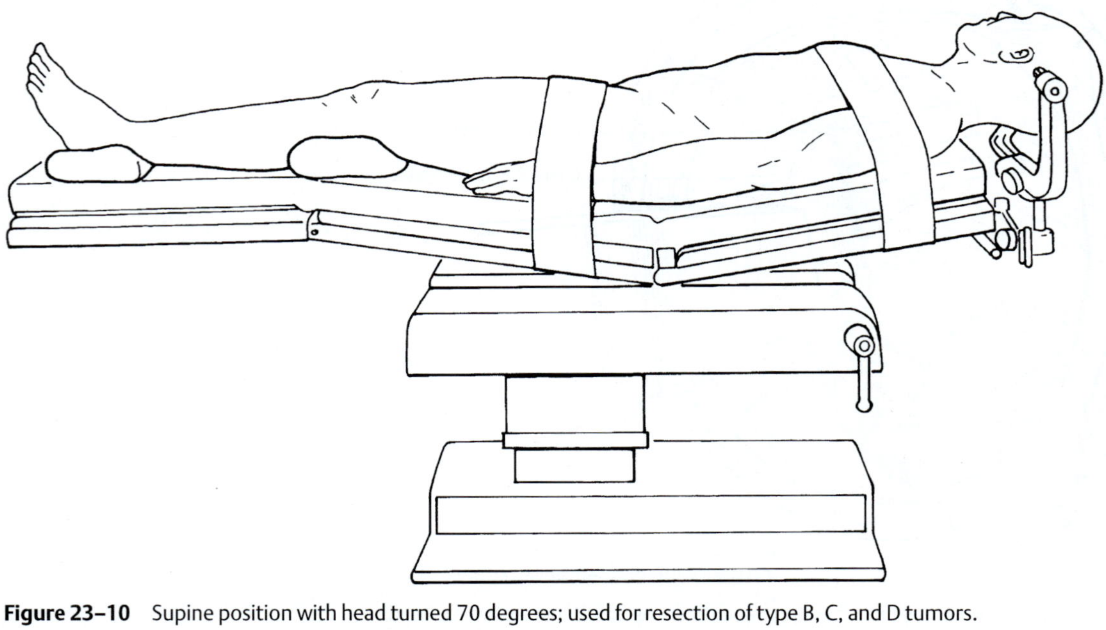

Figure 23–10 Supine position with head turned 70 degrees; used for resection of type B, C, and D tumors.

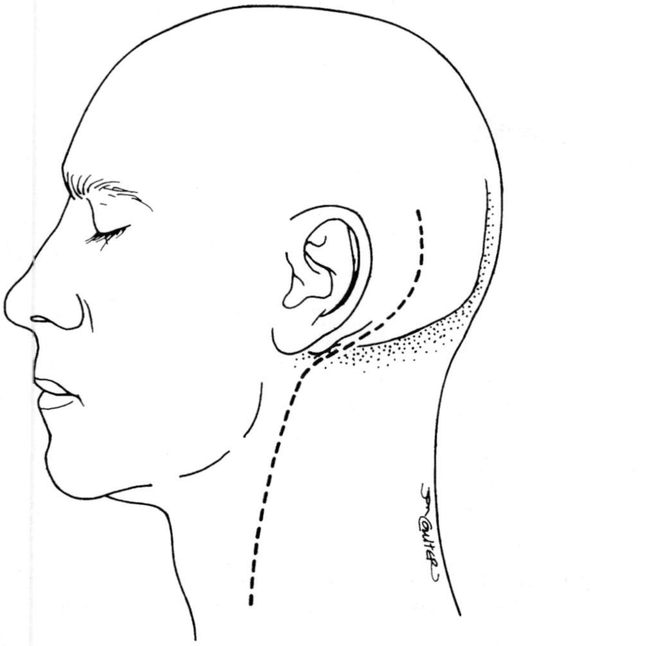

Figure 23–11 Retroauricular skin incision with extension into the upper cervical area; used for resection of type D tumors.

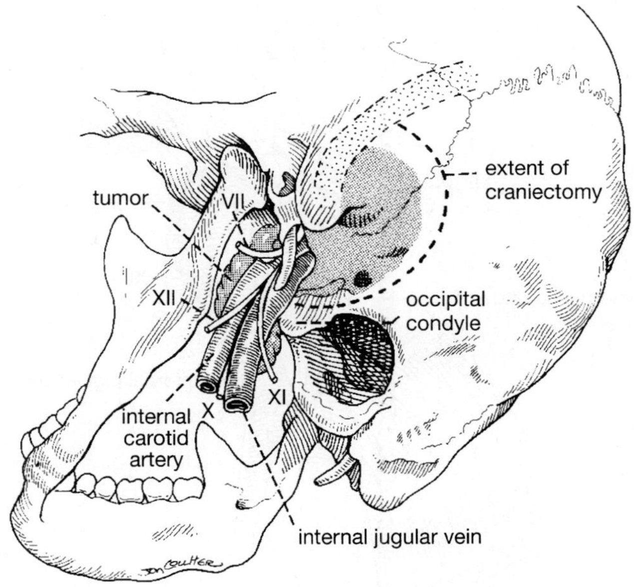

Figure 23–13 Drawing demonstrating the relationship of major vessels in the high cervical area to the mastoid hip, and the extent of craniectomy.

The mastoid and the adjacent suboccipital bone are exposed following mobilization of the sternocleidomastoid muscle and the posterior belly of the digastric muscles. Upper cervical dissection is then performed, identifying the lower cranial nerves, the internal jugular vein, and the carotid artery. All of these structures are followed cranially to the skull base. Lateral to the occipitomastoidal suture, a portion of the occipital squama, including part of the mastoid, is removed. At this point, a lateral suboccipital craniectomy, exposing the lower half of sigmoid sinus, is achieved **(Fig. 23–12).**

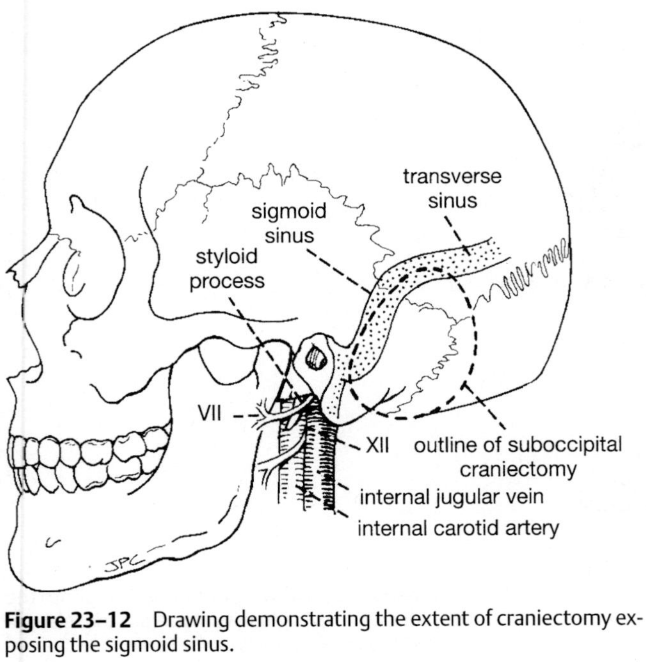

Figure 23–12 Drawing demonstrating the extent of craniectomy exposing the sigmoid sinus.

The sigmoid sinus is then mobilized from its bony groove caudally down to the jugular foramen. The mastoid is carefully removed without causing injury to the facial nerve. To further extend the exposure, the posterior portion of the occipital condyle may be removed, thus opening the jugular foramen dorsolaterally **(Fig. 23–13).** Once removal of bone is completed, the sigmoid sinus, the jugular bulb, the internal jugular vein, and the cervical portion of tumor (as seen in types C and D) are exposed at the area of the jugular foramen. The main stem of the facial nerve is exposed anteriorly to the origin of the digastric muscle, in the depth of the tympanomastoid fissure, as it exits the stylomastoid foramen **(Fig. 23–14).** The petrous bone is further drilled away up to the fallopian canal inferior to the labyrinth. Using a microsurgical technique, the extracranial portion of the tumor is resected. The intracranial portion of the tumor is then removed through the widened jugular foramen and the suboccipital craniectomy. Initially, the dura is opened posterior to the sigmoid sinus, extending the incision to the jugular foramen. The cerebellum is then covered with cottonoid and gently retracted upward and medially with a malleable brain retractor. For good relaxation of posterior fossa structures, CSF from the cerebellopontine cistern and the cisterna magna is drained. This exposes the intracranial portion of the tumor **(Fig. 23–15).**

The cranial nerves ventral to the tumor are identified and, if possible, are separated from the tumor. The tumor is then removed in a piecemeal manner using microsurgical techniques. In type D tumors, once the intracranial portion of the tumor is removed, tumor extension into the skull base outside the jugular foramen is followed. In this area, the tumor is gently separated from the caudal cranial nerves and then removed. In the majority of cases, the tumor is stuck to or arising from the nerve itself, so it is inevitable that some branches of the nerves will need to be resected. Schwannomas

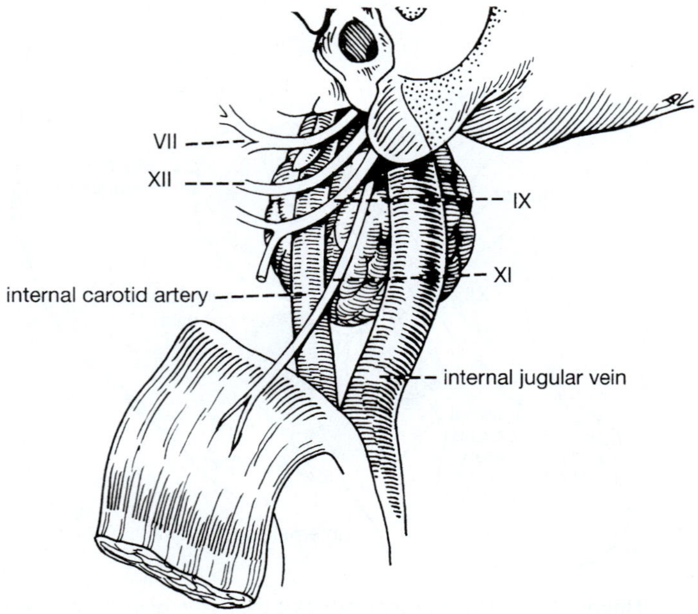

Figure 23–14 Drawing demonstrating the relationship of the seventh cranial nerve and the lower cranial nerves to the tumor.

of the jugular foramen usually displace the jugular bulb dorsally, and, in long-standing tumors, the jugular bulb is occluded. Unlike glomus jugulare tumors, schwannomas are outside of the lumen of the sinus, and hence the jugular bulb or the sinus is not sacrificed during tumor resection. To achieve a total cure, it is sometimes necessary to resect the tumor along with the distal portion of the sigmoid sinus and the proximal and distal stumps.

After tumor removal, the dura is closed watertight, as described for type A tumors. Prior to dural closure, when there has been extensive skull base bone resection involving mastoidectomy, exposure of the fallopian canal, and removal of the jugular tubercle (types B and D), a piece of fat obtained from the abdomen (treated with fibrin glue) is used to cover the area. To achieve a watertight seal of the dura at the jugular foramen, a piece of lyophilized dura or fascia lata is used to reinforce the posterior belly of the digastric muscle. The sternocleidomastoid muscle is sutured back and the remainder of the closure is completed after insertion of a Jackson-Pratt drain. Posterior fossa closure is similar to that described for type A tumors.

◆ Postoperative Management

Because the majority of patients with jugular foramen schwannomas have dysfunction of the lower cranial nerves prior to surgery, or are likely to sustain dysfunction during surgery, it is imperative not to extubate them immediately

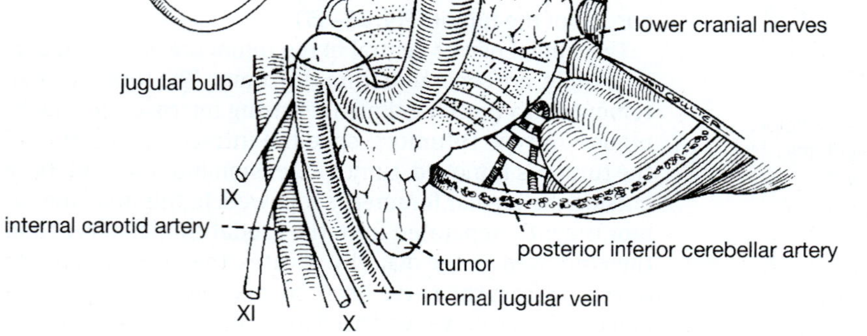

Figure 23–15 Drawing demonstrating both the intradural and extradural tumor. Note the relationship of the cranial nerves to the tumor.

following surgery. A thorough assessment of lower cranial nerve dysfunction indicates that any deficits are rarely permanent. However, it may be several weeks before the improvement occurs; hence, elective tracheostomy and gastrostomy are sometimes necessary. Postoperatively, patients are administered tapering doses of intravenous steroids and broad-spectrum antibiotics for a period of 72 hours, at which point the drains are removed.

◆ Complications

Injury to the lower cranial nerves and to the carotid artery can arise following the resection of large tumors in the jugular foramen. Injury to the lower cranial nerves is often inevitable in these nerve sheath tumors. However, careful neck dissection and identification and the separation and preservation of various structures, especially the nerves that are not giving rise to the tumor, aid in minimizing the deficit. Injury to the carotid artery generally occurs during upper cervical dissection, particularly on massive tumors where the carotid artery is completely incarcerated within the tumor. In these types of tumors, it is advisable to obtain proximal control caudal to the tumor and distal control in the petrous bone. In our experience, this scenario is more commonly seen in glomus tumors than in schwannomas. Intracranially staying within the tumor and the arachnoid, while debulking the tumor, would avoid injury to the neurovascular structures. Watertight dural closure with pericranium or fascia lata graft and tight muscle closure reduces the risk of CSF leak, pseudomeningocele, and seroma formation.

24

Surgical Approaches to Pineal Region Tumors

Alfred T. Ogden and Jeffrey N. Bruce

Although rare, pineal region tumors exhibit remarkably diverse histology. The many cell types that compose the normal anatomy of the pineal gland and adjacent structures can undergo the range of benign and malignant transformation. The midline, skull base location of the pineal region renders it among the preferred resting spots for ectopic tissue trapped during embryology that go on to form germ cell tumors. This histological diversity logically demands therapeutic intervention tailored to a specific histological diagnosis. For benign tumors and for some selected malignant tumors, radical resection offers the best promise for long-term survival. The diverse pathology and propensity for mixed tumors in the pineal region argues for surgical approaches capable of securing sufficient tumor sampling to maximize diagnostic accuracy. Open surgical approaches are preferred for most patients because they provide a representative sampling of what are often mixed tumors and offer the flexibility to perform an aggressive resection if indicated.

Open surgical approaches to the pineal region have attracted some of the great minds in neurosurgery over the last century, including Cushing, Dandy, Poppen, Jamieson, and Stein. Their efforts, combined with the evolution of modern neurosurgical techniques, have advanced open pineal region surgery to reasonable levels of safety. Of the numerous approaches developed, those that have withstood the scrutiny of time are the supracerebellar-infratentorial, the parietal interhemispheric, and the occipital transtentorial. The choice of surgical approach depends on the anatomical nuances of each tumor as well as the comfort level and personal preferences of the operating team.

Stereotactic and endoscopic approaches to procure small amounts of tissue offer different risks and benefits. Patients with medical contraindications to general anesthesia or prolonged surgery or patients with multiple lesions or extensive tumor invasion may be candidates for these alternatives.

◆ Patient Selection and Preoperative Preparation

Patients with pineal region tumors usually present with symptomatic hydrocephalus or visual disturbances, classically an upgaze palsy or other elements of Parinaud's syndrome. Initial diagnosis is often made with computed tomography (CT), but gadolinium-enhanced magnetic resonance imaging (MRI) is required to establish accurately the tumor's relationship to relevant anatomical structures such as the third ventricle, the quadrigeminal plate, the deep cerebral veins, and the tentorium **(Fig. 24–1).** Of particular importance is the degree of local tumor invasion, although in our experience this is often exaggerated by MRI. The presence of hydrocephalus will determine whether an initial procedure to divert cerebrospinal fluid (CSF) is required prior to craniotomy. Serum levels of germ cell markers, α-fetoprotein (AFP) and β-human chorionic gonadotropin (β-HCG), should be assayed because their presence indicates a malignant germ cell tumor that should be treated with either or both chemotherapy and radiation without the need for a biopsy. Although a CSF diversion procedure is sometimes obviated by removal of the obstructing tumor, significant hydrocephalus should be treated prior to open resection. Endoscopic third ventriculostomy (ETV) is preferred over placement of an indwelling shunt, but either procedure can give a satisfactory result. During diversion procedures, CSF should be sent for cytology and germ cell markers, which can in rare circumstances cinch a diagnosis when serum markers are negative or ambiguous.

◆ Operative Procedure

Patient Positioning

Numerous operative positions have been described and these may be interchangeable depending on the surgical approach **(Fig. 24–2).**

Sitting Position

The sitting position is usually preferred for the infratentorial-supracerebellar approach, although it can be used for supratentorial approaches as well. With the patient upright, gravity aids the surgeon by developing the natural surgical corridor between the tentorium and the cerebellum, pulling the tumor down into view and away from the deep venous structures, and preventing pooling of venous blood in the operative field. The attendant risks of subdural hematoma associated with cortical collapse, air embolus, and pneumocephalus can be anticipated and managed with proper precaution. Intraoperative monitoring of end-tidal expired carbon dioxide and vena cava Doppler ultrasound to detect the formation of small air emboli is critical. Emboli formation is quickly halted by flooding the operative field with

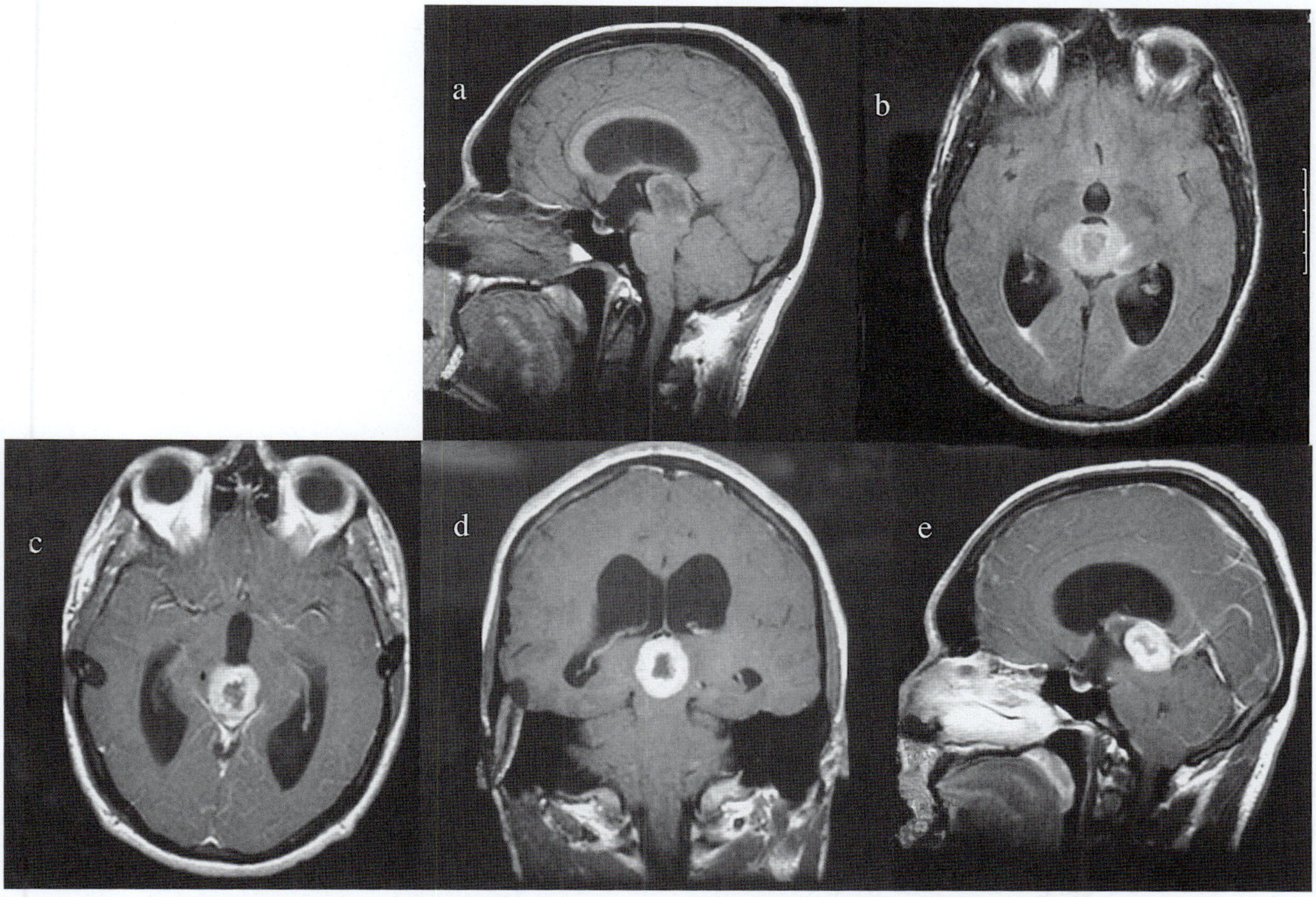

Figure 24–1 Magnetic resonance imaging sequences of a patient with a pineal region tumor. **(A)**, T1; **(B)**, FLAIR; **(C–E)**, contrast-enhanced T1. Histopathological analysis revealed a pineoblastoma.

irrigation and lowering the patient's head. If necessary, large air emboli can be retrieved via a central venous catheter, which should be placed preemptively in all patients prior to draping.

To bring the patient to the sitting position, the patient is first placed supine with the operative table in reverse orientation. After a three-point rigid headholder is placed, an assistant stabilizes the patient's head as the surgeon maneuvers the operating table to raise the patient's back and to flex the patient's legs, which also should be somewhat elevated to assist in venous return. Once the back is at the appropriate angle, the head is flexed so that the tentorium is approximately parallel to the floor. At least two fingerbreadths of space is needed between the patient's chin and sternum to avoid airway compromise and obstruction of venous return from the head. A Greenberg self-retaining retractor (Codman & Shurtleff, Inc., Raynham, MA) or similar retractor system frames the operative field to assist in cerebellar retraction.

Lateral Positions

Lateral positioning with the nondominant hemisphere down is generally preferred for supratentorial approaches. The patient is placed in a standard lateral position, with a three-point headholder and an axillary roll to keep weight off the downside shoulder. The head is fixed at a 30 degree angle above the horizontal in the midsagittal plane. If the occipital-transtentorial approach is to be employed, the head should be positioned with the patient's nose 30 degrees rotated toward the floor. The legs are flexed with a pillow between them and the patient is strapped down so that the table can be rotated at various times during the procedure to improve the exposure.

Often a more desirable variation is the three quarter prone position, especially for more posterior supratentorial approaches such as the occipital transtentorial approach. This is essentially the same as the standard lateral position, except that the head is extended and rotated to an oblique 45 degree angle. Additional support for the body is needed as the operating table is "airplaned" toward prone.

The advantage of lateral positioning over prone positioning is that the nondominant hemisphere is easily retracted with the help of gravity. Surgeon fatigue is reduced because the surgeon's hands are on a horizontal plane and the arms are not extended to the degree that they are for patients in the sitting position.

Prone Position

The prone position is simple and safe for supratentorial approaches and avoids the cumbersome aspects of placing a

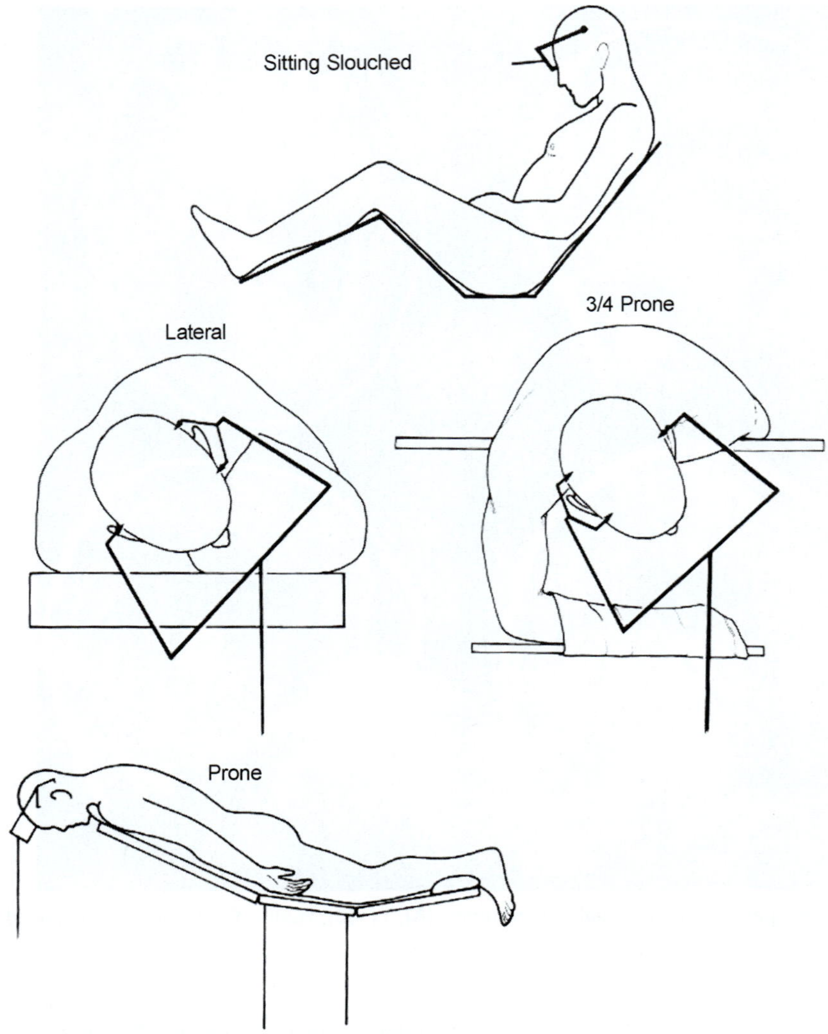

Figure 24–2 Patient positioning for pineal approaches.

patient in the lateral position. The steep angle of the tentorium, however, makes it impractical for the infratentorial approach. Although generally comfortable for the surgeon, the operative field is considerably elevated, which can make it difficult for the surgeon to be seated. This position enables the use of a bridge on the operating microscope, affording binocular vision to both the surgeon and the assistant. In a variation known as the Concorde position, the head is rotated 15 degrees away to facilitate occipital lobe retraction.

Operative Approaches

Widely accepted approaches to the pineal region are the infratentorial supracerebellar, the parietal interhemispheric, and the occipital transtentorial (**Fig. 24–3**). For most pineal region tumors there is no objective advantage to one approach over another, such that the choice of approach is dictated by the surgeon's comfort and expertise. There are important caveats to this rule, particularly with large tumors that extend supratentorially or laterally to the trigone of the lateral ventricle. Such tumors are generally more accessible via supratentorial approaches, which afford greater exposure; however, they have the distinct disadvantage of forcing the surgeon to work around the convergence of the vein of Galen, the basal veins of Rosenthal, and the internal cerebral veins. For this reason many surgeons prefer the infratentorial supracerebellar approach for all but the largest pineal region tumors or for tumors with a pronounced inferior projection.

The Infratentorial Supracerebellar Approach

The infratentorial supracerebellar approach was first described by Krause at the beginning of this century. The advent of the operating microscope and the development of microsurgical technique enabled its rediscovery and practical application by Stein in 1971.

The infratentorial supracerebellar approach is usually performed in the sitting position. In cases without previous CSF diversion, a ventricular drain can be placed into the trigone of the lateral ventricle through a bur hole in the midpupillary line at the lambdoid suture. A suboccipital exposure is begun through a linear midline incision extending

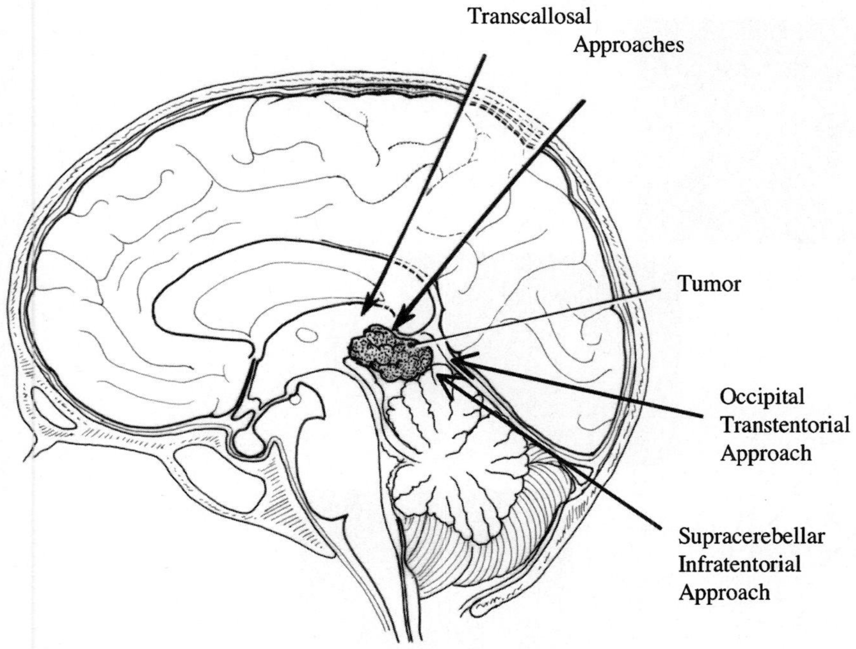

Figure 24–3 Trajectories of approaches to the pineal region.

from just above the inion down to the level of the spinous process of C4. The incision is brought through the nuchal ligament of the suboccipital musculature without detaching the muscles from the spinous processes of C1 and C2 and without exposing the foramen magnum. A single low-profile, self-retaining retractor contains the muscles and fascia of the suboccipital region, exposing the suboccipital bone. Although a craniectomy is a possible option, a craniotomy is preferred to reduce the incidence of postoperative pain, fluid collections, and aseptic meningitis. The craniotomy should be centered just below the inion and should be as generous as possible to provide working room for surgical instruments and adequate illumination. Four bone slots are drilled, one over the sagittal sinus just above the torcula, one over each transverse sinus, and a final slot in the midline 1 to 2 cm above the foramen magnum. A craniotome is used to connect the slots, allowing the bone flap to be elevated. There should be sufficient bone removed above the transverse sinus to ensure an unperturbed view down the tentorium. Bone edges should be carefully waxed, and venous bleeding controlled to avoid air emboli.

If the posterior fossa requires decompression, CSF can be removed through a ventricular drain or by opening the cisterna magna after dural opening. The dura is opened in a gentle semilunar curve, extending from the lateral aspects of the exposure. The dural flap is reflected upward and placed on some slight tension with tenting sutures and rubber bands. The amount of tension is defined by a balance between adequate superior tentorial retraction and maintenance of sinus patency. The inferior dura acts as a sling to support the cerebellar hemispheres.

To open the infratentorial corridor, the arachnoidal adhesions and bridging veins between the dorsal surface of the cerebellum and the tentorium are cauterized and carefully divided. As the cerebellum drops away from the tentorium, an excellent corridor reveals itself. The dorsal surface of the cerebellum should be protected with padding such as a Telfa sponge, and a small brain retractor placed if necessary to provide additional cerebellar retraction. Additional adhesions and bridging veins can be divided when they become visible near the anterior vermis. Deeper, the opalescent arachnoid covering over the pineal region can be seen.

The operating microscope is brought in at this time. It should be equipped with a variable objective and inclined eyepieces to accommodate the range of depths and angles required during this approach. A freestanding armrest is helpful to assist the surgeon and avoid fatigue.

Under the microscope, the arachnoid overlying the quadrigeminal plate is sharply opened. This is generally an avascular plane, and minimal cautery is necessary. Running from the anterior vermis to the vein of Galen, the precentral vein is identified, carefully dissected, cauterized, and divided (**Fig. 24–4A**). Although collateral cerebellar venous drainage enables sacrifice of this vein, it is not advisable to cauterize any of the other veins of the deep venous system. The retractor is now advanced to visualize the inferior portion of the tumor (**Fig. 24–4B**).

The central portion of the inferior pole of the tumor is cauterized and opened with a long-handled knife or bayoneted scissors. Specimens can be taken from within the capsule and sent for frozen sections, although the diagnostic inaccuracy inherent with frozen sections must be considered when making intraoperative decisions. The tumor is then internally debulked using a variety of instruments such as suction, cautery, tumor forceps, and an ultrasonic surgical aspirator if necessary. Most tumors are soft and generally deliver into a large-bore Japanese-style suction with variable control. After the tumor is decompressed, the capsule can be separated from the surrounding structures. The first step is to dissect the tumor capsule off the thalamus. Most vessels

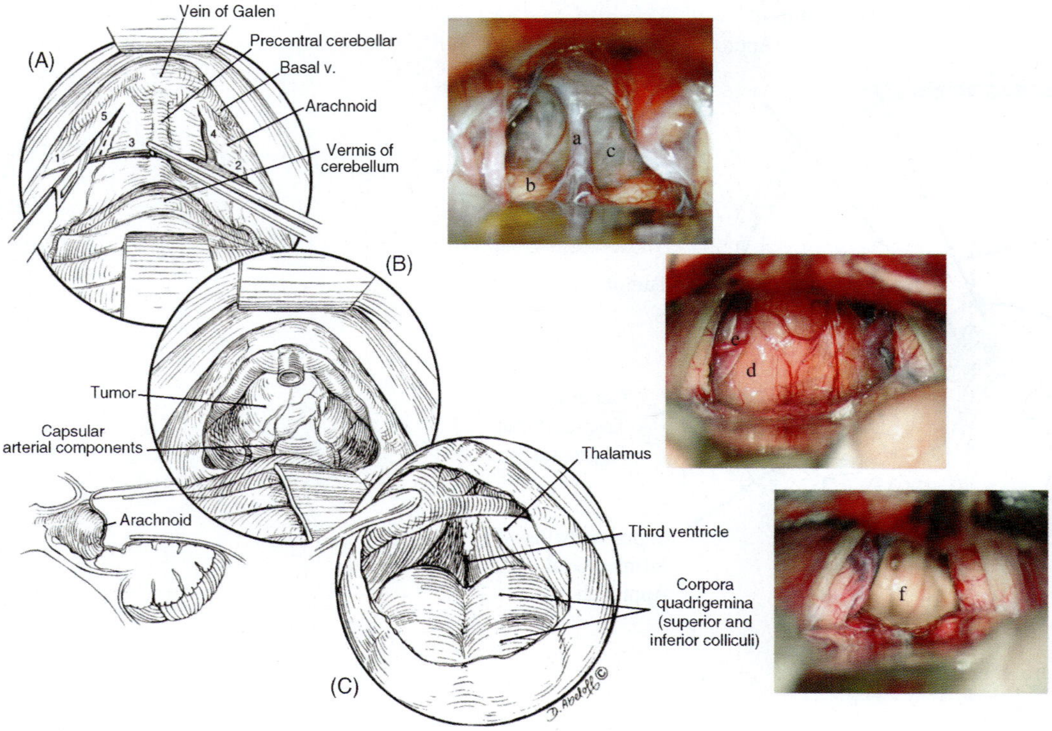

Figure 24–4 The supracerebellar infratentorial approach. **(A)** Exposure of the precentral vein; a, precentral vein; b, cerebellum; c, arachnoid. **(B)** Pineal tumor after precentral vein ligation and arachnoid dissection; d, pineal tumor; e, posterior choroidal artery. **(C)** View of the third ventricle after tumor excision; f, third ventricle.

encountered along the capsule wall are choroidal and need not be preserved. This segment of the dissection continues until the third ventricle is encountered. The inferior portion of the capsule is then carefully dissected off the brain stem. This is often the most difficult portion of the tumor dissection and can be facilitated by retracting the tumor superiorly, and bluntly dissecting it off of the brain stem under direct vision. The final portion of the capsule dissection involves separating the superior attachments along the velum interpositum and the deep venous system. These attachments must be carefully cauterized and sharply dissected without damaging the deep venous structures.

The intraoperative decision regarding the extent of tumor resection depends on the degree of tumor invasion and information from frozen sections. The relative benefit of radical resection depends largely upon histology and the ability to perform tumor removal with minimal morbidity.

Once the tumor is completely removed, the surgeon has an unobstructed view of the third ventricle **(Fig. 24–4C)**, the interior of which can be examined for clots or residual tumor using flexible mirrors. Hemostasis must be performed meticulously, without use of bulky hemostatic products like Gelfoam, which can float into the ventricular system causing obstruction or chemical meningitis. If necessary strips of Surgicel can be used to cover the cerebellar surfaces rarefied during retraction.

Once hemostasis is obtained and the retractors are removed, the dura is closed in as watertight a manner as possible and the bone flap is plated into place. The patient should be extubated with a reasonable degree of head gatch to avoid shifting of the decompressed brain within the cranial vault.

The Occipital-Transtentorial Approach

The occipital-transtentorial approach, originally described by Poppen and modified by Jamieson provides a wide exposure to the pineal region and is useful for large tumors. Because it utilizes an oblique trajectory for lesions that are essentially midline, this approach can be disorienting to surgeons who are not familiar with it. This problem can be minimized with stereotactic guidance. The surgeon is also hampered by having to operate around critical venous structures. Nevertheless, after division of the tentorium, unparalleled exposure of the quadrigeminal plate is achieved, making it particularly useful for tumors that extend inferiorly. A three quarter prone position is generally preferred for this approach because it utilizes gravity to aid downward retraction of the right occipital pole.

To begin, a U-shaped right occipital scalp flap is reflected inferiorly with the medial vertical limb beginning just to the left of midline at about the level of the inion. Two bur holes are drilled over or immediately adjacent to the sagittal sinus, one just above the torcula, and the second 6 to 10 cm above the first bur hole. A craniotome is then used to turn a generous right-sided craniotomy that extends 1 to 2 cm left of midline, and a dural flap is made toward the sagittal sinus.

Critical to the exposure during this approach is adequate nondominant occipital lobe retraction without causing a homonymous hemianopsia. Assisting in this retraction are the natural absence of bridging veins between the sagittal sinus and the occipital lobe and the effect of gravity if the three quarter prone position is used. Judicious use of mannitol and ventricular drainage can help minimize this danger as well.

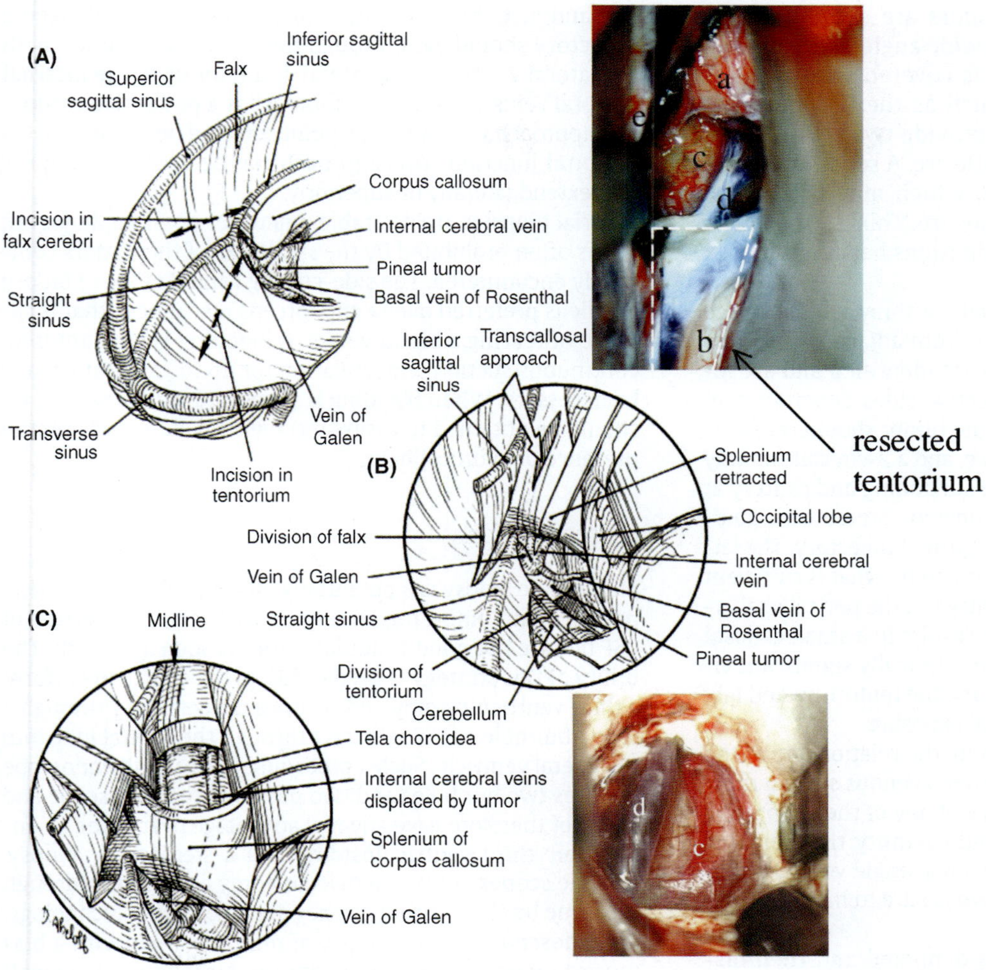

Figure 24–5 The occipital-transtentorial and interhemispheric approaches to the pineal region. **(A)** Relationship of the venous system, falx, and tentorium to the pineal region. **(B)** Exposure in the occipital transtentorial approach after resection of the tentorium and **(C)** after the interhemispheric approach. a, corpus callosum; b, cerebellum; c, tumor; d, internal cerebral vein; e, cauterized falx; white dotted line, resected tentorium.

Under the operating microscope, the straight sinus is identified so that the tentorium can be divided adjacent to it. A retractor can be placed over the falx and the inferior sagittal sinus for lateral exposure **(Fig. 24–5A,B).** If greater exposure of the contralateral tentorium is required, the falx and inferior sagittal sinus can be divided. At this point, the arachnoid overlying the tumor and the quadrigeminal cisterns can be seen. The tumor removal proceeds as already described, taking care to avoid injury to the deep venous system. The closure and hemostasis proceed as previously described.

Transcallosal-Interhemispheric Approach

The transcallosal-interhemispheric approach was first described by Dandy and has since been applied to deep-seated tumors in various locations around the third ventricle. Applying this approach to the pineal region involves the usual exploitation of interhemispheric fissure to generate a space accentuated by a corridor along the parieto-occipital junction on the nondominant side. This approach is usually reserved for pineal region tumors with anterior extension into the third ventricle. Any of the previously described patient positions can be used for this approach, although generally the prone or sitting position is preferred. Preparations for intraoperative stereotactic guidance can provide a useful adjunct.

Precise bone flap planning depends on the relationship of the tumor to the third ventricle, but the vertex is usually a reasonable target around which to center the craniotomy. Adequate exposure is provided by a U-shaped skin incision with the goal of extending the scalp flap across the midline to be reflected laterally. A craniotomy of ~8 cm in length is needed to provide options for surgical corridors between bridging veins. A bur hole is made over the sagittal sinus, both anteriorly and posteriorly, and a craniotome is used to turn a generous craniotomy, extending 1 to 2 cm to the left of the sagittal sinus.

The dura is opened in a U-shaped fashion and reflected medially toward the sagittal sinus. The bridging veins are inspected and an approach is chosen that will minimize the number of veins to be sacrificed. Usually sacrifice of one bridging vein is necessary to achieve the adequate exposure, although sacrifice of more than one vein is not recommended. Because the tumors are deeply seated, even a small opening provides a wide angle of deep exposure. The exposed hemisphere is covered with Bicol or Telfa and a retractor system, such as the Greenberg, is used to frame the opening and provide two retractors to retract the parietal lobe in a gentle arc. A separate retractor can be used along the falx, which may be divided inferiorly to provide further exposure. This is generally a nonvascular corridor with few adhesions between the falx and cingulate gyrus.

At the bottom of the surgical field, a shiny white surface distinguishes the corpus callosum from adjacent cingulate gyrus. Paired pericallosal arteries are identified and are retracted to one side or their respective sides depending on their natural course. At this point the tumor should reveal itself as a bulge in the callosal surface, and a 2-cm callosotomy should be performed using gentle suctioning and cautery at the point where the bulge is most obvious. Stereotactic guidance may be useful to identify the optimal trajectory. The lateral extent of the opening is determined by what is sufficient to expose the tumor and avoid damage to the pericallosal arteries. Following these guidelines results in a small callosal lesion that is unlikely to lead to any clinically significant visual or cognitive deficits. If necessary, the tentorium and falx can be divided to provide additional exposure.

Once through the corpus callosum, the relationship of the dorsal surface of the tumor to the deep venous system must be identified **(Fig. 24–5C)**. Sacrifice of any of the deep veins has met with variable success and calamity that remains anecdotal. Whereas sacrifice of even a single vein is undesirable and perilous, sacrifice of two is sure to have a devastating result.

Once a tumor is exposed, it is debulked and then dissected as previously described. Leaving a ventricular drain in place for 1 or 2 days is a prudent option.

Stereotactic Biopsy

Stereotactic biopsy carries a greater risk of hemorrhage in the pineal region than in other locations in the brain and therefore should be viewed with caution. The complexity and risk of stereotactic biopsy stem from the potential to encounter multiple ependymal surfaces along the needle trajectory, the proximity of the deep venous system to the target, and the lack of local tissue turgor to effect tamponade when bleeding occurs. Still, in experienced hands, stereotactic biopsy can be performed safely, and large series have shown that hemorrhages during pineal region biopsies are only rarely clinically significant.

Frame-based stereotactic systems are ceding to frameless systems that offer comparable levels of accuracy. For most tumors CT provides adequate resolution for localization and has as good or better spatial accuracy when using a frame-based system. For patients that have an obvious contrast-enhancing lesion, localization with CT is accurate, convenient, and economical. MRI provides better resolution and different imaging modalities, both of which can influence target selection and trajectory.

The most common stereotactic approach to the pineal region is anterolaterosuperior through a low precoronal entry point. An entry point is usually selected just behind the hairline and just above the superior temporal line. The needle trajectory should pass through the frontal lobe underneath the lateral ventricle and lateral and inferior to the internal cerebral veins. An alternate approach is a posterolaterosuperior approach with an entry point selected near the parieto-occipital junction. This approach can be useful for tumors that extend laterally or superiorly.

Serial biopsies are desirable whenever possible; however, this is often prohibited by the small size of the tumors commonly encountered. The side-cutting cannula type of biopsy needle is preferred over a cup forceps instrument that is capable of tearing a blood vessel. If bleeding is encountered, continuous suction and irrigation for up to 15 minutes may be necessary. When bleeding is suspected, an immediate CT should be obtained to assess intraventricular blood and the presence of hydrocephalus.

Endoscopic Biopsy

Endoscopic biopsy is a potentially elegant solution for many patients with pineal region tumors who require diversion of CSF but are not good candidates for an open approach. The utility of this strategy is predicated on the ability to perform a third ventriculostomy and secure a tissue biopsy through a single bur hole and single tract through the frontal lobe into the lateral ventricle. Such a procedure with a rigid endoscope requires two bur holes and two passes of the endoscope and does not therefore have any real advantage over doing an endoscopic third ventriculostomy and a stereotactic biopsy. Flexible scopes permit ventriculostomy and biopsy through the same bur hole, although they are an evolving technology. An endoscope permits biopsy of multiple areas with a bias toward biopsy of the tumor capsule. Although initial small series of pineal region tumors managed endoscopically show encouraging results, endoscopic biopsy carries a real risk of intraventricular hemorrhage—a potentially devastating complication for a biopsy—that is as of yet undefined.

◆ Postoperative Management

Appropriate postoperative care requires at least an overnight stay in an intensive care unit for proper, arterial line-directed blood pressure management and frequent monitoring of neurological function. Immediate postoperative confusion and agitation are usually a result of pneumocephalus, which requires no intervention and is self-limiting. Delayed neurological decline should raise concerns over development of hydrocephalus either as a result of an obstructive clot or cerebellar edema from venous congestion. To control for these possibilities we advocate a preliminary endoscopic third ventriculostomy in addition to placement of an extraventricular drain at the outset of the definitive procedure. Slow steroid tapers of approximately 10 days are appropriate to prevent chemical meningitis/posterior fossa syndrome, the frequency of which is diminished by craniotomy and replacement of the bone flap. Careful wound evaluation is important to catch CSF leaks as soon as they manifest. In our experience recovery from this surgery is usually uneventful, and patients are often discharged as early as postoperative day 3.

◆ Conclusion

Tumors in the pineal region can be safely accessed and resected using three approaches: the infratentorial supracerebellar, the parietal interhemispheric, and the occipital transtentorial. The choice of approach is sometimes influenced by the anatomical nuances of each tumor but is more often a function of the surgeon's personal preference.

Open surgery for pineal region tumors in the modern neurosurgical era is the treatment option of choice for benign lesions and facilitates maximal removal of malignant tumors to optimize diagnostic and prognostic capabilities. Stereotactic biopsy is preferred to an open approach in some selected cases. Endoscopic biopsy offers the ability to divert CSF and obtain tissue in a single operation but remains an evolving technology.

25

Surgical Approaches to Pediatric Midline Posterior Fossa Tumors

Sharad Rajpal and Bermans J. Iskandar

◆ Patient Selection

Pediatric tumors of the midline posterior fossa present a unique challenge for the neurosurgeon. Posterior fossa tumors (PFTs) include astrocytoma (pilocytic, fibrillary, and anaplastic), medulloblastoma, ependymoma, brain stem gliomas, and other, less frequent types. These tumors can be found incidentally or present with clinical symptoms for several days to months. Clinical manifestations are typically due to mass effect exerted by the tumor and depend on whether the lesion involves the cerebellum, the fourth ventricle, or the brain stem. Presentations usually include headache and vomiting, most often secondary to obstructive hydrocephalus, but may range from cranial nerve palsies to pyramidal and cerebellar signs. The goal for operative management of PFTs is twofold: obtain tissue for a histological diagnosis and reduce tumor burden. Knowledge of different tumor types and locations determines the extent of surgical resection and the need for adjuvant therapy.

◆ Preoperative Preparation

Once a PFT has been diagnosed, the time for surgical intervention must be determined. The danger associated with PFTs, in particular, is hydrocephalus secondary to obstruction of cerebrospinal fluid (CSF) drainage pathways. If the patient is stable, surgery can be scheduled for the next available operating time. However, if the patient develops acute hydrocephalus and mental status or vital sign changes, it may be necessary to place an external ventricular drainage (EVD) system and take the patient to the operating room sooner. Placement of an EVD must be exercised with caution because there is potential for upward herniation from posterior fossa mass effect. Controlled, gradual decreases in intracranial pressure (ICP) achieved through careful CSF drainage (15 to 20 mm Hg) relieves symptoms and minimizes the risk of upward herniation. Placement of a permanent CSF shunt prior to surgery is contraindicated because many patients benefit from definitive surgical management of the PFT and relief of the obstruction. Preoperative laboratory studies include a complete blood count with differential, partial thromboplastin time, internationalized ratio, electrolytes, and a type and cross-match for two units of packed red blood cells. Anticonvulsants are not indicated because seizures are uncommon from tumors in this location. Preoperative steroids are beneficial in reducing tumor edema and possibly alleviating the hydrocephalus. The dose of dexamethasone is dependent on the size of the child and consists of an intravenous bolus followed by a maintenance dose. Using mannitol (1 g/kg) or furosemide (1 mg/kg) is typically reserved for acute instances when the patient demonstrates deterioration, or immediately perioperatively to optimize brain relaxation.

Anesthesia

All attempts should be made to prevent elevated ICP prior to and during anesthetic induction. Once the patient is asleep, two peripheral venous catheters and an arterial line for blood pressure monitoring and blood sampling are placed. The use of a central venous catheter (CVC) is widely debated. Although CVCs are beneficial in monitoring volume status and the removal of a potential venous air embolism, their placement via the internal jugular vein or subclavian vein may cause pneumothorax, hematoma, or air embolism. We do not routinely place a CVC in our patients. The bladder is catheterized, and pulse oximetry, end-expiratory carbon dioxide, electrocardiography, blood pressure, body temperature, and precordial Doppler monitors utilized. For tumors that involve the brain stem, the use of motor, somatosensory, brain stem auditory evoked response (BAER), and direct electromyographic (EMG) stimulation of relevant cranial nerves may be beneficial. Cranial nerve monitoring at our institution involves placing EMG leads in the lateral rectus (CN VI), orbicularis oculi or ori (CN VII), pharyngeal (CN IX, X), sternocleidomastoid (CN XI), and tongue muscles (CN XII) **(Figs. 25–1A,B)**. It has also been customary at our institution to use frameless stereotactic guidance. Care should be taken to ensure the patient's core body temperature, especially in smaller children, remains within the 36° to 37°C range. Normothermia is maintained via heating lamps, heating blankets, and an elevated operating room temperature.

Patient Positioning

If the patient has hydrocephalus or the propensity to develop hydrocephalus postoperatively, placement of an EVD is recommended prior to initiation of the craniotomy. Some

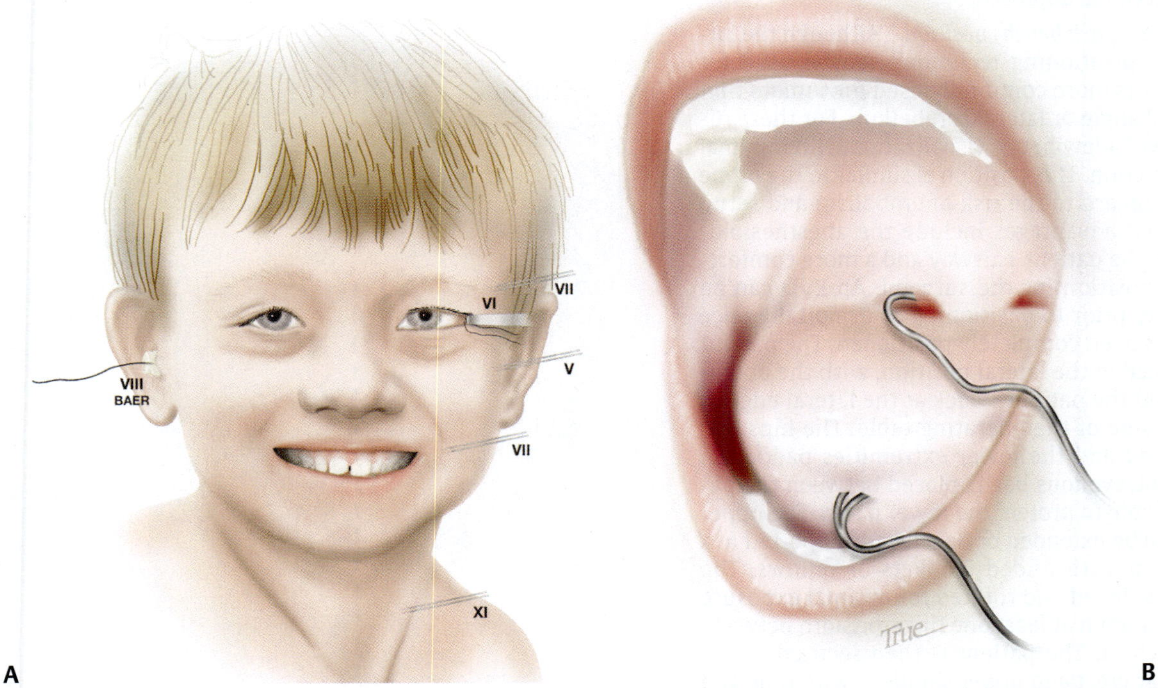

Figures 25–1 Motor, somatosensory, and brain stem auditory evoked response, and direct electromyographic stimulation of relevant cranial nerves are beneficial for brain stem tumor resection. Cranial nerve monitoring at our institution involves placing electromyographic leads in **(A)** temporalis or masseter muscles (CNV), the lateral rectus (CN VI), orbicularis oculi or ori (CN VII), sternocleidomastoid (CN XI), **(B)** pharyngeal (CN IX, X), and tongue muscles (CN XII).

patients require intraoperative ventriculostomy placement if the dura is noted to be under tension during surgery. EVD placement depends upon patient positioning (for specific EVD placement see individual positioning descriptions discussed in later sections).

Patient positioning depends upon surgeon preference and comfort level. Several positions exist, including the prone, seated, and lateral decubitus positions. Each position has its own advantages and disadvantages. Although the risk of air embolism is highest with the seated position, it is important to realize that this complication, though infrequent, can occur in *any* position in which the patient's head is elevated in relation to the heart.

- *Prone (Concorde and angulated Concorde) position* This is our preferred position because the risk of air embolism is low, the surgeon is able to work comfortably, and there is less risk of tearing bridging veins between the cerebellum and tentorium than in the seated position. Disadvantages to this position include venous engorgement in the operative bed resulting in more risk of bleeding, increased pressure on the facial structures throughout the procedure, and the anesthesiologist's decreased accessibility to the patient's airway. An EVD can be placed frontally prior to positioning or occipitally when positioning is completed. Once prone on the operating table, the patient is positioned with the majority of weight supported on rolls placed beneath the shoulders and pelvis. Pressure on the abdominal viscera and face should be avoided. The arms are then tucked to each side. The choice of head support depends upon the age of the child and skull thickness: patients older than 2 years of age can be placed in headholder pins with 30 to 60 lb of pressure, whereas infants and toddlers may do better without pin stabilization, although pediatric pins are available. Other techniques of cranial stabilization include the pediatric horseshoe, a specially folded bean bag, and others. The neck is flexed ~30 degrees in the Concorde position. There should always be at least one fingerbreadth between the patient's chin and chest. For cerebellopontine (CP) angle or lateral tumors, the head is also angled 30 degrees away from the midline, with the posterior fossa turned toward the surgeon (angulated Concorde).
- *Seated position* Although the seated position has been abandoned at our institution, it has several advantages, including improved blood and CSF drainage from the operative field. Disadvantages to the seated position include higher risk of air embolism and surgeon fatigue secondary to working with elevated arms. To position the patient, the shoulders are first placed at the end of the main section of the operating table. In older children, the head is placed in a three-pin headholder as already discussed. The arms are folded and supported on the patient's lap and the operating table gradually flexed to the sitting position. The head is kept vertical and slightly flexed with the chin approximately one fingerbreadth from the chest. The legs should be flexed at the hips and the knees, with the patient's back comfortable against the posterior support. With constant vigilance to avoid compromising the airway or venous drainage, the headholder is secured to the operating table.

Once the patient is positioned, an EVD catheter can be placed via an occipital approach.

- *Lateral decubitus (park bench) position* Although the lateral decubitus positioning technique can be used for midline PFTs, it is more commonly used for tumors that occur in the CP angle or lateral cerebellum. For these tumors gravity will allow better visualization with minimal cerebellar retraction. This position is similar to the prone position with regard to the risk of embolism and setup time. Additional advantages include the anesthesiologist's access to the patient's airway and a more comfortable working position for the surgeon. An EVD can be placed frontally prior to positioning or occipitally once the patient has been completely positioned. The patient is initially placed in the lateral position, with the operative side up and the patient's back at the lateral edge of the surgeon's side of the operating table. The hips and knees are flexed and the lower extremities padded. A towel roll or intravenous bag is placed between the patient and the table to protect the lower axilla. The upper extremities can be extended or flexed and supported in a neutral position with folded blankets or pillows. The head is slightly flexed and rotated for optimal exposure with care to maintain at least one fingerbreadth between the chin and chest. The patient is then secured to the table at the iliac crest and upper shoulder with tape and the head either taped to a doughnut in small children or placed in head pins (see earlier discussion) for older children. To improve exposure, the table can be tilted 5 to 10 degrees away from the surgeon. The back of the table is also elevated 20 to 30 degrees to help improve venous return and gravity drainage of blood and CSF away from the operative field.

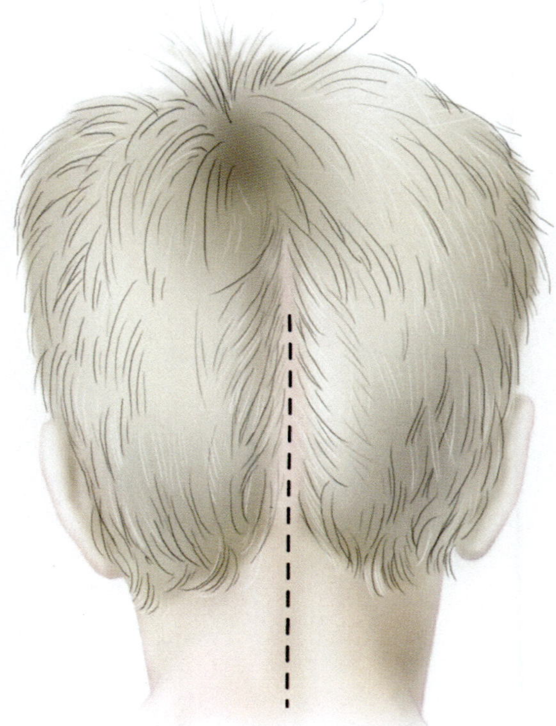

Figure 25–2 The skin incision is typically midline from the level of the inion to the level of C1–C2.

◆ Operative Procedure

Opening

A midline incision is used for both midline and paramidline tumors. For tumors in the lateral cerebellar hemispheres, the incision is made laterally over the bulk of the tumor mass between the midline and mastoid. The planned incision is typically from the inion to the C1–C2 level **(Fig. 25–2)**. After an appropriate prep and drape (including an area for possible intraoperative ventriculostomy placement), the skin is incised with a scalpel and the remainder of the subcutaneous tissues opened with a needle-tipped monopolar electrocautery down to the level of the occipital bone and most posterior aspect of the C1 arch. The muscle and fascia are cut just below their insertion, and the avascular midline through the ligamentum nuchae is developed to (1) minimize blood loss, (2) minimize postoperative pain, and (3) ensure a watertight closure **(Fig. 25–3)**. A T-shaped incision in the fascia allows the closure to be watertight by reapproximating all three limbs of fascia.

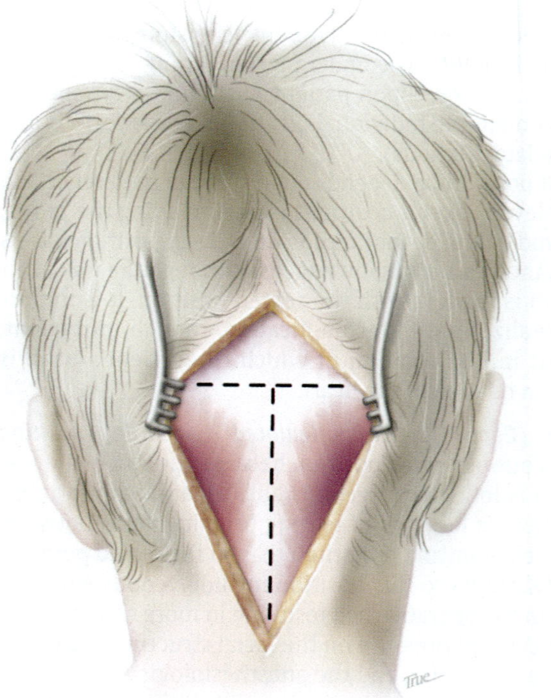

Figure 25–3 The skin is incised with a scalpel and the remainder of the subcutaneous tissues opened with a needle-tipped monopolar electrocautery down to the level of the occipital bone and the most posterior aspect of the C1 arch. The muscle and fascia are cut just below their insertion and the avascular midline through the ligamentum nuchae is developed. A T-shaped incision in the fascia allows the closure to be watertight by reapproximating all three limbs of muscle and fascia.

The subcutaneous tissues and muscles are dissected away from the calvarium and posterior arch of C1. Lateral dissection on C1 and C2 is limited to the width of the spinal canal to avoid injuring the vertebral arteries. Two self-retractors are then placed to maintain exposure **(Fig. 25–4)**. All emissary veins that are encountered are waxed and coagulated

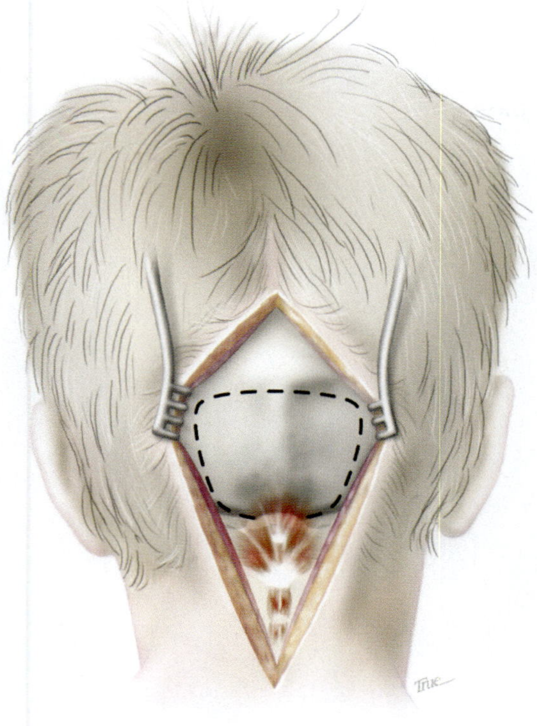

Figure 25–4 The subcutaneous tissues and muscles are dissected away from the calvarium and arch of C1. Lateral dissection on C1 and C2 is limited to the width of the spinal canal to avoid injuring the vertebral arteries. Two self-retractors are then placed to maintain exposure.

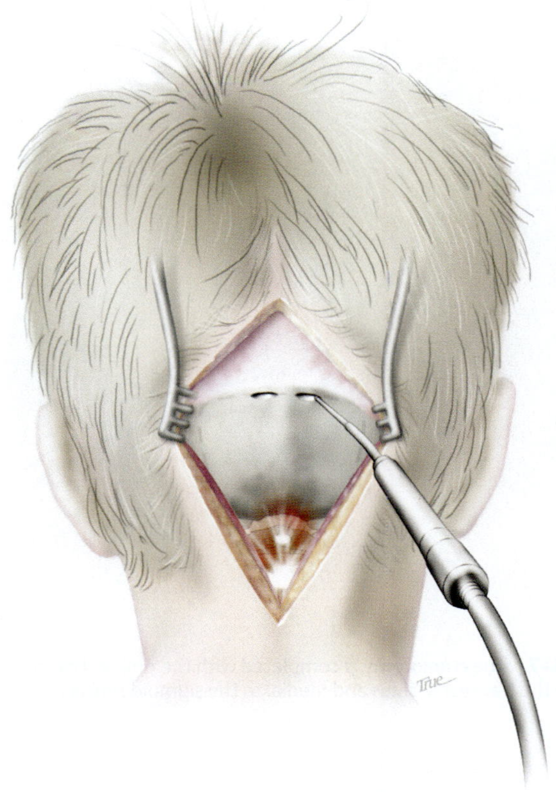

Figure 25–5 After exposure of the calvarium, two small bur holes are created on both sides of the midline at the most cephalad portion of the craniotomy flap.

to ensure hemostasis and minimize the risk of air embolism. Laminotomy is necessary if the tumor extends into the spinal cord.

We prefer performing a craniotomy rather than a craniectomy. Two small bur holes are first created on both sides of the midline at the most cephalad portion of the craniotomy flap **(Fig. 25–5).** This helps identify the midline strut, which is then drilled down carefully while connecting the two bur holes **(Fig. 25–6).** The remainder of the occiput is then removed with the drill **(Fig. 25–7).** The thickness of the occipital bone will vary and thus must be taken into account during any drilling to prevent injury to the underlying dura. The craniotomy is limited superiorly to the transverse sinus and laterally to the sigmoid sinuses. The dura is separated from the bone with a blunt instrument and the bone flap removed. All bone edges are waxed to reduce bleeding, and all sharp edges reduced with the rongeur or drill. Once hemostasis is achieved, the dura should be assessed for increased tension. If the dura is tight, several strategies can be employed before dural opening. If a tumor cyst is visible, it can be aspirated with a needle. If no cyst is visible, the patient can initially be hyperventilated or given a diuretic such as mannitol or furosemide. If the dura continues to remain tense despite employing these therapies, pressure can be reduced through controlled CSF drainage either through an already placed EVD or by placing one at this time. Drainage should occur slowly to prevent cerebellar herniation. The dura is opened in a Y shape, starting with the limbs and dissecting toward the midline. The occipital sinus needs to be properly occluded in the midline prior to its

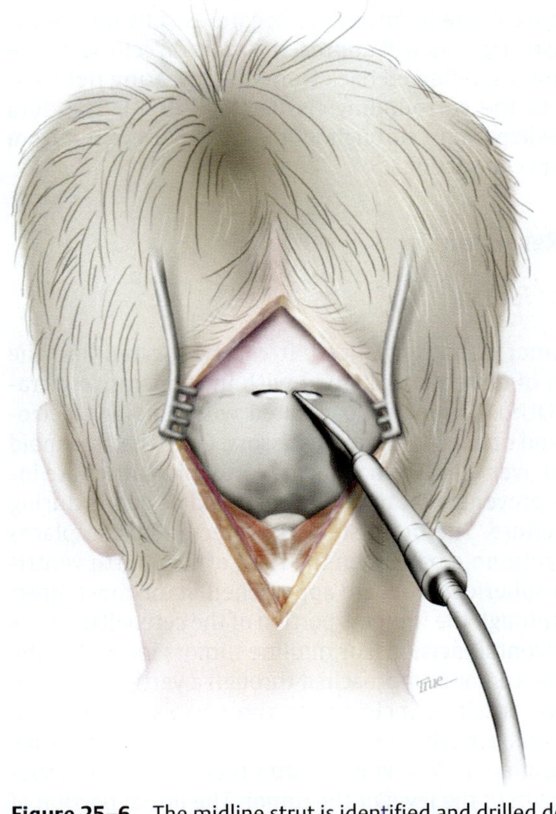

Figure 25–6 The midline strut is identified and drilled down while connecting the two bur holes. Care must be taken to avoid injuring the underlying transverse sinus.

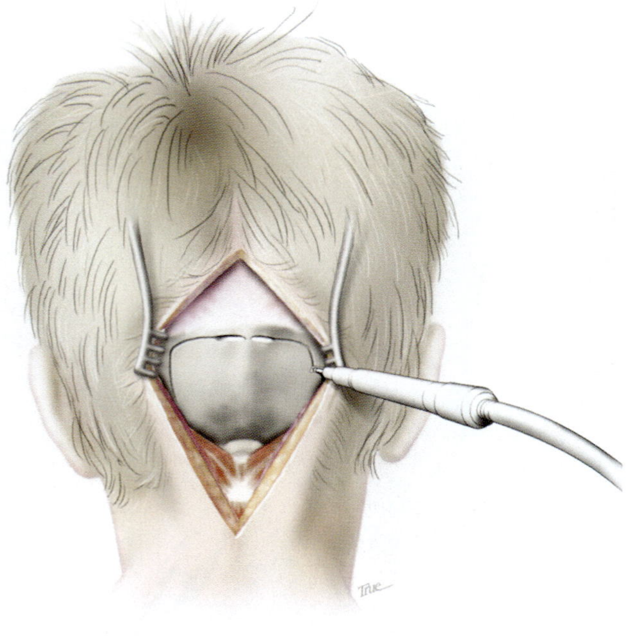

Figure 25–7 The craniotomy is completed with the drill and extends inferior to the transverse sinus and medial to the sigmoid sinuses.

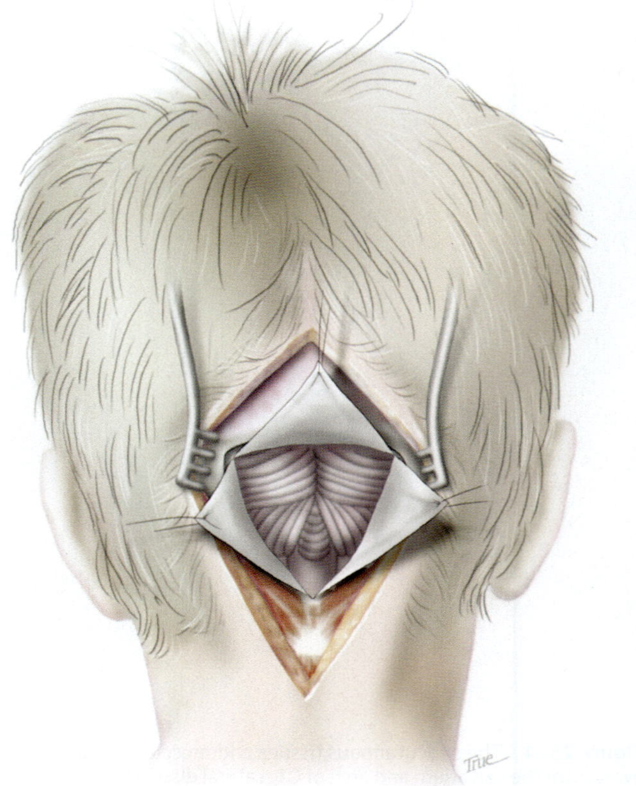

Figure 25–8 The dura is opened in a Y shape, starting with the limbs and dissecting toward the midline. The occipital sinus needs to be properly occluded in the midline prior to its transection. The inferior limb of the Y is then opened just off the midline down to the level of the inferior portion of the tumor.

transection. The inferior limb of the Y is then opened just off the midline down to the level of the inferior portion of the tumor. The inferior limb of the Y is sometimes placed laterally, directly over a cerebellar tumor if it is small and limited to a single hemisphere. Regardless of tumor location, most surgeons will approach it via a direct route. The dural flaps are reflected back from the operating field and sutured to the surrounding tissue **(Fig. 25–8)**. The dura should be kept moist throughout the case to prevent it from drying and contracting.

Tumor Resection

Cerebellar Tumors

If the tumor is not visualized, it can be located and the direction of dissection planned with intraoperative ultrasound (IOUS). The pia is coagulated with bipolar electrocautery and opened with microscissors. Once the arachnoid is opened over the cisterna magna, cottonoid patties are inserted to prevent any caudal flow of blood or debris during the procedure. The brain stem is protected by the placement of cottonoid patties on the floor of the fourth ventricle. Hemispheric tumors are approached in the most direct manner through the thinnest portion of the cerebellar cortex via a horizontal incision. For midline tumors located in the vermis, the tumor is approached through a vertical incision. Whenever possible, incisions in the vermis are avoided because this arguably increases the risk of postoperative cerebellar mutism. The white matter is coagulated and suctioned down to the level of the tumor. The initial portion of the tumor is sent to pathology for frozen section and preliminary diagnosis. The tumor is subsequently removed from its core to its periphery with bipolar electrocautery and suction or an ultrasonic aspirator (UA). The extent of tumor dissection depends on tumor size and histology (see later discussion). Most surgeons will continue with gross total resection until the tissue consistency changes to that of normal brain parenchyma. Tumors invading the floor of the fourth ventricle can be separated from the brain stem with gentle suctioning without injury to the brain stem. Hemostasis is achieved with bipolar electrocautery, Gelfoam, and/or Surgicel.

Fourth Ventricle Tumors

Tumor location will typically displace the cerebellar tonsils and vermis either laterally or inferiorly **(Fig. 25–9)**. Tumors are best approached down the midline through the midline aperture (foramen of Magendie). Incising the vermis is avoided in most cases by developing the cerebellomedullary (CM) fissure. The brain stem should be protected by placing cottonoid patties on the floor of the fourth ventricle whenever possible. The tumor is slowly mobilized laterally from the hemispheres, and the dorsal portions debulked along the way with suction and bipolar electrocautery or the UA. As the floor of the fourth ventricle is approached and visualized both caudally and rostrally to the lesion, the tumor is shaved off the level of the floor. This

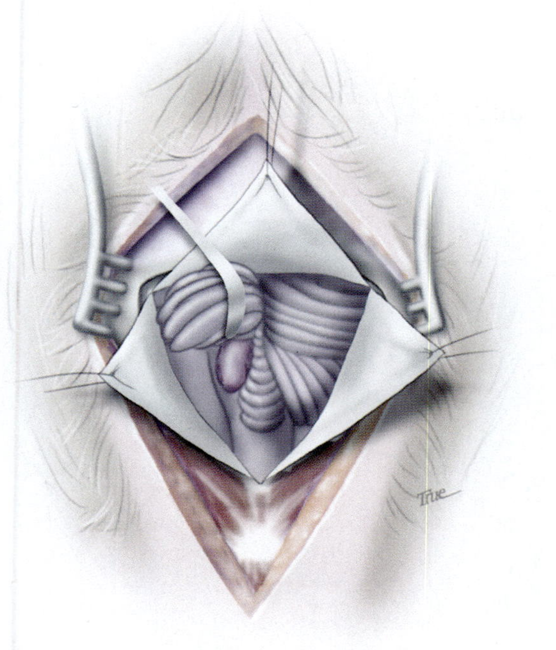

Figure 25–9 A tumor in the fourth ventricle will typically displace the cerebellar tonsils and vermis either laterally or inferiorly.

should represent the ventral margin of the tumor. The microscope often aids in dissection. The aqueduct of Sylvius, and the roof, floor, lateral recesses, and obex of the fourth ventricle are then checked to ensure adequate gross tumor resection. Important variations in extent of resection exist between the various types of fourth ventricular tumors, as described below.

- *Cerebellar astrocytomas* Cerebellar astrocytomas of the pilocytic, grade I, and grade II types can often be removed completely with minimal morbidity. When such tumors invade the brain stem, shaving them off the fourth ventricular floor is sufficient. Such residual tumors will often stay dormant or regress. If the brain stem residual tumor grows over time, a more aggressive secondary resection can be planned. At our institution, tumor resection involving the brain stem is assisted by intraoperative cranial nerve monitoring. A small, residual, low-grade astrocytoma of the cerebellum is acceptable and should be aggressively resected only when it demonstrates a tendency to grow over time.
- *Medulloblastomas* Resecting a medulloblastoma follows the same guidelines as low-grade gliomas, with the exception that a near-total resection is crucial to optimize prognosis. A near-total resection (greater than 90% resection) consists of leaving less than 1.5 cc of tumor tissue on postoperative magnetic resonance imaging (MRI). A partial resection (less than 90% resection or more than 1.5 cc of residual on MRI) is associated with a poor prognosis and should be avoided. A gross total resection (minimal tumor visible on MRI), however, has the same overall prognosis as a near-total resection. Increasing morbidity through a very aggressive resection of tumor that has invaded the brain stem is therefore not necessary.
- *Ependymomas* It is evident from large studies that ependymomas require a gross total resection for optimal long-term outcome. A near-total resection in such cases is insufficient. The extent to which tumor should be aggressively resected from the brain stem is controversial. At our institution, we have adopted an aggressive approach assisted by intraoperative cranial nerve monitoring.

Brain Stem Tumors

Surgery is only useful in patients with focal or exophytic brain stem tumors, which usually occur in the midbrain and at the cervicomedullary junction **(Fig. 25–10).** Patients with diffuse pontine gliomas, on the other hand, do not derive benefit from surgery. In fact, these malignant tumors are uniformly fatal regardless of treatment modality. Diffuse pontine gliomas are characteristic enough on MRI that biopsy is not usually indicated. Currently, such tumors are treated with various experimental protocols of chemotherapy and radiation therapy. Focal tumors of the medulla and cervicomedullary junction are resectable with a 70 to 80% long-term progression-free survival. Chemotherapy and/or radiation therapy are only indicated if surgical resection is not possible. One should exercise great caution during

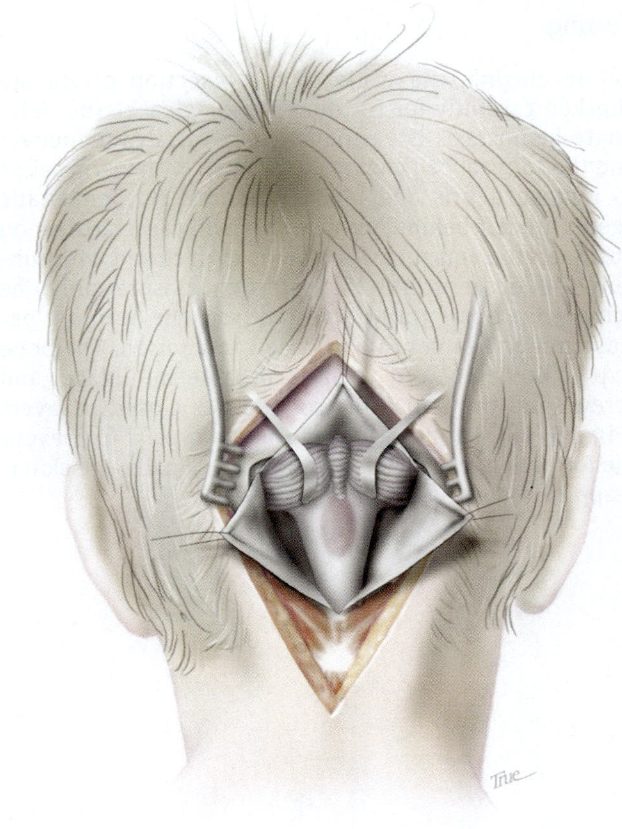

Figure 25–10 Dorsal view of a focal brain stem tumor with the fourth ventricle exposed.

brain stem tumor resections to avoid permanent cranial nerve deficits. Often, a partial resection or staged procedure may be more reasonable than an attempt at an aggressive removal. A tumor residual that demonstrates growth over time may then be approached in a more aggressive fashion.

To gain access to the fourth ventricle, the cerebellar tonsils are separated and the CM fissure developed. The vermis is rarely split for reasons described earlier. In dorsally exophytic brain stem tumors, the tumor presents itself before the fourth ventricle. In such cases, it is crucial to identify normal brain stem inferior and superior to the lesion prior to proceeding with the significant part of the resection. Starting with dissection at the superior pole of the tumor until the floor of the fourth ventricle is identified, the tumor is slowly separated until it is completely removed. Focal intrinsic brain stem tumors are challenging because, even though normal brain stem tissue is displaced inferiorly, superiorly, or laterally, tumor margins are close to important cranial nerve nuclei. We use intraoperative mapping with EMG stimulation to identify safe passages through the brain stem to reach the tumor. The remainder and majority of tumor resection within the brain stem is continued with the UA from the core to the periphery. Electrocautery should be used sparingly inside the tumor bed and only to coagulate specifically identified vessels; hemostasis is achieved primarily with thrombotic agents. The margin of the tumor is identified once the consistency of the tissue changes and, especially, if white matter is encountered. At this point the resection is halted.

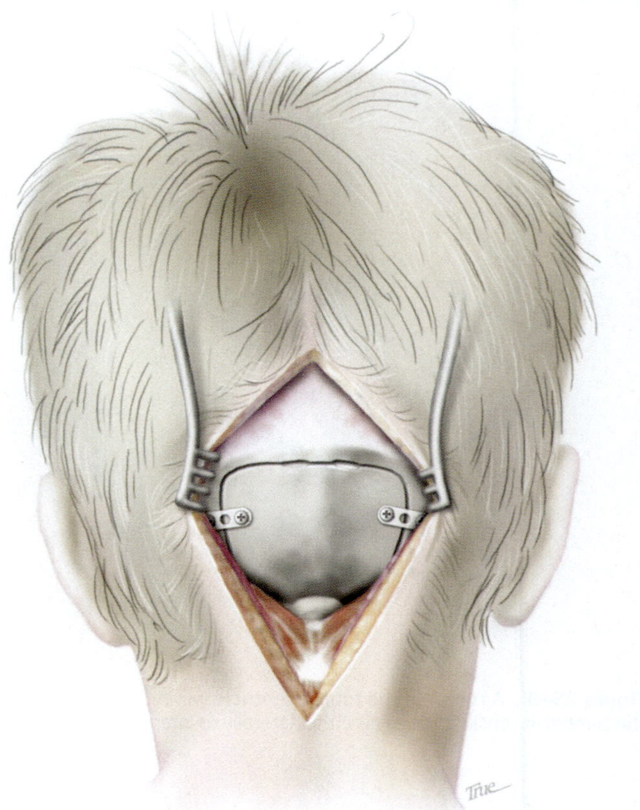

Figure 25–11 The bone flap is replaced with absorbable miniplates and screws.

Closing

Before closing, the walls of the resection cavity are checked carefully for residual pathological tissue. Adequate hemostasis is verified with a Valsalva maneuver and the surgical bed copiously irrigated with warm saline to remove debris and blood products. No hemostatic agents are left behind because they will cause artifact on postoperative imaging. The dura is then closed with running 4–0 Vicryl sutures. If a watertight closure cannot be achieved, a dural graft harvested from the occipital periosteum or ligamentum nuchae can be used. The bone flap is then replaced with absorbable miniplates and screws and the remaining soft tissues closed in layers **(Fig. 25–11)**. A tight fascial closure is crucial to prevent the formation of a pseudomeningocele. Finally, the skin is reapproximated.

◆ Postoperative Management

The location and extent of tumor resection determine the postoperative management. For tumors involving the medulla, patients remain electively intubated for 48 to 72 hours to prevent complications from postoperative edema, respiratory depression, and CO_2 retention. A nasal feeding tube is placed temporarily until an adequate gag reflex is identified. For patients with lesions outside the medulla, extubation occurs in the operating room and the patient is then transferred to the intensive care unit for 24 hours. Arterial $PaCO_2$ is monitored closely after extubation in patients who have undergone resection near the brain stem. An MRI scan is obtained on postoperative day 1 to assess the extent of tumor resection, evaluate for hydrocephalus, and provide a baseline for future imaging. If the patient has an EVD, it is initially drained at 0 to 5 mm Hg and gradually increased by 5 mm Hg over the ensuing few days, depending on the patient's clinical status and volume of CSF drained. We typically remove the EVD once the patient tolerates clamping for 24 to 48 hours. Steroids are continued for 2 to 3 days and tapered over the following 4 to 5 days. Patients who develop acute neurological changes postoperatively require a prompt noncontrasted head CT scan to evaluate for acute hemorrhage or hydrocephalus.

◆ Complications

Air Embolism

The risk for air embolism increases with elevation of the patient's head during the operation. If an air embolism is detected, the operative field is flooded with irrigating solution, the patient is placed on 100% oxygen and positive pressure ventilation, and the venous pressure is increased through a Valsalva maneuver, jugular venous compression, or lowering of the head of the table. The location of the venous site for venous air entry is located and occluded once the patient's condition is stabilized. If the patient is stabilized but no site is found, the operation can be completed with the patient's head lowered.

Venous Sinus Injury

Bleeding from the occipital, transverse, and sigmoid sinuses can be quick and devastating. Care must be taken to avoid sinus injury during bone flap removal. Additionally, brisk bleeding from the occipital sinus can occur during the dural opening because this sinus is often quite large in children. If bleeding occurs, it can be stopped with bipolar electrocautery of both dural leaflets. If this proves inadequate, a clip can be applied to the sinus until a suture can be placed. Removal of the clip is preferred to prevent future MRI artifact.

Postoperative Cerebral Spinal Fluid Leak

CSF leaks can be prevented by allowing CSF to drain from an EVD postoperatively. If no EVD is in place and the patient develops a CSF leak in the absence of obvious ventriculomegaly, the incision is initially oversewn. If there is a continued leak, strong consideration should be given to placing an EVD. Antibiotics are continued whenever a patient develops a CSF leak to prevent meningitis. The need for intraoperative wound exploration and revision is rare. Some patients may require a third ventriculostomy or placement of a ventriculoperitoneal shunt if there is progressive hydrocephalus despite tumor resection.

26

Surgical Approaches to Vestibular Schwannomas

Mark Pyle, Roham Moftakhar, and Behnam Badie

Vestibular schwannomas are one of the most common intracranial tumors, representing 8 to 10% of neoplasms. Most vestibular schwannomas arise from the neurilemmal sheath of the superior division of the vestibular nerve within the internal auditory canal, near the porus acusticus. Vestibular schwannomas present most commonly in the fourth and fifth decade of life. The incidence of vestibular schwannomas is increased in neurofibromatosis. Bilateral presence of these tumors is pathognomonic of neurofibromatosis type 2. An abnormality of chromosome 22, which codes for Merlin, a tumor suppressor gene, is felt to be responsible.

The most common presenting symptoms and signs are ipsilateral hearing loss, tinnitus, and balance difficulties. Larger tumors can cause facial numbness, weakness, or twitching. The majority of patients with vestibular schwannomas have a high-frequency hearing loss pattern, and word discrimination is usually affected. This chapter provides a description of three main approaches to vestibular schwannomas: translabyrinthine (TL), retrosigmoid (RS), and middle cranial fossa (MCF). These approaches are also useful for other neoplasms in the cerebellopontine angle, including meningiomas, epidermoids, lipomas, and others.

◆ The Translabyrinthine Approach

Patient Selection

The most common indication for TL surgery is a vestibular schwannoma of any size in an ear with nonserviceable hearing. Controversy persists in approach selection for patients with larger tumors (greater than 2 cm of cerebellopontine angle tumor component) who have good hearing. Some institutions may favor a TL approach for these tumors because the rate of hearing preservation is low. At our institution we will offer a hearing preservation approach even in patients with larger tumors (up to 3 cm in diameter) who have Gardner class 1 hearing preoperatively. Several variables, including patient characteristics, tumor size and location, patient preference, and the results of preoperative studies determine the feasibility of hearing preservation. All of these factors must be taken into consideration when deciding on a TL approach.

Advantages and Disadvantages

There are several advantages to the TL approach when compared with other routes to the posterior cranial base. In comparison to the retrosigmoid approach, it offers direct complete exposure of the internal auditory canal (IAC). The TL approach also offers better anterior and superior exposure than the classical retrosigmoid approach. Facial nerve decompression and mobilization are facilitated through this approach. Furthermore, the TL route offers excellent exposure for placement of an auditory brain stem implant if required. There is less cerebellar retraction, and all bone work is performed extradurally, which may limit postoperative headache. Cerebrospinal fluid (CSF) leakage is almost nonexistent in the TL approach.

The primary disadvantage of this approach is the obvious loss of hearing. In larger tumors, with a wide inferior brain stem attachment, a high jugular bulb can limit the surgical exposure. This route is contraindicated in patients with active chronic otitis media and mastoiditis.

Preoperative Preparation

A thorough otologic and neurotologic history and physical examination should be performed on all patients. The patient's subjective assessment of disequilibrium, imbalance, and tinnitus intensity is reviewed. A comprehensive neurological review of systems should be included, with particular attention to any cranial nerve symptoms. A past medical history of chronic ear disease or prior otologic surgery should be elicited. A family history of intracranial neoplasm or neurofibromatosis is of obvious importance. In addition to the standard otologic and head and neck examination, cranial nerve function and vestibular function should be assessed. Subtle physical findings may include a diminished corneal reflex, or drift and past-pointing to the ipsilateral side.

All patients undergo complete audiometric testing, including pure tone and speech audiometry. Electrocochleography (ECoG) and auditory brain stem response (ABR) testing are performed as a preoperative baseline if hearing preservation is being considered. Preoperative vestibular testing, including electronystagmography (ENG), is also useful. Preoperative evaluation by the balance physical therapy team, including platform posturography, may prove useful in selected patients who require vestibular retraining postoperatively. All patients undergo magnetic resonance imaging (MRI) with contrast enhancement. High-resolution computed tomography (HRCT) of the temporal bone is not required but may delineate anatomical abnormalities, including a high jugular bulb, sclerotic mastoid, or anteriorly placed sigmoid sinus. Widening of the IAC also correlates negatively with hearing preservation. The external canal is painted with gentian violet preoperatively.

Operative Procedure

The TL procedure should be performed in a large operating suite that provides ample room for equipment, including the operating microscope; intraoperative monitoring systems; dissection tools, including pneumatic drills; and cavitating ultrasonic aspirators. Increased room size is also needed for added personnel, including neuroanesthesia and nursing staff, the multidisciplinary surgical team, intraoperative monitoring personnel, and observers.

For the routine TL approach, the head is rotated 30 to 45 degrees to the contralateral side, with the chin gently flexed toward the shoulder. The surgeon is seated on the same side as the anesthesiologist, who is located toward the feet. The operating room nurse is positioned directly across from the surgeon. The first assistant and microscope base are positioned at the head of the table. Arterial line placement and facial nerve monitoring are always performed. Intravenous mannitol (0.5 g/kg) and dexamethasone are given for larger tumors.

A limited hair shave is performed and adhesive drapes are applied. A previous abdominal incision or the left lower quadrant is also prepared for harvesting an abdominal fat graft. The head is secured with tape and an incision is outlined **(Fig. 26–1)**. A fixation device is not required for the TL approach. The incision is infiltrated with 1% Xylocaine with 1:100000 epinephrine prior to the skin prep.

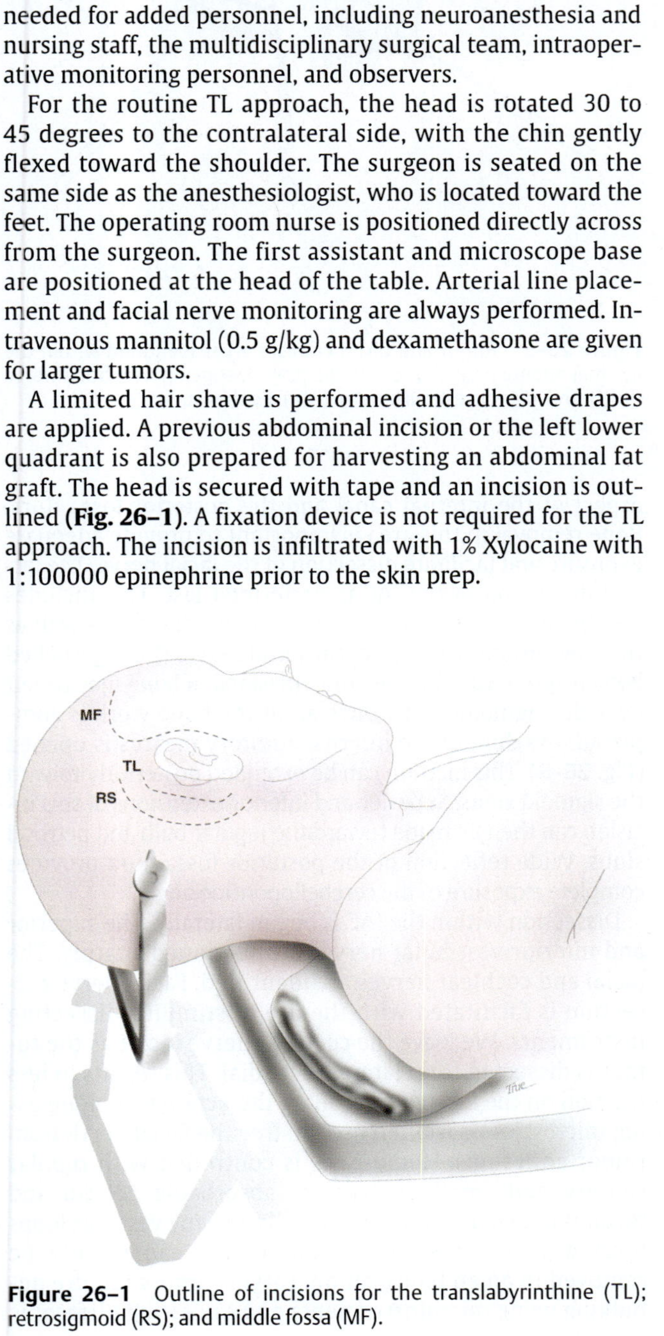

Figure 26–1 Outline of incisions for the translabyrinthine (TL); retrosigmoid (RS); and middle fossa (MF).

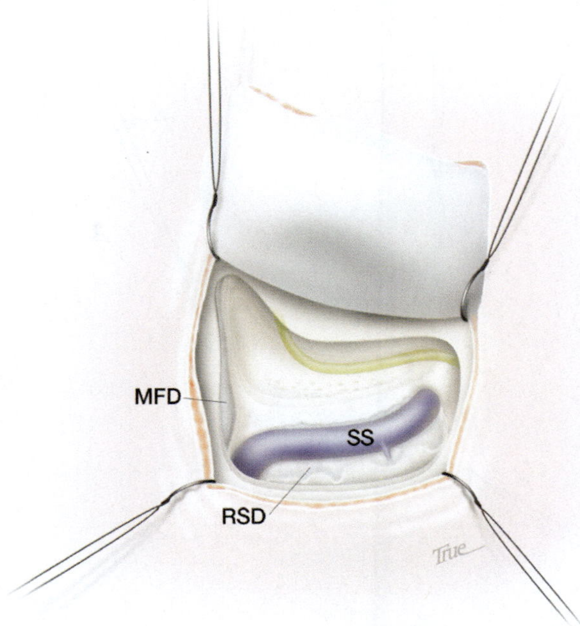

Figure 26–2 Initial TL bone work with skeletonization of sigmoid sinus (SS), middle fossa dura (MFD), and small amount of retrosigmoid dura (RSD).

The incision is made with a knife or an electrocautery device. The incision is normally beveled anteriorly to provide increased surface area for closure. Muscle and periosteum are incised and elevated using the cautery or periosteal elevators. All soft tissue is removed from the lateral cranial base to completely expose the mastoid process, digastric ridge, external auditory canal, and retrosigmoid region. The anteriorly based flap is retracted and held in position with fishhook retractors.

Bone work is begun with an extended mastoidectomy. Initial drilling may be done without microscopic control. The sigmoid sinus and a limited amount of retrosigmoid dura are completely skeletonized **(Fig. 26–2).** The mastoid tip is removed and the facial nerve, jugular bulb, and superior petrosal sinus are identified. All bone is removed from the MCF dura. The inferior limit of the dissection is the jugular bulb, which is completely exposed or down fractured. Usually the upper limit is the superior petrosal sinus and middle fossa dura, but the TL approach can be extended superiorly if needed **(Fig. 26–3)**.

A modified labyrinthectomy is performed. The posterior cranial fossa dura and the superior petrosal sinus are traced medially, followed by removal of the posterior canal, common crus, and superior canal. In this way the facial nerve is protected and the lateral semicircular canal is removed in the final portion of the labyrinthectomy. The vestibule is widely opened and the ampulated ends of the lateral and superior semicircular canals are removed. During anterior dissection, care must be taken to avoid injury to the tympanic segment of the facial nerve. Skeletonization of the facial nerve will significantly improve exposure, and the shoulder of a large diamond bur and continuous suction irrigation are used.

The next step in the bone work is the identification of the porus acusticus **(Fig. 26–4)**. A large trough is created

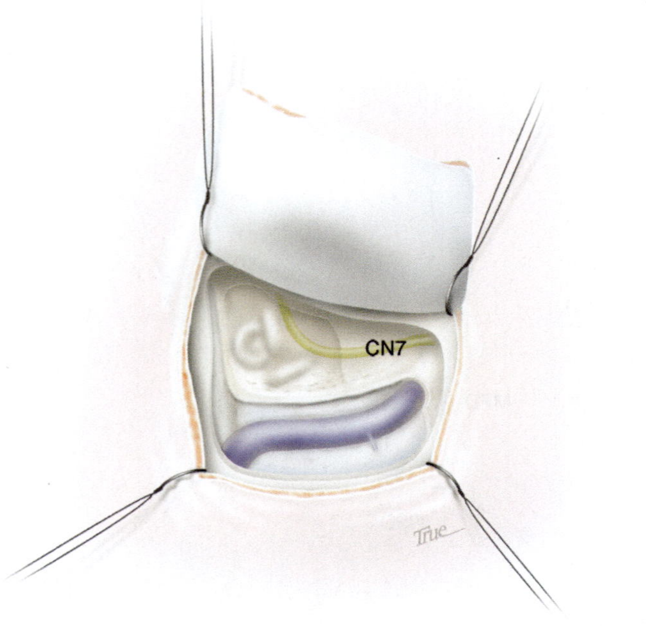

Figure 26–3 Further TL dissection with demonstration of semicircular canals and skeletonization of facial nerve (CN 7).

between the jugular bulb inferiorly and the IAC superiorly. The cochlear aqueduct is located in this region and is opened widely to allow egress of CSF. Once the inferior aspect of the IAC is identified dissection is continued superiorly with identification of the superior portion of the porus acusticus. There is a dense wedge of bone located between the superior

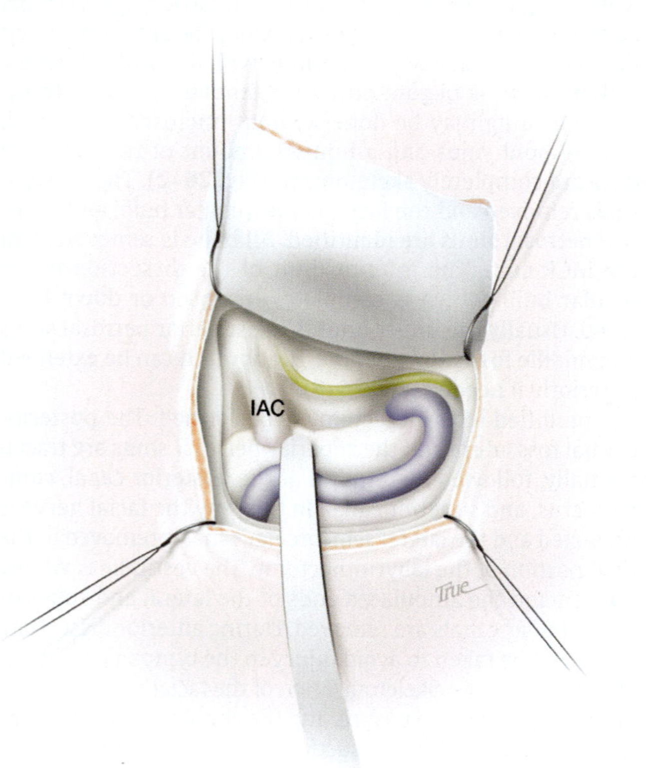

Figure 26–4 Internal auditory canal (IAC) and jugular bulb have been skeletonized. Retractor blade on presigmoid posterior fossa dura.

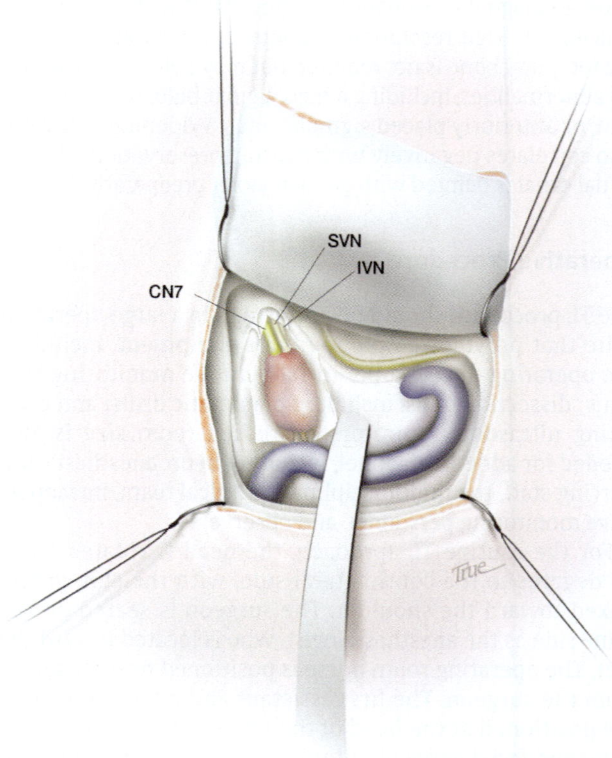

Figure 26–5 Tumor and distal cranial nerves identified within the internal auditory canal. Facial nerve (CN 7), superior vestibular nerve (SVN), and inferior vestibular nerve (IVN) are shown.

aspect of the internal canal and the posterior fossa dura. Bone removal in this area is important to provide adequate exposure and facilitate dissection of the facial nerve. The lateral dissection of the IAC is performed last. This includes identification of the vertical and horizontal crest as well as the labyrinthine segment of the facial nerve. The egg-shelled bone is removed from the dura. An island of bone may be left over the sigmoid sinus. Once all of the bone work is completed, the dura of the internal auditory meatus is opened **(Fig. 26–5)**. This incision can be extended posteriorly toward the sigmoid sinus. Superior and inferior extensions of this incision can then be made toward the jugular bulb and petrosal sinus. Wide reflection of the posterior fossa dura provides complete exposure of the cerebellopontine angle.

Dissection within the IAC is begun laterally. The superior and inferior vestibular nerves are sectioned sharply. The facial and cochlear nerves are identified. Facial nerve dissection is facilitated with the use of stimulus dissecting instruments. We leave the cochlear nerve intact as the tumor is dissected from lateral to medial. This results in less traction on the facial nerve. Sharp dissection technique using microscissors is often used to free the facial nerve from tumor adhesions. Hemostasis is controlled with bipolar cautery and small pledgets of absorbable gelatin and thrombin. Care must be taken to dissect any vascular loops located within the IAC. Small tumors can usually be removed in an en bloc fashion. Larger tumors require debulking using microinstruments or a cavitating ultrasonic aspirator.

Once tumor removal is complete and hemostasis has been assured, the abdominal fat graft is harvested. We also close the eustachian tube via the facial recess to prevent postoperative rhinorrhea. The middle ear and attic are closed with a muscle graft followed by bone wax through the facial recess. The abdominal fat graft is cut into bilobed strips. These strips are layered together to serially close the defect in the posterior fossa dura. A compressive mastoid dressing is placed for 48 hours. Hydroxyapatite cement may also be used to close the transtemporal defect with or without titanium mesh supplementation.

Bleeding during temporal bone dissection is usually easily controlled with bone wax, bipolar cautery, or diamond drill. However, hemorrhage from the sigmoid sinus and jugular bulb or superior petrosal sinus can be troublesome. Bleeding from the sinus can often be controlled with a large pledget of absorbable gelatin sponge moistened with topical thrombin and placement of a cottonoid followed by gentle pressure. The complex can be left in place and held with the arm of a self-retaining retractor while dissection is allowed to continue. Bleeding from the jugular bulb may require a firm oxidized cellulose pack. Care must be taken to avoid embolization of the packing material. Ligation of the internal jugular vein or complete occlusion of the sigmoid sinus has not been required in our experience. Bleeding from the petrosal sinus may be controlled with small clips posteriorly and with packing anteriorly. Bleeding from the subarcuate artery is easily controlled with the diamond drill.

Postoperative Management

In our experience, the TL approach to the IAC has the lowest rate of CSF leakage. In 200 consecutive operative cases of vestibular schwannoma reviewed at our institution from 1995 to 2001, only one of the 57 TL cases leaked. This is most likely due to the fact that we now close the eustachian tube through the facial recess approach in all cases. If it occurs, initial treatment of CSF leakage consists of bed rest and lumbar drainage.

The overall incidence of facial paresis has been dramatically reduced over the past decade. New techniques in tumor debulking, sharp dissection, and intraoperative facial nerve monitoring have led to excellent rates of facial nerve preservation. Despite these results iatrogenic injury to the facial nerve does occur. Complete facial nerve decompression of the labyrinthine segment and perigeniculate region is facilitated with the TL approach. Transtemporal rerouting of the facial nerve with direct anastomosis is rarely needed in schwannoma surgery. Intraoperative facial nerve monitoring may be useful as a predictor of postoperative facial nerve outcome.

◆ The Retrosigmoid-Transmeatal Approach

Patient Selection

The most common indication for this approach is the removal of vestibular schwannomas with hearing preservation. Presenting symptoms are similar to those mentioned in the previous section.

Preoperative Preparation

Studies determining a patient's candidacy for hearing preservation have already been described. ABR and ECoG are always performed as a baseline for intraoperative monitoring. It should be noted that MRI with gadolinium enhancement may not predict actual tumor extension into the IAC. The position of the vestibular labyrinth in relation to the posterior aspect of the porus acusticus is important in calculating the lateral extent of meatal bone removal. In those patients with more than 1 cm of tumor extension into the cerebellopontine angle and good hearing we perform the retrosigmoid-transmeatal approach. With larger tumors, patients are informed of the lower success rate with hearing preservation so that they do not have unrealistic expectations.

Operative Procedure

The patient is positioned supine with a large roll under the ipsilateral shoulder to facilitate rotation of the head and neck. In this approach we always use pin fixation of the head. The head is turned laterally at 45 degrees, the neck is flexed, and the vertex is tilted slightly down. In obese patients, or those with limited mobility of the cervical spine, a modified park bench or lateral position may be planned. All auditory and facial nerve monitoring electrodes are placed. The active electrode for ECoG can be placed on the tympanic membrane or middle ear promontory. Usually, direct eighth nerve monitoring, electrocochleography, and auditory brain stem response are used together.

There are some differences in surgical equipment between the TL and RS approaches. The pneumatic dissection tool should have a craniotome attachment in addition to the standard burs. The working distance for bone and tumor dissection is longer in the RS approach. We use a longer set of drill attachments and longer microinstruments for dissection.

The curved hockey stick incision is made and an anteriorly based flap is secured with fishhooks **(Fig. 26–1).** Initial bone work is performed, with complete identification of the sigmoid and transverse sinuses. The posterior emissary vein is identified, bipolared, and sectioned. The mastoidectomy is limited and as few air cells as possible are opened to lessen the possibility of CSF leakage. Skeletonizing the venous structures facilitates turning the bone flap, which is removed with the craniotome and preserved for later replacement **(Fig. 26–6).**

The dura of the posterior wall is coagulated and incised in a K-shaped fashion with a base at the medial aspect of the exposure. The dura is covered by moist collagen and retracted with sutures. Keeping the dura moist throughout the operation will not only help with its final closure but will also minimize the risk of sinus thrombosis, which may occur with lengthy surgeries. CSF is then drained from the cisterna magna to facilitate with cerebellar relaxation. In our experience, removal of normal cerebellum to expose the tumor has never been necessary. The rest of the operation is performed under a microscope. **(Fig. 26–7).**

For large neoplasms, tumor debulking is performed at this point. As tumor mass is reduced, tumor capsule can be freed

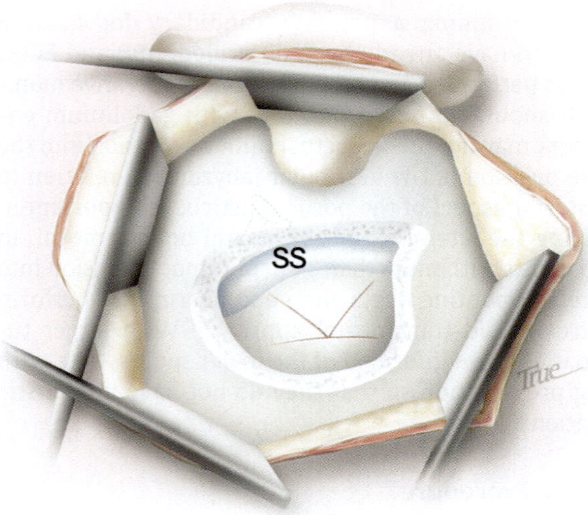

Figure 26–6 Sigmoid sinus (SS) exposure with K-shaped incision of posterior fossa dura.

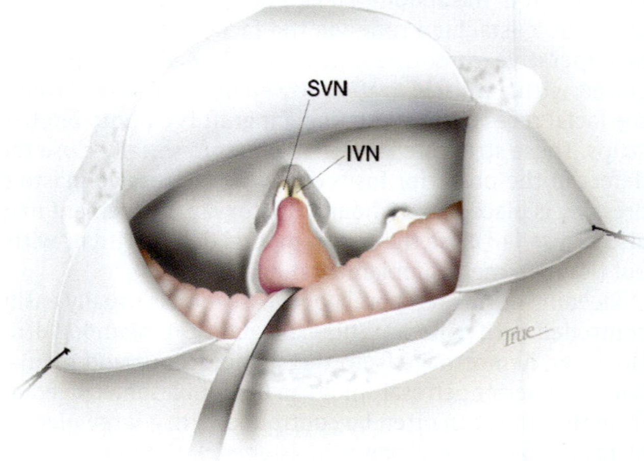

Figure 26–8 After transmeatal bone work distal cranial nerves superior vestibular nerve (SVN) and inferior vestibular nerve (IVN) are identified separated by transverse crest.

from the cerebellum and pons. Gentle pulling of the tumor capsule while carefully dissecting and peeling the arachnoid membrane between the tumor and normal central nervous system tissue is important in minimizing injury to the brain stem. We have found the SCANLAN *Advantage* Badie Bipolar (Scanlan International, Minneapolis, MN) to be especially helpful during this phase of tumor work because it allows for a "four-point" dissection technique.

Intermediate or small tumors are removed using an en bloc technique. Because hearing preservation is often the goal of these operations, the IAC is drilled prior to any tumor dissection. We believe that excessive manipulation of the cisternal component of the tumor may differentially affect the pressure in the IAC (intracanalicular pressure), thus compromising the blood supply to the cochlear nerve. For such tumors, the IAC is drilled first.

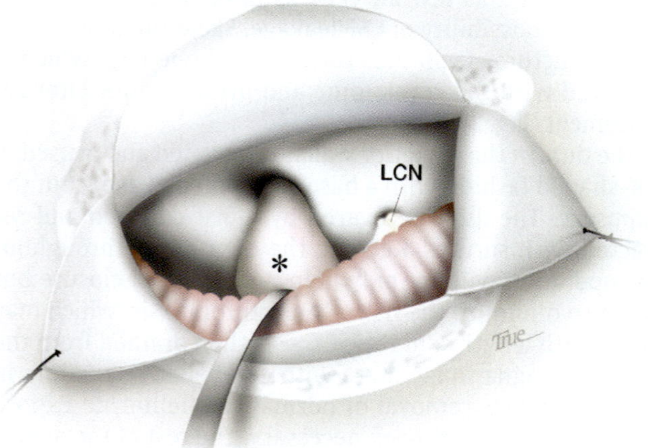

Figure 26–7 Small tumor (*) viewed from RS approach after cerebellar relaxation. LCN, lower cranial nerves.

The neurotologist returns to the operating room for the temporal bone dissection. A U-shaped incision is made in the dura extending from the jugular fold to below the level of the tentorium. Small pledgets of absorbable sponge are placed in the subarachnoid space to limit bone dust exposure. Labyrinthine landmarks, including the vestibular aqueduct and singular canal, are useful indicators during dissection. Once established, IAC dissection is continued from the porus laterally to the level of the vestibule. The vestibular labyrinth must be avoided. The common crus and posterior canal are at greatest risk. The endolymphatic sac is also left undisturbed. Normally, several millimeters of the IAC can be carefully exposed **(Fig. 26–8)**. It is very important to completely skeletonize the IAC circumferentially, at least 180 degrees, rather than simply unroofing the internal auditory meatus.

After the bone work is completed an inferior incision is made along the meatal dura, if distal tumor extent is present, lateral dissection may require the use of endoscopes and angled internal canal dissectors. Sharp dissection is required to identify the appropriate cleavage plane. Sharp technique is also important to limit traction on the cochlear nerve in hearing preservation. If the tumor is small it should be removed en bloc if possible. Identification of the normal proximal eighth nerve allows placement of an active electrode for direct eighth nerve monitoring. Frequent communication between the audiologist and surgeon is important during the tumor work. In larger tumors additional debulking is frequently required once tumor has been removed from the IAC and the course of the distal facial and cochlear nerves has been determined. This is a crucial part of the procedure and all significant vessels should be carefully dissected from the tumor in the proper plane and preserved. Again, sharp dissection technique is used as much as possible to free the tumor from the cochlear and facial nerves.

Closure is initiated with a careful search and occlusion of exposed air cells in the region of the meatus. Endoscopic visualization may reveal distal tumor or previously undiscovered air cells. The internal auditory meatus is sealed with a large piece of prepared free temporalis muscle. The dura is normally closed primarily but may require augmentation with autogenous grafts or manufactured dura substitutes. The bone flap is returned over a large pad of absorbable gelatin sponge and secured with miniplates. Routine closure is then performed. Primary cranioplasty is not usually required.

Postoperative Management

As previously mentioned, the incidence of complete facial paresis is now uncommon, although patients with larger tumors may have a significant delay in neural recovery. CSF leakage is somewhat more common in this approach than in the TL approach. If initial measures, including bed rest and short-term lumbar drainage, are ineffective in closing the leak, then a reoperation can be performed. If hearing has been maintained, a transmastoid approach without closure of the eustachian tube can be used.

Hearing loss may occur due to direct mechanical injury to the cochlear nerve or more likely due to interruption of the blood supply of the cochlea. Sharp dissection, preservation of microvasculature, intraoperative monitoring, one-piece tumor removal, and limiting cautery are all important in lowering the potential for hearing loss. As already mentioned, it is also possible that early bone work with decompression of the IAC may improve perfusion pressure during extended tumor dissection for larger schwannomas. Other serious complications, including stroke or hemorrhage, are rare. These may occur early in the postoperative period, and the surgeon must be vigilant and immediately evaluate any questionable change in mental status or the neurological examination. If sutures or staples are used for the skin closure, they are normally removed between 10 and 14 postoperative days. Facial function is assessed and eye care is initiated.

◆ Middle Cranial Fossa Approach

Patient Selection

The MCF approach is well suited for patients with small vestibular schwannomas (less than 1 cm cerebellopontine extension) and good hearing. Presenting symptoms are similar to those mentioned in the previous section.

Preoperative Preparation

Imaging analysis normally includes both MRI and computed tomographic (CT) techniques. Both modalities have the capability to be loaded simultaneously on the intraoperative navigation workstation. One can use the CT image during bone work and the neurosurgeon may refer to the MR images for intracranial work. When more extensive lesions of the middle cranial base are present, carotid artery status may need to be evaluated with preoperative test occlusion.

Operative Procedure

The patient is supine on the operating room table with the head turned 45 degrees. The final head position depends on tumor characteristics and individual patient mobility. Navigation may be useful to plan the surgical trajectory. Patient registration for the navigation system can be performed at this time. Accuracy may be improved through the use of pin fixation as well as bone-anchored anatomical markers. Intraoperative auditory electrodes and facial nerve electrodes are placed for monitoring. The surgeon and first assistant are positioned at the head with the microscope base near the side of the anesthesia team. Images for navigation can be observed at the workstation or as a heads-up display in the microscopic field.

The incision is made **(Fig. 26–1)** and carried down to the temporalis fascia. The frontotemporal branch of the facial nerve and the blood supply to the temporalis muscle are always preserved. There are several ways to divide the temporalis but in general the technique should preserve the integrity of the muscle for later use as a rotation flap if required.

Classically, a 4- × 5-cm rectangular flap extending two thirds anterior and one third posterior to the zygomatic root is removed. The creation of a rectangular flap with straight edges allowed use of the traditional self-retaining MCF retractor systems. We perform a wider, more anterior, craniotomy and utilize a lower profile retractor system with the dura retractors secured to a system applied to the headholder. This allows for a flexible approach and additional dural elevation if required **(Fig. 26–9).** Dura is elevated from the middle fossa floor in a posterior to anterior direction. The petrous ridge, superior petrosal sinus, arcuate eminence, greater superficial petrosal nerve (GSPN),

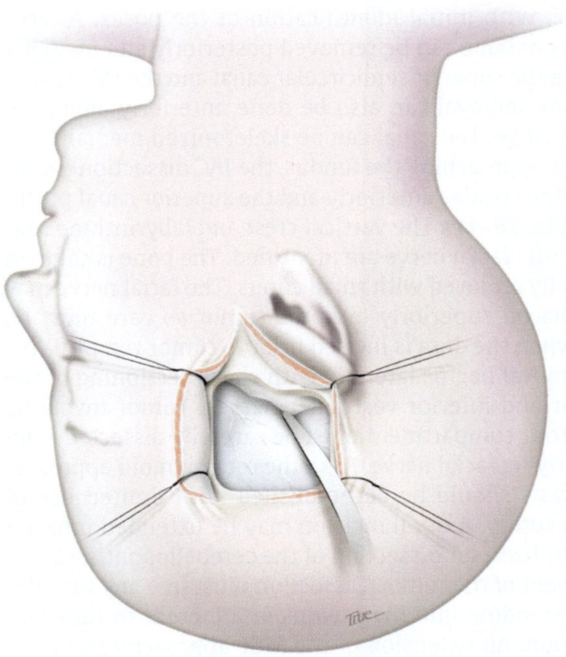

Figure 26–9 Initial extradural elevation of temporal lobe extending from posterior to anterior. Temporalis is retracted with fishhooks.

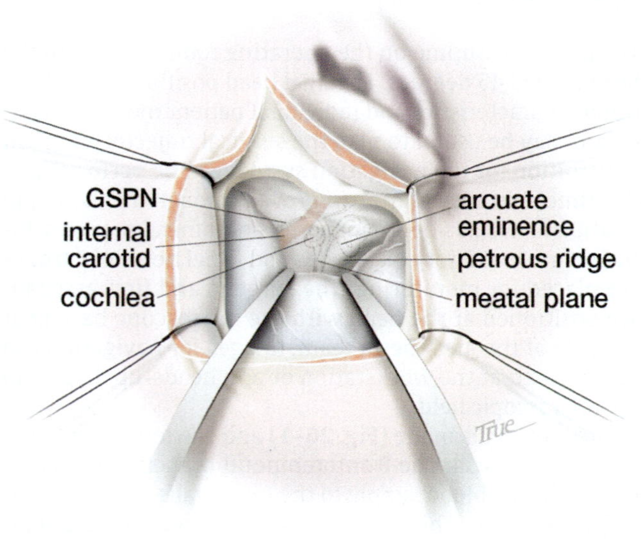

Figure 26–10 Middle fossa exposure with relative location of landmarks. GSPN, greater superficial petrosal nerve.

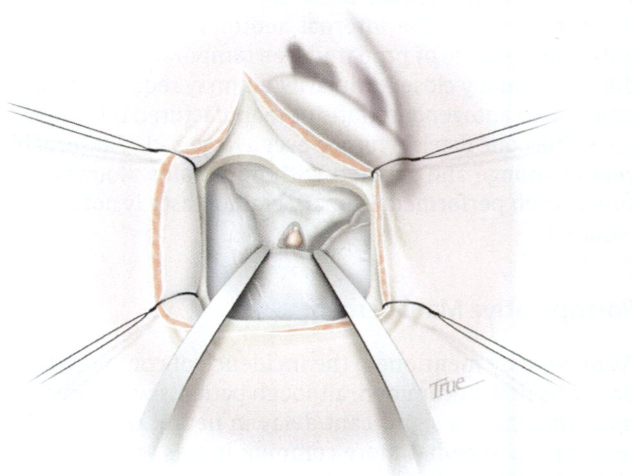

Figure 26–11 Tumor exposed in internal auditory canal (IAC). Note limited bone removal laterally near cochlea and vestibule.

and middle meningeal artery are all useful landmarks **(Fig. 26–10).** As the middle fossa dura is elevated, traction of the GSPN, and as a result the geniculate ganglion, should be avoided to prevent postoperative facial palsy. To accomplish this, the distal aspect of the GSPN is sharply dissected form the dura anteriorly. Furthermore, ligation of the middle meningeal artery as it exits the foramen spinosum may be necessary to improve dural elevation. Identification of the petrous carotid artery and dissection of the trigeminal ganglion may also be required for more anterior lesions of the petrous apex.

Drilling is begun on the meatal plane as medially as possible, with initial identification of the porus. A large quantity of bone can be removed posteriorly and medially between the superior semicircular canal and the IAC. Extensive bone removal can also be done anteriorly along the petrous ridge. The canal can be skeletonized medially but laterally, approaching the fundus, the IAC dissection is limited by the cochlea anteriorly and the superior canal posteriorly **(Fig. 26–11).** The vertical crest and labyrinthine segment of the facial nerve are identified. The bone is thinned and finally removed with small curets. The facial nerve may be displaced superiorly over the tumor so care must be taken when the dura is incised prior to tumor removal. Tumor removal begins laterally with sharp sectioning of the superior and inferior vestibular nerves. Tumor involving the inferior compartment must be carefully dissected from the overlying facial nerve. As in the retrosigmoid approach, hemostasis should be accomplished with limited use of electrocautery. A dural incision may be extended into the posterior fossa for dissection of the cerebellopontine angle component of the tumor. Dissection must free any vascular loops extending into the meatus or adherent to tumor in this region. An extension of the MCF approach can be accomplished with ligation of the superior petrosal sinus and incision of the tentorium. This allows for a more panoramic view of the posterior fossa and can be employed for larger tumors.

Bleeding can be a troublesome complication during middle fossa surgery. Methods for hemostasis have already been described. The middle meningeal artery can usually be controlled with bipolar cautery or firm packing of the lumen. In most other instances a combination of saline irrigation, careful cautery, gentle packing, and patience will result in adequate hemostasis. Vascular control of the carotid artery is not required for vestibular schwannoma surgery. Temporal lobe infarction or injury may occur as a complication during extended middle fossa surgery due to traction or damage to the vein of Labbé. The use of specialized retractor systems with extensive removal of bone along the floor of the middle fossa has limited the need for temporal lobe retraction. Lumbar drainage can be utilized to allow for additional relaxation if required.

Postoperative Management

Facial paralysis is an uncommon complication of MCF surgery. If an injury does occur, complete decompression, rerouting, or grafting is facilitated through the available exposure. Resection of facial nerve neuromas frequently requires end to end anastomosis with or without a cable graft. CSF leakage can occur following the MCF approach. Any exposed mastoid air cells must be thoroughly sealed with bone wax. Large defects may require bone grafts. We normally use a large sheet of autologous temporalis fascia supplemented with free or pedicled temporalis muscle held in place with fibrin glue. Persistent postoperative leakage that does not respond to bed rest and lumbar drainage may require reexploration through the middle fossa. Finally, injury to the labyrinth may cause sensorineural hearing loss and postoperative vertigo or dysequilibrium. The structures most at risk are the cochlea and the superior semicircular canal.

◆ Summary

The TL approach is appropriate for any size schwannoma in a patient with nonserviceable hearing. The advantages are the more direct exposure of the IAC, less cerebellar retraction, and almost nonexistent risk of CSF leakage. The disadvantages are loss of hearing and limitation of this approach in patients with chronic otitis media and mastoiditis.

The RS approach offers the best opportunity for preservation of hearing in larger tumors. The disadvantage of the RS approach is the difficulty in removing tumors from the lateral recess of the IAC without entering the vestibule and causing inner ear dysfunction as well as a higher incidence of headache and CSF leakage.

The MCF approach is well suited for patients with small vestibular schwannomas (less than 1 cm cerebellopontine extent) and good hearing. This approach may be associated with a higher risk in patients over 65 years of age and may have a slightly increased risk of cranial nerve VII paresis.

27

Surgical Resection of Lower Clivus–Anterior Foramen Magnum Meningiomas

Vallo Benjamin and Stephen M. Russell

Meningiomas are the most common of all benign intra- and extradural tumors of the foramen magnum. Among the intradural neoplasms, meningiomas are three times as prevalent as neurofibromas. Fewer than 20% of meningiomas arise from the posterior dura of the foramen magnum; surgical management of these tumors through suboccipital craniectomy and upper cervical laminectomy is fairly straightforward. However, the more common anterior variety is a surgical challenge and is the subject of this chapter.

There are two surgical approaches to the anterior foramen magnum: (1) the anterior (transoral or transcervical) and (2) the posterolateral (retrocondylar or extreme lateral transcondylar). Both approaches have advantages and disadvantages, with the optimal approach determined by tumor histopathology, its relationship to the dura (i.e., intra- or extradural), and its relationship to the brain stem and spinal cord.

The transoral and transcervical approaches provide direct access to the anterior foramen magnum, lower clivus, and cervical canal and are best suited for extradural lesions such as chordomas and metastatic tumors. When applied to intradural tumors, however, these approaches provide only a limited lateral exposure due to the presence of the atlanto-occipital joint. Furthermore, the difficulty of exposing the vertebral artery, medulla, spinal cord, and craniocervical nerve roots renders the anterior approach even less desirable. A high incidence of postoperative meningitis and incomplete tumor removal are well documented in the literature.

The strictly posterior midline approach through suboccipital craniectomy and C1–C2 laminectomy has long been used to resect foramen magnum meningiomas. Due to restricted anterior exposure of the lower clivus and foramen magnum, however, retraction and manipulation of the medulla and cord have often resulted in serious neurological morbidity and incomplete tumor resection.

Over the past 20 years, for anterior foramen magnum meningiomas, two posterolateral approaches have been used with excellent results: the transcondylar and the retrocondylar. The transcondylar approach requires mobilization of the vertebral artery from the foramen transversarium of C1–C2, with resection of the posterior one third to one half of the occipital condyle. This procedure carries a potential risk of injury to the vertebral artery and the twelfth cranial nerve, as well as possible instability of the craniocervical junction. This approach is valuable for the resection of some extradural and malignant tumors. We believe that when neoplasms such as chondromas, chondrosarcomas, and metastatic lesions have already destroyed the occipital condyle, the transcondylar approach may be the better choice. Surgeons undertaking this procedure should have special training in the anatomy of the region, as well as hands-on experience, before performing such surgery.

The retrocondylar approach, which involves opening the foramen magnum up to the dorsal limit of the occipital condyle and partial medial facetectomy of C2–C3, provides excellent exposure for resection of these tumors. In our experience, based on 18 consecutive cases of lower clivus–foramen magnum meningiomas resected through the posterolateral retrocondylar approach, there were no complications involving the vertebral artery or the twelfth cranial nerve, and no craniocervical instability.

◆ Pathological Anatomy

Meningiomas of the lower clivus and anterior foramen magnum have a surprisingly uniform site of origin and pattern of growth. The dural attachment in all of our cases was anterior and medial to the entrance and the course of one of the vertebral arteries. For this reason, almost all of these tumors, despite being ventral to the dentate ligament, are predominantly ventrolateral to the cord and medulla and rotate these structures along the longitudinal axis. As the neoplasm enlarges, the arachnoid of the premedullary and lateral medullary cisterns is stretched over it. With further growth, the ipsilateral vertebral artery is displaced laterally and may become completely encircled by tumor. The ninth, tenth, and twelfth cranial nerves are almost always elevated and stretched over the superior and dorsal aspects of the tumor. The spinal accessory nerve, the first and second cervical roots, and the first and second dentate ligaments are located in the inferior and dorsal aspect of the tumor.

These tumors rarely, if ever, grow beyond the vertebrobasilar junction. They invariably reach, but do not involve, the opposite vertebral artery. It is important to note that at the interface between any meningioma and an intracranial structure (i.e., the pia, a cranial nerve, or a vessel), a layer of arachnoid membrane is present. During microsurgical dissection, identification and preservation of this layer are crucial for minimizing injury to intracranial structures.

◆ Patient Selection

Patients who develop neurological deficits generally have tumors larger than 2 cm; these should be resected surgically to prevent further neurological damage and to restore function if possible. Incidentally discovered small neoplasms in asymptomatic patients should be followed carefully with serial magnetic resonance imaging (MRI). Obviously, the larger the tumor, the greater the degree of difficulty in resection because neurovascular structures become intimately involved with the lesion. In symptomatic patients who are elderly, radical subtotal resection with decompression of the brain stem may be the wisest course. Asymptomatic patients with incidentally discovered tumors or calcified tumors should, in general, not be subjected to surgery because the potential morbidity associated with resection is not insignificant. Otherwise, we feel that surgery should be the primary treatment, and patient age should not be a barrier except in those with serious anesthetic or medical risks. All patients should have a thorough medical examination and a careful evaluation of lower cranial nerve function preoperatively.

◆ Preoperative Preparation

MRI with intravenous gadolinium enhancement is the most valuable preoperative study. The three-dimensional spatial anatomy of the neoplasm, as well as its relationship to the vertebral arteries, medulla, cervical cord, and lower clivus, can be clearly seen **(Fig. 27–1)**. The outstanding degree of tumor enhancement and the dural "tail" sign with intravenous contrast enhancement serve to distinguish meningioma from neurofibroma, as well as epidermoid and arachnoid cyst. MRI is also the procedure of choice for monitoring the rate of lesion growth in nonoperated patients, as well as residual or recurrent tumor in operated ones. A computed tomographic (CT) scan with and without intravenous contrast, although having poorer resolution, clearly documents tumor calcification **(Fig. 27–2)**. Selective and superselective angiography is valuable in growths larger than 3 cm **(Fig. 27–3)**. The primary objective of angiography is to determine the presence and extent of blood supply to the tumor from the posterior inferior cerebellar artery. Angiography may also serve to assess the feasibility of embolizing the neuromeningeal feeders from the ascending pharyngeal artery and possibly from the transmastoid branches of the occipital artery.

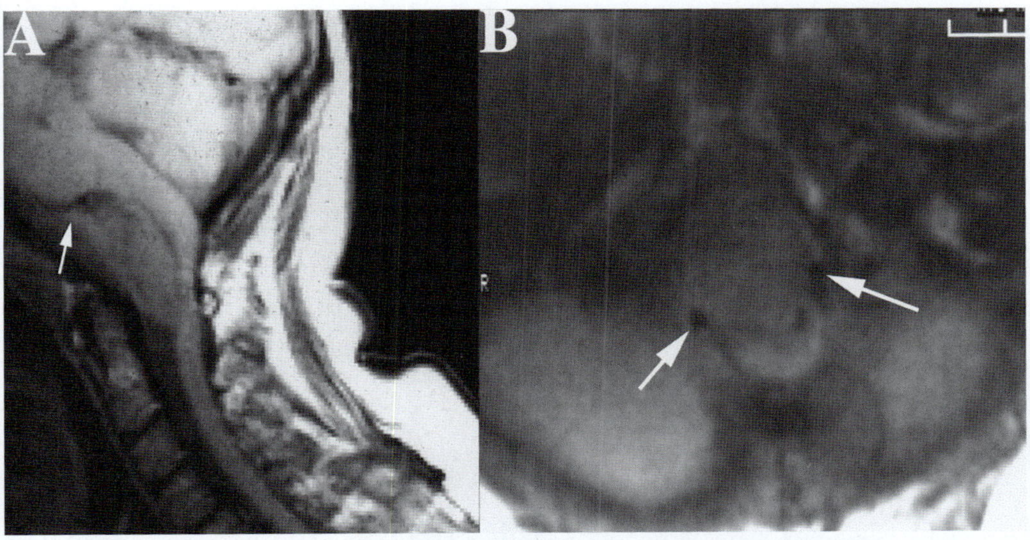

Figure 27–1 **(A)** Preoperative magnetic resonance imaging study in the sagittal and **(B)** axial planes in a patient with a large anterior foramen magnum meningioma that was eccentric to the right. A dural tail was present **(arrow in A)**. The tumor caused marked brain stem compression with displacement of both vertebral arteries **(arrows in B)**.

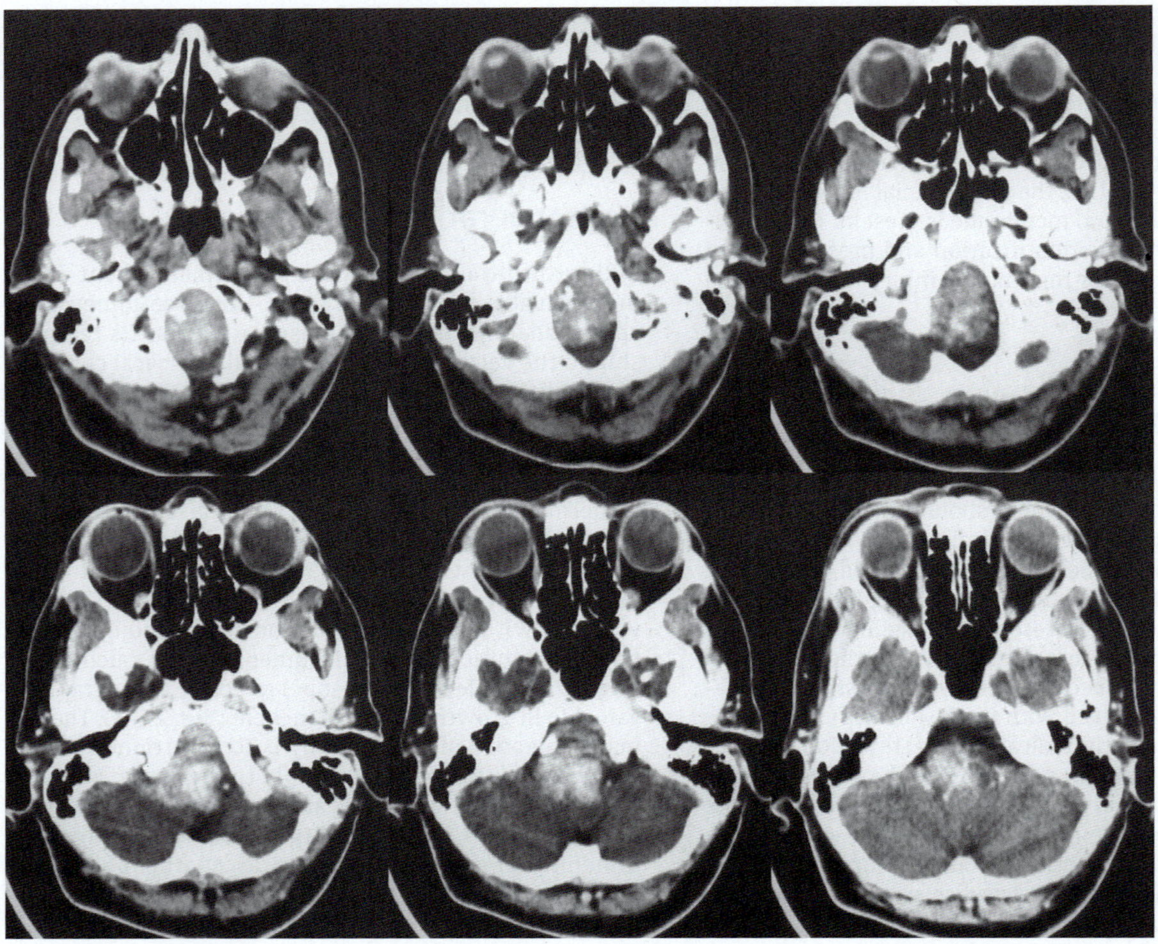

Figure 27–2 Serial preoperative computed tomographic scan images with contrast enhancement. Multiple areas of calcification within the tumor can be seen. Severe compression of the cervicomedullary junction was present.

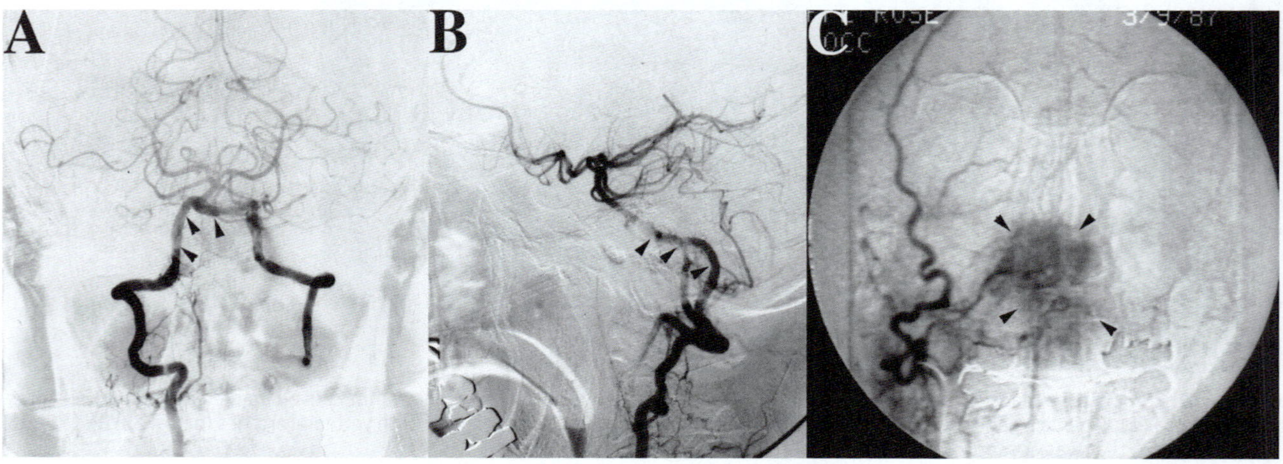

Figure 27–3 Preoperative cerebral angiography was performed, including **(A)** a right vertebral artery injection, frontal and **(B)** lateral views, as well as **(C)** a selective right external carotid artery injection, frontal view. Displacement of the lower vertebrobasilar complex by the tumor **(arrowheads in A and B)** is visualized. A distinct tumor blush can be seen on the external carotid injection **(arrowheads in C).** A significant portion of the vascular supply to anterior foramen magnum meningiomas is from the ascending pharyngeal artery, which can be embolized before surgery.

◆ Operative Procedure

Positioning

Patients are placed in a lateral decubitus position on the side opposite the predominant tumor growth. This carries less risk of air embolism and is more comfortable for the surgeon. It also offers a direct view of the posterior fossa as well as the upper cervical area. By rotating the table from side to side, the surgeon can see the posterolateral and anterior aspects of the foramen magnum.

Because this procedure may take several hours, the operating table should be well padded to prevent bedsores and nerve palsies. To minimize venous stasis, we routinely use pneumatic compression boots on the lower extremities throughout surgery. The head is fixed in a three-pin headholder, slightly flexed, and laterally bent toward the floor to provide an optimal view of the anterior and upper extent of the tumor. The entire table is tilted so that the head is 25 to 30 degrees upward. The patient is secured with tape so that the operating table can be rotated safely from side to side during surgery. Lumbar spinal drainage does not offer any added advantage because the cervical cisterns are easily accessible for direct drainage as soon as the dura is opened in the cervical spine at C2. The patient's head can be elevated above the level of the heart during opening to avoid excessive venous bleeding.

Skin Incision and Opening of Muscle

Because most tumors, despite their anterior location, grow predominantly on one side, the key to successful resection is a wide exposure of the lateral as well as the posterior aspects of the foramen magnum, with adequate access to the lower clivus and upper cervical canal. To achieve this goal, the most suitable skin incision in our experience is a step-like opening, used since 1982 **(Fig. 27–4).** The superior limb of the incision is started 3 cm medial to the mastoid process at the superior nuchal line, and brought down to the level of the foramen magnum. The incision is taken to the foramen magnum at an angle of 45 degrees to the midline. The inferior limb is then carried vertically over the spinous process of C1, C2, and C3. The suboccipital and cervical muscles are opened with electrocautery along the line of skin incision.

For anatomical orientation, it is best to first clear the muscles from the lamina and facet joints of C1, C2, and C3, then from the lateral aspect of the occipital bone toward the midline, and finally to expose the extradural course of the vertebral artery. Dissection of muscle attachment to the occipital bone at the foramen magnum and C1 and C2 on the side of tumor growth should be done with a blunt periosteal elevator. This minimizes the risk of injury to the vertebral artery at the posterior arch of C1. The posterior aspect of the occipital condyle, the atlanto-occipital articulation, and the facet joints of C1, C2, and C3 are then cleared. Exposure of bone on the side opposite the tumor need not be carried far laterally.

Suboccipital Craniectomy and C1–C2 Laminectomy

A suboccipital craniectomy, extending from the foramen magnum up to the occipital condyle, is performed on the side of the larger tumor growth **(Fig. 27–5).** It should be ~3 cm in the vertical dimension and 4 cm in the transverse. A C1–C2 laminectomy is done with the utmost care, and without introduction of a bone instrument under the lamina, so as to prevent injury to the already compromised medulla and cord. We prefer to use high-speed drills as much as possible for shaving the bone. The foramen magnum is opened with a drill until the atlanto-occipital articulation is seen. The posterolateral portion of C1 and C2, which includes part of the facet joint in line with the occipital condyle, is drilled in a similar fashion until the entrance of the vertebral artery into the dura and the C1 and C2 roots are clearly seen extradurally **(Fig. 27–4B).** In the same way, the posterior midline and lateral dura of the posterior fossa and the upper cervical canal are exposed. If mastoid air cells are entered, bone wax and fibrin glue with muscle are used for repair.

Dural Opening

The dura is opened along almost the same line of the skin and muscle incision. However, the cervical dura is first opened in the midline to remove cerebrospinal fluid, thus relaxing the posterior fossa contents. The dural incision is then carried laterally toward the cerebellar tonsil and hemisphere on the side of the tumor. The dura on the opposite side is opened for a short distance in a Y-shaped pattern for relaxation of the posterior fossa **(Fig. 27–5B).** The arachnoid overlying the spinal cord, the cisterna magna, and the cerebellum are preserved as much as possible. The incised dural edges are sutured tightly to the suboccipital and cervical muscles, exposing the floor of the posterior fossa, the lateral aspect of the foramen magnum, and the upper cervical canal as much as possible. The posterolateral and inferior aspects of the tumor can be seen immediately, without retraction of any neural structures.

Tumor Exposure

In virtually all meningiomas of the anterior foramen magnum, the first two dentate ligaments, the cervical roots, and the eleventh cranial nerve complex are stretched over the visible posterior inferior portion of the tumor **(Figs. 27–4C and 27–6A).** With the retrocondylar approach, as much as a fifth or a quarter of the tumor surface can be exposed without manipulation. In fact, except for a 1- to 1.5-cm elevation of the cerebellar tonsil and the lateral portion of the hemisphere, no retraction of the medulla or cord is necessary for complete resection of even the largest tumors. Further exposure of the neoplasm is achieved by opening the arachnoid at the cisterna magna and upper cervical canal **(Fig. 27–6B).** The arachnoid is held in place with metal clips or fine sutures to the dura laterally.

From this point on, the operating microscope is used until dural closure. Initially, the sensory roots of either or both C1 and C2 are cut at the point of dural exit. The first and second dentate ligaments are also cut near their dural attachment. The dentate ligaments and the cervical roots of C1 and C2 may be used to rotate the cord and the lower medulla along the longitudinal axis by suturing them into

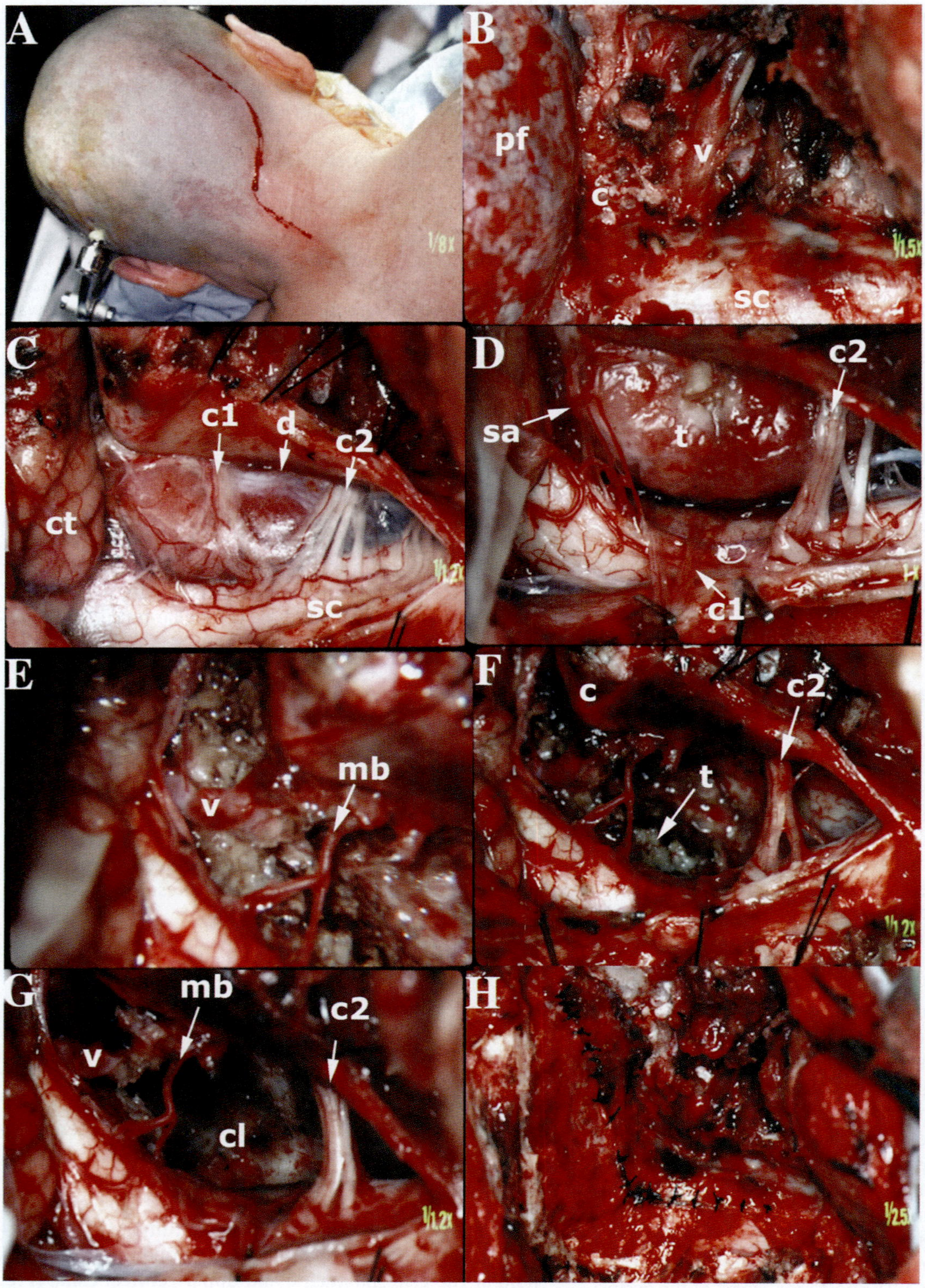

Figure 27–4 Serial operative photographs of a right-sided foramen magnum meningioma resected via a posterolateral approach. This is the same patient as in **Figs. 27–1 through 27–3 and 27–7.** Refer to the text for a step-by-step description. pf, posterior fossa; c, occipital condyle; sc, spinal cord; ct, cerebellar tonsil; c1, first cervical rootlets; c2, second cervical rootlets; d, dentate ligament; sa, spinal accessory nerve; v, vertebral artery; mb, medullary branch from vertebral artery; cl, clivus; t, tumor.

dura on the side opposite the tumor (**Fig. 27–4D**). Retraction of 3 to 4 mm or more of the lower medulla and upper cord can be achieved by this maneuver. The cervical rootlets of the eleventh cranial nerve are cut, and the nerve is mobilized superomedially away from the tumor. The medullary rootlets and the main trunk of the accessory nerve can be preserved even in large tumors (**Fig. 27–4E**). This exposure creates an inferior and lateral corridor adequate for removal

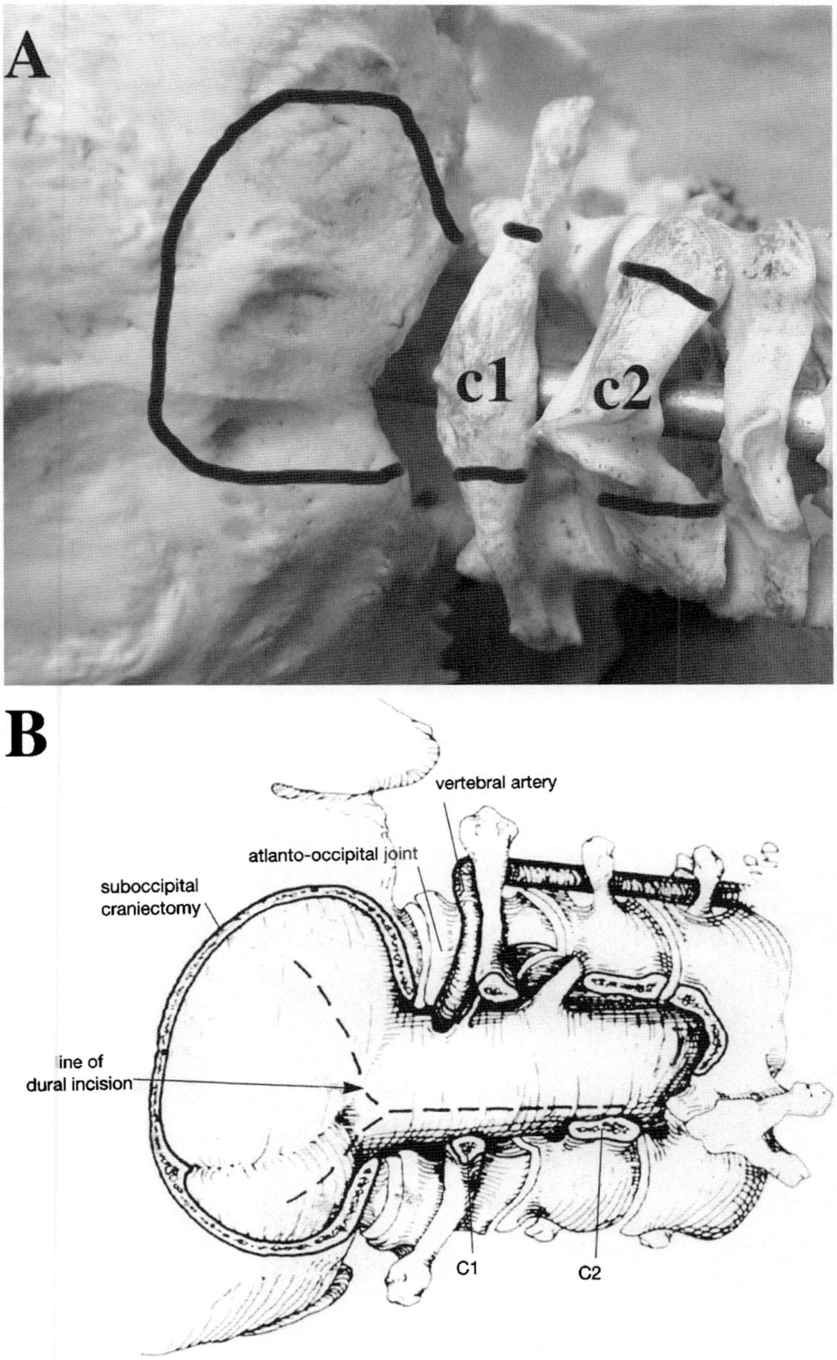

Figure 27–5 The extent of bone removal and dural opening for the posterolateral approach to the anterior foramen magnum. **(A)** The black line represents the extent of the craniectomy and laminectomies. Although the posterior occipital condyle is routinely exposed, it is not usually necessary to remove a portion of it. **(B)** The dura is opened in a Y-shaped fashion, more so on the side ipsilateral to the surgical approach. c1, first cervical lamina; c2; second cervical lamina.

of neoplasm of any size; there is excellent visibility under magnification and no need to manipulate the medulla or lower pons.

It must be remembered that the first dentate ligament is attached to the dura dorsal to and immediately above the entrance of the vertebral artery into the foramen magnum. This anatomical relationship should be used as a landmark for identifying the vertebral artery, which is easily seen when the first dentate ligament is cut. With large lesions, the vertebral artery may be completely embedded in the tumor. To avoid inadvertent injury to the vertebral artery, removal of the neoplasm should be started at its lower pole.

Tumor Resection

Tumor resection is accomplished in three successive stages. First, the inferior pole of the tumor at C1–C2, below the

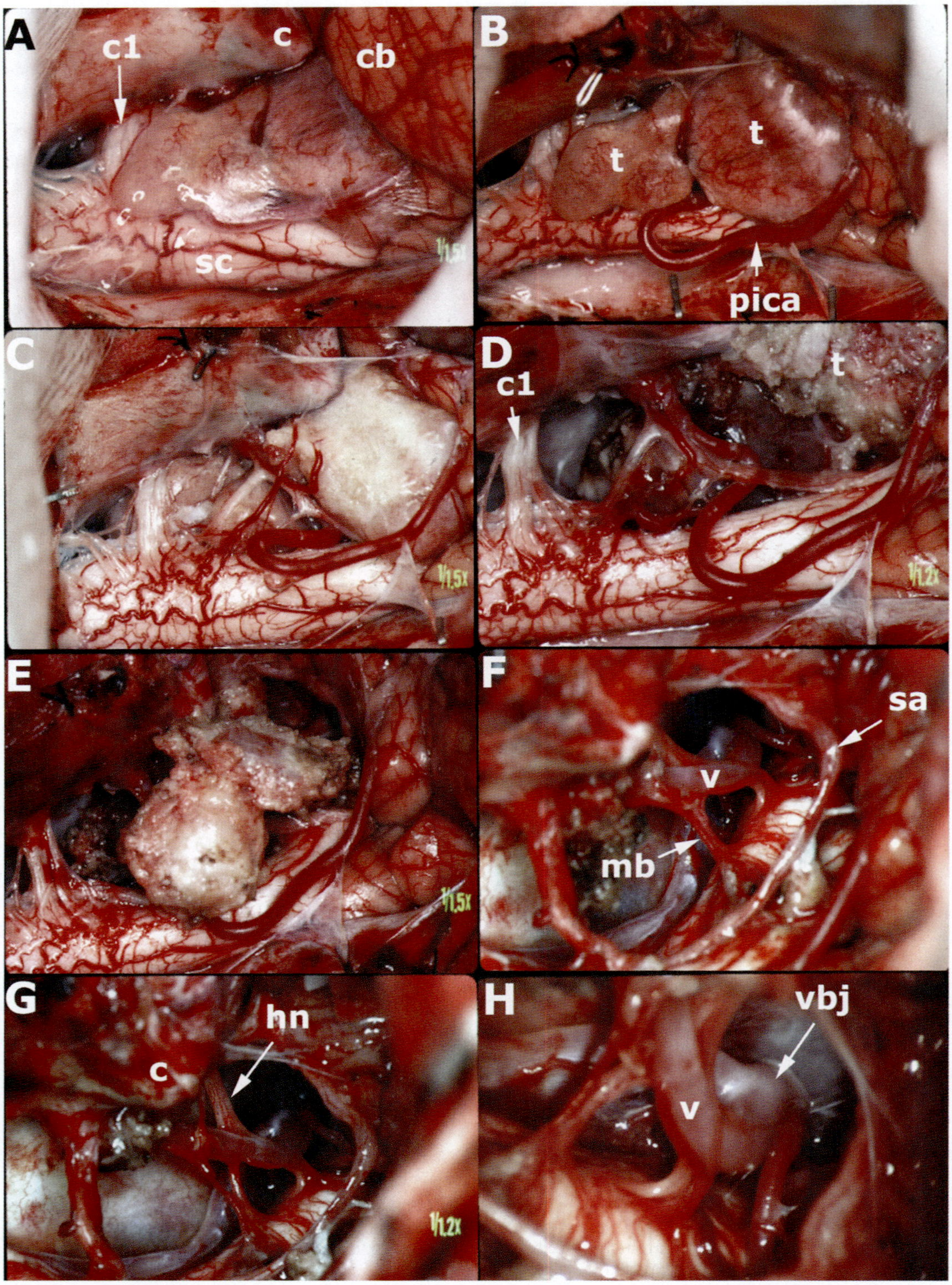

Figure 27–6 Serial operative photographs of a left-sided foramen magnum meningioma resected via a posterolateral approach. Refer to the text for a step-by-step description. c, occipital condyle; sc, spinal cord; c1, first cervical rootlets; pica, posterior inferior cerebellar artery; sa, spinal accessory nerve; v, vertebral artery; mb, medullary branch from vertebral artery; t, tumor; vbj, vertebrobasilar junction; hn, hypoglossal nerve.

entrance of the vertebral artery, is coagulated with bipolar forceps and removed **(Fig. 27–6C,D)**.

Second, the interior of the residual tumor is gutted in a piecemeal fashion, using bipolar forceps to coagulate the arterial blood supply from the ventral dura of the foramen magnum **(Fig. 27–6E)**. A 3- to 4-mm layer of tumor is left undisturbed at the interface between the vertebral artery dorsally and the pia of the upper cord and the medulla posteromedially **(Fig. 27–4F)**. As the interior of the tumor is debulked, the twelfth, tenth, and ninth cranial nerves become visible. In lesions with a large extension over the clivus, it is necessary to elevate the cerebellar tonsil with self-retaining retractors to identify the lower cranial nerves and the posterior inferior cerebellar artery (PICA). With large tumors, the PICA may be involved and provide direct blood supply to the neoplasm. In such cases, the arachnoid layer between the tumor and the PICA is used as a guide. The lesion is coagulated from the "subdural" side, and the tumor feeders are coagulated and cut, freeing the PICA. At this point, attention must be paid to the attachment of the neoplasm and its blood supply. Using the dura under magnification as a "road map," the clival arterial blood supply is coagulated and the lesion is detached from the dura. The arachnoid surrounding the base of the tumor attachment is carefully identified to expose the opposite vertebral artery. Tumor debulking is carried superiorly to the upper pole by angling the microscope upward toward the pons. At the end of this second stage of the operation, there should be little or no bleeding from the neoplasm and one half to two thirds of the ventral and inferior portion of the neoplasm will have been removed.

Dissecting the tumor inferiorly from the ventral aspect of the upper cord and the vertebral artery begins the third and final stage of removal **(Fig. 27–6F).** Because the arachnoid layer has been preserved, the tumor is retracted away from the pia of the upper cord and inferior medulla as well as the vertebral artery using micro-ring forceps. There should be enough empty space ventrally at this stage so that the devascularized lesion can be separated from the pia by the spring action of the microbipolar forceps. The arachnoid strands are cut with microscissors. Angled bipolar forceps may be used to coagulate the lateral attachment of the neoplasm immediately ventral to the entrance of the vertebral artery. Superiorly, the portion of tumor ventral to the twelfth, eleventh, tenth, and ninth cranial nerves is removed in a similar fashion, using microdissectors from above or below the vertebral artery **(Fig. 27–6G).**

The microscope is then adjusted, and the vertebral artery is followed toward the midline, exposing the opposite vertebral artery toward the vertebrobasilar junction **(Fig. 27–6H).** It is important to identify and preserve the anterior spinal artery and medullary branches of the vertebral artery **(Fig. 27–4G).** Because this area contains the largest diameter of tumor, causing maximum compression at the junction of the medulla and the cord, the anterior spinal artery may be attached to the neoplasm. Special attention must therefore be paid to this critical area. The last portion of tumor to be removed is the medial and superior segment at the upper medulla and vertebrobasilar junction. With large neoplasms, the basilar artery and the sixth cranial nerve are seen after resection.

Identification and preservation of the arachnoid are essential for safe management of this third stage of the procedure. The dural attachment of the tumor is coagulated with higher intensity bipolar current, and if necessary the meningeal layer of dura can be removed with microscissors or a no. 15 blade scalpel to decrease the risk of recurrence. After tumor removal, the lower medulla and upper cord will remain rotated and held in place to the opposite side, due to adhesions formed between the pia and arachnoid through longstanding compression. After release of the cervical roots and dentate ligaments from the opposite dura, the cord and medulla can be carefully dissected from the dura and brought into a more normal position in the foramen magnum. The second dentate ligament and the posterior arachnoid can be approximated to the dura with fine sutures.

Closure

The dura is closed with fine (5–0 or 6–0) nonabsorbable sutures. If the dura is kept moist throughout the operation, an almost watertight closure can be achieved **(Fig. 27–4H).** However, the most important aspect of closure is meticulous approximation of both the deep and superficial layers of the fascia and the obliquely cut suboccipital and trapezius muscles using interrupted sutures. The cervical muscles are sutured at the fascial layer without including a large portion of muscle in the needle. The superficial and deep cervical fascia are then carefully closed to keep the cervical and suboccipital muscles as close as possible to the foramen magnum and the posterior fossa, minimizing dead space and the formation of a pseudomeningocele. There is no need to leave a drain in this space. From this point, the rest of the closure is routine.

◆ Postoperative Management

Following surgery, the patient is taken to the recovery room with an endotracheal tube in place. With patients in whom the tumor was large, a thorough neurological examination should be performed as soon as the patient regains consciousness. Particular attention must be paid to respiratory function. Patients with preoperative swallowing or breathing difficulties, or those having had intraoperative manipulation of the medulla or inadvertent damage to the lower cranial nerves, the endotracheal tube should be kept in place for at least 24 hours. The tube is not removed until a patient is able to breathe spontaneously without the assistance of mechanical ventilation. Tracheostomy may be unavoidable in those with brain-stem dysfunction.

All patients are given nothing by mouth for 2 to 3 days, or until the swallowing function is found to be adequate. Some may require gastrostomy. Patients with unilateral permanent damage of the ninth or tenth cranial nerves will in time be able to swallow food without much trouble. In such cases, reconstruction of the vocal cords with a thyroplasty or injection of Teflon or both should be considered as soon as possible. However, in patients with anatomical preservation of lower cranial nerves, vocal cord reconstruction should be delayed for 6 to 9 months. The majority of these patients will make an excellent recovery.

Follow-up MRI with and without contrast enhancement should be obtained following surgery for general assessment and to rule out the possibility of residual tumor. Thereafter, MRI obtained annually for 5 years and then every 3 to 4 years is adequate for long-term follow-up **(Fig. 27–7).** Any residual tumor should be carefully monitored, both clinically and radiologically. If serial MRI shows regrowth, further surgery should be the first consideration. However, in elderly patients and in those with serious medical and neurological problems, stereotactic radiosurgery should be considered.

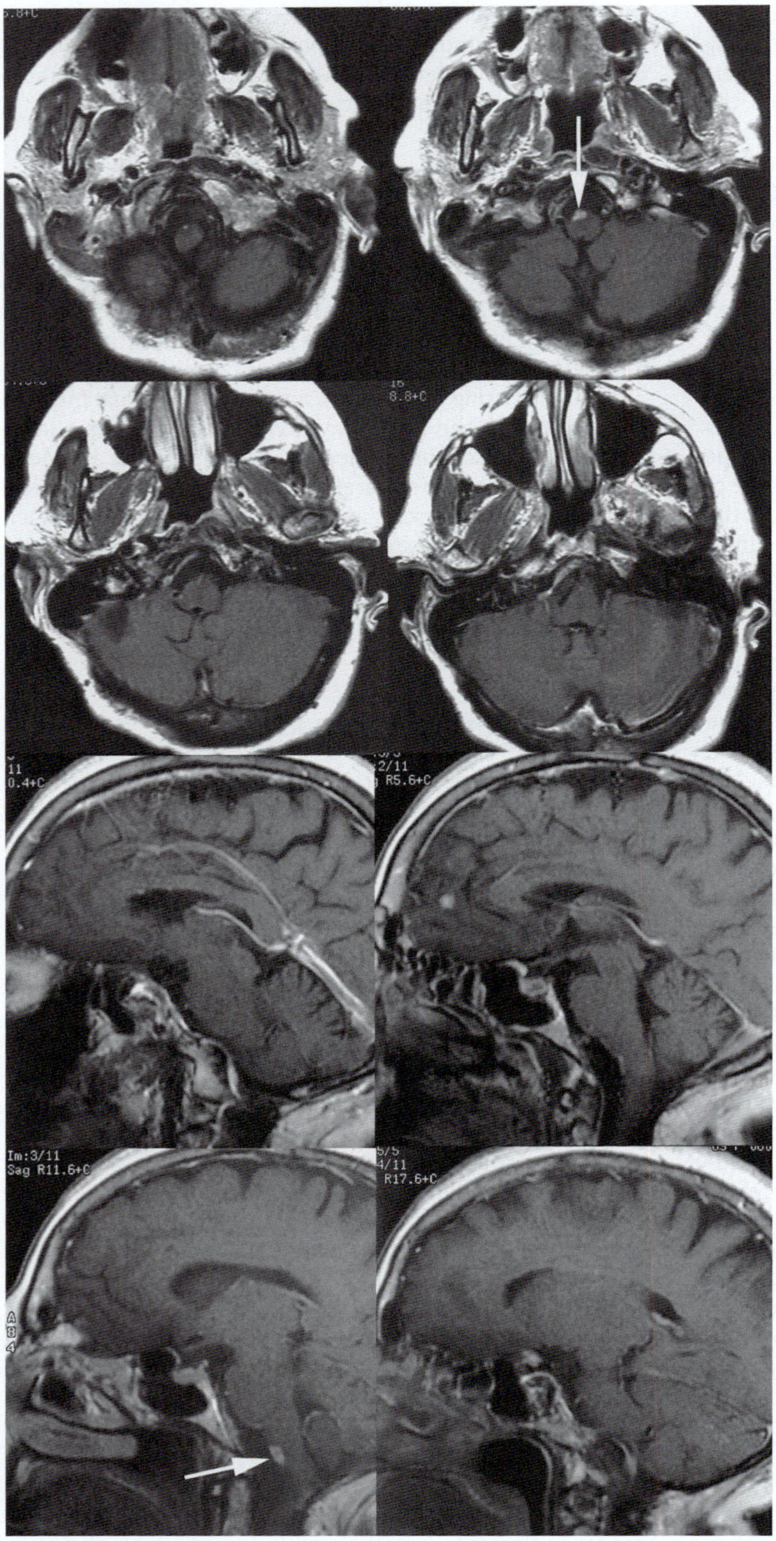

Figure 27–7 Postoperative contrast magnetic resonance imaging study performed in the axial (upper two rows) and sagittal (lower two rows) planes 9 years after surgery. A small tumor recurred just anterior to the medulla **(arrows),** but has not required additional treatment.

◆ Conclusions and Results

Surgical management of anterior foramen magnum meningiomas is complex, requiring intimate knowledge of the normal and pathological anatomy of this region. The use of meticulous microsurgical technique and careful postoperative management of respiratory and alimentary function can markedly improve the results of surgery.

We employed the posterolateral retrocondylar approach for 18 consecutive patients having anterior foramen magnum meningiomas ranging from 2 to 4.5 cm in size. Of these, 16 tumors were completely resected. No patients developed significant postoperative neurological deficits; however, two have permanent ninth–tenth cranial nerve palsy, and four have eleventh cranial nerve palsy secondary to surgery. One patient with neurofibromatosis and multiple brain tumors (i.e., bilateral large acoustic schwannomas, pineal tumor, and anterior foramen magnum meningioma) who was apneic and quadriplegic prior to surgery, died 4 months postoperatively from meningitis.

28

Surgical Management of Trigeminal Neurinomas

John Diaz Day

Neurinomas arising from the trigeminal nerve are rare lesions, accounting for 0.07 to 0.36% of intracranial tumors and 0.8 to 8% of all intracranial neurinomas. In the majority of reported cases they are not associated with other tumors in the head; however, patients with neurofibromatosis type 2 (NF-2) may harbor them in addition to vestibular neurinomas and meningiomas **(Fig. 28–1)**.

Trigeminal neurinomas have been classified according to their anatomical location and the apparent origin of the tumor within the nerve itself **(Fig. 28–2)**. In 1955, Jefferson proposed such a classification scheme that has been subsequently modified to include more extensive tumors that involve more than one basic segment of the nerve. This classification results in tumors being considered as one of four types. Tumors arising from the root of the nerve are generally confined to the posterior fossa **(Fig. 28–3)**. A second type of tumor is confined to the ganglion, within the lateral wall of the cavernous sinus **(Fig. 28–4)**. Tumors may also arise from one of the three peripheral divisions of the nerve and be located both intra- and extracranially. The fourth type is actually a combination of two or three of the previous classifications, being labeled "dumbbell" tumors **(Fig. 28–5)**. These tumors may span the posterior and middle fossae, the middle fossa, and extracranially, or they may extend from the posterior fossa to the extracranial space via the middle fossa. Classification has largely determined surgical strategy, especially with the employment of contemporary cranial base approaches.

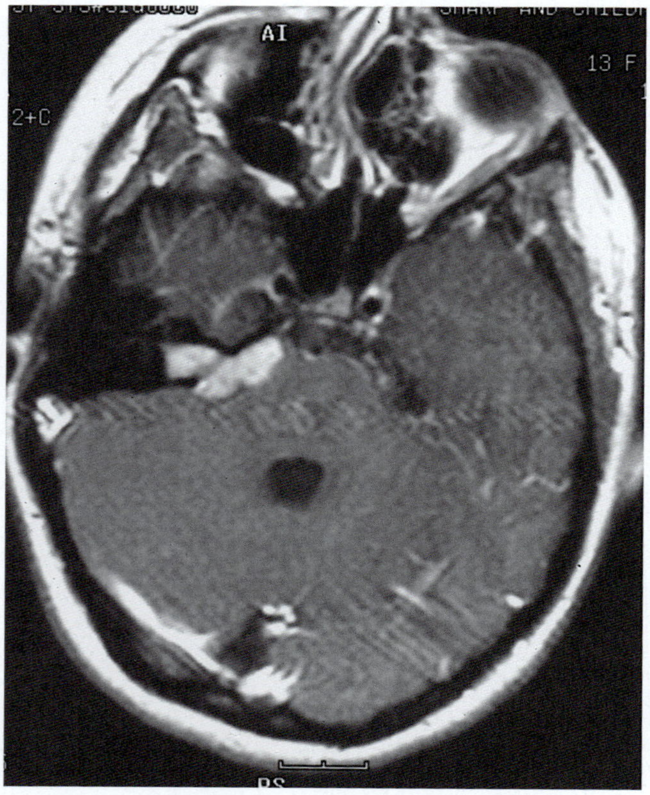

Figure 28–1 Axial contrast magnetic resonance imaging of a young patient with neurofibromatosis type 2 that demonstrates a small trigeminal neurinoma adjacent to the vestibular schwannomas present on the right side. Both tumors were removed at the same operation via an extended middle fossa type of approach.

◆ Patient Selection

The vast majority of patients with a trigeminal neurinoma present with symptoms of trigeminal nerve dysfunction. However, it has been reported that as many as 10% of patients may not have had trigeminal dysfunction as a presenting feature. Patients may present with diminished sensation in any one or a combination of the three divisions of the trigeminal nerve. The degree of sensory disturbance is highly variable in these patients. Diminished sensation also tends to occur over a long period of time, which is consistent with the slow-growing nature of these tumors. Possibly one of the most important features of diminished sensation is how it affects the corneal response in the individual patient. Certainly, diminished corneal sensation can lead to significant problems with an impaired blink reflex as well as neurotropic changes that may result in keratitis.

Pain may also be a classic presenting feature in these patients. In one series, the patients who presented with pain showed an almost 2:1 predominance of the ganglion type of tumor classification. However, the distribution of pain among tumor locations was even more in the series of Day and Fukushima. In that same series pain was a prominent complaint that at admission accounted for 43% of the 38 patients reported. It is important to recognize that the quality of pain in patients with trigeminal neurinomas differs from that in patients suffering from trigeminal neuralgia. This is despite the common description in the literature

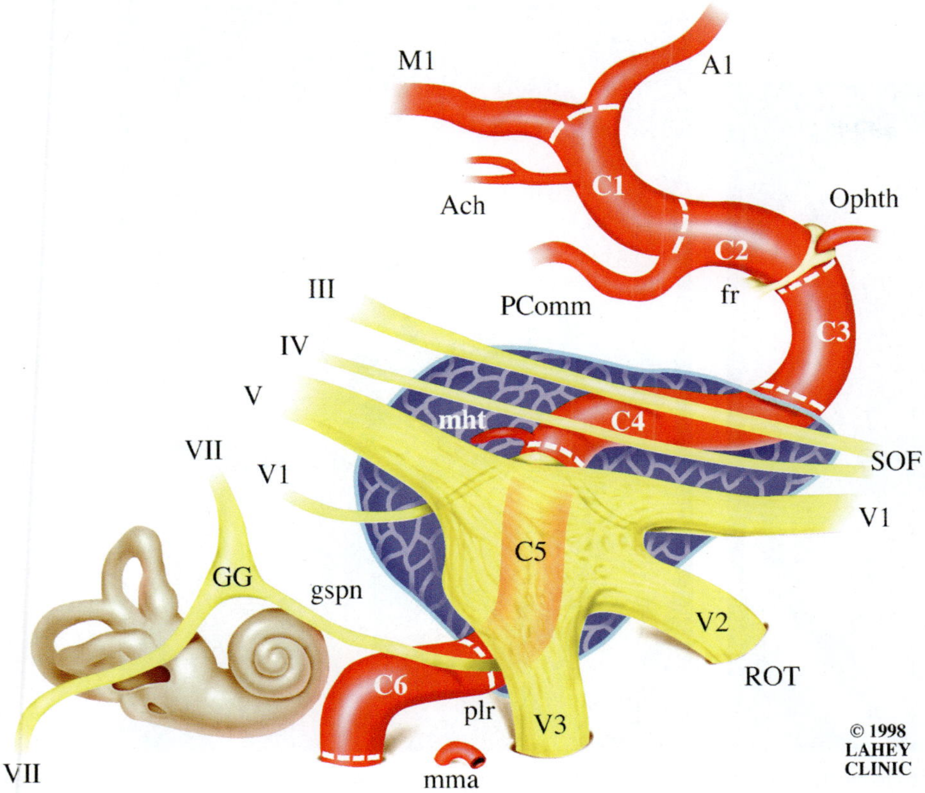

Figure 28–2 Anatomy of the trigeminal nerve in relation to the cavernous sinus venous plexus, carotid artery, and cranial nerves III, IV, and VI. Tumors may arise from the root, ganglion, or peripheral segments of the nerve. They may grow such that multiple segments of the nerve are involved by tumor. Ach, anterior choroidal artery; GG, genicular ganglion; GSPN, greater superficial petrosal nerve; Ophth, ophthalamic artery; PComm, posterior communicating arter; ROT, foramen rotundum; SOF, superior orbital fissure.

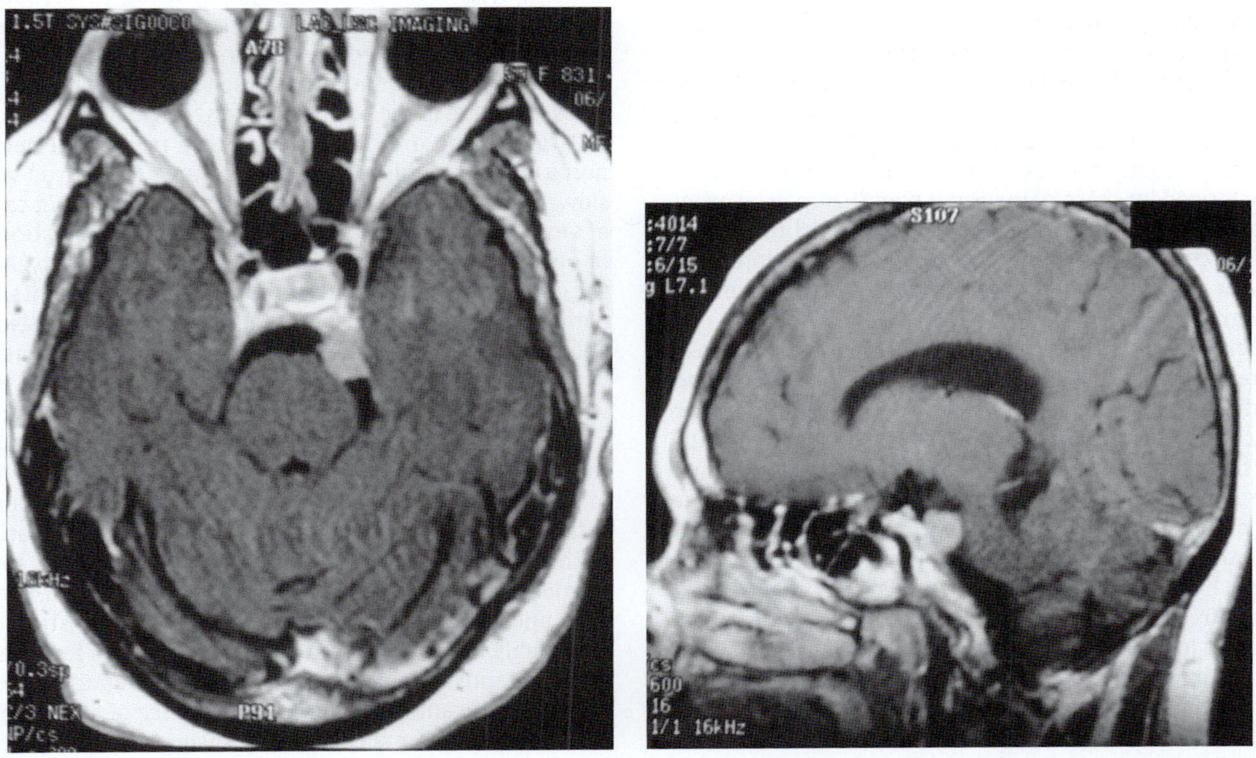

A B

Figure 28–3 **(A)** Axial and **(B)** coronal contrast magnetic resonance imaging of a typical small trigeminal neurinoma arising from the root segment of the nerve.

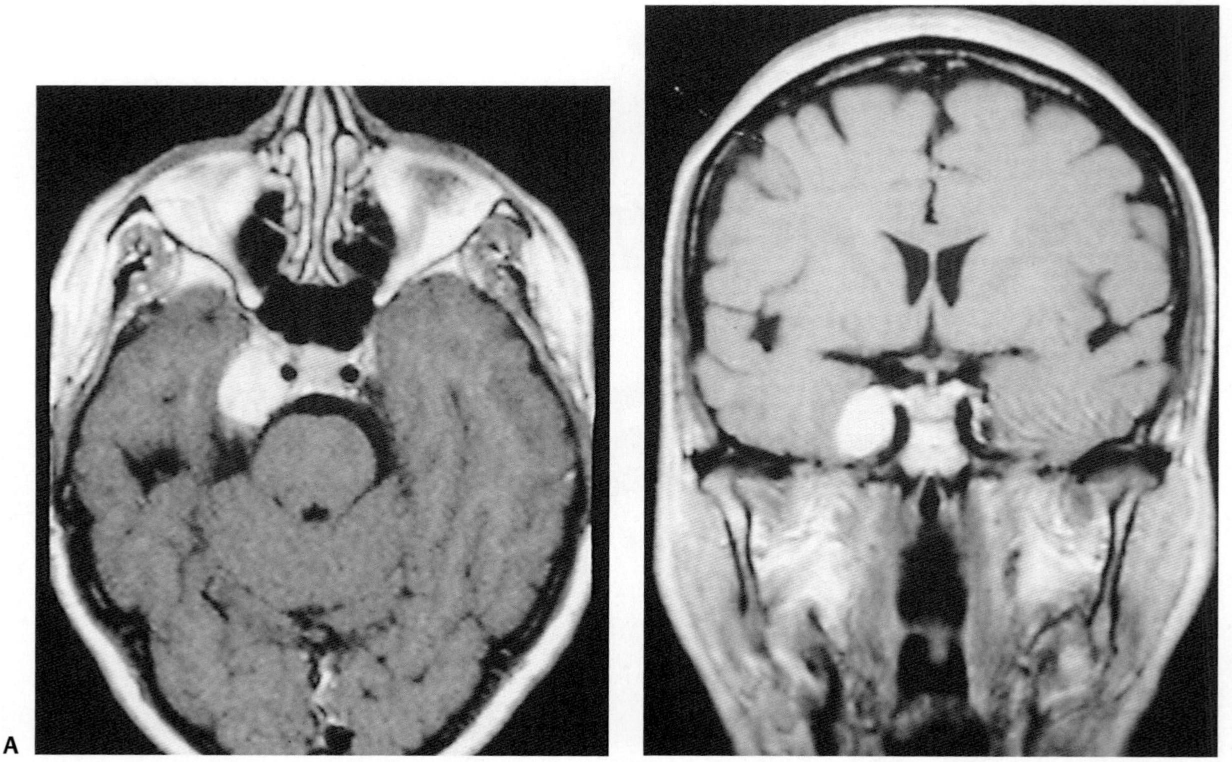

Figure 28–4 The most common location of trigeminal neurinoma is that confined to the ganglion, compressing the cavernous venous plexus and distorting the adjacent anatomy. **(A)** Axial and **(B)** coronal magnetic resonance images with contrast demonstrate such a tumor.

of ticlike pain in trigeminal neurinoma patients. Most patients with pain that is attributable to a neurinoma have facial pain episodes that tend to be more prolonged and are not always triggered by a specific stimulus. Pain in the patient with a neurinoma will not respond to medications that are commonly used for patients with tic doloureaux, such as antiseizure drugs. It is important to note, however, that a minority of patients will have pain syndromes that are more similar to classic trigeminal neuralgia. This is characterized by sharp paroxysmal pain that may be exacerbated by different stimuli. In a review of the literature, a small percentage of patients (approximately 13%) presenting with pain had complaints consistent with trigeminal neuralgia.

Patients have also been reported to present with diplopia, apparently attributable to nerve compression by the tumor. This diplopia may be secondary to compression of either the oculomotor or the abducens nerves. Patients with tumors that involve the ophthalmic division of the trigeminal nerve and extend into the orbit peripherally may also suffer from diplopia secondary to exophthalmos in addition to their cranial nerve dysfunction. The more common cause of diplopia has been oculomotor nerve palsy, reported to be as high as 50%.

Hearing loss and facial motor dysfunction have also been reported in association with these tumors. This has been observed most frequently in those patients who have NF-2. However, non-NF-2 patients may also present with these complaints. Large root-type tumors or dumbbell-shaped tumors may compress the eighth cranial nerve in the cerebellopontine angle and as the nerve enters the porus acusticus. A similar mechanical mechanism may be responsible for patients who suffer from imbalance owing to vestibular nerve dysfunction. Facial nerve dysfunction has also been reported in patients whose tumors have significantly involved the petrous bone and are then large enough to compress the nerve in the cerebellopontine angle.

Patients who are diagnosed with a trigeminal neurinoma have several options for therapy. Growth is very slow, quite similar to the natural history observed in cases of vestibular schwannoma. For this reason, one option is to observe the patient and obtain serial imaging to chart the rate of growth of the tumor. For older patients, or patients with small or asymptomatic tumors, it is reasonable to observe the patient with serial imaging at intervals of 6 to 12 months. Symptomatic patients, or those in whom early treatment is desirable to lessen the risk of morbidity with treatment, may be offered microsurgical resection with an attempt at complete removal. This has in general resulted in very low rates of recurrence when a total resection was possible. However, due to the location of these tumors in and around the cavernous sinus, total surgical resection is not always possible. Patients who have undergone a subtotal resection have demonstrated a reasonably high rate of recurrence within just a few years. Although most recent surgical series have reported a low risk of significant morbidity, the incidence of new cranial nerve deficits after surgery is not insignificant. Owing to these difficulties, a second treatment strategy has developed that has been based upon the satisfactory results

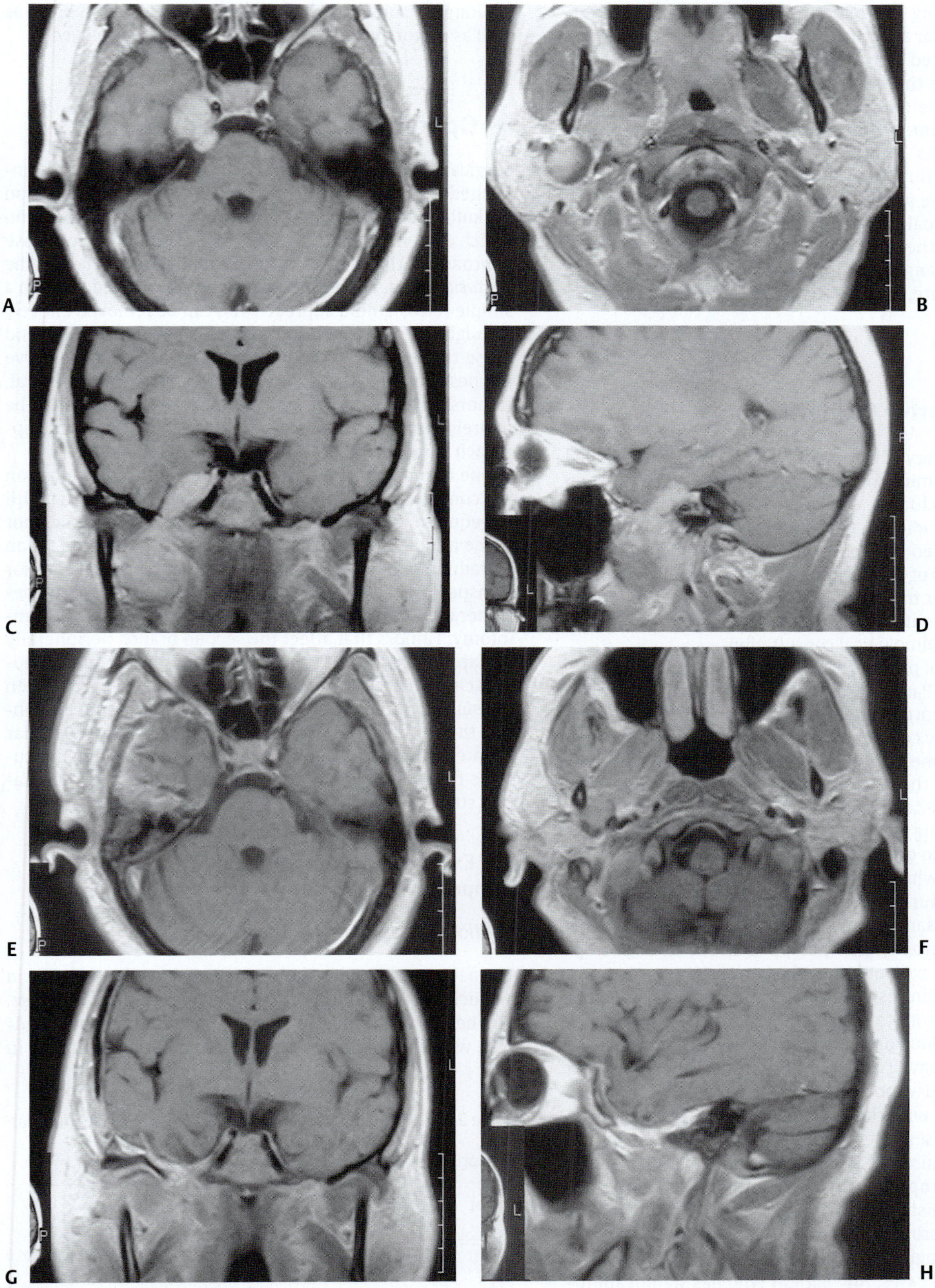

Figure 28–5 Large trigeminal neurinoma in a 54-year-old woman that extends from the posterior fossa to the infratemporal fossa, following V3 out the foramen ovale as seen in **(A,B)** axial, **(C)** coronal, and **(D)** sagittal sections. The tumor was removed via a combined preauricular infratemporal and anterior transpetrosal approach. Postoperative axial **(E–G)** and sagittal **(H)** images revealed a gross total resection.

obtained utilizing stereotactic radiosurgery in the treatment of vestibular schwannomas. Stereotactic radiosurgery has been suggested as a viable alternative treatment strategy in these patients that provides a low risk of complications and cranial nerve deficits with a documented short-term probability of tumor control. Patients should be presented with the various treatment options and appropriately counseled regarding their individual risks based upon tumor size, age, the patient's general medical condition, and the treatment goals of the patient. Many patients will accept the lack of the removal of the tumor offered by radiosurgery in exchange for a lower risk of new cranial nerve deficits. Therefore, treatment should be individualized for each patient.

◆ Preoperative Preparation

The medical history of the patient is obtained and a detailed neurological examination is completed. Fifth nerve function is observed, including the presence and quality of the corneal reflex. Grading on the abnormal side, using a 10-point scale, is compared with the normal side. This is quite important in terms of determining and tracking any postoperative decrease or improvement in sensory function. In the event signs of keratitis are detected, the patient is referred for neuro-ophthalmological consultation.

The majority of patients are diagnosed via magnetic resonance imaging. Particularly for those who will undergo a transpetrosal approach it is usually helpful to obtain a fine cut bone window computed tomographic (CT) scan through the temporal bone prior to surgery. Particular attention is directed toward the relationship between the cochlea, the internal auditory canal, and the carotid canal.

In the operating room patients are administered antibiotics and are also given steroids prior to the procedure. In those patients who will undergo a procedure where the supratentorial dura will be opened they are also loaded with anticonvulsants intravenously. In a majority of cases anticonvulsant prophylaxis is stopped on the tenth postoperative day if the patient has not had any seizures.

Patients are administered general endotracheal anesthesia. It is our custom to place a radial arterial line to invasively monitor blood pressure in each case. In addition, each patient should have two large-bore intravenous lines and receive a central venous line when medically indicated. Communication with the anesthesia team is critical, especially in those cases where significant temporal lobe retraction will be required. It is important that the intracranial pressure be appropriately managed utilizing hyperventilation, the administration of diuretic agents, and lumbar drainage of cerebrospinal fluid (CSF).

Neurophysiological monitoring is also employed in the large majority of cases. Any patient who has significant involvement of tumor in the posterior fossa will have monitoring of the facial nerve as well as brain stem auditory evoked responses. Monitoring of the trigeminal nerve itself has not been found particularly useful; neither has monitoring of the ocular motor nerves. In patients having procedures where brain retraction may be significant or prolonged, somatosensory evoked potentials (SSEPs) as well as motor evoked potentials (MEPs) are employed.

◆ Operative Procedure

Surgical removal of trigeminal neurinomas is largely accomplished in contemporary practice via one or a combination of skull base approaches. In general, the only tumor location which does not benefit from the utilization of a skull base approach is that confined to the root of the nerve in the posterior fossa. These tumors may be approached through a simple retrosigmoid approach and can be removed entirely through this strategy. Tumors that involve the ganglion and those that extend to the peripheral divisions of the nerve are best handled using a skull base approach. In general, tumors of the ganglion and peripheral branches may be entirely removed via an extradural strategy. The overall approach paradigm employed is listed in **Table 28–1.**

One of the important aspects of preoperative evaluation is a consideration of the extradural bone removal that will be required. Ganglion tumors that are confined to the floor of the middle fossa and cavernous sinus are removed via an extradural temporopolar approach or an extradural anterior transpetrosal strategy. Tumors that are located on the peripheral V1 branch are approached via a transorbital craniotomy. Tumors that affect the second branch peripherally are approached via a frontotemporal and extradural approach with access as well to the maxillary sinus between the superior orbital fissure and foramen rotundum. Peripheral third branch tumors are approached by a preauricular infratemporal fossa approach. In the case of extensive tumors that span two or more general locations a combination strategy is indicated.

The Extradural Frontotemporal Temporopolar Approach

Positioning

The patient is placed in the supine position with the table in a couched position to promote adequate venous drainage. The head is positioned with the Mayfield three-pin headrest, with the single pin arm placed such that the pin is in

Table 28–1 Selecting the Approach for Trigeminal Neurinomas

Location	Approach
Root	Retrosigmoid
Ganglion	Extradural subtemporal Extradural frontotemporal temporopolar
Dumbbell	Extradural frontotemporal temporopolar Combined petrosal Extradural subtemporal anterior transpetrosal
Peripheral branch V1	Frontotemporal orbitocranial
V2	Frontotemporal temporopolar
V3	Preauricular infratemporal

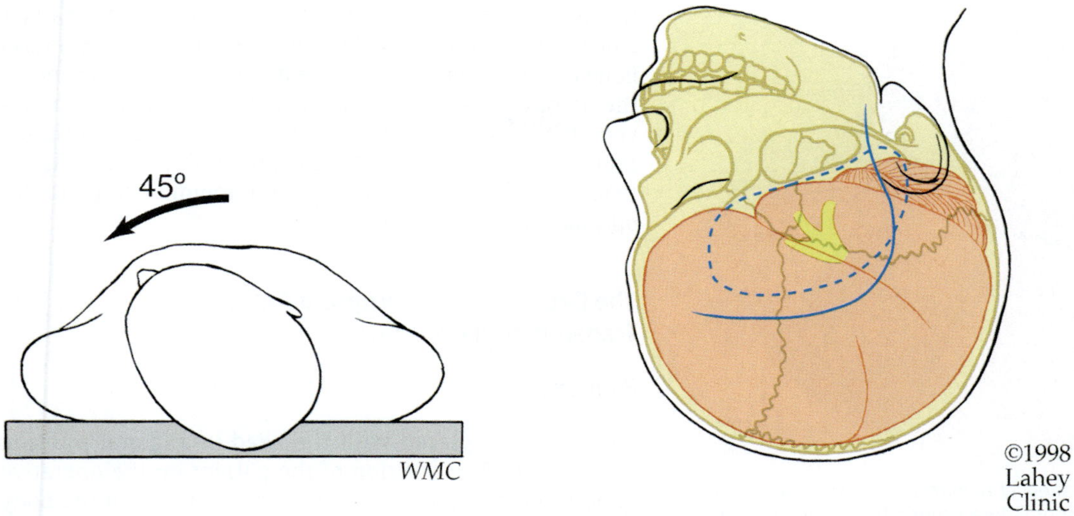

Figure 28–6 The patient is positioned supine with the head turned as shown for the extradural frontotemporal temporopolar approach. Most cases will require a routine frontotemporal craniotomy as outlined in the illustration.

the contralateral midpupillary line, within the hairline. The head is turned ~45 degrees toward the opposite shoulder **(Fig. 28–6).** A simple strip shave, or no hair shaved at all, is employed in these cases.

Surgical Technique

Beginning just anterior to the tragus of the ear and over the root of the zygomatic process the incision is started. The incision extends superior, within the hairline, and gently curves anterior to end at the midline. Utilizing an interfascial technique, the galeocutaneous flap is elevated and held anteriorly with blunt scalp hooks. To maximize anterior exposure, the temporalis muscle is rotated and deflected inferior and posterior. In most cases a vascularized pericranial flap medial to the linea temporalis is preserved. Elevation of soft tissue results in exposure of the superior and lateral orbital rims. The options for a routine frontotemporal versus transzygomatic versus orbitozygomatic bone flap are available with this opening, depending upon exposure requirements in the individual case.

Most cases of smaller ganglion type tumors will require nothing more than a simple frontotemporal craniotomy. This is illustrated in **Fig. 28–6.** A kidney-shaped bone flap is cut, centered approximately one third above and two thirds below the linea temporalis. The bone flap typically measures roughly 6 × 4 cm. In some cases a small temporal craniectomy is necessary to provide a view flat along the floor of the middle fossa. The dura is elevated away from the sphenoid ridge as well as the anterior fossa and middle fossa. Self-retaining retractor blades are used to hold the dura away from the skull base **(Fig. 28–7).** The extradural bone removal in these cases is variable in terms of the necessity of exposure of various elements. If maximal exposure is required, bone is removed over the optic canal, including removal of the anterior clinoid process. Bone also may be removed over the superior orbital fissure. V2 may be exposed by unroofing bone at the foramen rotundum. The third division of the nerve may be exposed by removal of bone over the foramen ovale. The extradural bone is removed at the cranial base such that the dissection plane between the temporal dura propria and the outer membrane of the cavernous sinus can be accessed **(Fig. 28–8).** This requires exposure of the interface between these two connective tissue layers so that they may be separated effectively.

At the superior orbital fissure, the cleavage plane between the temporal dura propria and periorbital fascia is separated using sharp dissection. The self-retaining retractor blade is placed such that posterior retraction pressure is applied over the temporal pole, between the dura propria and the outer cavernous membrane, which effectively splits the layers of the lateral wall of the cavernous sinus. With this dissection the tumor becomes gradually evident via the

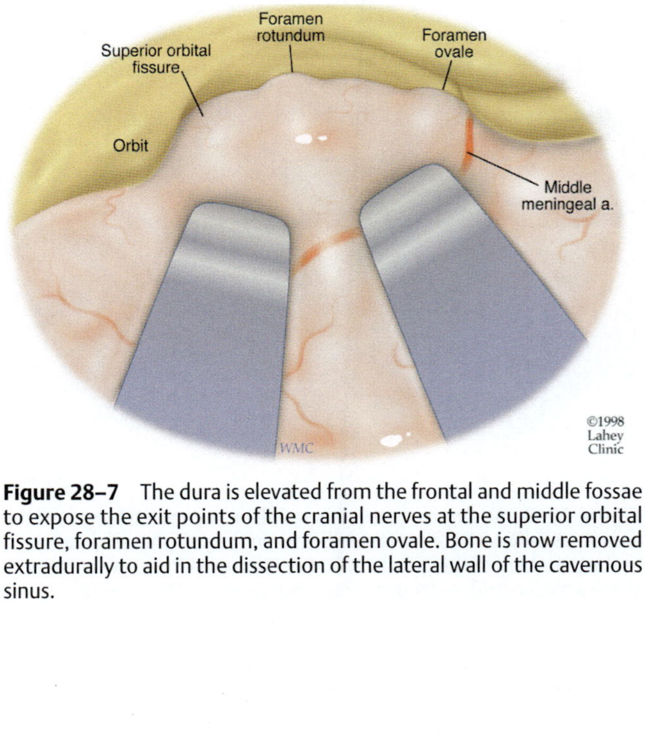

Figure 28–7 The dura is elevated from the frontal and middle fossae to expose the exit points of the cranial nerves at the superior orbital fissure, foramen rotundum, and foramen ovale. Bone is now removed extradurally to aid in the dissection of the lateral wall of the cavernous sinus.

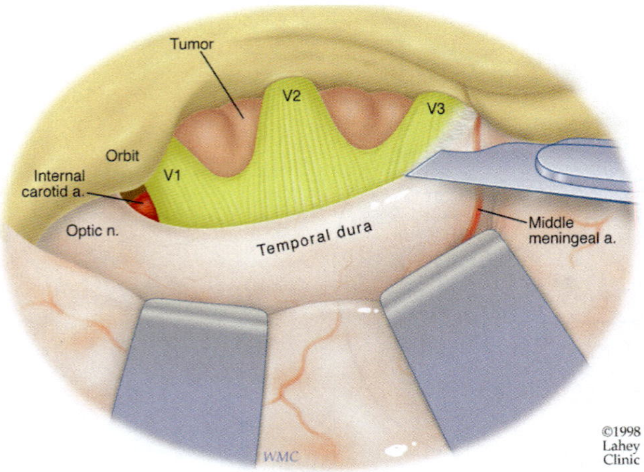

Figure 28–8 The critical maneuver to extradural cavernous dissection is separation of the temporal dura propria from the outer cavernous membrane. This allows a clear view of the nerves in the lateral wall and is the beginning point for tumor resection.

entirely extradural technique. Nerve fibers may be seen spreading over the tumor **(Fig. 28–9)**.

At this point tumor removal may proceed. The technique of tumor removal requires accessing the tumor capsule between fibers of the trigeminal nerve. Typically, access corridors are sought between major divisions of the nerve. The tumor capsule is opened and an internal debulking is performed. Tumor is sequentially separated from the surrounding nerve fibers and removed **(Fig. 28–10)**. In some cases, the nerve bundle that gives rise to the neurinoma can be identified because it seems to enter the tumor capsule. These small nerve fascicles when identified are divided. However, in the majority of cases no nerve fascicle of origin is identifiable.

After tumor removal the skull base defect is repaired. Any openings made in the dura are reconstructed in a watertight fashion. This may be done either by primary closure or

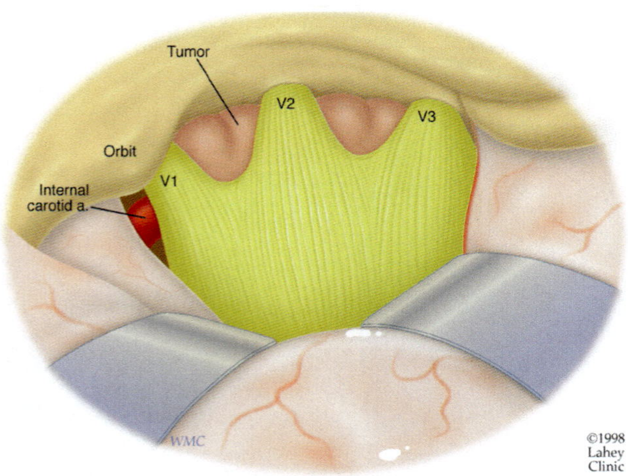

Figure 28–9 Trigeminal nerve fibers will be seen stretching over the tumor, usually with tumor visible between the peripheral branches or at the periphery of the ganglion. Tumor is entered from one or more of these access corridors for debulking and removal of the capsule.

the use of grafts as necessary. The situation in which an air sinus has been opened through the course of extradural bone removal requires closure with fascial grafts. In general, the nasofrontal duct is left open and is not occluded to prevent formation of a mucocele by promoting continued drainage. After the skull base is repaired, the bone flap is reapproximated and secured with titanium microplates for optimal cosmesis.

The Extradural Subtemporal Anterior Transpetrosal Approach

Positioning

The patient is placed with the head in a lateral position **(Fig. 28–11)**. The position of the patient on the operative table is either supine or lateral depending upon the body habitus of the patient, the flexibility of the neck, and the age of the patient. Some patients will not be able to tolerate full lateral positioning of the head while in the supine position due to cervical spondylitic disease. Prior to turning the patient's head therefore, the mobility of the patient's neck should be ascertained to determine the degree of resistance to placing the head in the lateral position. In some cases it is sufficient to place a shoulder roll to take pressure off of the neck and to minimize the chance of occlusion of the vertebral artery or internal jugular vein. The lateral position may be required to minimize strain upon the cervical spine and vessels.

The facial nerve is routinely monitored in this procedure because of the risk to the facial nerve during the exposure. Elevation of the dura in this procedure can place traction on the greater superficial petrosal nerve (GSPN), running across the middle fossa floor, which can damage the facial nerve. Therefore monitoring is indispensable in helping to minimize the chance of injury to the facial nerve.

Surgical Technique

The external landmarks that are important in planning the procedure are the zygomatic process and the tragus of the ear. The superior temporal line is additionally palpated. Two different incisions may be utilized. The predetermined size of craniotomy determines which incision is optimal. For the majority of small lesions that involve the ganglion or the peripheral V3 branch a straight incision with a small anterior curve is sufficient. This incision begins just anterior to the tragus of the ear at the inferior margin of the root of the zygomatic process. The incision continues superior in a straight line and curves slightly anterior as the superior temporal line is approached. The alternative incision is a question mark incision. This is performed when a larger craniotomy is deemed necessary. This incision also begins over the zygomatic process just anterior to the tragus and extends superior to the top of the pinna of the ear. The incision then curves posterior to the posterior extent of the pinna and then it curves anteriorly ending within the hairline just above the superior temporal line. With this technique the scalp flap is elevated and the temporalis muscle and fascia incised along the line of incision. The muscle is

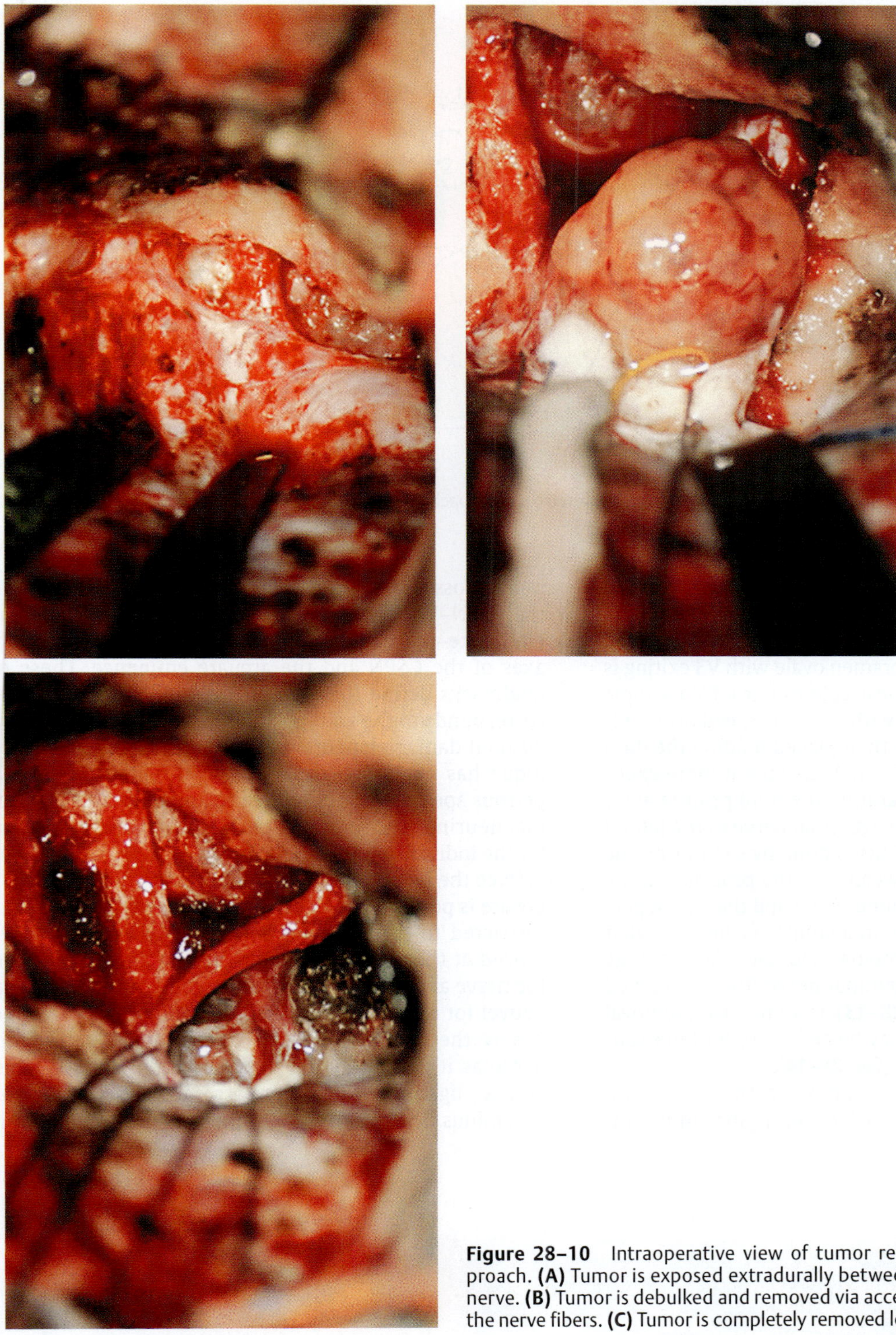

A B C

Figure 28–10 Intraoperative view of tumor removal via the temporopolar approach. **(A)** Tumor is exposed extradurally between the peripheral branches of the nerve. **(B)** Tumor is debulked and removed via access corridors between and around the nerve fibers. **(C)** Tumor is completely removed leaving the nerve fibers intact.

separated from the temporal squama and retracted anteriorly while being held in place with blunt scalp hooks.

A temporal craniotomy is then cut and is generally centered two thirds anterior and one third posterior to the external auditory canal. The typical size of the craniotomy is approximately 4 × 4 cm. Any remaining bone overhanging the middle fossa floor is then reduced with the high-speed drill. This results in the necessary flat viewing angle across the middle fossa floor. This is very important in terms of limiting temporal lobe retraction.

The dura is then elevated from the middle fossa floor beginning posterior at the petrous ridge **(Fig. 28–12)**. The sequence of dural elevation is quite important in terms of minimizing injury to the facial nerve. Working from posterior to medial exposing the petrous ridge and the arcuate eminence prior to the elevation anteriorly will result in elevation

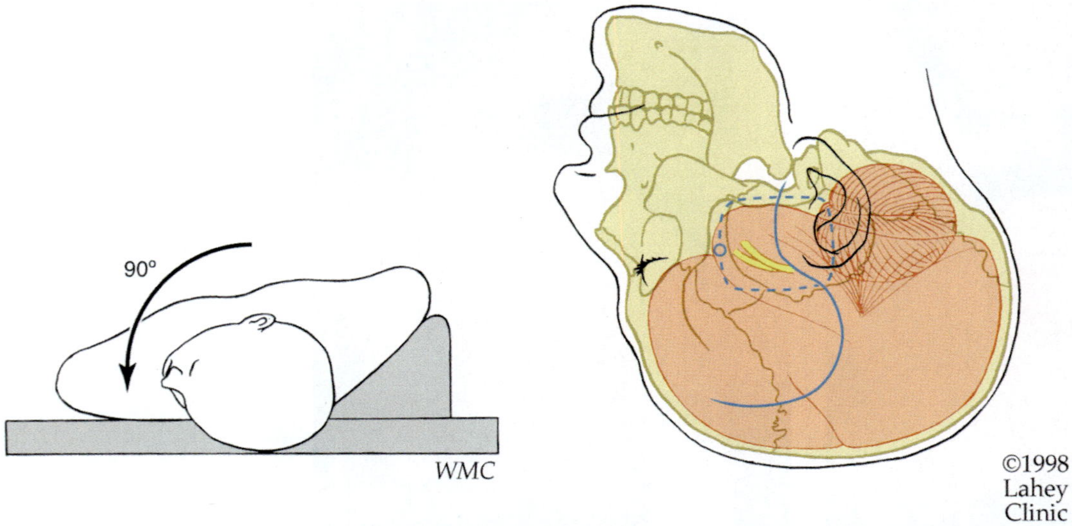

Figure 28–11 Position and incision for the extradural subtemporal transpetrosal approach.

of the dura without damaging the greater superficial petrosal nerve. Elevation proceeds anteriorly until the middle meningeal artery is exposed at the foramen spinosum. The artery is then coagulated and divided. The foramen ovale with V3 exiting is exposed. In some cases it is desirable to unroof V3 a short distance at the foramen ovale with the high-speed drill. Self-retaining retractor blades are then placed holding the dura away from the middle fossa floor. At this point more exposure may be obtained by separating the dura propria away from the lateral aspect of the trigeminal nerve in the lateral wall of the cavernous sinus. This is done by separating the cleavage plane identified between the dura propria and the connective tissue sheath surrounding V3 and the lateral portion of the gasserian ganglion in a similar fashion to what was described for the temporopolar approach. At this stage the exposure may reveal trigeminal nerve fibers stretched over the tumor capsule **(Fig. 28–13).** In some cases, removal of bone at the petrous apex may be necessary for full exposure and removal of the tumor **(Fig. 28–14).**

Bone removal at the petrous apex via this extradural trajectory is accomplished first by identifying important middle fossa floor landmarks. The important landmarks are the GSPN–V3 junction, the porus trigeminus, the arcuate eminence–petrous ridge junction, and the junction of the axes of the GSPN and the arcuate eminence. These four landmarks define the area of the middle fossa floor that corresponds to the volume of bone which may be removed without damaging neural or vascular structures. This technique has been well described in the literature. Radical petrous apex removal is seldom required in cases of trigeminal neurinomas; however, the approach must be tailored for the individual patient.

Once the bony removal that is necessary for adequate exposure is performed, the tumor is removed. Tumors that are restricted to the ganglion may be fully exposed and removed at this juncture. Tumor that extends to the root of the nerve and the posterior fossa requires an additional maneuver for adequate exposure. To obtain posterior fossa exposure the fibrous dural ring surrounding the trigeminal nerve as it enters Meckel's cave must be opened. This is done by ligating the superior petrosal sinus near the porus trigeminus. The root of the trigeminal nerve becomes visible

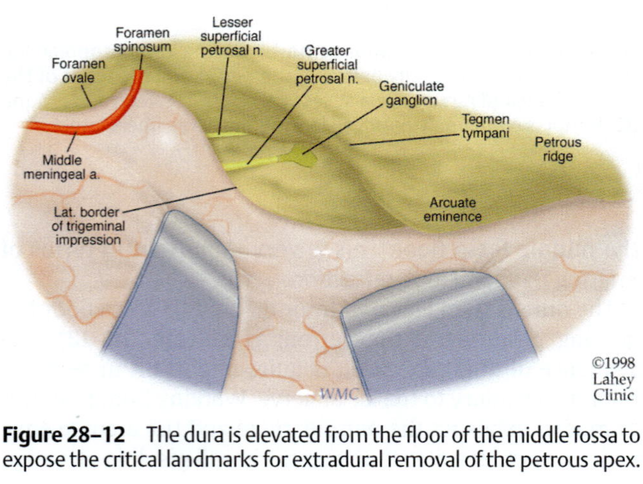

Figure 28–12 The dura is elevated from the floor of the middle fossa to expose the critical landmarks for extradural removal of the petrous apex.

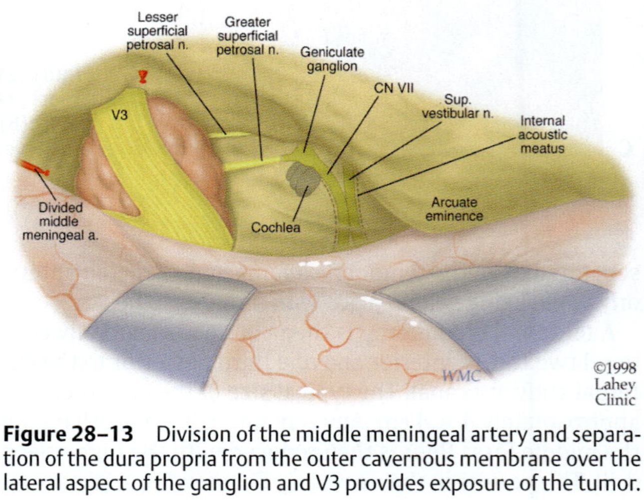

Figure 28–13 Division of the middle meningeal artery and separation of the dura propria from the outer cavernous membrane over the lateral aspect of the ganglion and V3 provides exposure of the tumor.

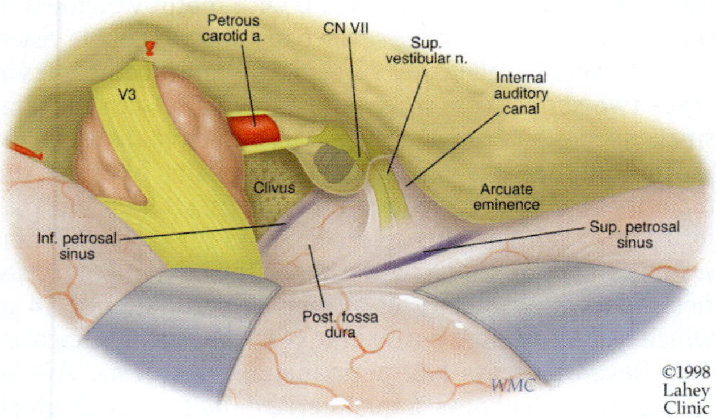

Figure 28–14 For improved and wider access the petrous apex may be removed extradurally. The dura may also be opened to access the posterior fossa and the root segment of the nerve.

in the posterior fossa. With the nerve in direct vision as it enters Meckel's cave the fibrous ring can then be opened and separated away from the nerve, which frees the nerve at this point and allows access into the posterior fossa. A suture is placed in the tentorium where the superior petrosal sinus has been ligated, and an incision directed posterior in the tentorium is made. This small tentorial flap is then retracted superior with the suture. Tumor is resected utilizing the same principles outlined earlier for trigeminal neurinomas. Once the tumor has been removed reconstruction of the cranial base is performed. Communication of spinal fluid through the petrous apex defect needs to be interrupted. Typically this is done utilizing an adipose graft, which seals off the posterior fossa compartment. This is augmented with fibrin glue in most cases. The bone flap is then resecured with titanium miniplates and the muscle, fascia, and galeal layers closed.

◆ Postoperative Management

Particular complications are common after the removal of a trigeminal neuroma via any surgical approach. Dysfunction of the trigeminal nerve can be expected in most cases in the early postoperative period. This may be in the form of hypesthesia, anesthesia, or pain. Many patients do not have resolution of these symptoms until some time after surgery. Most patients will have some resolution or a diminution of their hypesthesia. Those who present with pain typically experience good pain relief after surgery. In larger tumors and those that affect the third division, a large number of these patients will suffer trigeminal motor dysfunction after surgery. Certainly this is less common in those patients with small or medially situated ganglion type tumors and those with peripheral lesions of V1 and V2. Because of the high risk of motor dysfunction the rare patient with bilateral tumors is treated only on the side producing the majority of the symptoms. These tend to be patients with NF-2. The opposite side must be managed expectantly and stereotactic radiosurgery is a viable option in these patients.

Undoubtedly the most troublesome potential complication from removal of these tumors is keratitis suffered as a consequence of a diminished corneal reflex. Many patients present with a diminished corneal reflex due to diminished sensation over the cornea. Attention to proper eye care is extremely important beginning at the time of the patient's first presentation.

Diplopia is also a frequent presenting complaint that may or not be relieved after surgical removal of the tumor. The operation in or around the cavernous sinus carries with it the potential of injury to the ocular motor nerves. Though diplopia may be a consequence of surgical resection this is quite uncommon. It is more likely that the diplopia will be resolved with the pressure relieved from the nerves. Separation of the tumor capsule away from the third, fourth, and sixth cranial nerves in the cavernous sinus is the key to reducing the chance of permanent diplopia.

The seventh and eighth cranial nerves are particularly at risk when utilizing the extradural subtemporal transpetrosal approach. Traction on the GSPN during the elevation of the dura off the floor of the middle fossa may account for injury to the facial nerve. It is important that the dura be elevated from a posterior to anterior direction to reduce the chances of this complication. The seventh and eighth cranial nerves are further at risk during the bone removal phase of this procedure, especially when unroofing the internal auditory canal. The cochlea is also at risk during the drilling. Avoidance of the cochlea is achieved by mastering the anatomical relationship of the cochlea to the various surrounding structures.

Other anatomical structures that may be at risk are the carotid artery and temporal lobe. Anatomical structures are at risk both from direct damage from the high-speed drill and from the heat generated by using a diamond bur. For this reason bone removal is performed with continuous cooling irrigation, and these procedures should only be performed after adequate training and rehearsal in the cadaver laboratory.

◆ Outcomes

The results of both microsurgery and stereotactic radiosurgery have been presented in the neurosurgical literature. However, the results of surgical series are more prevalent due to the lack of long-term experience with stereotactic radiosurgery for trigeminal schwannomas in a large number of patients. Nevertheless, the initial results of stereotactic radiosurgery have been promising.

The largest series of trigeminal schwannomas treated by stereotactic radiosurgery reported to date has been sixteen (Huang et al). All patients presented with trigeminal sensory symptoms. Nine patients had ganglion-type tumors, six patients had tumors involving the root, and one patient had a peripheral mandibular branch tumor. Patients were treated with protocols that delivered 12 to 20 Gy at the margin of the tumor, which represented the 50% isodose curve. Average follow-up was 44 months with a range of 8 to 116 months. Nine of 16 patients had a decrease in size of their tumor after treatment. Seven patients demonstrated no further growth of the tumor at follow-up. The authors reported five of the 16 patients had improved clinical symptoms;

however, the report did not specify what deficits improved. The symptoms that patients presented with included 10 of 16 with decreased corneal response. Fifty percent of patients presented with an ocular motor abnormality, mostly abducens nerve paresis. Two patients presented with facial nerve involvement and three patients with deficits involving the vestibulocochlear nerve. Significantly, no new cranial nerve deficits were reported in any of the patients treated with radiosurgery. Two patients died of unrelated causes.

The treatment results of microsurgical series have varied to a significant degree depending upon the epoch in which they were collected. Contemporary series have largely utilized the extradural strategies for removing these tumors. The result of this shift in surgical philosophy has resulted in much better outcomes from microsurgical resection. In 1994, Dolenc reported the largest series to date of surgically treated trigeminal schwannomas by a single surgeon. He reported a 100% total resection rate in the over 40 patients that he treated. The series did not include any malignant tumors. Dolenc utilized an entirely extradural strategy for all tumors and reported excellent results. No patient died and there were no major surgical morbidities reported. Five of his patients had diplopia from abducens palsy, all of which were reported to have completely resolved. Regarding trigeminal function, 10 patients had slightly worsened hypesthesia, nine remained unchanged, and 11 improved. Day and Fukushima reported their series of 39 tumors in 1998, all of which were treated via an extradural strategy except for nine patients with root-type tumors in the series. As in Dolenc's series there was no perioperative mortality. The majority of patients presented with trigeminal hypesthesia. Of the 32 patients with decreased sensation, 25 remained with some degree of hypesthesia after surgery. Six patients had new hypesthesia after surgery. Thirteen patients prior to surgery had trigeminal distribution pain. Only one of these patients continued to have pain after surgery. Five patients were left with hypesthesia and 20 with motor weakness of the trigeminal nerve. Of the seven patients with double vision five experienced relief after surgery. The clinical outcomes in these two series were in general agreement with those in smaller series published recently. McCormick et al observed a greater number of new postoperative deficits; however, the majority of these resolved within weeks of surgery. The majority of patients in this series failed to realize significant resolution of trigeminal hypesthesia. The contemporary series reported by Pollack et al included 16 patients, 14 of which had immediate postoperative trigeminal dysfunction. Only seven patients had permanent hypesthesia. Five of their patients had new cranial nerve deficits, four of which improved within 6 months. In general, complications reported in contemporary microsurgical series have been uniformly low, with a low chance of recurrence.

◆ Summary

Trigeminal neurinomas are uncommon tumors that have traditionally been treated by microsurgical removal. The results of treatment in contemporary series have generally demonstrated low complication rates with a low chance of recurrence. Recurrent tumors have also been treated with microsurgical removal. The surgical approach is dictated by the tumor classification, which is based upon anatomical location. More recently a growing number of patients are being treated with stereotactic radiosurgery. The number of reports has been limited, with short follow-up periods; however, the morbidity and mortality figures with this strategy are exceptionally low. Patients are currently best treated by considering the available options and applying the appropriate strategy that will result in the lowest morbidity in the individual case.

29

Surgical Management of Intracranial Glomus Tumors

L. Madison Michael II, Wayne Hamm, and Jon H. Robertson

Glomus jugulare tumors pose a formidable challenge to the treating surgeon. Because they typically arise from glomus bodies positioned in the dome of the jugular bulb, the neoplasm is intimately associated with critical neurovascular structures. A clear understanding of the anatomy of the jugular foramen and the natural history of glomus jugulare tumors is necessary for successful treatment of these lesions.

Over the past 5 decades, continual efforts have focused on total surgical removal. Earlier treatments focused on limited resection secondary to the relative inaccessibility of the jugular bulb region, the potential for harming the surrounding neurovasculature, and the extremely vascular nature of these tumors. As experience was gained, innovative surgical procedures were developed, most notably the combined lateral skull base approaches and the infratemporal approach. In addition to the advancements in surgical approaches, the implementation of adjunctive therapies, such as selective embolization, and the aggressive treatment of postoperative neurological deficits have resulted in dramatic improvements in long-term outcomes.

◆ Patient Selection

Achieving an optimal treatment outcome is directly related to the proper choice of a management strategy unique for each patient. A multidisciplinary team utilizes a comprehensive and selective approach in defining the appropriate treatment regimen for a particular lesion. Risk factors considered include age, general medical condition, extent of tumor, and the presence of neurological deficits.

Symptomatic elderly patients or those with significant medical conditions are best treated with palliative radiotherapy, despite the lack of conclusive data establishing its efficacy. In extensive tumors in which it is felt significant postoperative morbidity will occur, subtotal resection with or without postoperative radiation may be the treatment of choice. This decision changes with the skill of the surgeon; we have found increasing confidence in treating larger tumors as experience is gained. In selected patients with static cranial nerve deficits and no evidence of brain stem compression, observation alone may be warranted.

Once the decision is made for surgical treatment, judgment must be used with regard to subtotal versus gross total resection. Infiltration of surrounding structures and abolition of anatomical planes occur with this neoplasm and make complete extirpation difficult. If surgical planes are preserved, then total resection may be accomplished with minimal morbidity. However, if surgical planes are obliterated, then subtotal resection may be the treatment of choice. This is especially true in patients with no preoperative cranial nerve deficits who may not be able to compensate postoperatively.

◆ Preoperative Preparation

The surgical removal of glomus jugulare tumors requires a complete and thorough preoperative evaluation involving a multidisciplinary team. Careful attention is given to the medical condition of the patient, extent of disease and involvement of the surrounding neurovascular structures, vascular supply of the tumor, and the presence or absence of catecholamine secretion.

Plain skull x-rays are of limited benefit, but they may show enlargement of the jugular foramen. A computed tomographic scan with thin cuts defines the extent of temporal bone involvement by the tumor and the altered anatomy of the jugular foramen **(Fig. 29–1)**. Magnetic resonance imaging with and without contrast reveals excellent definition of the soft tissue component of the tumor at the level of the skull base and extracranial space **(Fig. 29–2)**.

Four-vessel cerebral angiography should be performed in all cases as a definitive diagnostic study to allow proper treatment planning. One often finds rich arterial contributions to the tumor, mostly from the ascending pharyngeal and caroticotympanic arteries **(Fig. 29–3)**. In large tumors, a significant arterial contribution may be found from the internal carotid vessel wall when the artery is encased by tumor growth. An examination of the late venous phase is mandatory to determine the patency of the sigmoid–jugular venous system and to identify unusual collateral venous outflow, which has developed in response to the tumor. The contralateral jugular vein should also be visualized because it may be blocked in cases of multicentric tumors. The sigmoid–jugular venous system may be blocked at any level from compression or intraluminal invasion by tumor. Evaluating the intraluminal extent of the tumor aids in determining the proper level for ligation of the sigmoid sinus and jugular vein in the surgical removal of the tumor.

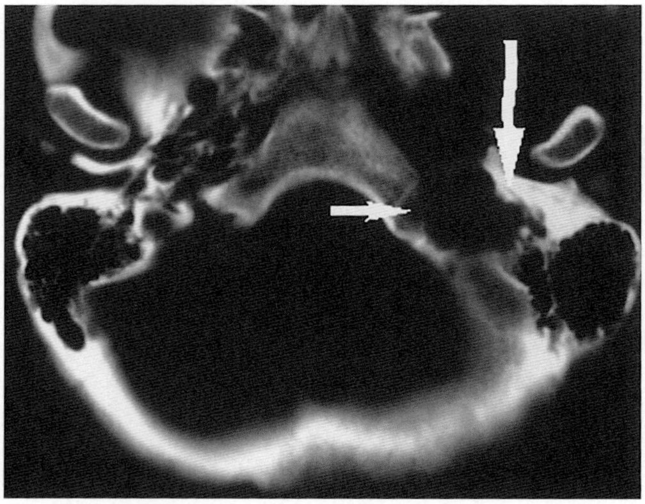

Figure 29–1 Axial computed tomographic scan without contrast reveals a destructive lesion of the left jugular foramen region consistent with a glomus jugulare tumor. Note expansion of the jugular foramen **(straight arrow)** and obliteration of the jugular spine **(curved arrow).**

Patients with tumors that encase or displace the carotid artery must be evaluated for the possibility of arterial sacrifice or bypass. An assessment of the collateral circulation during the arterial phase of the angiogram gives one some initial insight into whether the patient would tolerate permanent occlusion of the artery. The gold standard for determination is temporary balloon test occlusion, which may be performed during the angiographic study. Temporary occlusion of the internal carotid artery identifies the majority of individuals tolerant of carotid artery sacrifice intraoperatively. However, there is no single test or combination of tests that can absolutely insure the absence of a cerebrovascular accident following occlusion of an internal carotid. Therefore, ligation of the carotid artery is a feasible option if the patient tolerates disruption of flow, but not without risk. If the patient fails the test occlusion, then a bypass or subtotal resection of tumor is recommended.

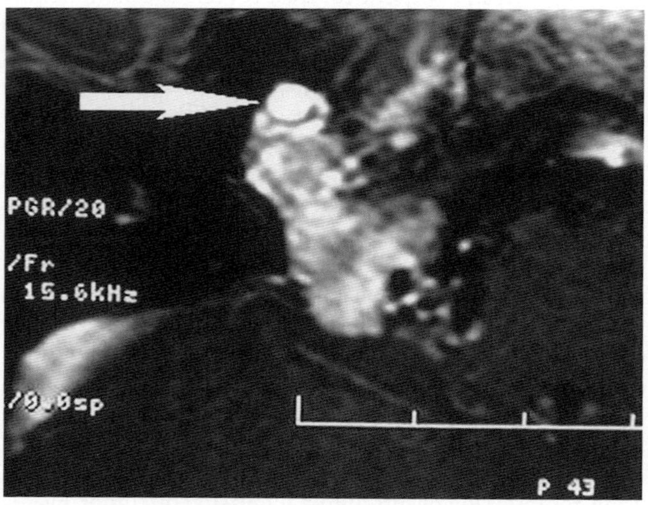

Figure 29–2 Axial magnetic resonance imaging with contrast shows an intensely enhancing, lobulated mass in the right jugular foramen with extraforaminal extension. The carotid artery is seen anteriorly to the mass **(arrow).**

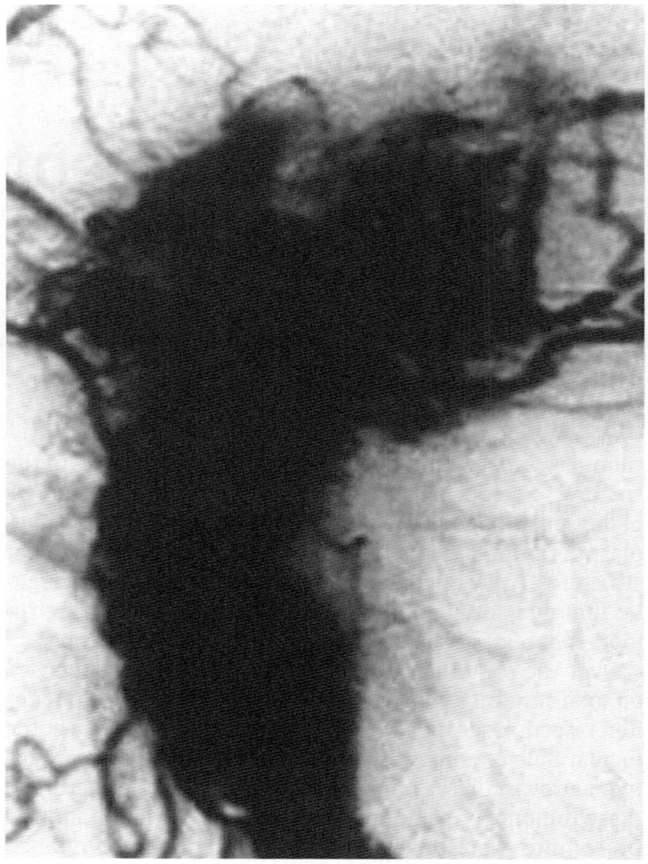

Figure 29–3 An intense vascular blush reveals the rich arterial supply to the tumor after carotid artery injection.

A major advancement in the surgical treatment of glomus jugulare tumors over the past 2 decades has been the development and application of preoperative superselective embolization. Performed by the interventional radiologist 24 to 48 hours prior to surgery, embolic materials or coils are used to selectively occlude the arterial feeders of these complex vascular tumors. The current state of technology and expertise in interventional radiology has significantly reduced the incidence of stroke and cranial nerve injury experienced during the early years of application. The dramatic reduction in blood loss following successful embolization of a glomus jugulare tumor results in less chance of injury to vital structures because less coagulation or packing is required to control bleeding.

In a minority of cases, glomus jugulare tumors secrete catecholamines. An excess of catecholamines can elevate the blood pressure. Manipulation of the tumor during surgery may result in significant intraoperative hypertension, which may be uncontrollable. A preoperative 24-hour urine specimen is performed to detect the presence of vanillyl-mandelic acid, metanephrines, and free catecholamines. If present, a pharmacological blockade is performed with the use of an α-blocker, and this is usually initiated 2 weeks before the operation. A β-blocker is given ~24 hours before surgery to avoid tachycardia.

Other testing completed during the preoperative period includes routine audiometry to establish the function of the hearing apparatus. Routine laboratory studies should include a peripheral blood count and coagulation panel because of the highly vascular nature of these tumors with anticipated blood loss.

◆ Operative Procedure

Anesthesia and Monitoring

The goal of general anesthesia for glomus jugulare tumors is to provide a quiet surgical field and ample working space for multiple surgical teams. One must be prepared for a lengthy operation with multiple stages that may involve considerable blood loss and cranial nerve dysfunction. A thorough discussion of the anesthetic plan, to include prolonged intubation and invasive monitoring, should precede surgery.

A smooth induction with a one-time dose of a nondepolarizing muscle relaxant facilitates intubation with a reinforced tube. After the airway is secured, a nasogastric tube is placed. Continuous systemic monitoring is essential and includes placement of an arterial line (in the contralateral radial artery), a central line (placed in the femoral vein), a Foley catheter, and a rectal temperature probe. Facial nerve monitoring is performed routinely. Glossopharyngeal and vagal nerves are monitored in selective cases, only if the size of the tumor suggests the potential for injury. Blood gases and electrolytes are evaluated periodically as well as blood sugars when indicated. Maintenance of anesthesia is accomplished with a continuous infusion of narcotic (Sufenta) plus a lowered concentration of inhalation agent.

Emergence from anesthesia should include rigid blood pressure control. Strict maintenance of blood pressure control should occur in the first 12 hours in the postoperative period. We commonly use a continuous infusion of the calcium channel blocker Cardene for its ease of titration and short-acting effects.

In tumors involving the jugular fossa, in the absence of preexisting lower cranial nerve deficit, conservative airway management immediately postoperatively with continued intubation during the initial 12 to 24 hours is encouraged. In patients with long-standing cranial nerve deficits, with a surgery ending in less than 8 hours, and with no comorbidity considerations, a more aggressive approach to extubation may be considered. Patients with brain stem compression should be managed conservatively with regard to extubation.

Positioning

Positioning of the patient has two main goals **(Fig. 29–4)**. First is optimal surgical access by multiple surgical teams.

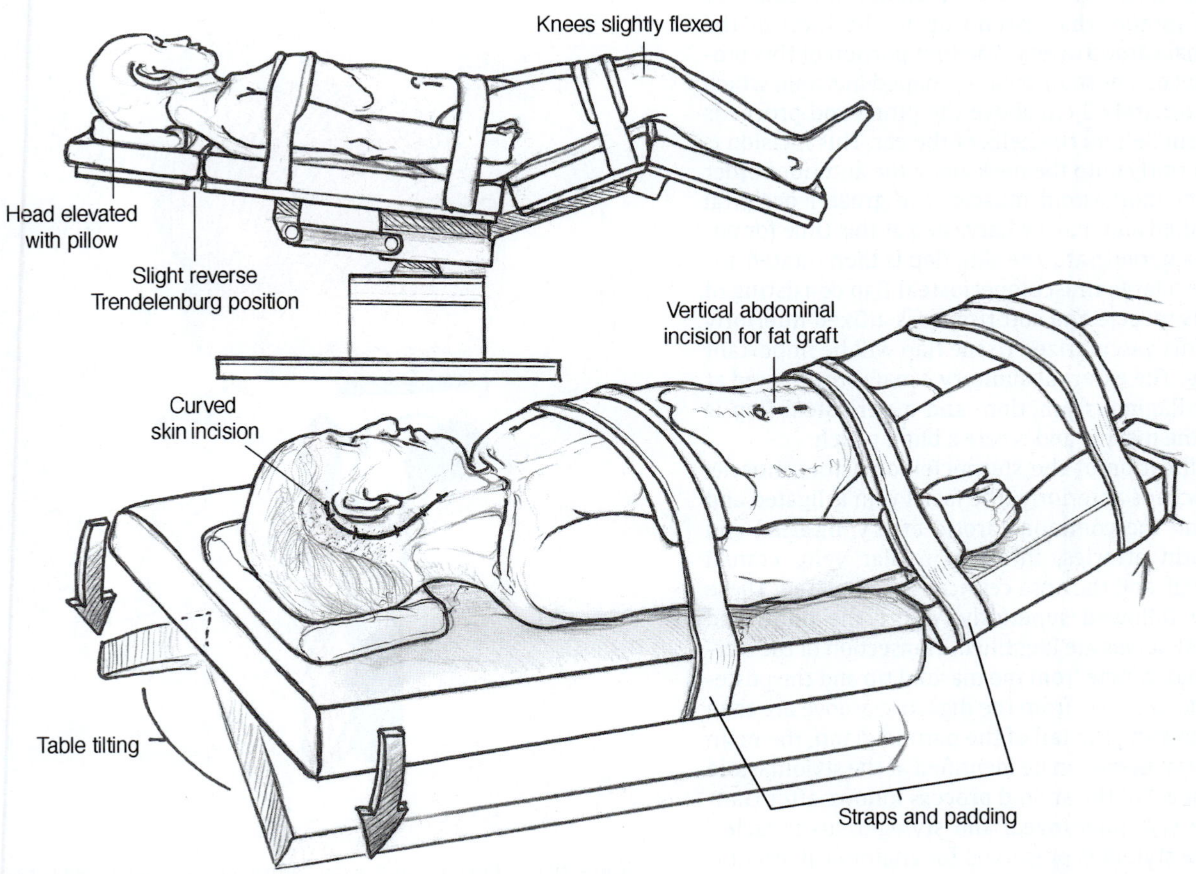

Figure 29–4 Positioning of the patient. The head is not placed in a fixed headrest so that the surgeon is able to turn the head and neck as desired. Additional rotation in either direction can be accomplished by turning the bed.

The second goal is to facilitate venous drainage. We accomplish these goals by placing the patient supine in a flexed position, head up, with the legs slightly bent at the knees. The head is not placed in a fixed headrest; instead, the head and neck are available for turning according to surgeon preference. The arms are tucked at the patient's side after each arm is placed in slight flexion at the elbow with the hands open and flexed. Straps are padded with cushioning and placed across the patient's chest, hips, and legs to allow for full tilt of the table in any direction.

Operative Approaches

The operative approach is dictated by the extent of the tumor mass. In glomus jugulare tumors, the size of the tumor and the need for control of the carotid artery mandate individualization of the surgical technique. Three techniques are described here: the combined lateral skull base approach, the modified lateral skull base approach, and the infratemporal fossa approach. Modifications of these approaches may be used for tumors with intracranial extension. These include a retrosigmoid, presigmoid, retrolabyrinthine, translabyrinthine, or transcochlear approach.

The Combined Lateral Skull Base Approach

High Cervical Exposure

This approach is the procedure of choice for small or medium-size tumors that extend up to the level of the petrous internal carotid artery. The first portion of this procedure consists of a postauricular C-shaped incision, which begins approximately 3 cm above the pinna and proceeds posteriorly 3 cm behind the helix of the ear. This incision is continued inferiorly onto the neck along the anterior border of the sternocleidomastoid muscle. The greater occipital nerve is identified and may be harvested at this time for potential use as a nerve graft. The skin flap is then rotated anteriorly, while a large musculoperiosteal flap consisting of the temporalis muscle and soft tissues is affixed inferiorly with hooks. This vascularized tissue flap will be important during closure. The external auditory canal is transected at the bony–cartilaginous junction, and a periosteal flap is used to close the meatus and create a blind pouch.

After identification of the sternocleidomastoid muscle, dissection proceeds anteriorly. The facial vein is ligated and transected, and the common carotid artery, internal and external carotid arteries, internal jugular vein, cranial nerves X and XII, and the ansa cervicalis are isolated. These structures are followed superiorly, where the ninth and eleventh cranial nerves are identified. Transection of the sternocleidomastoid muscle from the mastoid tip and the posterior belly of the digastric from the digastric groove are then completed. Elevating the tail of the parotid gland, the main trunk of the facial nerve can be identified at the stylomastoid foramen. Removal of the styloid process follows after transection of the stylopharyngeal and styloglossus muscles. The base of the styloid is preserved for anatomical orientation, and direct access to the high cervical carotid artery and jugular foramen region is now possible. Removal of the styloid process also allows identification of the ninth cranial nerve turning forward, crossing the lateral surface of the internal carotid artery.

Palpation of the transverse process of the first cervical vertebra, the base of the styloid process, and the mastoid tip provides constant bony landmarks for orientation with respect to the jugular foramen.

The jugular vein is found resting on the rectus capitis lateralis muscle, which extends from the transverse process of C1 to the posterior bony margin of the jugular foramen. The transverse process of the first cervical vertebra may be removed for exposure; however, care should be taken to identify and protect the vertebral artery. The eleventh cranial nerve is usually identified as it crosses over the anterior surface of the jugular vein at or above the level of the transverse process of C1 to turn posterior to enter the sternocleidomastoid muscle. Soft tissues surrounding the jugular foramen may be removed, allowing a 270 degree control of the jugular vein **(Fig. 29–5).** The medial margin of the jugular foramen is not violated in the dissection to protect the lower cranial nerves as they exit the skull base.

Temporal Bone Exposure

The initial step involves a simple mastoidectomy. The bone of the external ear canal is removed followed by disarticulation

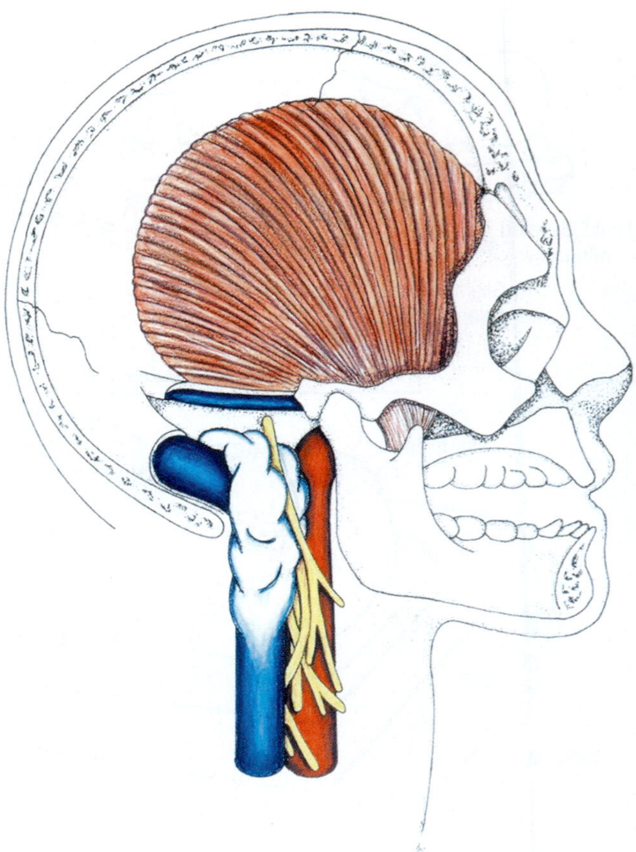

Figure 29–5 Proximal and distal control of the jugular vein is obtained. A 270 degree exposure of the jugular foramen provides the surgeon excellent visualization of the neurovascular anatomy.

of the incostapedial joint. This allows removal of the tympanic membrane, malleus, and incus. Care is taken to protect the stapes. If tumor is present in the middle ear, it is mobilized inferiorly. One must take caution to remain below the labyrinth to avoid loss of hearing. In patients with nonserviceable hearing, removal of the cochlea and labyrinth may be necessary for tumor exposure. Skeletonization of the mastoid and tympanic segments of the facial nerve ensues, and the nerve is traced superiorly to the geniculate ganglion and drilled from the fallopian canal. Fibrous attachments along the course of the nerve are then cut sharply. Depending upon the size and extent of the tumor, the greater superficial petrosal nerve and the chorda tympani may be sectioned, and the facial nerve mobilized anteriorly. Drilling of the anterior epitympanum to soft tissue depth forms a tangential notch where the facial nerve can be placed. The proximal nerve lies within this groove and the distal portion within the parotid gland. Care is taken for the remainder of the procedure to protect the nerve from manipulation. If it is found that the nerve is directly involved with tumor during the exposure, the diseased portion may be resected, and an interposition nerve graft placed.

Bone overlying the sigmoid sinus is drilled away, and the presigmoid and retrosigmoid bone is removed to expose the posterior fossa dura. With the skull base cleared of attachments (as performed during the high cervical exposure), drilling is continued to reveal the tumor as well as the jugular bulb. This involves removal of all bone between the posterior end of the digastric groove and the jugular foramen.

Attention is then turned to obtaining distal control of the carotid artery. The bony tympanum, hypotympanum, and roof of the glenoid fossa may be drilled away. The mandibular condyle is displaced anteroinferiorly or resected, depending on the need for exposure. In our experience, resection of the condyle produces less postoperative pain with little restriction on range of motion. Drilling continues beginning at the entrance of the internal carotid artery into the carotid canal. The artery is followed superiorly to the genu adjacent to the eustachian tube and cochlea. If the horizontal segment needs to be exposed, the eustachian tube is divided, inverted, and obliterated with muscle graft, bone wax, and fibrin glue.

Tumor Removal

The jugular vein inferior to intraluminal tumor extension is ligated with a silk suture and sharply divided **(Fig. 29–6).** This maneuver is necessary to prevent embolization of tumor present in the jugular vein distally into the superior vena cava as the tumor is manipulated in its removal. The sigmoid sinus is closed with a silk suture ligature distal to the entry of the superior petrosal sinus into the junction of the transverse and sigmoid sinuses **(Fig. 29–7).** Closure of the sigmoid sinus in this manner will allow venous drainage from the superior petrosal sinus in a retrograde fashion. The lateral wall of the sigmoid sinus is resected and mobilized toward the jugular bulb. Working from above and below the bulb, the tumor is removed piecemeal. It is very important to maintain the medial wall of the vein at this point to protect the lower cranial nerves. Profuse bleeding can occur within the jugular bulb from the inferior petrosal sinus, often from multiple channels. Gentle packing with Surgicel or soft

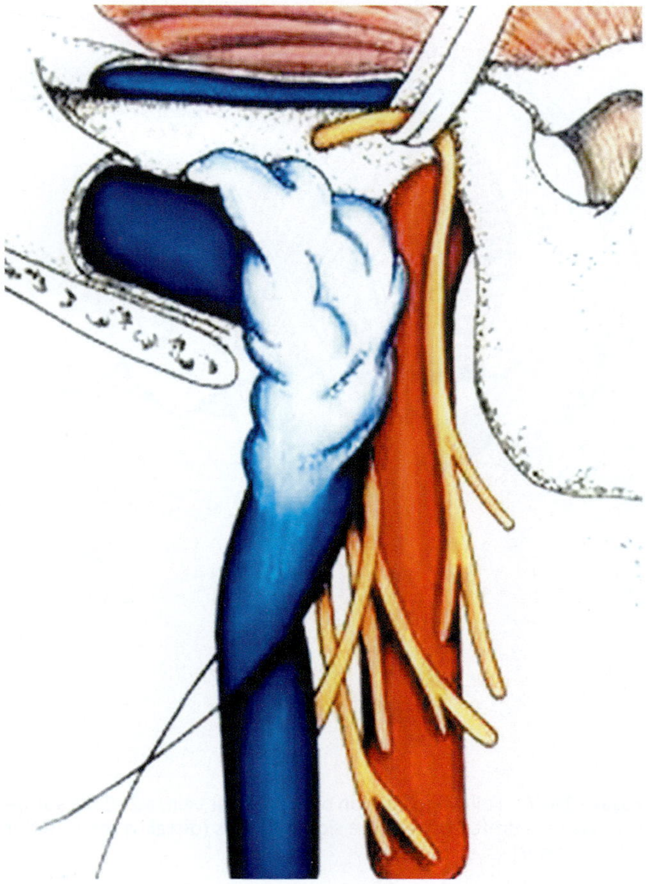

Figure 29–6 The facial nerve has been transposed anteriorly. Ligation of the distal jugular vein is performed inferior to the level of tumor extension.

bone wax will usually control this bleeding, which is predominantly venous in origin, if preoperative embolization of the tumor has been successful. Care must be taken to avoid using bipolar cautery or excessive compression with cottonoid pledgets to control bleeding along the medial wall of the jugular bulb. Failure to do so will often result in lower cranial nerve injuries. During the final steps of tumor dissection, one must directly visualize the carotid artery and the lower cranial nerves to avoid injury **(Fig. 29–8).**

Most tumors that invade the posterior fossa tend to preserve dural integrity and push it medially. Taking care to maintain this layer can help reduce the risk of postoperative cerebrospinal fluid (CSF) leakage. Occurring less often, however, there is no layer of dura between the tumor and the contents of the posterior fossa.

Wound Closure

The facial nerve remains in the anterior position. If a dural defect is present, it is either repaired primarily or with the use of a graft in a watertight fashion. Fat harvested from the abdomen is then placed into the dead space of the wound **(Fig. 29–9).** The vascularized musculoperiosteal flap developed earlier is then placed over the fat and tacked down to the soft tissue edges. Lumbar drainage is occasionally used in the postoperative period to avoid CSF leakage.

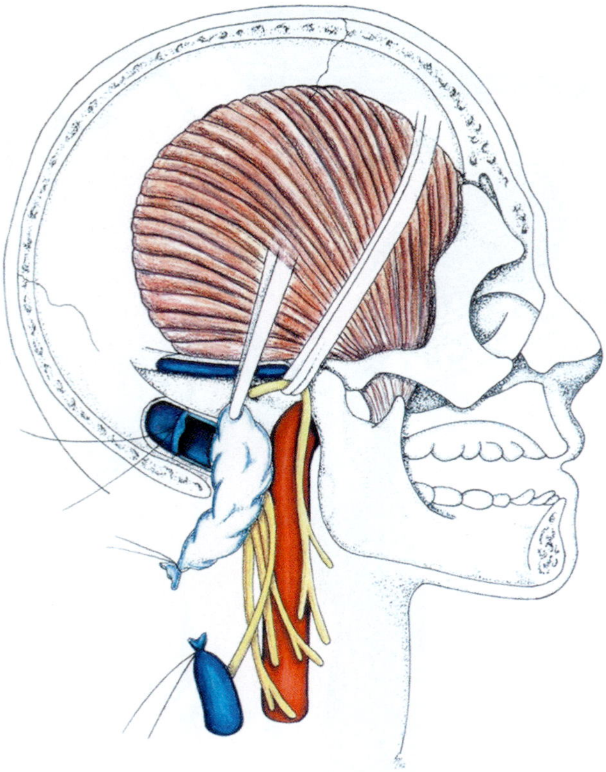

Figure 29–7 Following ligation of the jugular vein, a 2–0 silk suture is passed circumferential to the sigmoid sinus (distal to the superior petrosal sinus).

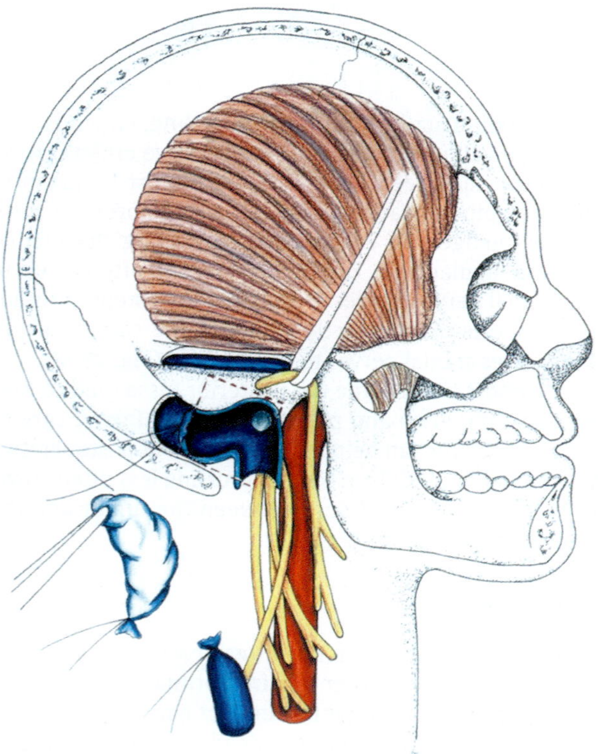

Figure 29–8 Tumor removal. Care must be taken to preserve the medial wall of the jugular bulb to ensure protection of the lower cranial nerves. The lateral wall of the sigmoid sinus is resected and mobilized toward the jugular bulb.

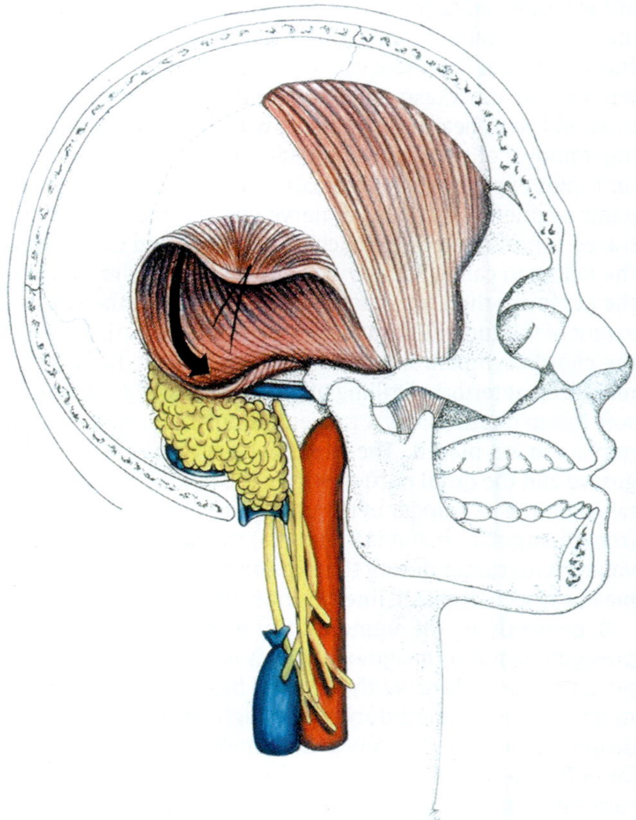

Figure 29–9 Fat harvested from the abdomen is placed within the dead space of the wound. The vascularized musculoperiosteal flap is then mobilized and placed over the fat. Sutures are then used to affix the flap to the soft tissue edges.

The Modified Lateral Skull Base Approach

This approach is used for patients with small tumors localized to the region of the jugular bulb. Often, this select group of patients has functional preoperative hearing, and it is necessary to preserve middle ear function. The initial phase of the operation involves the high cervical dissection as described earlier. However, only the posterior half of the external canal is incised. One proceeds with a simple mastoidectomy but limits the bone removal to preserve the posterior bony canal, tympanic membrane, and ossicles **(Fig. 29–10)**. The mastoid segment of the facial nerve is mobilized and may be manipulated anteriorly or posteriorly as needed for tumor resection. Tumor that is present in the middle ear may be removed through the facial recess.

The Infratemporal Fossa Approach

The infratemporal fossa approach is used for larger tumors with extensive involvement of the petrous carotid artery. Further dissection is performed anterior to the ear canal to expose the infratemporal fossa. Bone removal is similar to the combined lateral skull base approach, but continued work is focused anteriorly to expose the carotid artery to the cavernous sinus.

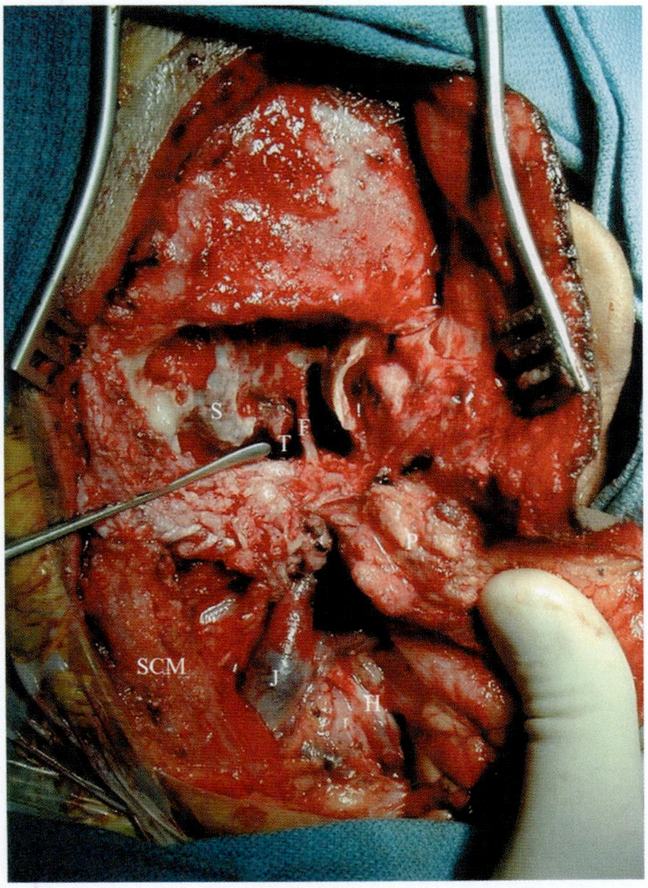

Figure 29–10 Intraoperative photograph illustrating the modified lateral skull base approach. A simple mastoidectomy has been performed, and the mastoid segment of the facial nerve (F) is skeletonized. The parotid gland (P) is mobilized anteriorly. With the exception of the hypoglossal nerve (H), the lower cranial nerves are hidden deep to the jugular vein (J). Tumor (T) is visualized in the region of the jugular bulb. SCM, sternocleidomastoid.

◆ Postoperative Management

Cranial Nerve Palsy

Growth of a glomus jugulare tumor may result in direct compression or invasion of cranial nerves in the region of the jugular bulb or jugular foramen. Most commonly affected are the lower cranial nerves, and less frequently the facial nerve. Lack of preoperative cranial nerve dysfunction may not correlate with the finding at surgery of tumor invasion of a particular cranial nerve. An acute loss of lower cranial nerve function can be devastating if not properly managed, whereas those patients with chronic loss of function can usually compensate for the deficit. The aggressive management of postoperative cranial neuropathies is absolutely critical to a successful surgical outcome.

Injury to the lower cranial nerves is one of the primary risks when operating on glomus jugulare tumors. Acute loss of a single lower cranial nerve is usually tolerated, but loss of multiple lower cranial nerves or the vagus nerve may cause a sudden incoordination of swallowing and lead to life-threatening aspiration pneumonia. An acute glossopharyngeal and vagal palsy should be aggressively treated with early placement of a gastrostomy tube. Immediately following the operation, the patient may not manifest symptoms of aspiration secondary to swelling of the vocal cord from the endotracheal tube. However, as the swelling resolves, the patient is at increased risk for aspiration. If the nerve is expected to recover, injection of the vocal cord with Gelfoam will suffice to temporarily protect the patient. If it is not expected to recover, permanent medialization of the vocal cord is recommended. Most patients with preservation of the anatomical continuity of the cranial nerves compensate for swallowing dysfunction and improve in phonation over a 3-month period, at which time the gastrostomy tube can be removed. There is the rare patient that presents with regurgitation through the nose secondary to paralysis of the palate, and a palatoplasty will effectively correct this. Persistent dysphagia resulting in recurrent aspiration despite aggressive therapy may require a cricopharyngeal myotomy.

Protection of the eye in a patient with facial nerve palsy is paramount. In the acute postoperative period, a protective eye patch and lubrication are necessary. If the patient's facial palsy is anticipated to persist for beyond 2 months, augmentation of eyelid closure with implantation of a gold weight is recommended. As long as there is anatomical continuity of the nerve, recovery should ensue. In patients in whom the continuity is not preserved, a facial to hypoglossal anastomosis is performed during the early postoperative period as the patient's condition permits.

Cerebrospinal Fluid Leakage and Wound Healing

CSF leakage following resection of glomus jugulare tumors is related to several factors; namely, the size of the tumor and involvement of the dura, nutritional status of the patient, and the state of CSF dynamics.

Careful attention is paid to achieving a watertight closure of the dura with either a primary repair or a fascial graft. However, at the level of the jugular foramen, there is usually a dural defect. This is repaired using a fat graft to obliterate the dead space, placement of a vascularized graft over the surgical defect, followed by a multilayered tissue closure. A postoperative lumbar drain may be used. Rhinorrhea and otorrhea are prevented by closure of the eustachian tube and external auditory canal.

Early nutritional supplementation is mandatory to promote tissue healing. If the patient is not able to tolerate feedings by mouth, a small-diameter feeding tube is inserted within the first 24 hours. Alimentation is begun immediately.

Altered CSF dynamics may lead to postoperative hydrocephalus and resultant CSF leakage. This may be due to blood, bone dust, or occlusion of the venous circulation at the level of the jugular bulb. The use of continuous lumbar drainage for 3 to 7 days after surgery aids in the normalization of intracranial pressure and prevents accumulation of fluid under the wound flap. This promotes sealing of the dural defect and healing of the wound. We have found that the impairment of CSF absorption is usually transient; thus obviating the need for permanent CSF diversion.

Vascular Injury

In larger tumors that encase the internal carotid artery, there is a risk of injury to the artery itself. Every patient that demonstrates involvement of the carotid artery undergoes temporary balloon test occlusion to determine the adequacy of collateral circulation. Surgical removal of tumor proceeds with the intent of preserving the internal carotid artery. If injury to the carotid artery should occur, temporary occlusion of the artery followed by a primary repair is attempted using 9–0 Prolene. If this can't be performed, then the results of the balloon occlusion test dictate whether the artery is sacrificed or whether an arterial bypass is utilized. We use a saphenous vein interposition graft if a bypass is necessary.

◆ Conclusion

Although appearing histologically benign, glomus jugulare tumors are characterized by unpredictable biological behavior. Because they originate in the jugular bulb region, the neoplasm presents a significant surgical challenge. Successful treatment of glomus jugulare tumors mandates a clear understanding of the anatomy of the jugular foramen and the natural history of glomus jugulare tumors. With the significant advances in surgical approaches to the lateral skull base, surgeons can now accomplish complete extirpation of glomus jugulare tumors with low morbidity rates and good long-term outcomes.

Section VII

Skull Base Approaches

30

Preauricular Transzygomatic Subtemporal and Infratemporal Approaches to the Skull Base

Amin B. Kassam, Arlan H. Mintz, Ajith Thomas, Carl H. Snyderman, Paul A. Gardner, and Ricardo L. Carrau

Subtemporal approaches can provide direct access to lesions located deep within the middle cranial fossa, tentorial notch, interpeduncular cistern, cavernous sinus, upper third of the clivus, petrous segment of the carotid artery, and infratemporal fossa. Dr. Charles Drake first popularized the subtemporal approach for posterior circulation aneurysms by demonstrating its usefulness in exposing aneurysms with low-lying necks below the posterior clinoid process. In addition to posterior fossa aneurysms, a wide variety of neoplastic lesions involving this area can also be removed, including epidermoid cysts, cholesterol granulomas, meningiomas, and chordomas.

To best understand these corridors it is imperative to have a thorough understanding of the complex anatomy in this space. We find it useful to segregate the anatomy into osseous, soft tissue, and vascular elements. This chapter discusses the preauricular and transzygomatic approaches to the middle cranial and infratemporal fossae. We will review these approaches by discussing the relevant anatomical relationships, then focusing on patient considerations, followed by a more detailed description of individual approaches.

◆ Anatomy

Accessing the deep portion of the middle cranial fossa, upper portion of the clivus, and petroclival junction can prove to be challenging and requires a thorough understanding of the regional anatomy. A variety of anatomical corridors have been created to reduce the amount of brain and neurovascular manipulation required to access lesions in this space.

Osseous Elements

Anatomical corridors needed to access the subtemporal and infratemporal space require the segmental removal of the osseous framework that protects the region. The key osseous anatomical boundaries surrounding this space can be divided into lateral and medial elements. The lateral osseous framework consists of the superior and lateral wall of the orbit anteriorly, the arch of the zygoma anterolaterally, the root of the zygoma and temporomandibular joint posterolaterally, as well as the squamous temporal bone **(Fig. 30–1A).** The medial osseous framework consists anteriorly of the posterior clinoids and dorsum sella as it transitions to the upper third of the clivus; the medial margin posteriorly is formed by the petrous bone **(Fig. 30–1B).** The middle cranial fossa then sits like a saddle within these boundaries, separating itself from the infratemporal fossa below. It is very useful to consider the medial and lateral pterygoid plates as the anterior and inferior boundary of the middle cranial fossa as it transitions into the infratemporal fossa **(Fig. 30–1C).**

Soft Tissue and Vascular Elements

The critical soft tissue components of this space consist of the temporalis muscle as it envelops the zygoma attaching to the temporal bone, as well as the masseter and pterygoid muscles below as they attach to the pterygoid plates. Within this soft tissue lies the pterygopalatine plexus, which represents a rich venous plexus that can bleed significantly. Finally, where the temporal bone curves inferiorly and begins to transition to the infratemporal fossa just deep to the level of the pterygopalatine plexus are found the great foramina of the middle cranial fossa **(Fig. 30–1B).** Starting anteriorly these are represented by the foramen rotundum (V2), foramen ovale (V3), and foramen spinosum (middle meningeal artery). It is important to note that the foramen rotundum emerges from the middle cranial fossa obliquely at approximately a 45 degree angle, whereas the foramen ovale emerges in the same plane or parallel to the middle cranial fossa **(Fig. 30–1B).** Just medial to foramen ovale is the lateral wall of the carotid artery within its canal as it courses horizontally from the posterior genu toward the cavernous sinus.

Anatomical Corridors

In designing a corridor for accessing a lesion in this location we find it useful to conceptualize the location of the lesion in three axes: lateral to medial in the axial plane (x-axis), anterior to posterior in the axial plane (y-axis), and superior to inferior in the coronal plane (z-axis, **Fig. 30–1A,B).** Osseous elements required to generate the corridor will depend on these considerations.

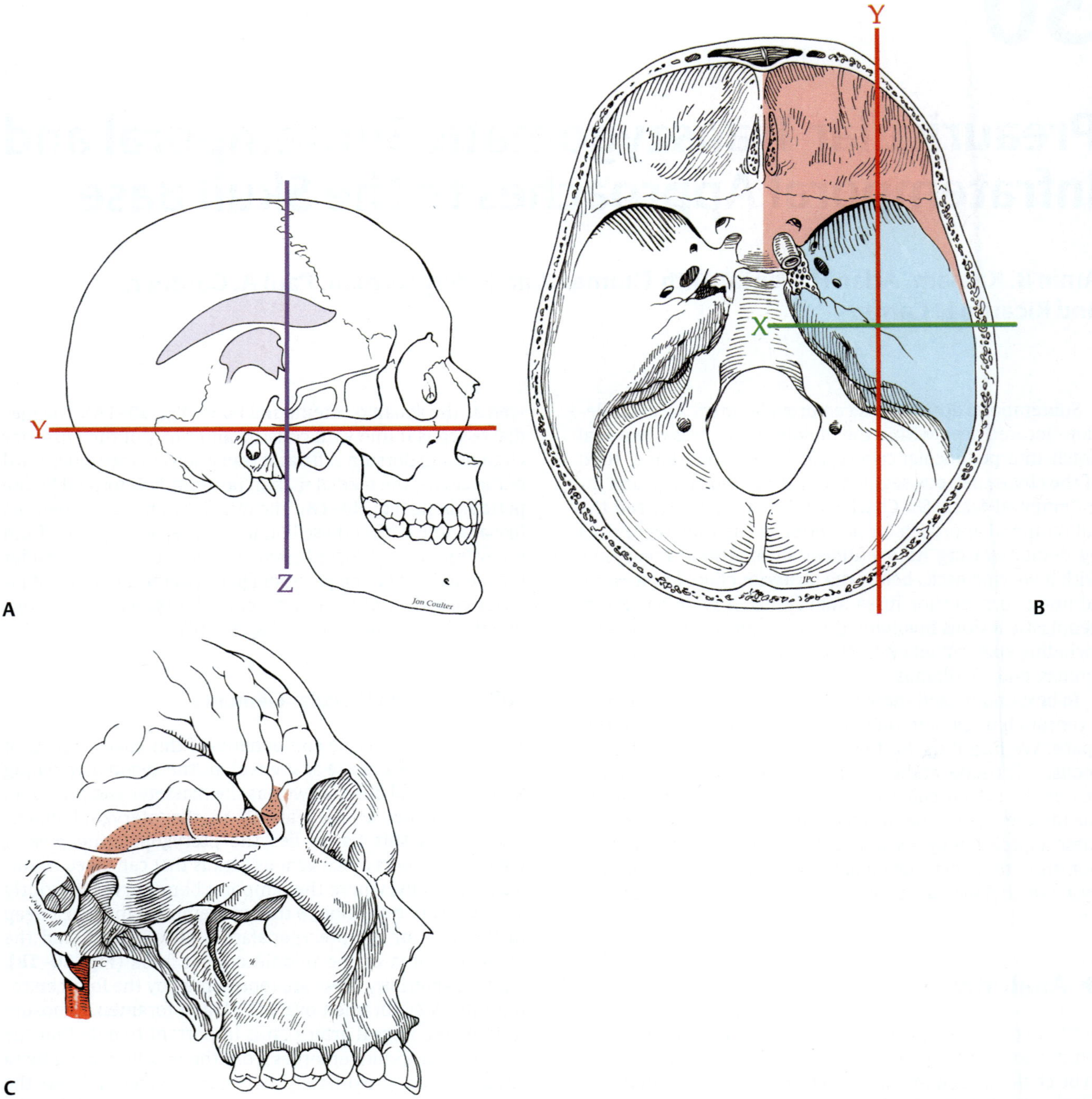

Figure 30–1 **(A)** The *y*- and *z*-axis relationships on a lateral skull projection. Note the *z*-axis provides access along the superior-inferior plane as demonstrated by the osseous and intracranial structures, whereas the *y*-axis is along the anterior-posterior plane. **(B)** An axial skull showing the *x*- and *y*-axis along with the osseous framework. The anterior and middle cranial fossae are highlighted. The course of the internal carotid artery (ICA) through the cavernous sinus and the location of the important middle fossa foramina are illustrated. **(C)** A lateral skull in an oblique view from below. The infratemporal is outlined as well as the course of the ICA from the vertical portion to the supraclinoidal portion.

In general, removal of the zygoma primarily provides for access along the *z*-axis (i.e., along the axis of the third ventricle, clivus, and infratemporal fossa in a superior-inferior plane) **(Fig. 30–2A).** The removal of the lateral wall of the orbit provides for increased lateral to medial access along the *x*-axis, minimizing the retraction to reach the medial osseous framework, in particular the transition between the anterior and middle cranial fossa **(Fig. 30–2B,C).** To gain progressive anterior to posterior access along the *y*-axis of the middle cranial fossa, the zygomatic osteotomies can be extended from the frontozygomatic suture to the temporomandibular joint (TMJ) as needed **(Fig. 30–2A,C).** This essentially provides access along the course of the carotid artery from the transition of the vertical segment into the posterior genu under the TMJ and glenoid fossa through the horizontal segment as it turns into the cavernous sinus at the anterior genu **(Fig. 30–2A).** The simultaneous removal of the lateral orbital wall and the entire zygoma: orbitozygomatic

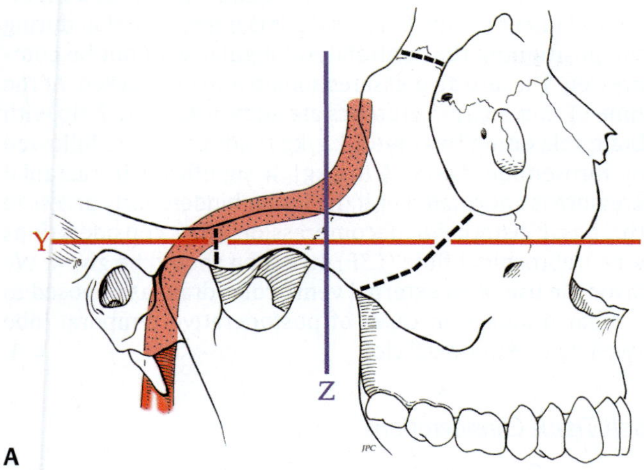

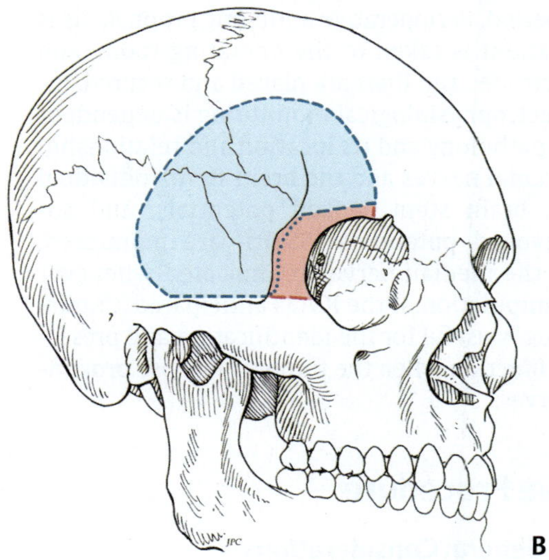

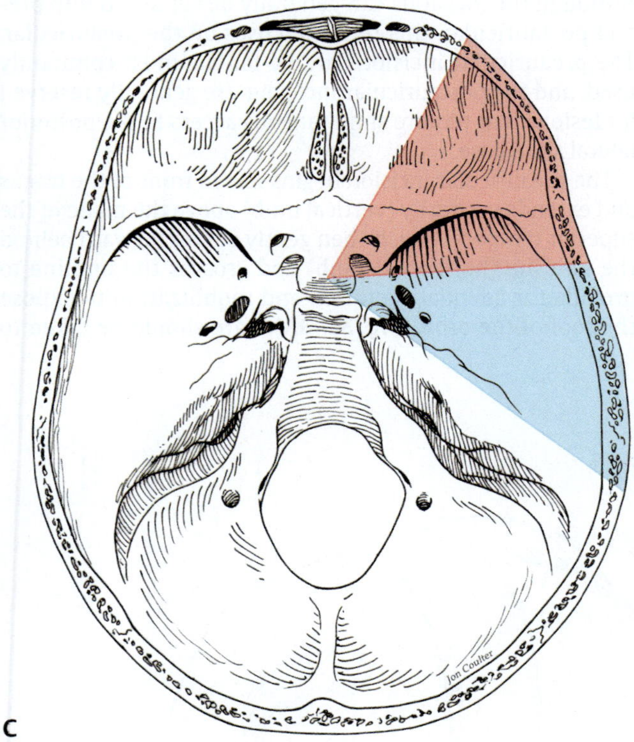

Figure 30–2 **(A)** The lateral skull focusing on the zygoma and supralateral orbit. The location of the osteotomies used to complete an orbitozygomatic approach from the supralateral orbit to the zygomatic process is shown. The *y*- and *z*-axes are shown in overlay to identify the intra- and extracranial regions that can progressively be accessed as osseous elements are removed. **(B)** The skull with the location of the pterional craniotomy and the supralateral orbitotomy. The removal of the lateral orbital wall allows for access in a medial to lateral plane. **(C)** The axial skull base showing the intracranial locations that can be accessed with specific bone removal. The supralateral orbitotomy allows for access in a medial to lateral direction along the *x*-axis anteriorly, whereas the addition of the zygotomy allows for further access in both the *y*-axis (anterior-posterior) and *z*-axis (superior-inferior).

osteotomy (OZ) combines these two modules, providing for complete exposure of the anatomical framework already described in all three axes (*x*, *y*, and *z*) **(Fig. 30–2C)**. Obviously, these are not absolute, but they are good general considerations when designing an anatomical corridor.

◆ Preoperative Preparation

In addition to the customary history and physical examination, imaging studies include a computed tomographic (CT) scan utilizing bone windows and a magnetic resonance imaging (MRI) scan with and without gadolinium enhancement. Intraoperatively, we have found the use of computed tomographic angiography (CTA) to be the most useful study for stereotactic navigational planning because it provides simultaneous correlation between the osseous, lesional, and vascular anatomy.

Cranial nerve dysfunction needs to be carefully evaluated during the initial examination for designing an anatomical corridor and in planning the postoperative rehabilitation for these patients. If the internal carotid artery (ICA) is involved by the tumor and at significant risk for intraoperative sacrifice, then a balloon test occlusion and cerebral blood flow studies should be considered. We in general do not electively sacrifice the ICA to improve the degree of tumor resection. Instead we prefer to leave residual tumor in the case of carotid encasement to be treated by adjuvant therapy. However in the event of inadvertent carotid sacrifice it is important to have a preoperative indication of collateral blood flow, or lack thereof, which would determine the need for cerebral revascularization in such circumstances.

If significant manipulation of the temporal lobe or subpial dissection is anticipated, prophylactic anticonvulsants are administered preoperatively and continued in the postoperative period. Perioperative antibiotic prophylaxis is utilized. The patient is taken to the operating room, and monitoring electrodes and lines are placed and secured. Intraoperative electrophysiological monitoring is dependent on the specific pathology and its location and relationship to individual cranial nerves and the brain stem. Individual cranial nerves, brain stem evoked potentials, and somatosensory evoked potentials (SSEPs) are monitored. SSEPs utilizing the median nerve are indicated whenever the surgical manipulation of the ICA is anticipated. Cranial nerve monitoring is useful for the identification and preservation of nerve function when the tumor is in close proximity to cranial nerves.

◆ Operative Procedure

Exposure and General Considerations

Patient Positioning

The location of the pathology determines the approach and lateralization. For midline structures such as basilar aneurysms, the nondominant side is preferred. The presence of cranial nerve deficit or focal deficit would be an indication to lateralize the approach to the affected side. The vein of Labbé is also a consideration in laterality because an anteriorly located vein places it at a higher risk during retraction.

The patient is positioned with the head turned to the contralateral side such that the squamous part of the temporal bone is directly horizontal. The vertex is tipped 20 degrees below the horizontal. Often this requires the use of a shoulder roll under the ipsilateral side. It is imperative that during the positioning the contralateral jugular vein not be compressed. The airway pressures should also be checked. At the time of skin incision diuretics are administered to help with brain relaxation [mannitol 1 g/kg is administered followed by furosemide (Lasix) 1 mg/kg]. If significant intracranial pressure is anticipated or if the lesion hinders early access to the basal cistern for decompression then considerations for cerebrospinal fluid (CSF) diversion should be given. We favor the use of an external ventricular drain as opposed to lumbar drainage in cases of postoperative temporal lobe swelling or extra-axial clot.

Soft Tissue Considerations

Although the incisions can generally be classified into pre- and postauricular, this report focuses on the preauricular. The preauricular incisions are by far the most commonly used, and the postauricular incisions are generally reserved for lesions that require simultaneous access to the posterior lateral skull base.

The preauricular incision begins just in front of the tragus and extends vertically (vertical limb) above the plane of the superior temporal line. It then gently curves forward behind the hairline (horizontal limb) and crosses the midline to provide for adequate rotation and mobilization to expose the roof of the orbit **(Fig. 30–3A).** Care should be taken to

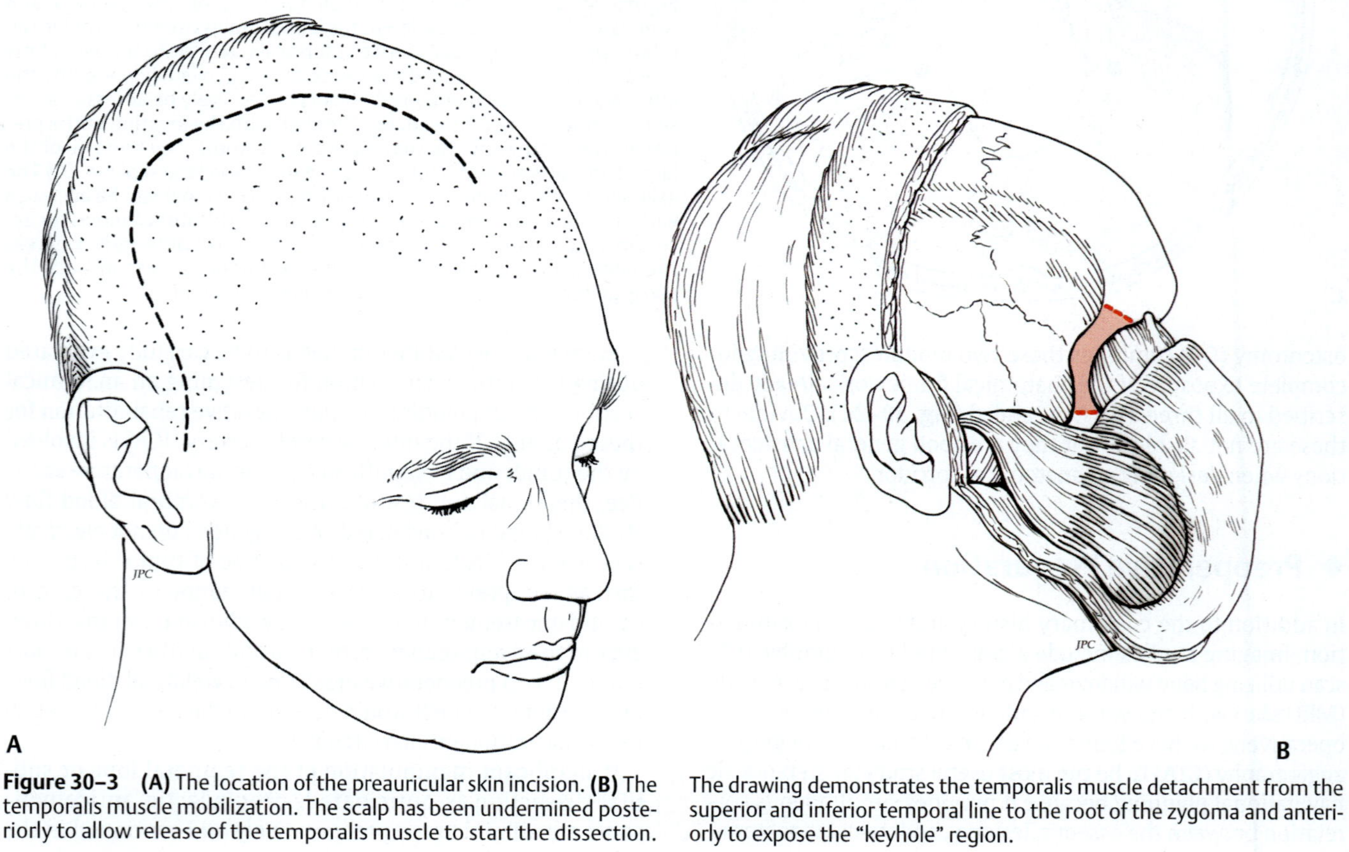

Figure 30–3 **(A)** The location of the preauricular skin incision. **(B)** The temporalis muscle mobilization. The scalp has been undermined posteriorly to allow release of the temporalis muscle to start the dissection. The drawing demonstrates the temporalis muscle detachment from the superior and inferior temporal line to the root of the zygoma and anteriorly to expose the "keyhole" region.

dissect in a plane at the level of the fat pad within the temporalis fascia to avoid injury to the frontalis branch of the facial nerve. This incision provides complete access to the frontotemporal region as well as the zygoma and frontozygomatic suture. In situations where only posterior exposure along the *y*-axis is required, only the vertical limb of the incision is needed, such as is the case for middle cranial fossa exposure of the internal auditory canal.

We prefer to mobilize the temporalis muscle from a posterior to anterior direction rather than splitting and transecting the muscle. We believe that this may reduce the incidence of postoperative scarring, pain, truisms, and atrophy. Undermining the scalp posteriorly and identifying the posterior attachment of the muscle to the temporal and parietal bones initiates this. The muscle is then dissected from the bone subperiosteally in an attempt to preserve the blood supply. Superiorly, the muscle is detached from the superior temporal line, and the inferior detachment continues to the level of the root of the zygoma. Finally, the temporalis is then detached from the pterion, exposing the "keyhole," and the differential flap separating it from the fat pad above allows the muscle to be mobilized downward to the level of the zygoma **(Fig. 30–3B)**. If additional exposure is required along the *z*-axis, the muscle needs to be detached from the zygoma (see Zygotomy Module).

Osseous Considerations

The craniotomy over the temporal fossa can be tapered based on the exposure required. For example, for a combined frontotemporal approach a larger pterional-type craniotomy crossing the sylvian fissure is used. In comparison, for isolated temporal fossa or combined infratemporal approaches a small craniotomy below the sylvian fissure directly over the temporal lobe is made. We prefer to utilize a craniotomy that is initiated with a single trough/entry hole made inferiorly and use a high-speed drill to turn the bone flap.

Specific Anatomical Modules

One can divide the preauricular and transzygomatic approaches into three anatomical corridors based on the removal of specific osseous elements: supralateral orbit, zygoma, and TMJ. We will discuss these approaches individually and briefly comment on the more posterior approaches.

Supralateral Orbit Module

This approach is based on a standard pterional craniotomy with additional removal of the supralateral orbit from just medial to the supraorbital notch to the frontozygomatic suture inferiorly. This approach allows for increased exposure in the *x*-axis (medial-lateral) and for simultaneous access to the anterior cranial fossa floor to the anterior portion of the middle cranial fossa.

Following the general soft tissue exposure described earlier, additional soft tissue needs to be mobilized to initiate this module. The orbital notch is identified as the medial border for the bone removal and rarely does one need to dissect medial to this. The periorbita is dissected under the orbital roof and laterally along the lateral wall of the orbit. Care should be taken to preserve the periorbita to minimize herniation of the orbital fat. The lacrimal gland is identified at the apex of the superior portion of the orbit as it transitions to the lateral wall and should be preserved. The inferior lateral soft tissue dissection continues to the level of the inferior orbital fissure (IOF).

Once this is completed, a pterional craniotomy is done to expose the orbital roof and allow for separation of the overlying dura. The dura is then stripped away from the lateral orbital roof, exposing the orbitomeningeal artery, which provides an important landmark between the superior orbital fissure (SOF) and optic canal. This vessel is often hypertrophied in the case of meningiomas and can be taken. Next, an osteotomy using a reciprocating saw is then made lateral to the supraorbital notch along the orbital roof **(Figs. 30–2A,B, 30–4A)**. This is then followed by an osteotomy along the lateral orbital wall at the level of the IOF. Once this is completed, a trough along the deep portion of the orbital roof, across the pterion and along the lateral orbit is made, connecting the osteotomies already described. The supralateral orbit is then fractured along this trough and removed **(Figs. 30–2A, B, 30–4A)**. The remainder of the orbital roof can be rongeured back to the level of the clinoid (which can be removed extradurally if needed). Similarly the lateral wall of the orbit can be further resected to the level of the SOF and cavernous sinus.

Intradural Considerations

The dura is opened in a "sunburst fashion" based on the pterion. CSF is released from the opticocarotid cistern to further aid in brain relaxation. The sylvian fissure is opened widely to allow the temporal lobe to be displaced laterally, which is facilitated by taking the anterior temporal bridging veins. This provides excellent access to the lateral cavernous wall and anterior middle cranial fossa along the sphenoid wing **(Fig. 30–4B)**.

If further exposure is required along the *x*-axis (medially) to access the tentorial notch and interpeduncular fossa, the uncus must be identified because this represents a critical landmark for this exposure **(Fig. 30–4B)**. The uncus can be mobilized to expose the underlying third nerve or can be gently resected subpially to allow exposure of the tentorial notch. During this stage great care should be taken to avoid injury of the anterior choroidal artery (ACha).

Once the uncus is elevated or resected, the third cranial nerve along the medial border of the tentorium can be seen as it forms the oculomotor triangle and enters the cavernous sinus **(Fig. 30–4B)**. At this point, the tentorial edge and the cerebral peduncle can be seen. Opening the arachnoid just inferior to the third nerve now provides access to the interpeduncular cistern. After the egress of CSF, the proximal posterior and superior cerebellar arteries are seen. Access to the interpeduncular fossa and its contents will vary depending on the relative position of the tentorial notch, posterior clinoid, and the position of the basilar apex and peduncle.

Several maneuvers can be performed to occasionally augment this view along the *z*-axis. The first is to drill away the posterior clinoid and the second is to retract the tentorium

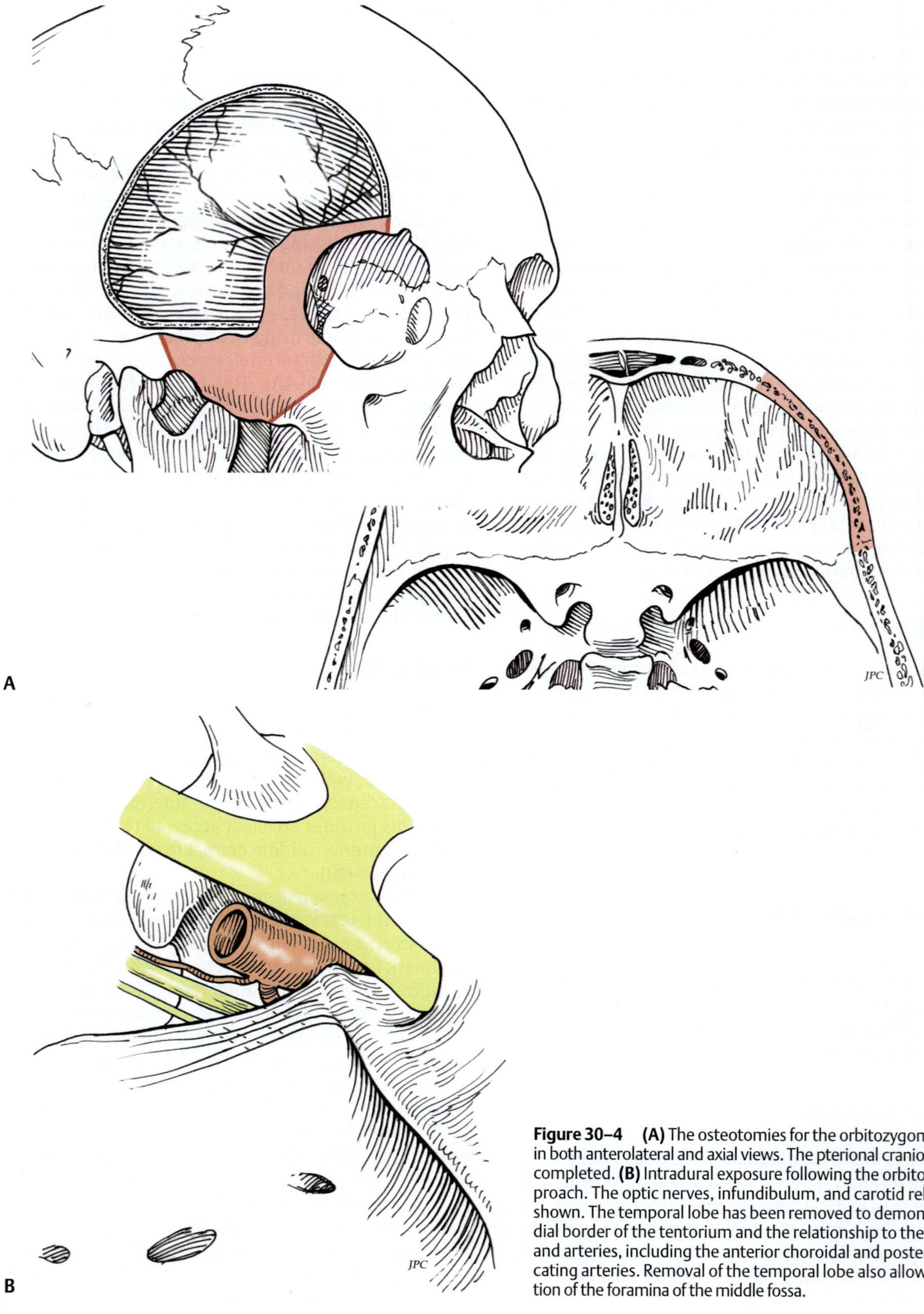

Figure 30–4 **(A)** The osteotomies for the orbitozygomatic approach in both anterolateral and axial views. The pterional craniotomy has been completed. **(B)** Intradural exposure following the orbitozygomatic approach. The optic nerves, infundibulum, and carotid relationships are shown. The temporal lobe has been removed to demonstrate the medial border of the tentorium and the relationship to the cranial nerves and arteries, including the anterior choroidal and posterior communicating arteries. Removal of the temporal lobe also allows for visualization of the foramina of the middle fossa.

laterally with a stitch (see Transtentorial Approach section). The posterior cerebral artery is followed back to the basilar trunk where proximal control can be obtained when clipping basilar artery aneurysms. The posterior cerebral artery is deep behind the hippocampal gyrus, and often vigorous retraction is required to expose this, particularly in the case of a high basilar apex. For this reason, the superior cerebellar artery is the preferred vessel used to find the basilar trunk.

Visualization of the contralateral posterior cerebral artery and its perforators is difficult through this approach. However, after the ipsilateral posterior cerebral artery is dissected away, it is possible to visualize the contralateral posterior cerebral artery.

Zygoma Module

Removal of the zygoma provides for increased access in the *z*-axis (superior-inferior). Following the general soft tissue exposure described earlier, the musculature, including the temporalis and masseter overlying and enveloping the zygoma, are removed in layers and displaced anteriorly **(Fig. 30–3B).** This is done by exposing the root of the zygoma posteriorly and then undertaking a subperiosteal dissection, separating the fascia of the muscles enveloping the zygomatic arch to the level of the frontozygomatic suture **(Fig. 30–3B).**

The anterior osteotomy is tailored based on the required exposure along the *y*-axis. It can be made at the level of the frontozygomatic suture by an osteotomy made with the reciprocating saw. The anterior osteotomy can also be made where the zygomatic arch transitions into the lateral orbit **(Figs. 30–2A,B and 30–4).** Care should be taken during the anterior osteotomy not to extend too deep and injure the vascular supply to the temporalis muscle.

Inferiorly, an osteotomy is made obliquely across the zygomatic bone from the inferior orbital fissure to the center and inferiorly to the bottom of the zygomatic bone to form a V **(Figs. 30–2A,B and 30–4).** The arch is removed, including the zygomatic process up to the capsule of the temporomandibular joint. Once this is complete, the transition point of the middle cranial fossa and the infratemporal fossa can be exposed. This requires dissecting the soft tissue extracranially along the temporal fossa and exposing the attachment of the pterygoid plate anteriorly. The pterygopalatine plexus can be packed with hemostatic agents to deal with the venous bleeding. The previously described focal craniotomy over the temporal fossa is then extended using rongeurs. The key feature in these exposures is that the inferior edge of the craniotomy should be flush with the floor of the middle fossa. Even a 5-mm lip of bone can dramatically reduce the exposure.

This exposure allows for access to the great foramen of the middle fossa, including the foramina rotundum, ovale, and spinosum. Specifically, the middle cranial fossa is drilled along its lateral curve until the foramen ovale is identified **(Figs. 30–1B and 30–5A).** Directly posterior to the ovale the foramen spinosum can be seen and the middle meningeal artery is isolated and ligated. Traveling anteriorly along the *y*-axis toward the lateral pterygoid plate attachment, additional bone along the middle fossa floor is removed. This then exposes the foramen rotundum, which emerges at a 45 degree angle from the horizontal plane when compared with the foramen ovale, which emerges at a 90 degree angle **(Figs. 30–1B and 30–5A).** At this point the respective branches of the trigeminal nerve can be unroofed and mobilized or transected as is appropriate to expose the lateral carotid canal.

Exposure of the Horizontal Petrous Internal Carotid Artery

The greater superficial petrosal nerve (GSPN) is identified medial to the foramen ovale and it is followed to the geniculate ganglion **(Fig. 30–5A).** The horizontal portion of the petrous ICA lies parallel and inferior to the GSPN. It also lies posterior to the foramen ovale and the mandibular branch of the trigeminal nerve (V3). The GSPN is sectioned to avoid traction on the geniculate ganglion. The eustachian tube lies lateral to the horizontal portion of the ICA and can

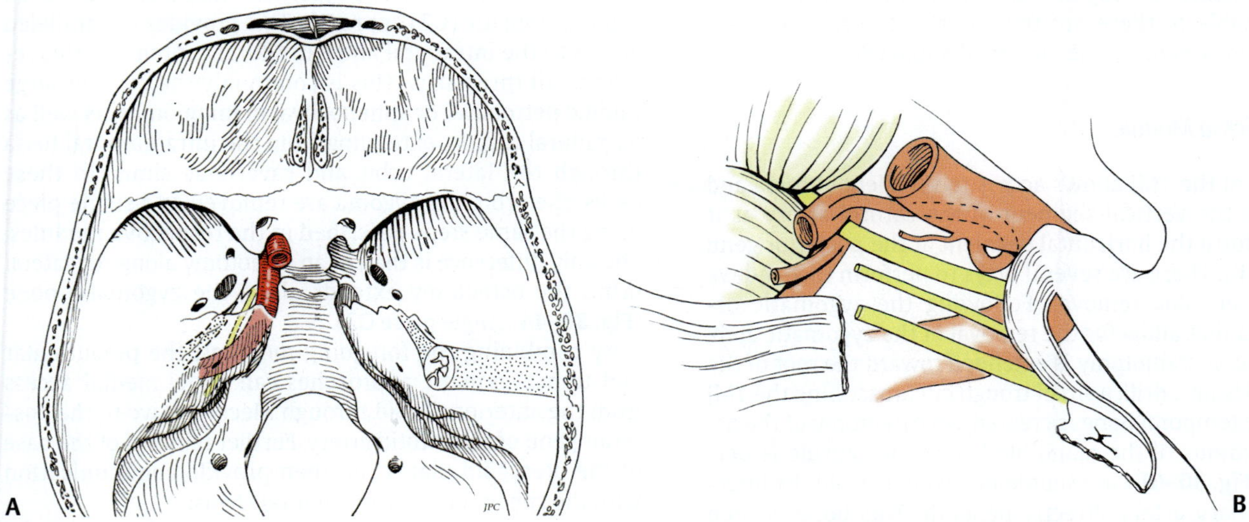

Figure 30–5 **(A)** The middle fossa. The major foramina of the middle fossa are illustrated along with the course of the internal carotid artery (ICA). The greater superficial petrosal nerve is seen medial to the foramen ovale running parallel to the horizontal portion of the ICA to the geniculate ganglion. The eustachian tube is seen lateral to the ICA. **(B)** The transtentorial approach demonstrating the tentorial incision and resulting flap. Once the tentorium is incised cranial nerves III, IV, and VI can be identified along with the ICA and its branches, the posterior communicating and anterior choroidal arteries. The posterior communicating artery travels posteriorly to the posterior cerebral and basilar arteries. Note the visualization of the brain stem and the third cranial nerve origin.

be injured in this location. The lateral carotid canal can then be drilled away with a diamond drill bit under magnification **(Fig. 30–5A).** If the ICA needs to be transposed, then the posterior genu may need to be released, which can then provide access to the petroclival region (see Glenoid Fossa Module).

Intradural Considerations

The osseous removal previously discussed allows for intradural access from the anterior recess of the third ventricle through to the middle third of the clivus. The inferior reach to the middle third of the clivus is somewhat dependent on the individual patient anatomy and medial osseous framework of the temporal fossa. Several maneuvers can be instituted to augment the inferior exposure along the *z*-axis to access the midclival region with variable success, the most important of which is incising the tentorium (see Transtentorial Approach).

Transtentorial Approach

The transtentorial approach is initiated by the identification of the entry of the fourth nerve into the tentorium. The tentorium is sharply incised starting just behind the entry point of that nerve in a medial to lateral direction for ~1 to 2 cm, staying parallel to the petrous bone **(Fig. 30–5B).** The dura is often quite vascular and requires bipolar coagulation. The anterior leaf is then sutured to the floor of the middle fossa. The arachnoid along the anterior border of the cerebellum is opened and the petrosal vein cauterized and sectioned. Gentle retraction of the pons is often necessary to visualize the midline. The sixth cranial nerve is located in close proximity to aneurysms of the midbasilar and often has to be dissected free. The degree of visualization of these structures will be contingent upon patient-specific anatomy and can prove to be disappointing. To compensate for these limitations, several posterolateral approaches have been developed, which are beyond the scope of this chapter. The most notable of these are the anterior transpetrosal approach and variants of the far lateral approach.

Glenoid Fossa Module

Removal of the TMJ allows access to the glenoid fossa and therefore the vertical segment of the carotid artery as it turns to form the horizontal segment at the posterior genu **(Fig. 30–6).** There are several ways to perform this and we favor an en bloc removal. Following the zygomatic osteotomies that allow for the removal of the zygomatic arch, the temporal craniotomy is extended toward the root of the zygoma. Using a drill, a small trough circumscribing the TMJ along the temporal bone is created. An osteotomy of the ascending ramus of the mandible below the capsule is performed **(Fig. 30–6).** Care should be taken to avoid the internal maxillary artery directly beneath. This bone is then fractured and removed as a single piece. The bone is drilled further along the posterior portion of the middle cranial fossa under magnification connecting the horizontal portion of the ICA and the posterior genu. The eustachian tube is transected and the bone overlying the vertical segment is removed. The fascial band over the carotid is released allowing for mobilization.

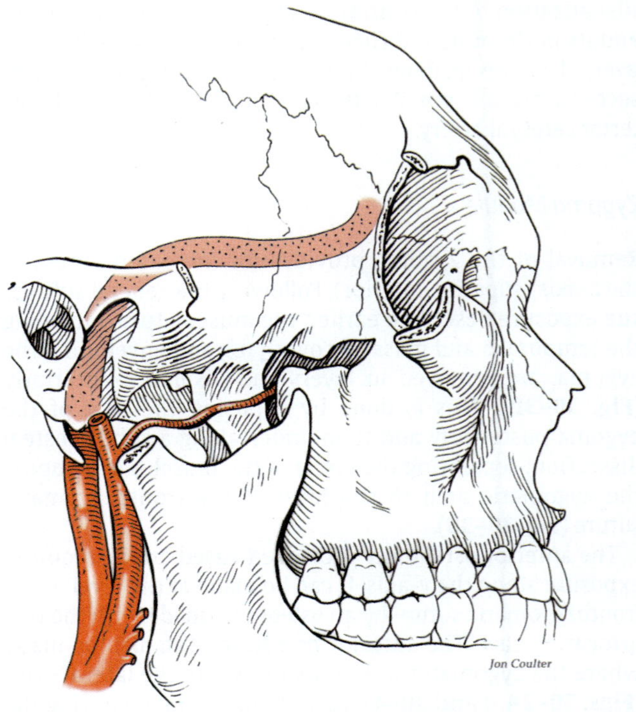

Figure 30–6 The anatomy seen in the glenoid fossa module. Removal of the temporomandibular joint allows access to the vertical portion and posterior genu of the internal carotid artery through the glenoid fossa. The relationship to the internal maxillary artery can be visualized because the ascending ramus of the mandible has been removed.

Combined Modules

Occasionally, there is a need to combine the supralateral orbitotomy module with the zygomatic module, creating the orbitozygomatic (OZ) approach. This provides unparalleled access to the intradural and extradural contents of this region in all three axes. This is commonly the case for large middle petroclival or sphenoclival meningiomas, as well as extradural tumors extending from the infratemporal fossa through the lateral orbit and cavernous sinus. In these cases, the orbit and zygoma are removed as a single piece using the same steps described in the respective modules. The only difference is that, in an osteotomy along the lateral orbit, the osteotomy extends along the zygomatic bone (**Fig. 30–4A**: single piece OZ).

By combining the foregoing modules, the preauricular and transzygomatic approaches can allow medial access from the anterior clinoid through Meckel's cave to the posterior genu of the carotid artery. Further removal of the base of the pterygoid plates can then provide communication with the sphenoid sinus and ventral clivus.

Posterior Middle Fossa Approaches

The middle fossa approach to the IAC via a subtemporal route and the subtemporal anterior transpetrosal approach are two important approaches to be considered when accessing the posterior portions of the middle cranial fossa. It is beyond the scope of this chapter to discuss the most posterior portion of the middle cranial fossa as it transitions to the body of the petrous bone (posterior *y*-axis). However, in the present modules we have discussed key concepts that have common characteristics with the posterior approaches that will familiarize the reader with the nomenclature and anatomy related to these modules.

◆ Postoperative Management

The complications vary with the areas approached. When the interpeduncular cistern is exposed the two most frequently reported complications are hemiparesis and third nerve palsy. Other complications include cerebral contusion or hematoma, ICA occlusion or injury, postoperative infection, and cranial nerve palsies. Temporal lobe edema and contusion are important complications that need to be closely monitored in the postoperative period. Attempts should be made to preserve the venous drainage of the temporal lobe because loss of venous drainage, especially the vein of Labbé can result in hemorrhagic infarcts. CSF leakage can occur from the eustachian tube. When intraoperative cranial nerve injury is recognized, immediate resuture or graft reconstruction is done. Complications resulting from an orbitotomy include ecchymosis, diplopia, and ptosis. Although these usually resolve spontaneously, treatment includes steroids and intraocular pressure monitoring.

◆ Discussion

Access to lesions located deep within the middle cranial and infratemporal fossae can be obtained using a variety of techniques. We have outlined our technique using the preauricular and transzygomatic approaches. Our modular approach is based on a three-dimensional construct using the standard stereotactic axes. Each module is designed to gain progressive access in specific planes, which can be used individually or in combination based on the anatomical location of the lesion. Despite extensive removal of bone the transzygomatic approaches can still be limiting, especially along the lower portion of the *z*-axis to the level of the midclivus. More extensive posterior lateral approaches can be used to help gain access in this region.

To best understand these modules, it is imperative to have a thorough understanding of the regional anatomy. The anatomy has been segregated into osseous, soft tissue, and neurovascular considerations, and their relationships have been outlined. Our approach often focuses on the location and course of the ICA, which defines and controls access to structures in this region.

31

Combined Craniofacial Resection of Anterior Skull Base Tumors

Gregory Karl Hartig

Resection of benign and malignant lesions involving the paranasal sinuses and anterior skull base began with the development of the radical maxillectomy with orbital exenteration procedure in the 1940s. In the 1950s, the use of a combined approach utilizing both a transfacial and an intracranial exposure was described for the management of frontal sinus cancers. In the1960s, the approach and rationale for a combined transfacial and intracranial approach became better defined and established. The anterior craniofacial resection has become the standard procedure for the management of anterior skull base lesions. In recent years we have begun to see a shift from the use of open approaches to those that employ greater use of endoscopic techniques. Although early results are encouraging, the efficacy of strict endoscopic excisions of anterior skull base tumors without the use of a craniotomy is not yet well established. Furthermore, the availability of surgeons experienced in these extensive endoscopic resections remains limited.

The anterior craniofacial resection allows the combined exposures of the extracranial paranasal sinuses and orbit as well as intracranial exposure of the frontal lobes, cavernous sinuses, and optic nerves. Most such lesions addressed are malignant and include adenocarcinomas, squamous cell carcinomas, and sinonasal undifferentiated carcinomas (SNUCs) originating in ethmoid sinuses, or olfactory neuroblastomas arising in the superior nasal vault. When describing olfactory neuroblastomas, the Kadish system is most often employed. Kadish A lesions are confined to the nasal vault, B lesions extend into the ethmoid, and C lesions extend into the orbit or anterior cranial fossa.

Other lesions within the differential diagnosis include various sarcomas, lymphomas, malignant melanomas, adnexal malignancies of ocular origin, and various benign lesions such as olfactory groove meningiomas and fibrous dysplasia (**Table 31–1**).

Patients with lesions in these areas are best evaluated and managed in the context of a multidisciplinary team, which typically includes a neurosurgeon and otolaryngologist. Occasionally, other surgical specialists such as oculoplastic and plastic surgeons play a role as well. Nonsurgical specialists such as a radiation oncologist, medical oncologist, neuroradiologist, and pathologist complete the multidisciplinary team. Indeed much of the improvement in oncological outcomes for these patients has come about with advances in nonsurgical treatment such as intensity modulated radiotherapy (IMRT) and tomotherapy, which both allow millimeter accuracy in the delivery of radiotherapy to critical areas.

This chapter focuses on the critical surgical components of optimizing the oncological resection while minimizing risk for the anterior craniofacial resection.

Table 31–1 Neoplastic Differential Diagnosis

Neoplasm
Benign
Fibrous dysplasia
Meningioma
Paraganglioma
Inverting papilloma
Hemangiopericytoma
Neurofibroma
Malignant
Carcinoma
Squamous cell
Adeno carcinoma
Adenoid cystic
Sinonasal undifferentiated
Neuroendocrine
Renal cell
Basal cell
Mucoepidermoid
Melanoma
Olfactory neuroblastoma
Sarcoma
Osteogenic
Rhabdomyosarcoma
Leiomyosarcoma
Fibrosarcoma
Neurofibrosarcoma

◆ Preoperative Preparation and Patient Selection

Presenting Symptoms

Neoplastic lesions originating in the nose and paranasal sinuses often present at a later stage because the symptoms produced by these tumors early on are similar to those of benign rhinosinusitis. Early symptoms include nasal congestion, anterior and posterior nasal drainage, facial pressure, decreased olfaction, and headache. As tumors progress, asymmetric sinonasal symptoms, such as complete unilateral nasal obstruction and more profound obstructive sinusitis, often with epistaxis, constitute a more typical scenario at the time of diagnosis. Unfortunately, patients with still more advanced tumors may present with signs and symptoms related to progression of tumor into the adjacent orbit such as proptosis, diplopia, and obstruction of nasolacrimal outflow. Lesions with intracranial extension often have few symptoms of dural or frontal lobe involvement. Cranial nerve loss due to lateral extension to the cavernous sinus or foramen rotundum/ovale involvement can be seen with larger and typically unresectable lesions.

Brain invasion by itself is not a contraindication for surgery, but it does decrease the probability of cure and increase the morbidity associated with the resection. The patient's age, overall medical condition, tumor type, and opportunity for postoperative radiotherapy will all play a role in determining whether a patient with frontal lobe involvement should undergo surgery.

Tissue Diagnosis

Biopsy of sinonasal tumors is usually performed only after adequate cross-sectional imaging has excluded the rare possibility of a benign meningocele or encephalocele. Occasionally, routine histopathology is inadequate in fully defining lesions. For example, when dealing with undifferentiated malignancies, immunohistochemical markers for neuroendocrine tumors can provide prognostic hope when compared with undifferentiated SNUC lesions.

Radiographic Evaluation

Both computed tomographic (CT) and magnetic resonance (MR) imaging are helpful in defining lesions of the anterior skull base. Axial and coronal CT provides better definition of bone anatomy such as subtle erosion, or enlargement of skull base foramina. Both CT and MR now offer multiplanar orientation, angiography (CTA, MRA), and the potential for stereotactic imaging for intraoperative use. However, MRI has superiority in identifying peritumor inflammatory changes, meningeal involvement, and nerve involvement, and in distinguishing between retained secretions and tumor within the paranasal sinuses. T2-weighted images will typically show retained secretions to enhance relative to solid tumor where these same secretions will appear dark as compared with enhancing tumor on gadolinium-enhanced T1-weighted images. Proton density sequences will produce better definition of the dark cerebrospinal fluid (CSF) component as compared with normal T2-weighted images. For malignancies of the paranasal sinuses or orbits, regional nodal disease should be evaluated and, in addition to the more commonly evaluated deep cervical lymph nodes, the lateral nasopharyngeal lymph nodes, which often serve as first echelon drainage for these lesions, should be assessed. With CT and MR imaging of the skull base and neck, further metastatic survey can consist of chest x-ray, and in cases with higher distant metastatic potential, fluorodeoxyglucose positron emission tomography–CT (FDG-PET-CT) fusion is often the most straightforward and sensitive metastatic survey option.

Overall Treatment Planning

Although the surgeon typically serves as the primary and directing member of the treatment team, review of such patients in the forum of a multidisciplinary tumor board conference is invaluable. The ability to have a skilled neuroradiologist review the patient's films with both the treating surgeons and the radiotherapist in attendance is best in arriving at a plan of combined therapy. Discussion of the balance between a safe oncological resection and the often necessary postoperative radiotherapy can best be accomplished in this setting. Also, surgical reconstruction of anticipated defects can be discussed as well as the need for prosthetics from an anaplastology specialist. Reconstruction of most defects of the anterior cranial fossa can typically be accomplished with local vascularized tissues such as the pericranial fascial flap. Larger defects occasionally necessitate the use of vascularized free tissue transfers such as the rectus abdominis myofascial flap. This robust vascularized muscle can effectively seal the dura and separate the intracranial and extracranial spaces.

◆ Operative Procedure

Anesthetic Considerations

Standard preparation includes the placement of a larger-bore venous catheter, placement of a urinary catheter, and placement of lower extremity intermittent compression stockings. When the planned resection is to include total maxillectomy, the anticipated blood loss will be greater, and an arterial catheter is placed as well. In general, the use of a lumbar drain for CSF decompression is not required. Use of lumbar drains has its own inherent hazards, most typically related to overdrainage during the postoperative interval. This increases the risk of postoperative pneumocephalus and rarely more serious complications such as herniation. Neuromuscular relaxing agents are favored to minimize the potential for patient movements during the procedure, and conservative hyperventilation and osmotic agents such as mannitol (0.5 mg/kg) reduce the CSF pressure to acceptable levels to decompress the frontal lobes and minimize potential for inadvertent dural tears during formation of the craniotomy flap and also to minimize the need for frontal lobe retraction during tumor removal. The use of a properly placed craniotomy is much more important in minimizing the need for frontal lobe retraction than is the use of dehydrating agents; this will be discussed in greater detail shortly.

Patient Positioning and Preparation

Once the patient is asleep, placement of neurosurgical cottonoids soaked in oxymetazoline or phenylephrine will help reduce later bleeding from nasal mucosa.

Next, use of a three-point pin fixation of the head within a Mayfield head frame is the best way to avoid unexpected head movement during the procedure. Also, this allows a more optimally positioned bicoronal incision line (i.e., more posterior) than does positioning on a typical horseshoe headrest. The three-pin Mayfield also allows stationary positioning if intraoperative image guidance is being utilized; however, image guidance is typically not necessary for this operation. The head is positioned in a neutral to slightly flexed position (i.e., 20 to 30 degrees from horizontal) because this optimizes the head location for both the transfacial and transcranial approaches. If the patient is having a concurrent tracheotomy, placing the head in a more neutral position works for most patients. Those with an obese or short neck are better served by beginning with a tracheotomy and then placing the patient in the three-pin head frame. Tracheotomy has been favored by some as a protective measure in avoiding postoperative pneumocephalus. In our experience with standard anterior craniofacial resection, tracheotomy is not necessary. In those who are having a more extensive resection, including total maxillectomy, significant postoperative pharyngeal secretion output and the potential for oropharyngeal swelling make tracheotomy the safest option for managing the airway. In those rare patients who are anticipated to need a free tissue transfer reconstruction of the resulting dural/soft tissue defect, good neck exposure for microvascular anastomosis is required. Likewise, neck dissection for overt regional nodal disease will occasionally be required. In these situations, carefully repositioning the head with the neck in an extended position after completion of the craniofacial ablative component of the operation works best.

The eyes can be protected with lubricating ointment and either corneal shields or an occlusive dressing. However, both of these can be displaced. In our experience, use of a simple "frost stitch" between the upper and lower lids along the gray line using a small nonbraided suture (i.e., 5–0 nylon or Prolene) works best. With mobilization of the bicoronal flap over the facial tissue for much of the procedure, the eyes are not in view; therefore a foolproof method of avoiding corneal abrasion is best.

The scalp is typically shaved along a 2- to 3-cm path of the planned incision, but the remainder of the hair-bearing scalp is not shaved. The hair anterior to the incision is banded if it is longer.

The prep solution may vary with surgeon preference. After careful degreasing of the face with isopropyl alcohol swabs, we prep the face with half-strength Betadine paint and use a more vigorous prep on the scalp. The half-strength Betadine offers less chance for ocular irritation.

Intraoperative antibiotic therapy usually consists of a third-generation cephalosporin with good CSF penetration such as ceftriaxone. If the patient is penicillin sensitive, vancomycin and metronidazole can be used in combination. A throat pack is also typically placed to limit blood accumulation in the hypopharynx and larynx.

Incision

A bicoronal incision is created behind the coronal suture and typically across the vertex of the cranium **(Fig. 31–1).** The inferior extent of each side falls within the lower portion of the temporal hairline and would follow the path of the preauricular crease if extended inferiorly. The incision is scored in three locations to simplify closure alignment. Raney clips are placed to minimize dermal bleeding, and the anterior flap is elevated between the plane of the galea fascia and the underlying pericranium. The anterior flap is elevated down over the supraorbital rims, with identification and preservation of the supraorbital neurovascular pedicles. Blunt mobilization at this level helps delineate the orbital rim perimeter without injury to the pedicle. One should also avoid injury to the supratrochlear vessels located at the medial extent of the brow. Preservation of these vessels improves the vascular supply to the pericranial flap. Good exposure at this level is important for an optimally positioned craniotomy. Laterally, one needs to avoid injury to the frontal branches of the facial nerve passing over the zygomatic arch into the frontalis muscle. Although the temporalis muscle fascia can be elevated with the galea/skin flap to offer an additional barrier to frontal branch injury, this is not necessary and dissection in the plane below the temporalis fascia can result in temporal muscle wasting.

Pericranial Flap Development

The pericranial flap is based on the supraorbital and supratrochlear vessels already described. It is an outstanding source of easily harvested, well-vascularized tissue, which is used to form a healthy barrier between the anterior fossa and sinonasal cavity below. This tissue is elevated as a rectangular flap pedicled inferiorly. The lateral aspect of the flap width is defined by the medial edge of the temporalis muscle. The superior extent is typically taken 3 to 4 cm posterior to the bicoronal flap incision. With elevation posteriorly between the galea and pericranium, this extra length is obtained. Once the perimeter of the flap has been defined with an incision through the pericranium using a no. 15 blade, the flap is separated from the underlying cranium with a periosteal elevator. Careful elevation at this stage helps avoid tears in the flap; however, small tears can be easily repaired. Once the pericranial flap is developed, it is separated from the scalp flap with moist gauze. Moist gauze is also placed over the pericranium to prevent desiccation.

Frontal Craniotomy

The medial aspect of the temporalis muscle can be elevated such that the lateral bur holes can be placed just under the

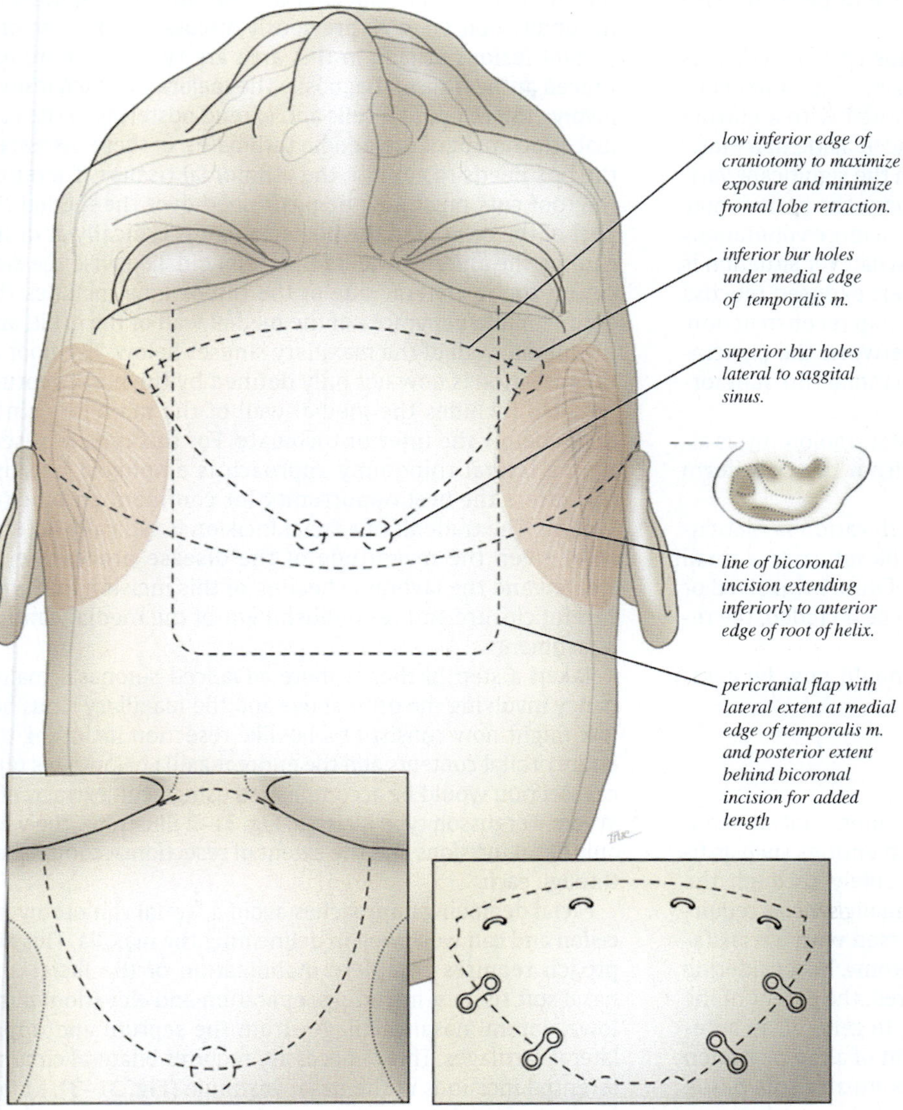

Figure 31–1 Bicoronal incision.

medial edge of the muscle and in this way is hidden. The medial bur hole can be placed in the midline from 3 to 5 cm above the supraorbital rims **(Fig. 31–1).** Care is taken to avoid trauma to the underlying sagittal sinus. The dura is then stripped and the bone cuts connecting the bur holes are created. The bone plate is then further separated from the underlying dura and removed and preserved for later replacement.

Alternatively, a fronto-orbital bone flap can be developed as illustrated in the **Fig. 31–1** inset. The advantage of this technique is in avoiding the lateral bur holes and in creating an even lower craniotomy, which further limits the need for frontal lobe retraction. The disadvantage is in the potential for loss of the orbital rims if the bone flap becomes infected or fails to heal. However, in our experience, this has not occurred. With this later approach, the midline bur hole is used to extend cuts down through the orbital rims just medial to the supraorbital pedicles. In addition, a cut is required at the frontal bone–nasal bone suture line because this bone is fairly thick and cannot be easily fractured. The final divisions of the orbital roof bone between the lateral divisions of the supraorbital rims and the bone cut through the base of the nasal bones is created by gently retracting the bone flap downward and allowing this remaining thin bone to fracture. Again the flap is then carefully separated from the dura and the periorbita along the orbital roof.

In our experience, it is not necessary to drain CSF prior to the bone cuts. We have not experienced tearing of the dura if careful technique is employed. The most important component of the bone flap design is creating an inferior margin just above the orbital rims. This low position of the flap allows the best exposure posteriorly with minimal retraction of the frontal lobes. The fronto-orbital flap design is lower still but requires more experience to perform with confidence.

The posterior wall of the frontal sinus is removed, as is the mucosa within the sinus. Sharp edges of the inner contour of the frontal sinus are also smoothed with a cutting bur. Once cleaned the bone plate is placed aside in a moist sterile local for later replacement. Given the significant variability in frontal/ethmoidal sinus anatomy, the patient may have only a simple frontal sinus duct, or a more voluminous supraorbital ethmoidal complex. With whatever situation is encountered, one must remove or invert exposed mucosa such that, with the final perichondrial flap reconstruction, one does not have mucosa trapped between the pericranium above and the remaining medial cranial rim/supraorbital rim below.

Next, after performing the low bifrontal craniotomy as already described, the dura is divided from the cribriform back to the planum sphenoidale.

The dural defect present after such elevation is meticulously repaired using interrupted 4–0 silk suture on a small tapered needle. If a larger component of dura is involved or if an anterior frontal lobe resection is to be included, the resection is modified as appropriate.

The anterior fossa floor exposure should now be complete.

Facial Exposures

Next, depending on the extent of the tumor, a facial exposure may or may not be required. Benign entities such as fibrous dysplasia might be addressed solely through the frontal craniotomy exposure. However, malignancies requiring a visualized margin are best addressed with a transfacial exposure to complement the craniotomy. In considering the type of extracranial approach required, the extent of the tumor resection needs to be evaluated. In general, an anterior craniofacial resection can be thought of as an operation that removes a rectangular "box" of bony and soft tissue from the central anterior fossa floor and sinonasal tissues below. If the roof of this "box" is defined by the four cuts through the anterior fossa floor, there remain the sidewalls of this box and the floor cut of the box, before the resected specimen can be removed. As with any oncological resection, the execution of an en bloc resection requires careful planning of which tissues will be removed. For example, consider a small olfactory neuroblastoma, which has arisen from the olfactory epithelium high on the septum or cribriform. Assuming this lesion is anterior and medial to the cranial attachment of the middle turbinate, the roof cuts laterally would be through the fovea ethmoidalis above into the ethmoidal cells below. The anterior and posterior roof cuts would be located anterior and posterior to the crista galli. In this instance, an endoscopic approach might be adequate for guiding the remaining extracranial components of the resection. The lateral sides of the " box" would consist of the lateral surface of the middle turbinates. These surfaces could be easily mobilized with bilateral endoscopic ethmoidectomy. The anterior and posterior side cuts would be through the anterior and posterior septum carried down from the roof cuts above and guided by the endoscopic view below. The floor cuts of the box would consist only of a cut through the inferior aspect of the septum, again guided by the endoscopic view. As previously discussed, however, malignant lesions arising in this area are typically more advanced at the time of diagnosis. The majority of such lesions involve the ethmoidal cells and extend posterior to the cranial attachment of the middle turbinates. In these instances, the box needs to contain the ethmoidal tissues. Therefore the roof cuts must now be positioned over the medial aspect of the orbit, and the posterior cut is typically at or including the anterior wall of the sphenoid. Likewise the side cut on the ipsilateral side of the tumor now includes the entire lamina papyracea of the medial wall of the orbit, and the medial wall of the maxillary sinuses below. The floor of the resection is now not only defined by the nasal septum but also includes the medial wall of the maxillary sinus taken below the inferior turbinate. For this type of resection, a lateral rhinotomy approach is employed because this offers the best opportunity for confident en bloc resection. The tradeoff of a facial incision is typically acceptable, given the magnitude of the disease process being treated and the favorable healing of this incision line with careful closure and reestablishment of the medial canthal attachment.

Taken a step further, a more advanced sinonasal malignancy involving the orbit above and the maxillary sinus below might now consist of a boxlike resection including the entire orbital contents and the entire maxilla below. This type of resection would be accomplished using a full extracranial Weber-Fergusson type incision. **Fig. 31–2** illustrates the variable facial incisions and the extent of resection accomplished through each.

Facial degloving approaches avoid a lateral rhinotomy incision and can work well in delineating the maxilla. This approach requires complete mobilization of the facial and nasal soft tissues, including separation and elevation of the lower lateral nasal cartilages from the septum and upper lateral cartilages. This of necessity requires bilateral circumferential incisions in the nasal vestibule **(Fig. 31–3).** Mobilization of the infraorbital nerves or even division of these nerves improves visualization of the medial orbital walls. With this full mobilization, the exposure approaches that achieved with the Lynch or lateral rhinotomy without the need for facial incisions/scars. In our opinion, somewhat poorer visualization and the potential morbidities of nasal vestibular soft tissue cicatrix/stenosis, and cheek anesthesia make this a less favorable option.

Highpoints of Typical Craniofacial Excision Using Bifrontal Craniotomy and Lateral Rhinotomy Approaches

The most common extent of operation would be performed for an olfactory neuroblastoma or ethmoidal malignancy, which necessitates a resection to include the ipsilateral medial maxilla as well as the entire anterior fossa floor up to the contralateral fovea ethmoidalis. Starting with the steps already described for a bifrontal craniotomy and assuming a lateral rhinotomy incision on the ipsilateral side of the tumor, the following highpoints are required to minimize morbidity and assure a sound resection.

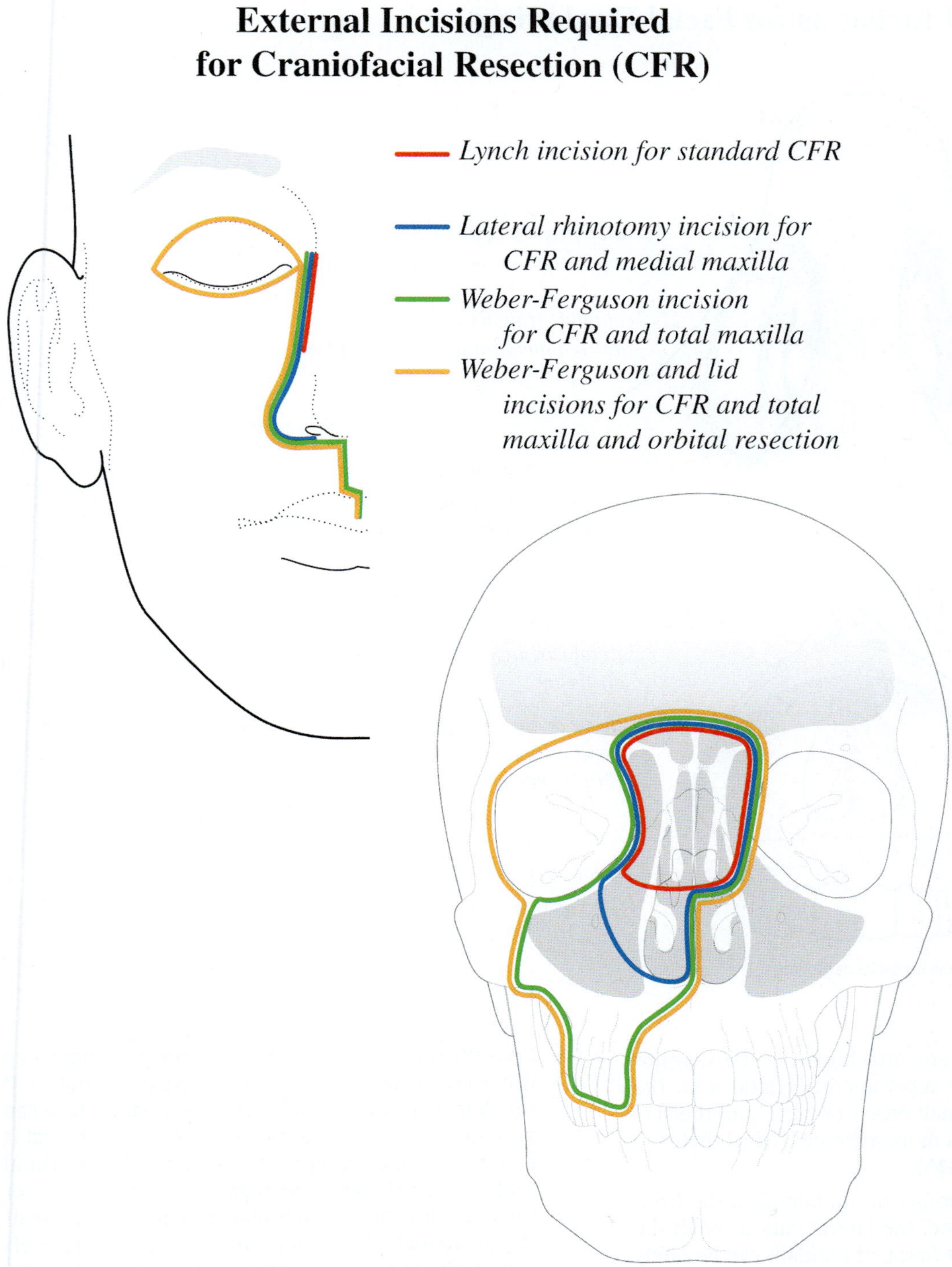

Figure 31–2 External incisions required for craniofacial resection.

The lateral rhinotomy incision is shown in **Fig. 31–2.** This incision typically begins at a point 1 cm above the medial canthus to a point halfway down the facial–alar crease.

1. Elevation of the periosteum with the soft tissue in the medial canthal area allows a clean elevation of the medial canthal ligament attachments for later replacement. After elevating the lacrimal sac away from its fossa, division of the lacrimal sac low in the fossa and subsequent fishmouthing of the distal end minimizes the chance of postop lacrimal sac dysfunction and epiphora.
2. With further elevation of the periorbita away from the lamina papyracea and fronto-ethmoidal suture line, one should avoid periorbita disruption, particularly in the area of the anterior ethmoidal artery where the periorbita will be dehiscent. This minimizes the chance for postoperative herniation of orbital contents into the ethmoidal void, which can result in diplopia and enophthalmos.

Intranasal Incisions for Facial Degloving

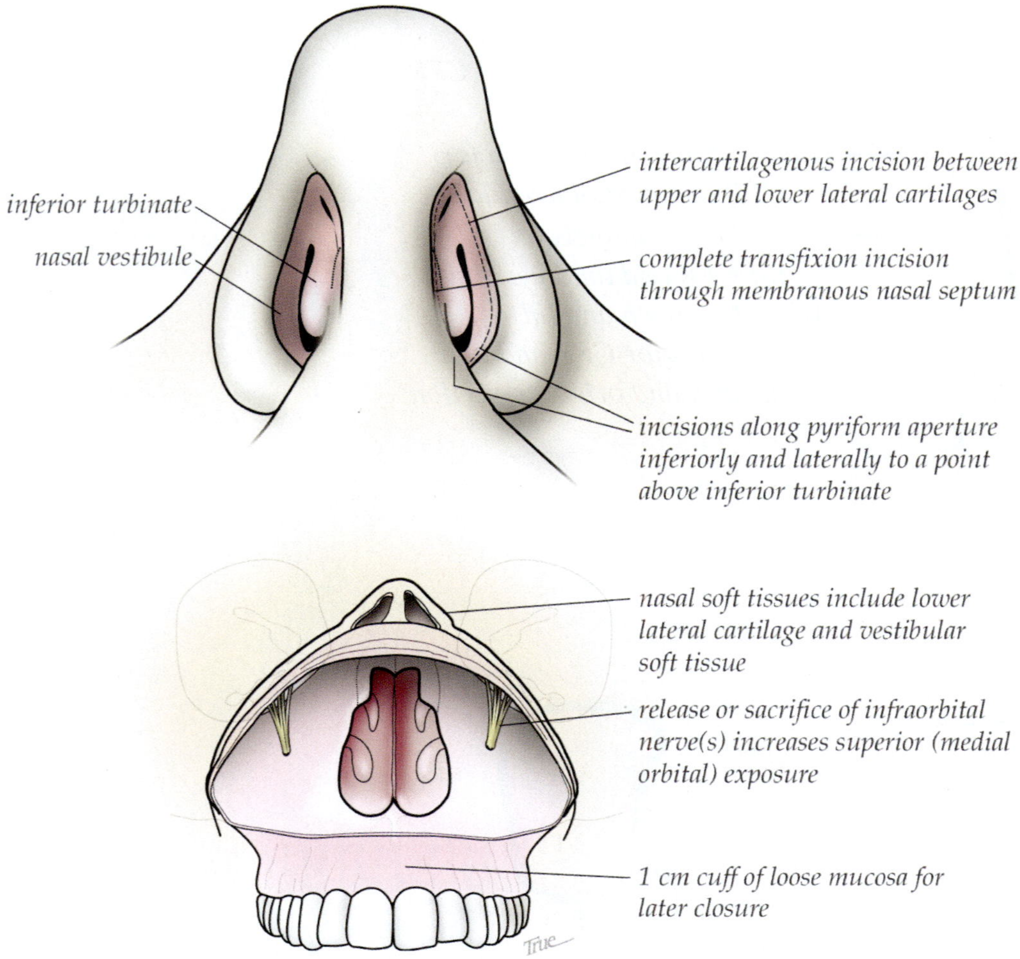

Figure 31–3 Intranasal incisions for facial degloving.

3. Preserve the trochanteric attachment of the superior oblique muscle in the superomedial orbital wall. The trochanter sits in a small recess of bone, and the surrounding periorbita is more adherent, which helps in identification **(Fig. 31–4A).**
4. With separation of the periorbita lateral to the frontoethmoidal suture line, the lateral cuts through the bone just lateral to the fovea ethmoidalis can be safely made without injury to the periorbita. **Fig. 31–4B** illustrates the relevant bony floor anatomy.
5. Likewise the anterior, posterior, and contralateral cranial base cuts can be created because these simply enter the sinonasal cavity
6. Next the cuts for a medial maxillectomy can be performed. These will vary based on the extent of the tumor.
7. Finally, the inferior cut across the septum can be created.
8. Typically it is easier to mobilize the specimen downward and extract it through the lateral rhinotomy approach incision because the inferior aspect is wider than the rectangular cuts in the anterior fossa floor.
9. Once the tumor has been removed, the pericranial flap is used to provide two-layer coverage of the defect. If the defect is small (usual case) the nasal surface can be allowed to heal by secondary intent. If the defect is larger (i.e., more lateral involvement of the orbital roof), a split-thickness skin graft can be placed over the periorbita and the pericranial flap to hasten sealing of the defect and minimize scar contracture effects. Only with large defects, which might include orbital contents, orbital roof, and maxilla, will consideration of additional vascularized tissues be needed.
10. After a typical reconstruction of the floor with pericranium, the sinonasal cavity is packed with water-soluble antibiotic-coated strip gauze. The packing is layered to avoid displacement into the nasopharynx. The packing is snug but not tightly packed against the surrounding orbit and pericranium above **(Fig. 31–5).**
11. Before replacing the bone flap, three to four small titanium plates are placed on the perimeter of the bone flap, securing the plates to the flap with monocortical screws

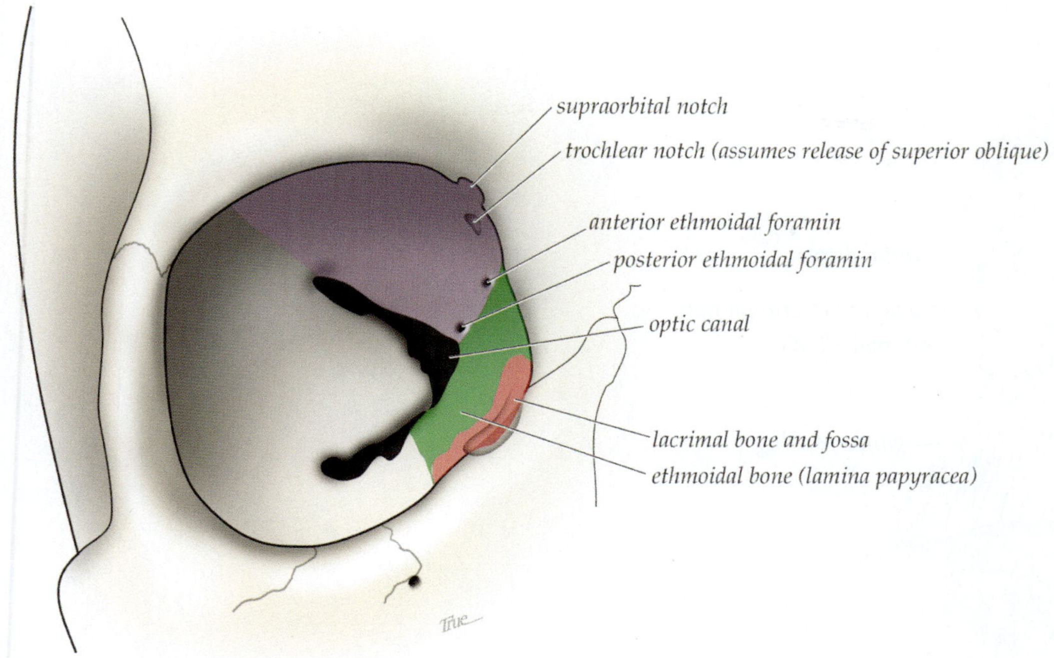

A

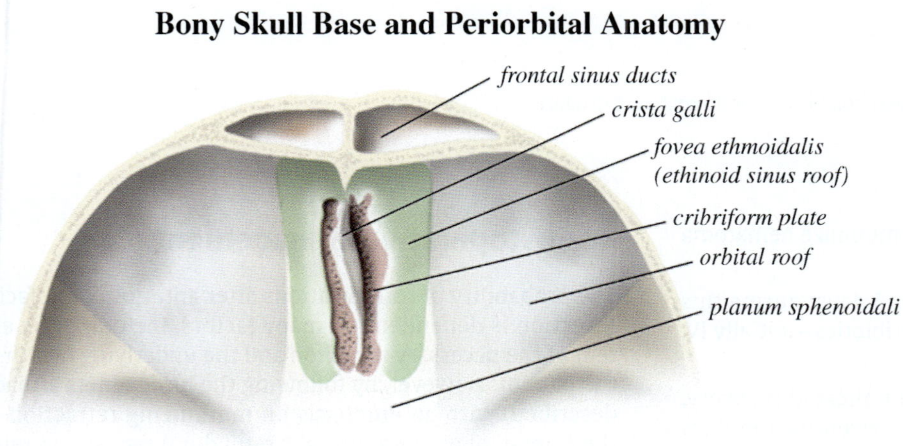

B

Figure 31–4 **(A)** Preservation of the trochanteric attachment of the superior oblique muscle in the superomedial orbital wall. **(B)** Bony skull base and periorbital anatomy.

prior to replacing the flap. We have found that "dog-bone"–style plates with only one hole on either side work well. Placing these plates (typically 1.3 to 1.5 mm in thickness) prior to replacing the bone flap simplifies the process. In addition, eight small holes (four sets of two closely spaced holes) are created 1 cm above the lower edge of the frontal bone plate or 1 cm above the supraorbital rims in the case of a fronto-orbital flap. Again these holes are placed prior to replacing the flap. These will allow placement of four tacking sutures between the frontal dura and the bone plate **(Fig. 31–1)**.

12. Next, before replacing the bone plate, the four tacking sutures composed of 4–0 silk must be placed but not tied. With the free ends of these sutures exiting through the four pairs of inferior bone plate holes, the bone plate can now be replaced. The remaining screw fixation is accomplished, and the four tacking sutures are gently brought forward and tied. These sutures have now brought the dura forward and eliminated much of the pneumocephalus that would otherwise be present.
13. Prior to closing the lateral rhinotomy incision, the distal end of the nasolacrimal duct is enlarged by splaying the distal 5 mm of the duct and everting the inner mucosa outward with resorbable suture in an effort to avoid postoperative epiphora secondary to scarring and stenosis of the distal duct.
14. Closure of the facial incisions follows. Careful reapproximation of the medial canthal tendon attachments is required to prevent blunting and lateral displacement of the canthus. The facial incisions are dressed with antibiotic ointment, which is continued twice daily until the sutures are removed.
15. The bicoronal incision is typically closed simultaneously and, although a drain is not typically placed, a

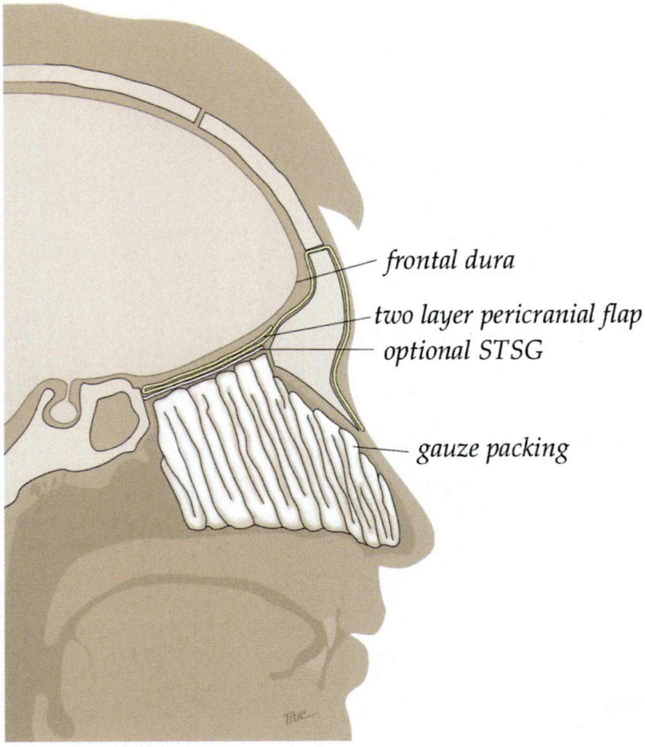

Figure 31–5 Sinonasal cavity packed with water-soluble antibiotic-coated strip gauze.

light pressure dressing is applied to minimize hematoma risk.

16. Packing is typically left in place for 5 days; during this time the patient is covered with antibiotics—initially IV, and oral after discharge.
17. Assuming the patient has an uncomplicated recovery, discharge is usually reasonable between postop days 2 to 4, but with older individuals or those who might have some mild frontal lobe edema, hospitalization may last 1 to 2 weeks.

◆ Postoperative Management

The probability of complications after anterior craniofacial resection is dependent on many factors, including the extent of the necessary resection and the underlying health of the patient. However, by following the basic tenets already described, with an emphasis on minimizing retraction of the frontal lobes, obtaining a careful dural repair, and reinforcing the cranial base with a healthy pericranial flap, problems can be minimized.

32

Surgical Resection of Esthesioneuroblastoma

Aaron S. Dumont, John A. Jane Jr., Jay Jagannathan, Nader Pouratian, and John A. Jane Sr.

Esthesioneuroblastoma is an uncommon malignant neoplasm arising from olfactory neuroepithelial cells high in the nasal vault that frequently invades the cranial base, orbit, and cranial vault **(Fig. 32–1).** Since its first description in 1924 by Berger and Luc, experience with this pathological entity has increased, although limited numbers of reported case series have accrued over different eras of treatment consequently limiting the quality of data available. Advances in imaging technology and widespread availability coupled with improvements in pathological diagnosis have led to an apparent increase in the incidence of esthesioneuroblastoma. Recent data suggest that treatment of esthesioneuroblastoma by a multidisciplinary cranial base team employing a standardized treatment protocol can achieve excellent long-term outcomes.

◆ Patient Selection

Patients with esthesioneuroblastoma most commonly present to an otolaryngologist with nasal obstruction or epistaxis. There appears to be no sex predilection, and tumor incidence demonstrates bimodal peaks in the second and fifth decades of life. Regardless of the mode of presentation, all patients undergo a thorough history and physical examination complemented with imaging studies, including computed tomographic (CT) scanning and magnetic resonance (MR) imaging, to determine the extent of disease. An otolaryngologist typically assesses the extent of sinus and potential metastatic cervical disease and obtains a tissue diagnosis. A neuro-ophthalmologist evaluates visual function preoperatively.

Staging by the Kadish system is an important component of patient selection for treatment. Patients with stage A disease exhibit tumor confined to the nasal cavity, patients with stage B disease demonstrate tumor confined to the nasal cavity and one or more paranasal sinuses, whereas patients with stage C disease demonstrate tumor extending beyond the nasal cavity, including involvement of the orbit, cranial base, intracranial cavity, cervical lymph nodes, or distant metastatic sites. The patient's stage determines the approach to treatment, including the use of preoperative adjunctive therapy (chemo- and/or radiation therapy as will be discussed). In general, at our institution, patients with Kadish A and B disease receive preoperative radiation therapy (50 Gy) followed by craniofacial resection 6 weeks later. Patients with Kadish C disease receive preoperative radiation therapy as

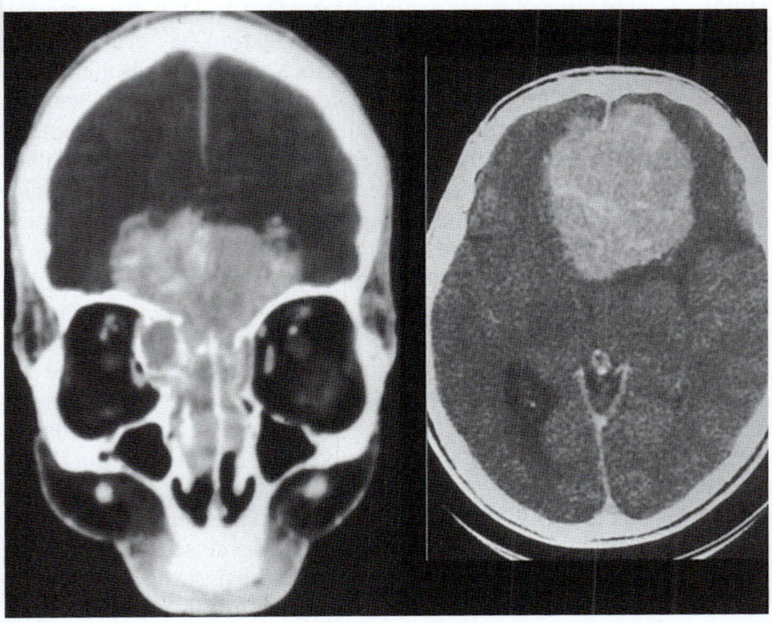

Figure 32–1 Coronal and axial contrast-enhanced computed tomographic images demonstrating an esthesioneuroblastoma with significant intracranial, orbital, and paranasal sinus extension.

above; however, they also receive a cycle of intravenous chemotherapy (usually vincristine and cyclophosphamide). For responders, another cycle of chemotherapy is administered followed by craniofacial resection in 6 weeks. For non-responders, patients proceed to surgical resection in 6 weeks following completion of radiation therapy.

In general, any patient harboring an esthesioneuroblastoma should be considered for aggressive treatment. Severe medical comorbidities and diffuse metastatic disease precluding aggressive management are contraindications to craniofacial resection. Potential risks of surgery are similar to other cranial base resections, including bleeding, infection, and cerebrospinal fluid leakage. Patients should also be informed that they will be permanently anosmic following surgery.

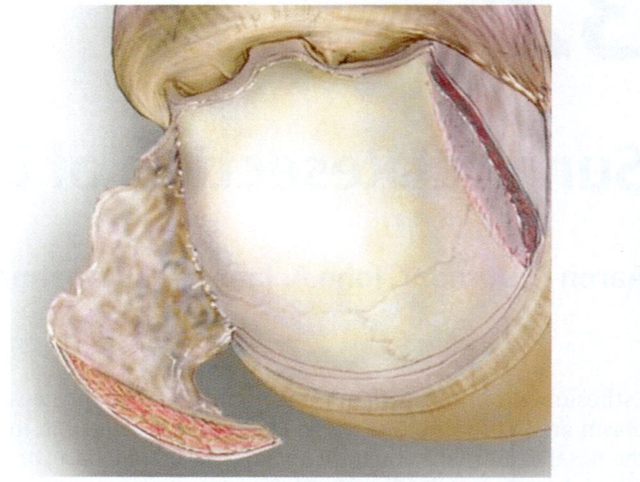

Figure 32–2 The pericranial flap is harvested separately from the scalp flap with its pedicle based laterally on the temporalis muscle.

◆ Preoperative Preparation

A multidisciplinary team composed of neurosurgeons, otolaryngologists, neuro-ophthalmologists, and medical and radiation oncologists is involved in the preoperative preparation of each patient. In addition to the imaging evaluation already outlined, patients undergo a 6-ft Caldwell projection skull x-ray, which can be used as a template during the surgery should the frontal sinus be of sufficient size for surgical access.

All patients receive preoperative antibiotics (typically nafcillin and ceftriaxone), which are continued postoperatively until the nasal packing is removed (usually within 5 days). Patients with significant intracranial extension are given a loading dose of phenytoin and are maintained on this for 1 week following surgery in the absence of seizures. Patients with significant intracranial extension and mass effect receive preoperative dexamethasone, which is rapidly tapered off in the early postoperative period.

A lumbar drain is routinely placed to facilitate atraumatic frontal lobe elevation and may be removed in the early perioperative period. Appropriate peripheral intravenous lines are placed and a central line generally has not been necessary. An arterial line and Foley catheter are also placed. The patient is intubated orotracheally and a combination of inhalational and intravenous anesthetic is administered throughout the case. The end-tidal CO_2 is maintained at 25 to 30 mm Hg for the transcranial portion of the procedure when frontal lobe elevation is required. Mannitol is not routinely administered and induced hypotension is not utilized.

◆ Operative Procedure

The patient is placed in a supine position on the operating table under general anesthesia after placement of the lumbar drain and other preparatory measures as already listed. Rigid skull fixation is generally not performed, which permits small movements of the head that facilitate the transfacial component of the procedure. Temporary tarsorrhaphies are performed in both eyes. The head is prepped and draped ensuring adequate exposure for both the transcranial and transfacial components of the procedure. The abdomen and lateral thigh are also prepped and draped for possible harvest of fat, fascia, and skin.

The transcranial approach is performed through a bicoronal incision. The scalp flap is reflected forward to the level of the orbital rims, leaving the pericranium in situ. The posterior portion of the incision can be undermined for additional length of pericranium to be harvested. The pericranium is usually harvested based laterally on the temporalis muscle **(Fig. 32–2),** although it may be based inferiorly above the orbital rims. The pericranium is protected in a moist sponge for later reconstruction.

The size of the frontal sinus, in part, determines the subsequent steps for tumor exposure. In the case of a small frontal sinus, a single bur hole is placed at the glabela (which will be covered with a bur hole cover plate at closure for cosmesis), providing access into the sinus. The sinus mucosa is then exenterated and a bifrontal craniotomy is performed **(Fig. 32–3).** In the case of a larger frontal sinus, the 6-ft Caldwell skull film is sterilized and placed onto the skull **(Fig. 32–4A).** The edge of the sinus is then traced and opened using a thin side-cutting drill bit. Alternatively, frameless stereotactic neuronavigation has proven to be useful for tracing the frontal sinus and facilitates identification of the optic canals in cases with extensive involvement by tumor. The anterior wall of the frontal sinus is then removed and its mucosa is exenterated. The posterior wall of the frontal sinus is then removed in its entirety **(Fig. 32–4B).** If additional exposure is necessary a bifrontal craniotomy can then be fashioned.

The dura over midline and laterally over the medial orbital roofs is then elevated. The lumbar drain may be opened at this point to minimize frontal lobe retraction. The crista galli is removed using a drill and/or rongeurs **(Fig. 32–5).** The anterior ethmoidal arteries are coagulated. The dural sheaths overlying the olfactory fibers are sharply divided as close to the cribriform plate as possible **(Fig. 32–6A).** The dural dissection is carried as far posterior as necessary for exposure. In cases without significant intracranial extension, these two parallel linear dural openings can be closed in watertight fashion using a running suture once hemostasis is confirmed. When the tumor exhibits significant intracranial extension,

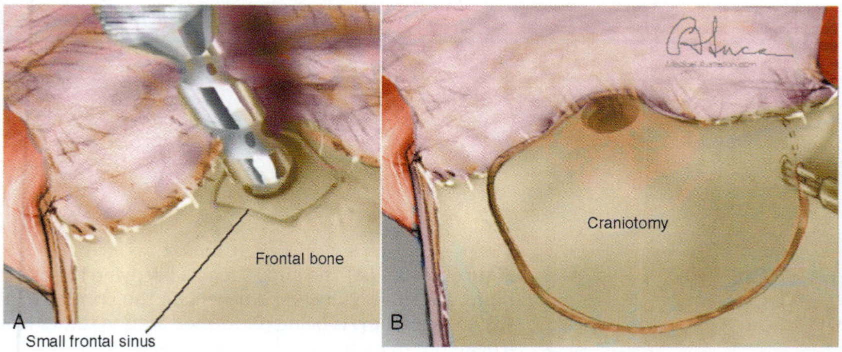

Figure 32–3 **(A)** In the case of a small frontal sinus, a single bur hole is placed over the glabela and **(B)** a subsequent bifrontal craniotomy is performed.

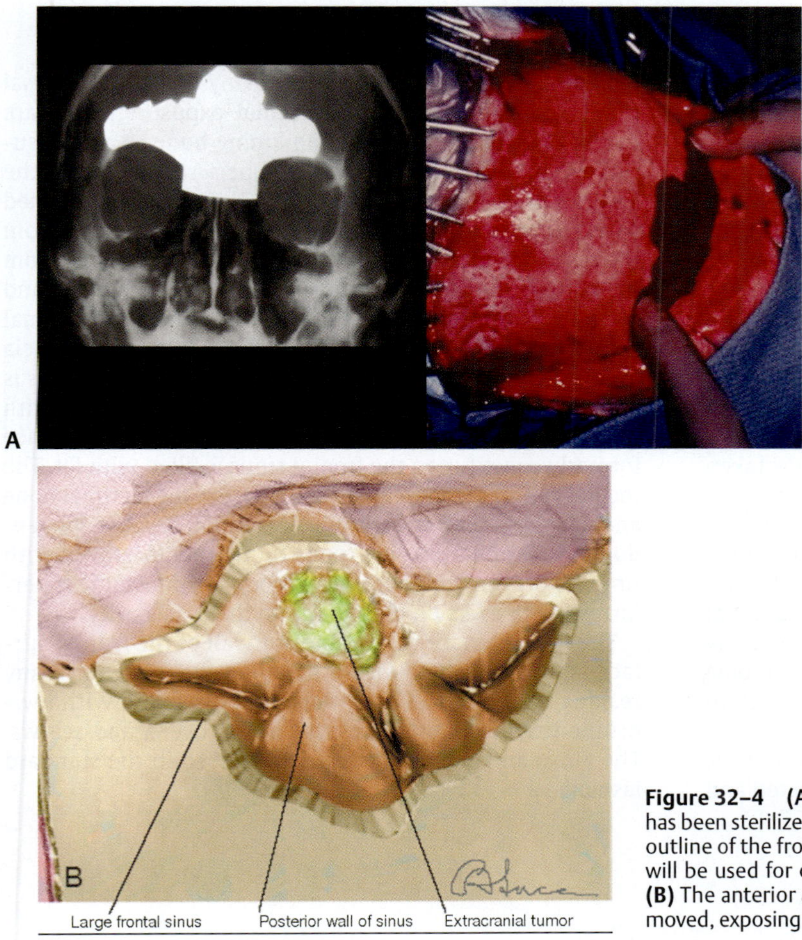

Figure 32–4 **(A)** A 6-ft Caldwell skull film has been performed. The x-ray has been sterilized and the frontal sinus has been cut out from the x-ray. The outline of the frontal sinus from the x-ray is being placed over the skull and will be used for opening of the frontal sinus using a side-cutting drill bit. **(B)** The anterior and posterior walls of the frontal sinus have now been removed, exposing the tumor and anterior cranial fossa floor.

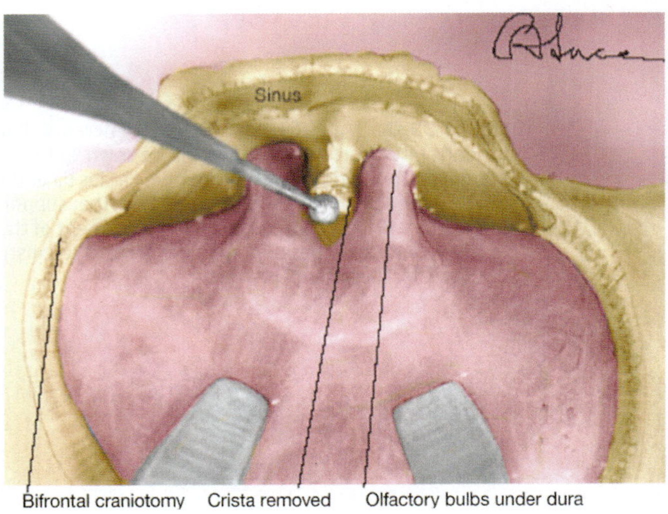

Figure 32–5 The dura over the anterior cranial fossa floor has been elevated and the crista galli is being removed using a combination of rongeurs and a high-speed drill.

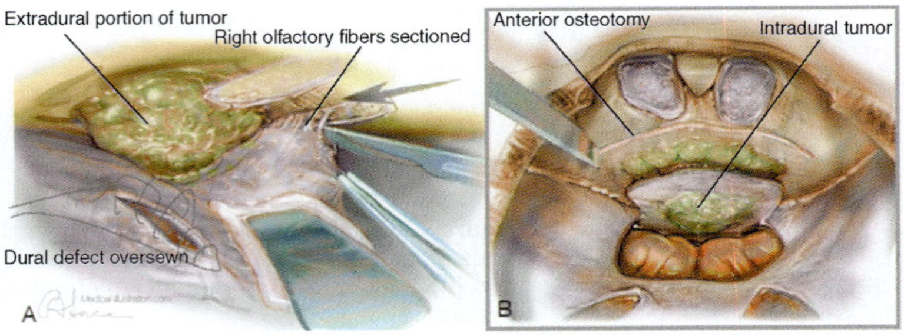

Figure 32–6 **(A)** The dural sheaths overlying the olfactory fibers are sharply divided adjacent to the cribriform plate **(B)** An osteotomy is being performed around tumor leaving a generous margin around the perimeter.

this portion of the tumor and the involved dura are radically removed. A duroplasty is then performed with a graft (usually fascia lata) that is sewn in a running watertight fashion.

Osteotomies are performed along the anterior cranial base around the tumor margins because the tumor will be removed en bloc **(Fig. 32–6B).** Cottonoid patties are placed along the inferior dura to assist identification during the transfacial portion of the procedure.

The transfacial exposure is performed through a lateral rhinotomy incision starting within the eyebrow and extending down halfway between the nasal dorsum and nasomaxillary groove. The lacrimal system may be spared if not involved by tumor. The medial canthal tendon is marked for identification at closure. A lateral osteotomy is undertaken to allow medial mobilization of the nasal structures to allow opening of the maxillary sinus. The periorbita is elevated following sectioning of the lacrimal duct. The ultimate extent of orbital bone and periorbital resection is determined by the extent of tumor involvement. Additional osteotomies are performed to allow a medial maxillectomy and delivery of the tumor and invaded structures en bloc from above. Frozen intraoperative sections are sent to pathology to verify tumor-free margins.

Meticulous attention to closure is necessary to prevent CSF fistula and infection. The frontal sinus is inspected and a diamond bur is used to remove bony crypts of mucosal remnants. Through the transcranial exposure, holes are placed long the edge of the remaining bone to accept sutures that will secure the pedicled pericranial graft to the anterior cranial fossa floor **(Fig. 32–7).** The graft is planned so as to extend beyond the edges of the bony defect. From the transcranial exposure the fat and fascia harvested from the abdomen are placed beneath the pericranial graft and secured to adjacent bony edges. An additional abdominal split-thickness skin graft is placed below the fat and fascia with the epidermal side facing the nasal cavity, and this is reinforced by Gelfoam. The nasal cavity is then packed with gauze covered in petroleum jelly and bacitracin. The space formerly constituting the frontal sinus is filled with fat. The medial canthal tendon is suspended from the lacrimal bone and overcorrection is generally performed because the tendon on the operated side tends to migrate inferiorly with time. To prevent epiphora, a dacryocystorhinostomy is performed with eversion of the sac into the nasal cavity.

The inner surface of the anterior wall of the frontal surface is also polished with a diamond bur to remove any residual mucosa. The bone flap is then secured with low-profile titanium miniplates, bur hole covers, and screws. The facial and cranial incisions are closed in the standard fashion.

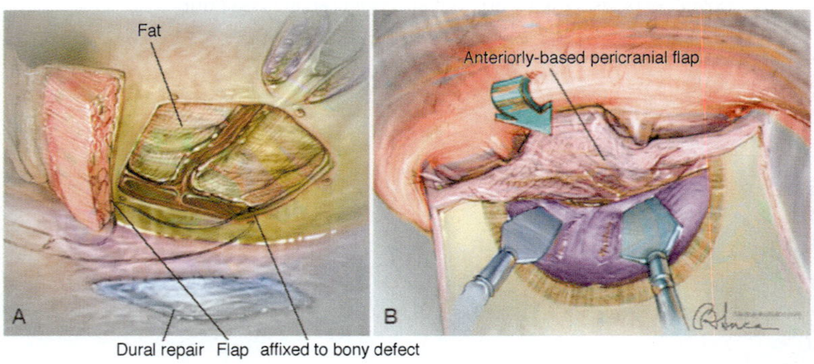

Figure 32–7 **(A)** The vascularized pericranial flap is brought into position. Its edges will be sewn to the bony margin surrounding the resection bed. Fat fascia and skin will be placed below this layer to provide further support to the closure. **(B)** Appearance following placement of the alternative anteriorly based pericranial graft to reconstruct the defect of the anterior cranial base.

◆ Postoperative Management and Complications

The lumbar drain may be removed in the operating room or left closed and removed within 24 hours. Pneumocephalus can develop with postoperative lumbar drainage and we now routinely remove the lumbar drain early. The patient is extubated and observed for 24 hours in the neurosurgical intensive care unit. The patient undergoes a routine postoperative CT scan the morning following surgery. The nasal packing is removed within 3 to 5 days following surgery. Antibiotics are discontinued following removal of the packing. Steroids, if administered perioperatively, are rapidly tapered. Phenytoin, if administered before surgery, is continued for 1 week if no seizures have occurred. Of note, steroids and anticonvulsants are rarely used in our practice.

Complications may arise from treatment of esthesioneuroblastoma. Radiation-induced optic neuropathy, retinopathy, or keratoconjunctivitis has been reported. Radiation-related wound complications have also been reported but are infrequent. Complications related to chemotherapy, including peripheral neuropathy, herpes zoster, and vocal cord palsy are occasionally encountered. Surgical complications including cerebral contusion, stroke, blindness, CSF fistula, epidural abscess, meningitis, and visual complications (blindness, decreased acuity, diplopia, etc.) have been reported. Systemic complications, including hyponatremia, myocardial infarction, and deep vein thrombosis/pulmonary embolism may also occur.

◆ Conclusions

Esthesioneuroblastoma is an uncommon neoplasm arising from the olfactory epithelium high in the nasal vault. Using a standardized treatment protocol applied by a multidisciplinary cranial base surgical team excellent long-term tumor control and survival are possible. Judicious use of adjuvant therapy combined with aggressive surgical resection, based on Kadish staging, has proved to be efficacious. Surgical treatment of esthesioneuroblastoma incorporates en bloc resection through combined transcranial and transfacial corridors and subsequent meticulous reconstruction to avoid postoperative complications.

33

Transmaxillary Approaches to the Clivus

Patrick J. Gullane, Michael J. Odell, Peter C. Neligan, and Christine B. Novak

The term *clivus* was introduced by Johannes Blumenbach to describe the anatomical region in the midline of the face between the root of the dorsum sellae and the anterior margin of the foramen magnum. Because of the anatomical location of the clivus, it is a region that is difficult to surgically access for tumor resection. Advances in radiology and surgical techniques have led to a more aggressive approach in the treatment of clival tumors and with the development of multidisciplinary skull base teams, including otolaryngologists, neurosurgeons, ophthalmologists, anesthesiologists, and allied health professionals, improving the assessment and management of patients with clival pathology. Knowledge of the anatomical region and the surgical approaches, including their limitations, is essential to the successful treatment of the patient requiring clival surgery.

Several approaches have been described for surgical exposure of the clivus. The transmaxillary approach to the clival region provides excellent exposure with minimal patient morbidity.

◆ Anatomy

The clivus is a complex three-dimensional anatomical structure that occupies the area in the midline of the face, immediately inferoposterior to the nasopharynx. It is composed of the occipital and sphenoid bones and the medial aspects of the petrous apices of the temporal bones. The clivus is divided into the basisphenoid component above (forms the posterior wall of the sphenoid sinus) and the basiocciput component below (inferior rim defines the anterior lip of the foramen magnum). The petrous apices of the temporal bones contribute to the superolateral segment of the clivus.

◆ Preoperative Preparation and Patient Selection

Imaging

Preoperatively, all patients undergoing clival surgery require evaluation with either or both computed tomography (CT) and magnetic resonance imaging (MRI). The complementary nature of the images obtained from the CT and MRI scans provides valuable information to the surgical team. This assists in defining the differential diagnosis and in identifying potential difficulties that may arise during the surgical procedure.

Angiography is not routinely performed in these patients because in general the necessary preoperative information can be obtained from CT or MRI scans or both. However, angiography is done on patients with lesions that will benefit from preoperative endovascular therapy. Because of the continuing modifications and improvements in radiological imaging, communication with the radiologist is essential to obtain the most accurate preoperative information.

Dental Evaluation

Because the dental status of the patient may affect intraoperative decisions, evaluation of dentition should be included in the preoperative patient assessment. Treatment of nonviable, infected teeth before surgery will minimize the risk of postoperative wound infection. Knowledge of the patient's dental status will also assist in surgical decision making regarding the site of osteotomy placement. Preoperative dental restorations and extractions are also important in patients who are likely to require postoperative radiotherapy.

General Medical/Anesthetic

All patients should undergo preoperative anesthesia evaluation. Patients with medical comorbidities should be referred to the appropriate medical service for management of these conditions to reduce the risk of perioperative complications. Preoperative evaluation also provides the anesthesia team with a baseline assessment to assist in treatment during the postoperative hospital stay.

◆ Operative Procedure

Patient Positioning

The patient is placed in a supine position. Mayfield stabilizing pins are generally not employed because it may be necessary to reposition the patient's head during surgery. Depending on the anticipated size of the defect, potential reconstructive donor sites (abdomen, thigh, forearm, temporalis muscle) are appropriately exposed, positioned, and prepped.

Tarsorrhaphy

To prevent corneal abrasions, tarsorrhaphy sutures are placed bilaterally using fine (5–0 or 6–0) nylon sutures. These sutures are placed prior to facial cleaning to avoid corneal injury during the facial antiseptic cleansing and to minimize the amount of antiseptic solution that comes in contact with the cornea and conjunctiva.

Tracheostomy

The decision to perform a planned tracheostomy is based upon several factors, including the surgical approach, the anticipated amount of postoperative upper airway edema, and the patient's ability to swallow effectively and to clear the airway postoperatively. Routine tracheostomy to minimize the risk of postoperative pneumocephalus during coughing or sneezing has been recommended. However, individual patient assessment regarding the need for a tracheostomy is preferable.

Lumbar Cerebrospinal Fluid Drainage

To minimize the risk of a postoperative cerebrospinal fluid (CSF) leak, some surgeons routinely advocate a lumbar drain. However, this decision should be based upon individual patient risk factors and in collaboration with the neurosurgical team. Patients who have a craniotomy with a significant intradural tumor resection are more likely to require a lumbar drain.

Prophylactic Antibiotics

Prophylactic antibiotics are administered 30 minutes prior to incising the skin or mucosa. These operative cases are classified as clean contaminated and therefore at least three antibiotic doses are administered postoperatively to minimize the risk of wound infection. The duration of antibiotic coverage is determined by the nature of the surgical defect, the type of reconstruction, and whether alloplastic material has been used.

Corticosteroids and Mannitol

The decision to administer corticosteroids and/or mannitol is made on an individual patient basis. In general, however, cases involving a craniotomy or significant intradural dissection should be considered for a course of these pharmacological agents.

Transmaxillary Surgical Approaches

Transmaxillary approaches provide excellent surgical exposure for tumor removal in the clival region. This can be accomplished using a variety of incisions and osteotomies. A midface degloving incision or a modification of the lateral rhinotomy with an upper lip split and a lateral subciliary incision is often employed (Weber-Fergusson incision). The most commonly used approaches include a lateral rhinotomy

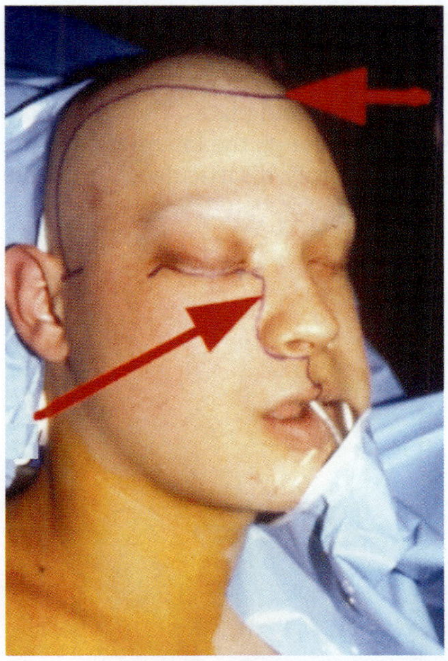

Figure 33–1 Outline of lateral rhinotomy incision (lower arrow) with planned subciliary extension (Weber-Fergusson incision). This patient also required a frontal craniotomy to expose the superior intracranial extension of the neoplasm (upper arrow).

with medial maxillectomy, a LeFort I osteotomy, and a maxillotomy. The optimal approach will depend on the location and complexity of the neoplasm.

Lateral Rhinotomy ± Medial Maxillectomy

A lateral rhinotomy approach with or without a medial maxillectomy is frequently used to expose clival tumors via an incision extending from the upper lip and nasolabial fold to the infrabrow region (**Fig. 33–1**). Osteotomies of the nasal process of the maxilla and of the nasal bones are performed using osteotomes and the medial walls of the maxilla and anterior and posterior ethmoid sinuses are removed. The posterior aspect of the nasal septum and the face of the sphenoid sinus are also removed. A dacryocystorhinostomy and repair of the medial canthal ligament is performed after tumor excision. The limitations of this approach include inadequate exposure of the neoplasm that extends inferiorly below the level of the soft palate or far laterally.

LeFort I Osteotomy

The LeFort I osteotomy approach for access to the clivus is performed using sublabial incisions. The advantage of this approach is the avoidance of external facial incisions. The exposure is accomplished by extending a sublabial incision from tuberosity to tuberosity into the piriform apertures. This incision is combined with a complete transfixion and an intercartilagenous incision to allow for nasal degloving.

With adequate exposure, the maxillary osteotomy sites are planned. For accurate restoration of maxillary position and dental occlusion, the necessary screw holes are drilled and microplates applied to the maxilla, prior to performing the osteotomies. The first osteotomy is performed using a reciprocating saw and usually extends from the piriform aperture of the nose laterally and posteriorly through the maxillary sinus toward the base of the pterygoid plates. The second osteotomy extends posteriorly through the lateral nasal wall. The nasal septum is then sharply disarticulated from the hard palate, which allows downfracture of the maxillary infrastructure once the pterygoid plates are separated from the maxilla. This is accomplished by placing a curved osteotome into the pterygopalatine fissure and gently cleaving the plates from the maxilla. The maxillary infrastructure is then pedicled on both greater palatine arteries **(Fig. 33–2A–G).**

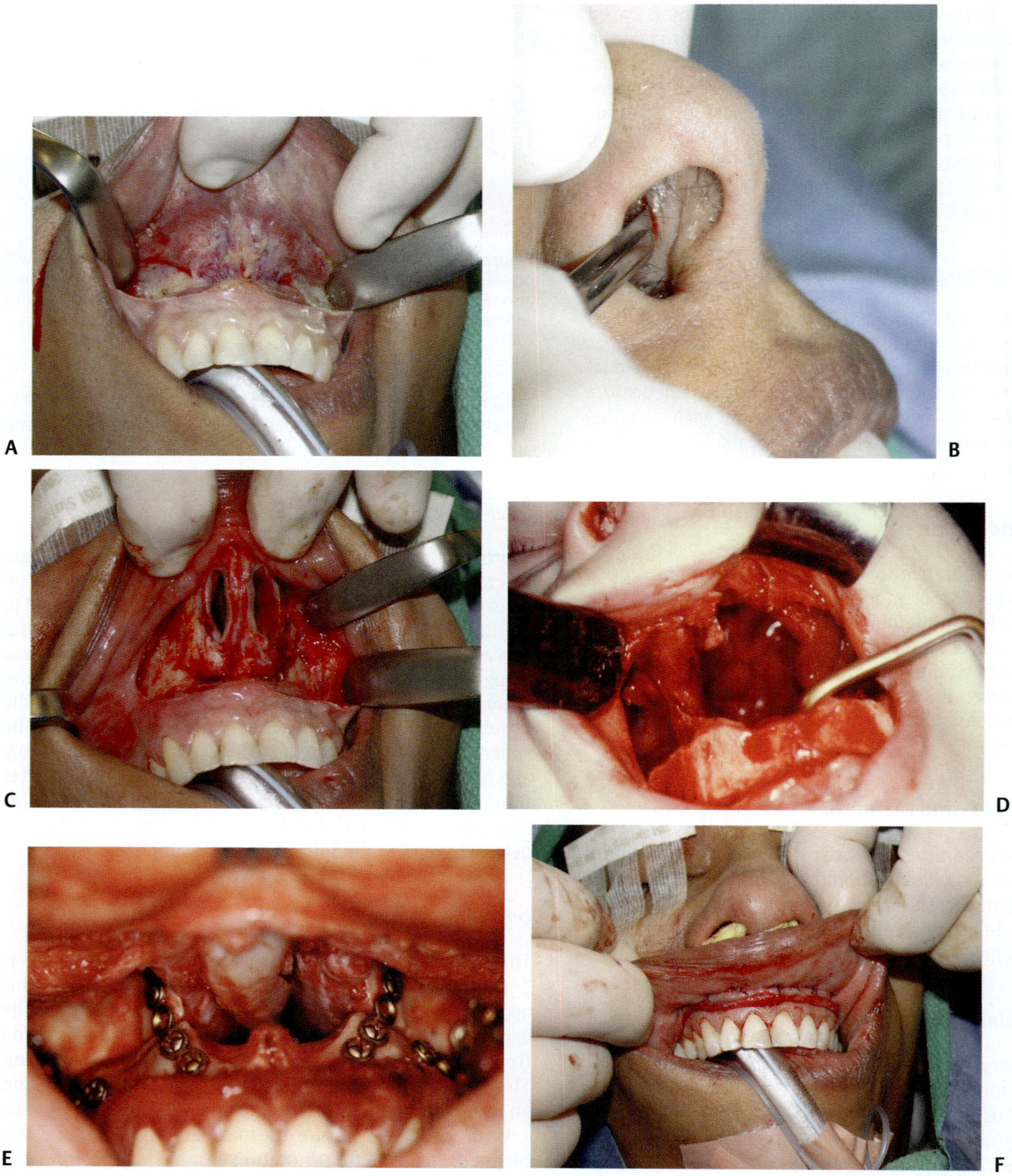

Figure 33–2 **(A)** A sublabial incision is performed. **(B)** Planned transfixion incision. **(C)** Degloving approach exposing the septum. **(D)** The osteotomy is completed with intraoperative downfracture of the palate. **(E)** Plate reapproximation of the osteotomies. **(F)** The closure is completed.

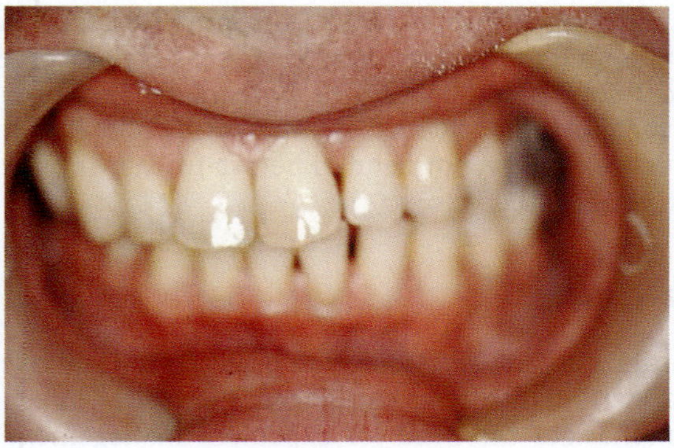

G

(*Continued*) **Figure 33–2** **(G)** At 6 months postoperative, there is excellent occlusion with no loss of dentition.

If more exposure is required, a midline palatal division may be performed, leaving each maxilla pedicled on its respective greater palatine artery. This maneuver permits a more inferior dissection than a LeFort I osteotomy alone, although restoration of the maxillary position is more difficult.

A LeFort I osteotomy is closed using standard surgical techniques. The microplates are reapplied and the sublabial and intranasal incisions approximated using absorbable sutures. The nose is lightly packed with antibacterial gauze, which is generally removed within 24 to 48 hours following surgery.

Maxillotomy

Maxillary translocation can achieve wide surgical exposure from the contralateral eustachian tube to the ipsilateral carotid artery and can be used to approach the ipsilateral cavernous sinus and the infratemporal fossa. Further exposure of the skull base, orbit, and middle cranial fossa is readily accomplished by adding an orbitozygomatic osteotomy.

This approach is performed using a Weber-Fergusson incision. Although degloving approaches can provide exposure of the maxilla and removal of some segments, more extensive approaches generally necessitate facial incisions. With adequate exposure of the lateral maxilla, the anterior fibers of the masseter muscle are detached from the zygoma, exposing the coronoid process. If necessary, the coronoid process can be removed to facilitate exposure and subsequent ligation of the internal maxillary artery. The lateral pterygoid process can now be identified and detached from its muscular attachments, which will allow adequate visualization of all necessary osteotomy sites. Microplates are applied as described previously prior to performing the osteotomies, which include the maxilla, zygoma, palate, and pterygoid plates. The maxilla is then swung laterally and pedicled on the cheek flap and the greater palatine vessels. This provides superior exposure to the clivus **(Fig. 33–3)**.

Bony and soft tissue closure is achieved by reapproximating the bony osteotomies using microplates and with subcutaneous absorbable sutures. Because the lacrimal duct is routinely transected, the lacrimal sac is marsupialized prior to closure. At the end of the procedure, the airway is evaluated and if significant edema is present, a temporary tracheostomy is performed.

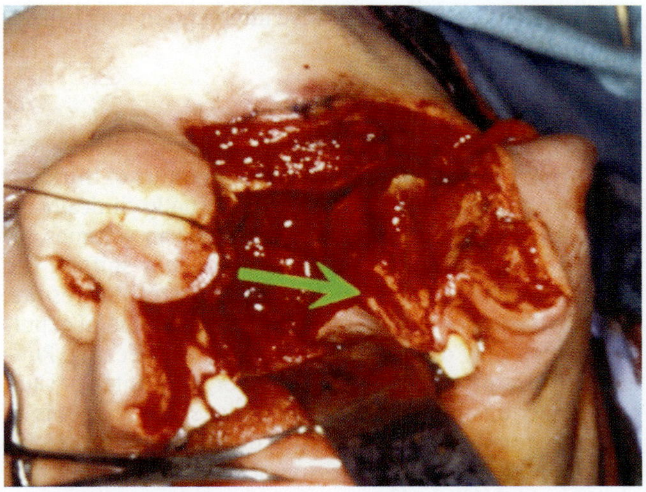

Figure 33–3 Maxillotomy exposure with excellent visualization of the clivus. The pterygoid plate is indicated by the arrow.

◆ Postoperative Management

Tracheostomy

Tracheostomy tubes are generally removed 3 to 5 days postoperatively following downsizing and corking. However, patients with significant dysphagia or aspiration symptoms remain tracheostomy dependent until these symptoms abate.

Antibiotics

Postoperative antibiotics are continued for 48 hours or until nasal/sinus packing is removed. With evidence of postoperative infection, appropriate cultures are obtained and antibiotic therapy is continued.

Lumbar Drain

Lumbar drains are rarely used during the resection of clival tumors. However, patients who develop a postoperative CSF leak are treated conservatively with bed rest and avoidance of straining. If the leak persists then a lumbar drain is inserted temporarily.

◆ Complications

Cerebrospinal Fluid Leak

With a large dural resection or an increased area of dural exposure, the postoperative risk of a CSF leak increases. To prevent this complication, it is necessary to ensure a watertight closure of the dura and on occasion the use of vascularized tissues for dural repair. In the majority of patients, a CSF leak will resolve spontaneously with appropriate conservative management (head elevation, lumbar drainage, and the avoidance of Valsalva maneuvers). However, in cases that fail to resolve, operative intervention may be necessary.

Pneumocephalus

Following cranial base surgery, small amounts of intracranial air commonly accumulate and are usually clinically insignificant. However, with large intracranial air volumes, increased intracranial pressure can produce a shift of the intracranial contents with potentially catastrophic results. Air from the upper airway likely results from forceful expulsion, which may occur during coughing or sneezing. Routine tracheostomy for all patients undergoing anterior skull base resections has been advocated by some surgeons to minimize the risk of postoperative pneumocephalus. However, individual patient assessment of the extent of dural exposure and dural resection prior to tracheostomy is recommended. If a tension pneumocephalus occurs, any obstructive dressings or nasal packing should be removed, followed by immediate intracranial decompression with needle aspiration and/or reexploration.

Meningitis

The incidence of meningitis has been significantly reduced with improved surgical techniques including flap repair and prophylactic antibiotics. However, if symptoms of meningitis occur, a lumbar puncture, culture, and appropriate antibiotics are utilized.

Wound Infection

Wound infection in skull base surgery is relatively uncommon. Simple wound infections are managed with drainage of suppurative collections and the appropriate culture-directed intravenous antibiotic(s). In those cases where the oral or nasal cavities have been breached, prophylactic antibiotic therapy (broad spectrum cephalosporin and an anaerobic agent) is indicated.

Dysphagia

Dysphagia or aspiration can result from injury to those cranial nerves that control glossopharyngeal function, particularly cranial nerves IX, X, XII. Some surgeons have recommended prophylactic gastrostomy tube placement or vocal cord medialization or both in these patients. However, postoperative assessment of swallowing and voice function is recommended before further intervention is instituted.

Palatal Fistula

Oronasal or oroantral fistulae can occur from local tissue breakdown. This is often a consequence of wound infection and emphasizes the need for expedient management of postoperative infections. Once a fistula has occurred, treatment is determined by the fistula site and individual patient factors. Many patients with small oronasal/oroantral fistulae remain asymptomatic and require no further treatment. Fistulae that are persistent or symptomatic can be managed with obturation or surgical repair, depending on the site and size of the defect.

Serous Otitis Media/Eustachian Tube Dysfunction

Serous otitis media or eustachian tube dysfunction or both often occur following extensive eustachian tube manipulation or resection that may be necessary for tumor exposure and extirpation. Although many patients can be managed conservatively, some will require tympanostomy tubes for long-term middle ear ventilation.

◆ Conclusion

The development of the multidisciplinary skull base surgery team over the past 10 to 15 years combined with improved radiological evaluation and a better understanding of the limitations of each surgical approach has resulted in improved exposure, the ability to resect extensive neoplasms, and a reduction in surgical complications. Although the described transmaxillary approaches provide excellent exposure with minimal morbidity, we feel that improved technology using minimally invasive techniques, including endoscopic equipment and intraoperative guided imaging, will likely replace some of the current surgical methods and improve patient outcome.

34

Surgical Management of Cholesterol Granulomas of the Petrous Apex

Mark B. Eisenberg and Ossama Al-Mefty

Cholesterol granulomas (CGs) are benign expansile lesions most commonly found in either the middle ear or the mastoid region in association with some type of inflammatory ear disease. Petrous apex cholesterol granulomas (PACGs), however, have been described less often and in many cases have been erroneously grouped with epidermoid tumors, which are etiologically and histologically distinct from PACGs.

PACGs are the end result of chronic obstruction of the normal aeration to the petrous air cells. This obstruction leads to the development of negative pressures within the air cells causing mucosal engorgement. The mucosal hemorrhage that ensues sets the stage for a cycle of hemorrhage and inflammation ending in the formation and growth of a CG. Because this progression from hemorrhage to granuloma formation is an ongoing process, these lesions will have varied clinical and radiographic characteristics depending upon what stage of formation they are in.

In the past, most of these have been drained by otolaryngologists via either a transtemporal or transsphenoidal route followed by placement of a small Silastic tube to reestablish aeration. Unfortunately, the recurrence rates following these approaches have been reported in the literature to be as high as 60%, with some patients requiring multiple revisions. An alternative approach is complete excision of the lesion, including the mucosal lining, followed by obliteration of the cavity with vascularized tissue.

◆ Patient Selection

The presenting signs and symptoms of PACG are largely dependent upon the size and extent of the lesion. Smaller lesions that are asymptomatic may only be discovered during the evaluation of an unrelated complaint (e.g., headache, dizziness). As the PACG grows it has a compressive effect upon the surrounding neurovascular structures. The trigeminal and abducens nerves are particularly vulnerable because of their proximity to the petrous apex. As such, many patients first present because of either diplopia or facial numbness/pain. Larger lesions may present with hearing loss and facial nerve dysfunction. Although there is no pathognomonic symptom of a PACG, the time course of symptoms often gives a clue as to the diagnosis. The cyclical pattern of hemorrhage and inflammation often leads to periodic worsening of symptoms rather than a steady progression as in a neoplastic growth.

Small asymptomatic or minimally symptomatic lesions in a compliant patient may be safely followed with serial magnetic resonance imaging (MRI) studies. A small subset of these patients will have an arrest of the progressive cycle and will therefore not require further treatment. Patients with progressive symptoms or enlarging lesions will obviously require treatment. Patients who present with either significant symptoms (regardless of lesion size) or large lesions (regardless of symptoms) will also require intervention. The traditional mode of therapy involved a drainage procedure via either a transtemporal or a transsphenoidal route. Because the recurrence rate for these types of procedures was relatively high, we have approached these lesions via an extended middle fossa approach, which allows complete removal of the granuloma and pseudocapsule. This is then followed by obliteration of the cavity with vascularized tissue in the form of a pedicled strip of temporalis muscle.

Because of the frequent involvement of the VI and VIII cranial nerves, all patients should undergo formal neuro-ophthalmological examination as well as an audiogram and brain stem auditory evoked responses (BAERs). The radiographic evaluation consists of an MRI with and without contrast to confirm the diagnosis. Petrous apex cholesterol granulomas most often display a high signal characteristic on both T1- and T2-weighted images with only meager peripheral enhancement **(Fig. 34–1A,B)**. Depending upon the age of the lesion, however, this "classic" appearance may not always be present. The MRI scan also provides information regarding the extent of the lesion and whether there is any intradural extension. A computed tomographic (CT) scan with bone window settings should also be performed to evaluate the extent of erosion of the petrous apex and temporal bone. Any involvement of the middle ear will also be readily seen on the CT.

◆ Preoperative Preparation

The extended middle fossa approach is an extradural, subtemporal approach to the petrous apex. Although the dissection is entirely extradural, there is a small risk of postoperative seizures as a result of the temporal lobe

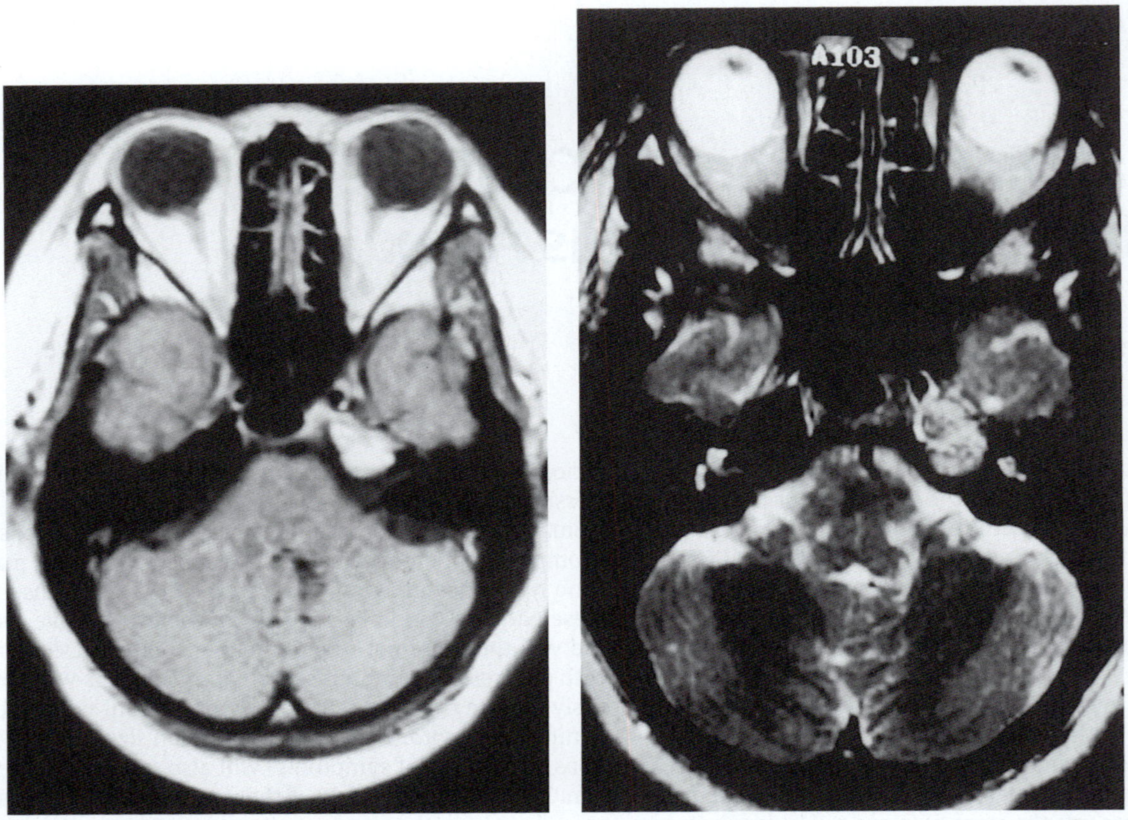

Figure 34–1 **(A)** T1-weighted axial magnetic resonance imaging (MRI). Note high signal of left petrous apex cholesterol granuloma. **(B)** T2-weighted axial MRI. Note high signal of left petrous apex cholesterol granuloma.

elevation. Patients are therefore started on an anticonvulsant medication the night prior to surgery. This is continued for 3 to 6 months following surgery. No other special preparations or medications are required apart from the routine preoperative evaluation and preparation for surgery.

◆ Operative Procedure

Following the induction of general endotracheal anesthesia, a lumbar drain is placed to allow cerebrospinal fluid (CSF) drainage during the extradural subtemporal dissection. The patient is also maintained in a hypovolemic state and hyperventilated. These maneuvers are important in maximizing brain relaxation. Electrodes are then placed to allow for monitoring of somatosensory evoked potentials (SSEPs) and facial nerve electromyography (EMG). In addition, an earphone is placed in each external auditory canal and scalp electrodes are inserted for monitoring of brain stem auditory evoked potentials. During the exposure, excessive traction or manipulation on the greater superficial petrosal nerve (GSPN), which runs along the floor of the middle fossa, may result in traction injury to the facial nerve via the geniculate ganglion. This complication has been minimized by continuously monitoring the facial nerve EMG. The patient must therefore not receive any muscle relaxants following induction and intubation.

The patient is positioned supine and the head is fixed in a three-pin head clamp. The head of the bed should be elevated to bring the patient's head above the level of the heart, thus maximizing venous drainage and brain relaxation. The head is turned to bring the zygoma nearly horizontal, and a roll is placed under the ipsilateral shoulder to keep the neck in a neutral position **(Fig. 34–2).** Alternatively, the patient may be placed in the true lateral position with a subaxillary roll in place. The operating microscope is then balanced and brought over to the field to check that it will be in a comfortable operating position prior to draping. The ipsilateral frontotemporal region is then shaved, prepped, and draped in a standard manner. For cases where there is suspected intradural extension, the lateral thigh is also exposed and prepared should the need for a fascial or fat graft arise.

A preauricular curvilinear incision is made **(Fig. 34–2)** and the scalp flap is elevated along the subgaleal plane. Care is taken to preserve the superficial temporal artery. At the anterior third of the temporalis muscle, the superficial layer of the deep temporal fascia is incised down to the muscle and reflected anteriorly with the scalp flap, thus sparing the frontalis branches of the facial nerve. The zygomatic arch may then be safely dissected in a subperiosteal manner and sectioned at its most anterior and posterior ends. This allows downward displacement of the arch along with the temporalis muscle. This maneuver provides access along the middle fossa floor with less than 1 cm of

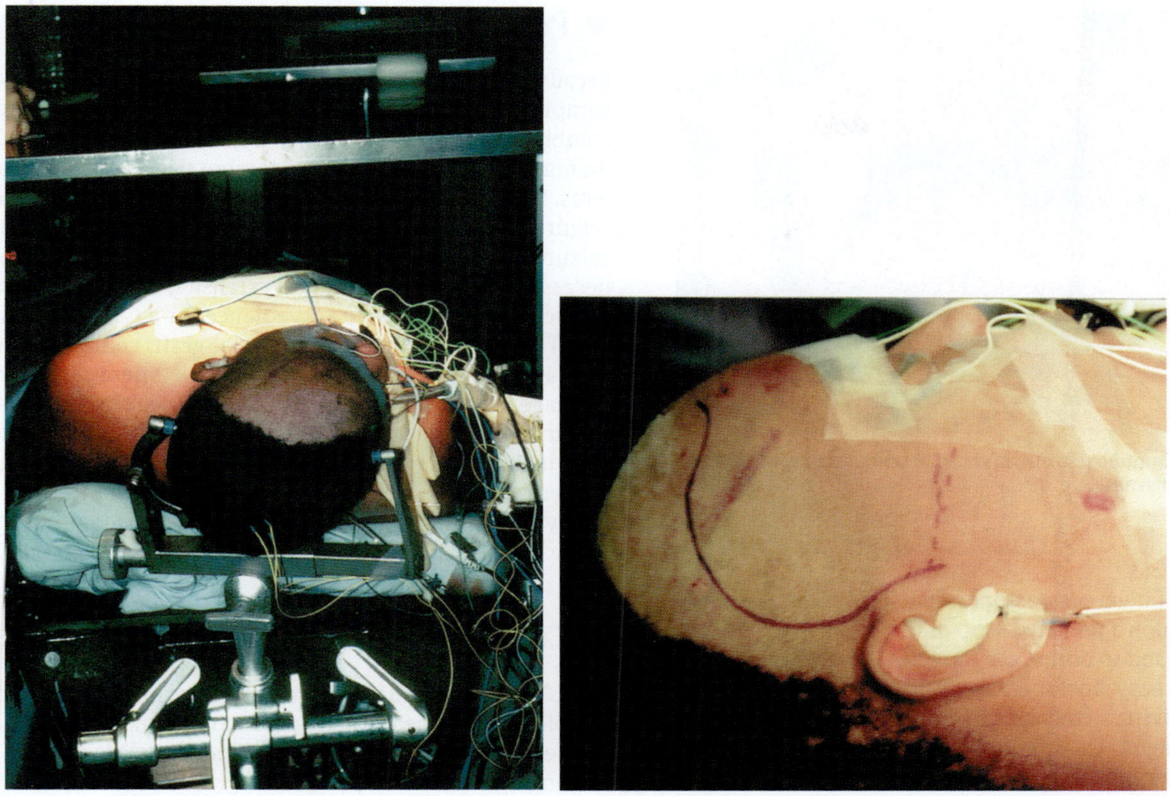
A B

Figure 34–2 **(A)** Patient positioning and **(B)** scalp incision for an extended middle fossa approach to the petrous apex.

temporal lobe elevation. A limited temporal craniotomy abutting the floor of the middle fossa is performed. It is important to drill the edge of the craniotomy flush with the middle fossa floor to avoid unnecessary temporal lobe retraction **(Fig. 34–3).**

At this point the operating microscope is brought into the field and the remainder of the surgery is performed under the microscope. The lumbar drain is opened and 30 to 50 mL of CSF are allowed to drain. The temporal lobe is supported extradurally with a malleable retractor, and the

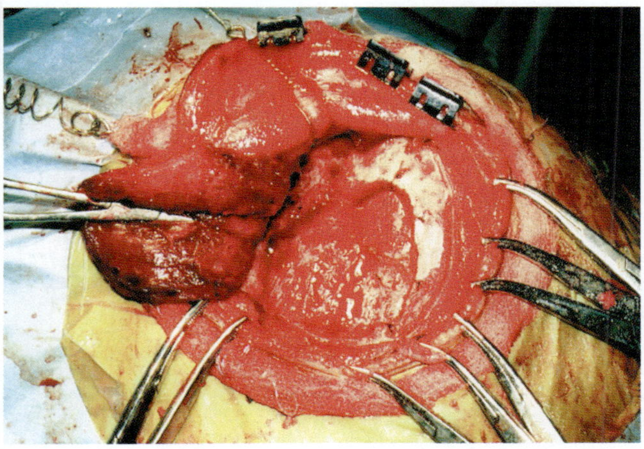

Figure 34–3 Temporal craniotomy flush with the middle fossa floor to avoid retraction of the temporal lobe.

extradural dissection is carried medially until the middle meningeal artery (MMA) is identified at the foramen spinosum. Small dural vessels traversing the middle fossa floor are easily controlled with either direct bipolar coagulation or bone wax. The MMA is coagulated and sectioned sharply, and the foramen is packed with bone wax or oxidized cellulose. The foramen ovale anteriorly and the GSPN medially are then identified. The lesser superficial petrosal nerve (LSPN) may be seen lateral to the GSPN. The GSPN is sharply dissected from its dural attachment and preserved; in some cases, the GSPN must be divided to avoid traction injury to the facial nerve. Further medially, the petrous portion of the internal carotid artery (ICA) can be seen deep to the posterolateral border of the third division of the trigeminal nerve, and, depending upon the size of the PACG, may be deviated superolaterally. Care must be taken in exposing this region because the bone over the carotid canal is often thin or even dehiscent. Once the PACG is identified and entered, the fluid is drained and the soft tissues, including the pseudocapsule, are completely excised. This is most often done with a combination of microdissectors, bipolar forceps, and smooth ring curets. When using the ring curets it is important to be sure that they are smooth to avoid injury to the carotid artery. Very often a portion of the remaining petrous apex must be removed with a high-speed drill to gain access to all areas of the cavity. If this is necessary a diamond bit is used to minimize the chance of injuring any surrounding structures (e.g., dura, ICA). Obliterating the resultant cavity with fat fragments makes follow-up MRI arduous because of the difficulty in distinguishing the signal

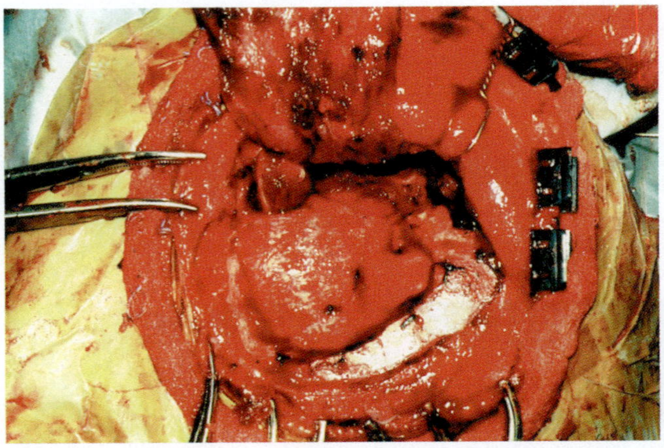

Figure 34–4 Emptied petrous apex cavity obliterated with pedicled strip of temporalis muscle.

intensities of fat versus postoperative fluid collections. We therefore fashion a pedicled strip of temporalis muscle that can then be used to obliterate the PACG cavity **(Fig. 34–4).** This permits easy postoperative MRI follow-up, with the muscle flap giving a consistently hypointense signal on T1-weighted images. The bone flap is returned and secured with titanium miniplates and screws and the remainder of the flap is closed in a standard fashion. No subgaleal drain is utilized. The lumbar drain is removed prior to the patient being reversed from anesthesia unless a dural repair was necessary, in which case it is usually left in place for 24 to 48 hours.

Patients are reversed from anesthesia in the operating room and observed overnight, either in the neurosurgical intensive care unit or in the recovery room. They are kept on dexamethasone for 1 to 2 days followed by tapering doses, and antibiotics are maintained for 48 hours. All patients receive antiseizure medication for 3 to 6 months and are then tapered off if they remain seizure-free.

◆ Postoperative Management

Because this is an extradural approach, primary neurological complications are rare. Maximal brain relaxation using a combination of hypovolemia, hyperventilation, and CSF drainage has nearly eliminated temporal lobe–related problems. Despite this, however, there is a risk of postoperative seizures, and patients are therefore maintained on antiseizure medication for 3 to 6 months. If a dural repair was necessary because of intradural extension of the granuloma, then close postoperative surveillance for a CSF leak is crucial. The use of either a fat or fascial graft, combined with the vascularized temporalis flap and postoperative lumbar drainage, helps minimize the risk of a CSF leak in those cases requiring a repair. If it should occur, all efforts to stop the leak, including reexploration, must be taken. As mentioned earlier postoperative facial weakness is related to traction injury via the superficial petrosal nerve. This is prevented with careful intraoperative monitoring of facial nerve EMG.

◆ Conclusions

1. CGs of the petrous apex are distinct lesions resulting from blockage of the normal aeration of the petrous apex air cells, which in turn, leads to a repeating cycle of mucosal engorgement, hemorrhage, and granuloma formation.
2. The extended middle fossa approach provides a safe, shallow, extradural exposure of the petrous apex. It enables the surgeon to radically remove the granuloma and obliterate the cavity with vascularized tissue.
3. Complications related to temporal lobe retraction are minimized by combining a zygomatic osteotomy and drilling of the temporal squama flush with the middle fossa floor with adequate brain relaxation through the use of hyperventilation, hypovolemia, and CSF drainage.
4. Ipsilateral facial nerve function is protected by attention to the GSPN and intraoperative EMG monitoring.

35

Transbasal Approaches to the Skull Base and Extensions

Iman Feiz-Erfan, Robert F. Spetzler, Randall W. Porter, Stephen P. Beals, Salvatore C. Lettieri, and Edward F. Joganic

The transbasal approach is a transcranial extradural approach to the anterior skull base through a bifrontal craniotomy and involves sacrifice of olfaction by resection of the olfactory fila at the cribriform plate. This approach allows transcranial access to the sinonasal cavity. It is primarily designed for sinonasal and nasopharyngeal tumors involving the anterior skull base. Tumoral extensions to the clivus can also be addressed through this approach. Several variations of this approach with extensions involving osteotomies of the orbit and nasal bone allow further exposure of anterior and central skull base structures in the midline.

◆ Patient Selection

Patients with midline anterior or central primarily extradural tumors are the typical candidates for a transbasal procedure. Magnetic resonance imaging (MRI), computed tomography (CT), or both are used to identify such candidates. The usual indication is a symptomatic primary tumor that fails to respond to nonoperative treatment. Lymphomas, plasma cell neoplasms, nasopharyngeal carcinomas, rhabdomyosarcomas, and neuroendocrine carcinomas are usually responsive to nonoperative management. Hence all lesions considered for a transbasal procedure must be biopsied to exclude tumors that can be treated with radiation or chemotherapy and do not require resection.

◆ Preoperative Preparation

Because the sinonasal cavity must be opened, antibiotics should be administered to patients before surgery. Usually gram-positive and -negative coverage and coverage for anaerobic organisms are recommended. A spinal subarachnoid drain can be placed to relieve retraction pressure on the brain. If dural resection and reconstruction are required, lumbar drainage can help to reduce a leakage of spinal fluid. Patients should be informed that they will lose olfaction unless a cribriform plate osteotomy is performed (see cribriform plate osteotomy). Pneumatic compression boots are placed at the time of general anesthesia to reduce the risk of deep venous thrombosis. The endotracheal tube should be wired to the lower teeth to protect the airway in case a separate transfacial procedure is required during surgery. Temporary tarsorrhaphies should be performed to protect the cornea.

◆ Operative Procedure

Indications for the Transbasal Approaches and Their Modifications

For tumors involving the upper nasal vault and anterior skull base with no extensions into the orbit, a transbasal approach is sufficient. If tumors are benign, a subcranial transbasal approach with a cribriform plate osteotomy is necessary to save olfaction. Otherwise, for most craniofacial resections, the transbasal approach is adequate when combined with a transfacial approach.

For extensive tumors that significantly involve the frontal fossa, with or without orbital involvement, an extended transbasal approach is preferred. This exposure provides access to the orbit, minimizes brain retraction because the orbital rim is osteotomized, and enhances skull base exposure. A subcranial or a radical transbasal approach is best suited for tumors intensively involved with the nasal cavity and possibly with the maxillary sinus. Removing the nasal bone enhances access to the nasal cavity. Furthermore, exposure of the maxillary sinus from above is increased by removal of the nasal bone. To maximize exposure of the maxillary sinus, a radical transbasal approach allows the easiest and safest retraction of the globes **(Fig. 35–1),** improving the angle of approach into the maxillary sinus from above.

For tumors that also involve the sphenoid sinus and clivus, an extended transbasal approach and a subcranial transbasal approach are superior to the standard transbasal approach because the angle of approach is increased. These procedures require osteotomies of the cribriform plate either to preserve olfaction or to sacrifice the cribriform plate. Removal of both ethmoidal sinuses on each side allows the sphenoid sinus to be entered. From there the clivus can be exposed further.

The foramen magnum is the limit of exposure in the midline; the lateral limits are the hypoglossal nerves. The cavernous portions of the carotid arteries are the lateral limits

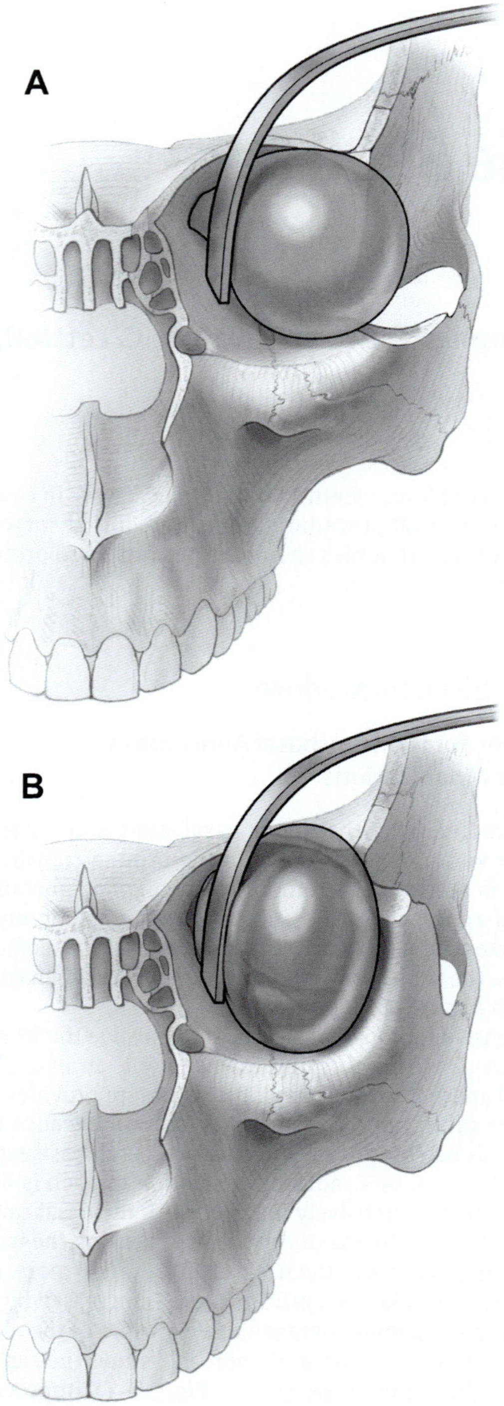

Figure 35–1 **(A)** In the subcranial transbasal approach, the lateral orbital wall is not osteotomized. Therefore, if the orbital contents are retracted laterally, pressure is exerted on these structures while they are pushed against the lateral orbital wall. **(B)** This retraction pressure can be minimized by osteotomizing the lateral wall. (From Feiz-Erfan I, Han PP, Spetzler LF. The Radical Transbasal Approach for Resection of Anterior and Midline Skull Base Lesions. J Neurosurg 2005;103:486, with permission.)

of the transbasal approaches and their extensions. If structures off midline, lateral to the cavernous portions of the carotid arteries and lateral to the cranial nerves, must be exposed, then lateral or anterolateral approaches are needed.

Cribriform Plate Osteotomy

A cribriform plate osteotomy in which the cribriform plate is spared can preserve olfaction. The cribriform plate must be osteotomized circumferentially. The lateral and anterior cuts are part of the osteotomy used to remove the orbital bar. The posterior cut along the posterior edge of the cribriform plate is performed with a reciprocating saw. A no. 1 Penfield dissector or a periosteal elevator is used to peel the dura from the planum sphenoidale. The reciprocating saw is inserted, and its tip is placed in the midline of the posterior edge of the cribriform plate. A cut aimed anterolaterally from midline on each side frees the cribriform plate **(Fig. 35–2A)**.

Mucosal and bony cartilaginous attachments to the cribriform plate are cut with curved heavy scissors **(Fig. 35–2B)**. At least 1 to 2 cm of nasal mucosa must be left attached to the surface of the cribriform plate. After the mucosa is cut from the nasal cavity toward the back of the cribriform plate, the freed olfactory unit can be retracted upward while attached to the frontal dura **(Fig. 35–2C)**. Dural rents around the cribriform plate are stitched extradurally using either loupe or microscopic magnification. If an extradural repair is too difficult to achieve, an intradural approach can be used. If a cribriform plate osteotomy is desired to preserve olfaction, the nasal bone must be incorporated in the supraorbital bar as it is in the subcranial or radical transbasal approach. Otherwise, there will not be enough room to cut a sufficient nasal mucosal cuff below the cribriform plate. For closure, drill holes are placed anteriorly or laterally at the cribriform plate and at the corresponding osteotomy rims in the frontal fossa. The cribriform plate is then wire twisted into place using 28-gauge wires. The pericranium must be divided in the midline to allow incorporation of the cribriform plate. The remainder of the closure is the same as described earlier.

Transbasal Approach

The patient is positioned supine with the neck flexed (15 to 30 degrees) and the head extended slightly. Three-point fixation of the head is achieved with a Mayfield headholder. The pins must be positioned behind the ears so that enough pericranium can be harvested for later reconstruction of the anterior skull base. Hair is usually shaved in a coronal plane. On each side the skin incision begins in front of the tragus and continues in a coronal plane. Either a curvilinear incision or a "wave" incision can be used. The latter offers a better cosmetic outcome because it is better concealed than the former after the hair regrows.

Next, a plane is developed while leaving the pericranium intact. The scalp flap is reflected anteriorly using either sharp dissection with a scalpel or monopolar cautery dissection. The pericranium must be preserved so that an intact layer of vascularized tissue is available for skull base reconstruction. Fishhooks can be used to retract the skin flap. Dissection usually extends no more than 1 cm above the orbital rims to prevent damage to the supraorbital arteries, which provide the vascular supply of the pericranial flap.

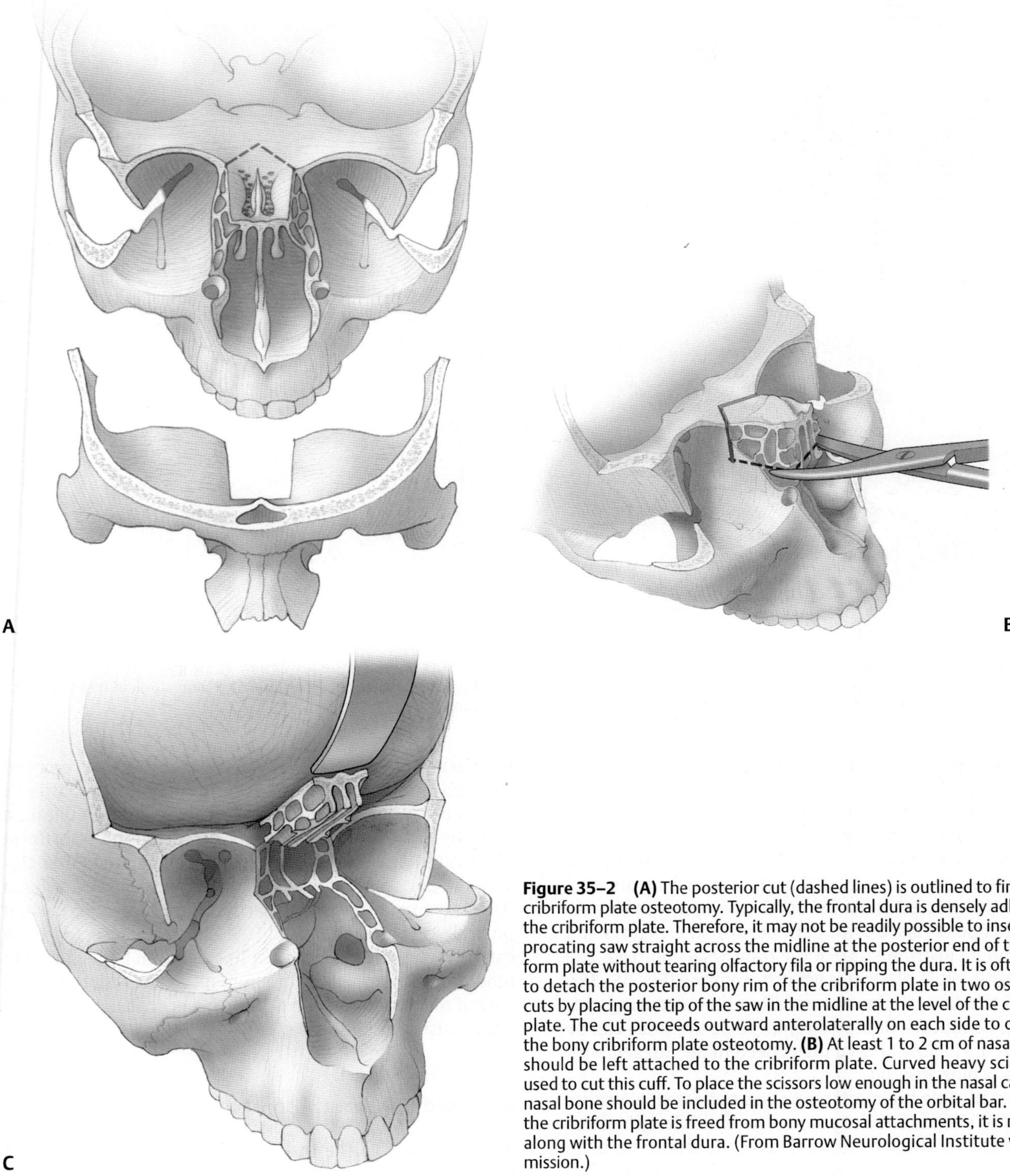

Figure 35–2 **(A)** The posterior cut (dashed lines) is outlined to finalize the cribriform plate osteotomy. Typically, the frontal dura is densely adherent to the cribriform plate. Therefore, it may not be readily possible to insert a reciprocating saw straight across the midline at the posterior end of the cribriform plate without tearing olfactory fila or ripping the dura. It is often easier to detach the posterior bony rim of the cribriform plate in two osteotomy cuts by placing the tip of the saw in the midline at the level of the cribriform plate. The cut proceeds outward anterolaterally on each side to complete the bony cribriform plate osteotomy. **(B)** At least 1 to 2 cm of nasal mucosa should be left attached to the cribriform plate. Curved heavy scissors are used to cut this cuff. To place the scissors low enough in the nasal cavity, the nasal bone should be included in the osteotomy of the orbital bar. **(C)** Once the cribriform plate is freed from bony mucosal attachments, it is retracted along with the frontal dura. (From Barrow Neurological Institute with permission.)

Laterally, the interfascial dissection over the temporalis muscle should be performed carefully to protect the frontalis branch of the facial nerve. Interfascial dissection should begin as soon as the subcutaneous fat pad over the temporalis muscle is visible.

Next, the posterior cutaneous flap is undermined slightly with sharp or blunt dissection. The pericranium is usually harvested 13 to 15 cm from the orbital rim. The pericranium is cut using electrocautery or a scalpel, and the flap is elevated with periosteal elevators until the orbital rim is approached. Again, the supraorbital arteries supplying the pericranial flap must not be damaged. The pericranium is reflected with the scalp flap, which can be retracted with fishhooks. The temporalis muscle is released bilaterally, and

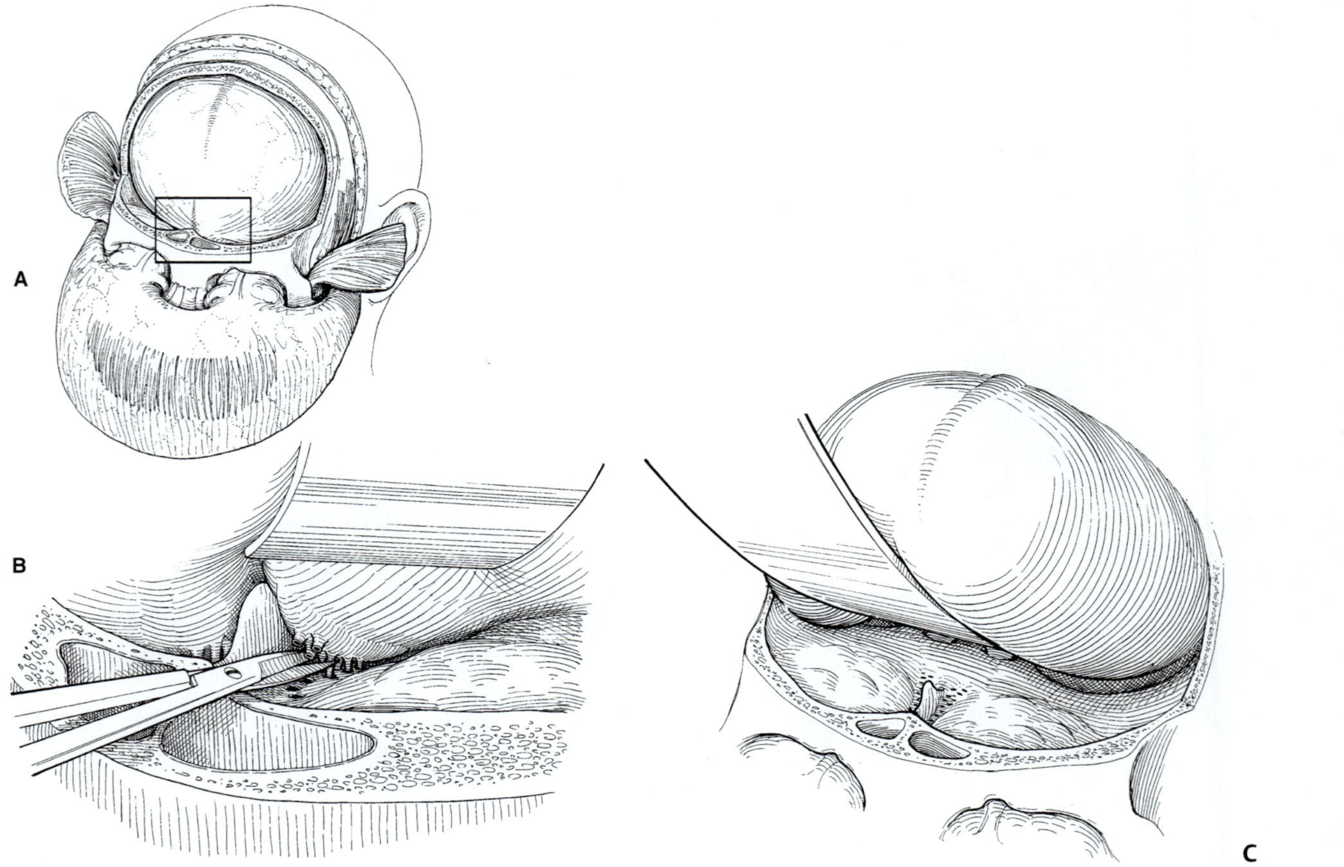

Figure 35–3 **(A)** The frontal dura is exposed after elevation of the bifrontal craniotomy bone flap. **(B)** Enlargement of area framed in **(A)**. The dural sheath around the olfactory nerve bundles is cut with microscissors under gentle retraction. **(C)** Extradural exposure of the frontal fossa is obtained. (From Barrow Neurological Institute with permission.)

an anterior rim of muscle fascia cuff is left attached for later reanastomosis. The rest of the muscle can be detached from the bone with periosteal elevators and retracted posteriorly.

Next, four bur holes are drilled using the air drill. Two bur holes are placed on each side of the vertex, flanking the parasagittal suture at the level of the coronal suture. The footplate is inserted and a bifrontal craniotomy is turned. The bone flap is raised with both periosteal elevators and no. 3 Penfield instruments. For the transbasal approach, the orbital bar is left in place; it is not osteotomized **(Fig. 35–3A).** Because the frontal sinus is usually entered during craniotomy, its mucosa has to be removed or the sinus can be cranialized. The frontonasal ducts need to be plugged with autologous muscle or fat.

Next, malleable brain retractors and periosteal elevators are used to elevate the dura along the entire length of the frontal fossa. To access the frontal fossa, the cribriform plate is exposed by bipolar cauterization of the olfactory fila, which are then incised with microscissors **(Fig. 35–3B).** Alternatively, the dura can be excised circumferentially around the cribriform plate, leaving a small dural defect that must be repaired later. At this point the frontal fossa is completely exposed to the level of the lesser sphenoid wing, anterior clinoid process, tuberculum sella, and planum sphenoidale **(Fig. 35–3C).**

The orbits and the sinonasal cavity can be entered using osteotomes or drills. Sinonasal and nasopharyngeal tumors with extensions to the skull base and orbit can be removed through this approach. For reconstruction, the patient's pericranium or temporalis fascia can be used to obtain a watertight closure of the dural defect at the cribriform plate. Alternatively, dural substitutes can be used. After closure the pericranium is placed on top of the anterior fossa defect to provide a vascular barrier to prevent infection and possible cerebrospinal fluid (CSF) leakage. Resected bone can be reconstructed with a split calvarium bone graft and other implants, including titanium mesh. If a watertight closure of the dura cannot be achieved, a ventricular or lumbar drain must be used to drain CSF.

Extended Transbasal Approach

An alternative to the transbasal approach, the extended transbasal approach consists of the bifrontal craniotomy as performed for the transbasal approach and osteotomies of the supraorbital bar **(Fig. 35–4A,B).** Compared with the standard transbasal approach, this extended approach provides a more basal exposure of the skull base **(Fig. 35–4C),** which lessens retraction of the frontal lobes. Clival and orbital exposure is also enhanced. Osteotomies of the orbital roofs and orbital bar facilitate access to both orbits. The positioning and initial approach are performed as for the transbasal approach.

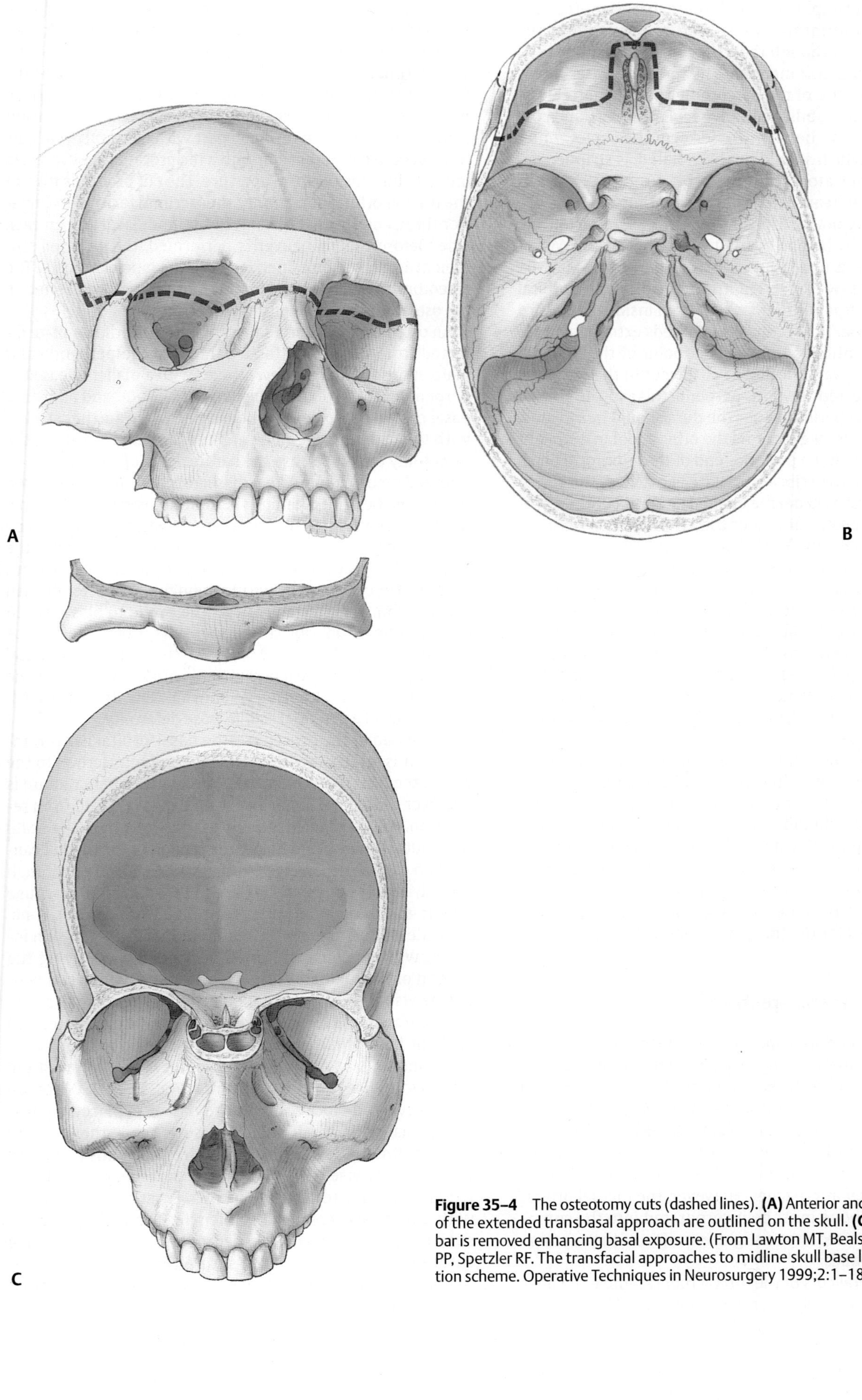

Figure 35–4 The osteotomy cuts (dashed lines). **(A)** Anterior and **(B)** superior views of the extended transbasal approach are outlined on the skull. **(C)** The supraorbital bar is removed enhancing basal exposure. (From Lawton MT, Beals SP, Joganic EF, Han PP, Spetzler RF. The transfacial approaches to midline skull base lesions: a classification scheme. Operative Techniques in Neurosurgery 1999;2:1–18, with permission.)

Once the bony exposure for the transbasal approach is achieved, a reciprocating saw is used to osteotomize the supraorbital bar. Although the drill can be used instead of the saw, it is not recommended. The former creates larger bone gaps at the site of the osteotomy than the latter. The gaps decrease the stability of bony reconstruction, and cosmetic outcomes can be poor. To perform the osteotomies, the periorbita, which should not be violated, is stripped using periosteal elevators from the orbital roof. This task is difficult and small tears can be left without repair.

Once the periorbita is stripped from the roof, retractors are inserted into the orbit and overlying the frontal dura. While the tip of the saw is under direct visualization, the orbital bar is cut. First, the saw is inserted inside the orbit. The orbital roof is cut in a perpendicular fashion from inside out toward the temporal fossa. The second cut proceeds extracranially to intracranially continues from the endpoint of the first cut, and is directed upward. It begins at the cut in the temporal fossa and is directed upward, perpendicular to the frontal fossa. Neither the periorbita nor the dura should be violated. The cut continues straight across the orbital roof in a straight line drawn to match the posterior end of the cribriform plate. When the end of the cribriform plate is reached, the saw is turned forward at a 90 degree angle. The third cut then proceeds from the posterior end of the cribriform plate to the anterior end of the cribriform plate, crossing the anterior rim of the cribriform plate to the contralateral side.

Next, an external cut is made across the nasion. The orbital bar is loosened. The supraorbital nerve is freed from the orbital bar. If a supraorbital canal is present, it must be released with osteotomes. Periosteal dissectors designed to elevate soft tissue are used to remove the supraorbital bar. The frontal sinus is exonerated from the supraorbital bar using forceps. If needed, an air drill is used to bur out the remaining mucosa.

After surgery, the supraorbital bar is reattached with miniplates and screws. After the orbital bar is repositioned, the vascularized pericranium is laid over the frontal fossa. The pericranium should not be squeezed between the bifrontal craniotomy flap and supraorbital bar. If necessary, a rongeur can be used to remove bone from the bifrontal craniotomy flap to create plenty of room for the pericranium to be rolled into the frontal fossa. The closure is the same as that used for the transbasal approach.

Subcranial Transbasal Approach

The subcranial transbasal approach is a further modification of the original transbasal approach. It offers more extensive exposure because it involves osteotomies of the entire nasal bone along with a supraorbital bar **(Fig. 35–5A)**. Exposure of the nasal cavity is facilitated **(Fig. 35–5B)**, and basal exposure extends to the clivus. The osteotomies and craniotomy are similar to those used in the transbasal and extended transbasal approaches. However, the medial orbital walls and nasal bone must be incorporated into the supraorbital bar, which requires a slight variation of the supraorbital bar osteotomies.

The initial lateral cuts of the orbital roof resemble the ones performed in the extended transbasal approach. However, the cut across the nasion is not performed. Rather, the tendon of the medial canthus is detached from its bony insertion (called the dacryon) just in front of the lacrimal fossa on each side. The lacrimal sac is completely released from the lacrimal fossa and retracted with periosteal elevators. The nasal bone is dissected until the cartilaginous vault is reached. The vault is then detached from the bony part with elevators. Two cuts (one on each side) are made with a reciprocating saw inserted laterally into the piriform aperture. The cut proceeds toward the medial orbital bar, crosses the lacrimal fossa in its superior third, and stops at the anterior ethmoidal artery on each side. Before this maneuver is performed, the anterior ethmoidal artery can be cauterized with the bipolar and cut. The osteotomies involving the orbital roof are then connected to the osteotomy from the piriform aperture.

An osteotome is inserted in front of the cribriform plate directed from the frontal fossa parallel to the perpendicular plate of the ethmoids. A few strokes with a mallet release the perpendicular plate from the bony nasal vault and allow the nasal orbital bar to be loosened. If necessary, further strokes with the osteotomes can be applied laterally and along the osteotomy cuts to release the bar further. Soft tissues can be released by using periosteal dissectors. For the closure, two holes must be drilled behind the superior end of the lacrimal fossa on each side. A 28-gauge wire is passed through each hole for medial canthopexy, which must be performed at the end of the procedure. The medial canthal tendons are thereby overcorrected by wiring them further posterior than the dacryon. This strategy allows the eyelid to be stretched out and offers superior cosmetic results. Holes can also be drilled at the border of the bony nasal and cartilaginous nasal vaults so they can be reapproximated with 2–0 Polydioxanone (PDS; Ethicon Inc., Johnson & Johnson, New Brunswick, NJ) stitch to avoid a potential saddle-nose deformity.

At the end of the procedure, the nasal-orbital bar is reinserted. It is attached with miniplates and miniscrews to the rest of the facial bony elements. Vascularized pericranium is laid over the frontal fossa. The scalp flap is released from retraction. An 18-gauge needle is used to perforate the scalp from outside above and below the tendon of the medial canthus on each side. The two 28-gauge wires inserted through both drill holes on each side are fed through the 18-gauge needle to the outside of the scalp flap **(Fig. 35–5C)**. A no. 15 blade is used to make a circumferential C-shaped skin incision with its convexity oriented medially, overlying the tendon of the medial canthus. The tendon, which can usually be visualized in subcutaneous tissue, is a whitish structure. Care should be exerted to avoid cutting the tendon with the knife while performing the C-shaped incision.

On one side, an empty needle holder is used to twist the wires clockwise three to four turns **(Fig. 35–5D)**. Wires are always twisted clockwise. A wire passer is placed against the medial orbital wall under pressure. While the pressure is maintained, the contralateral wires are pulled out and twisted clockwise **(Fig. 35–5E)**. The wires on each side are trimmed with wire cutters. The final twist of the two wires with a hemostat creates a semicircle. The twisted wire is sunk in the subcutaneous tissue, and the small incisions are sutured with a 5–0 chromic suture **(Fig. 35–5F)**. The remainder of the closure follows that of the extended transbasal procedure.

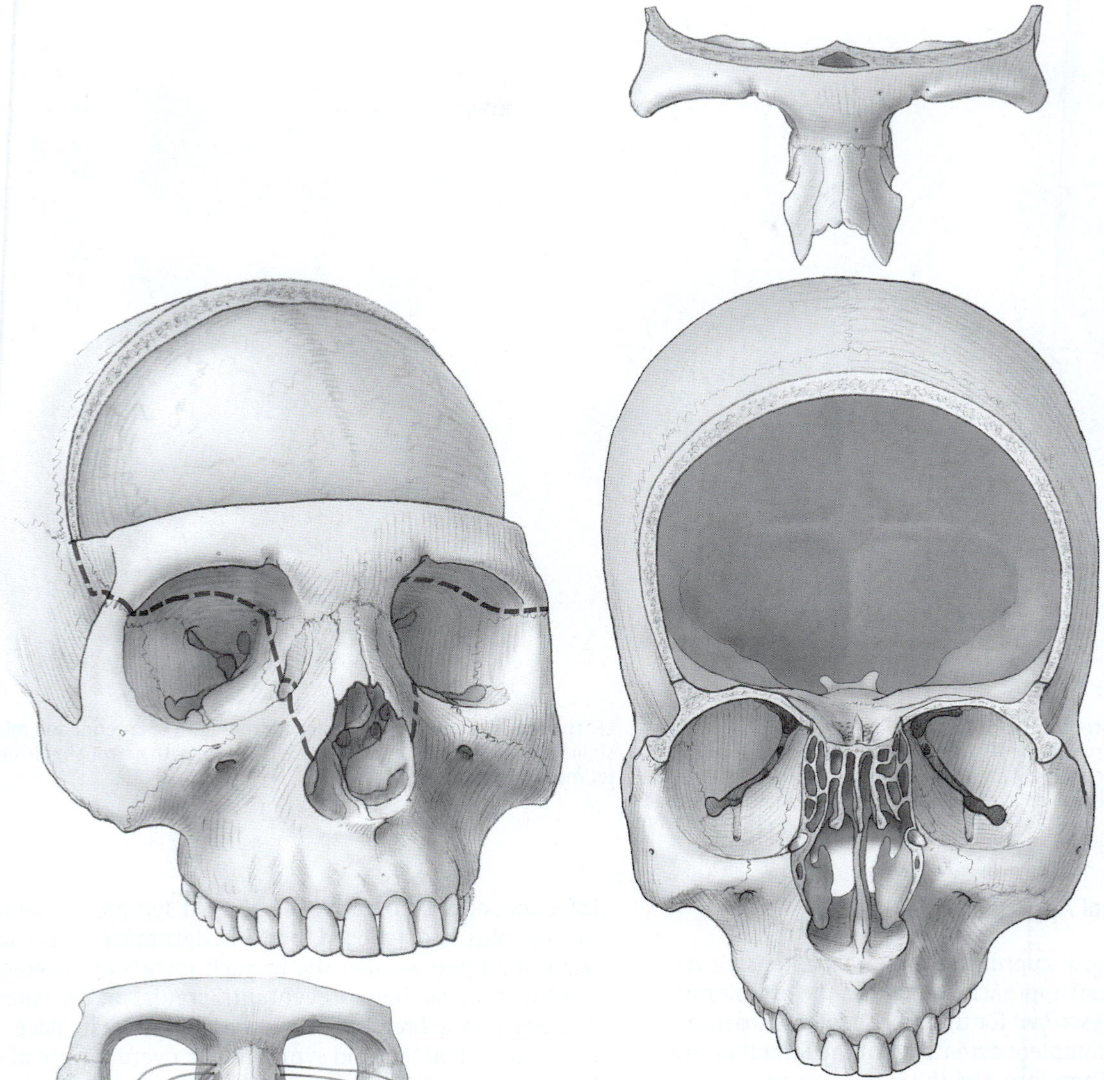

A

B

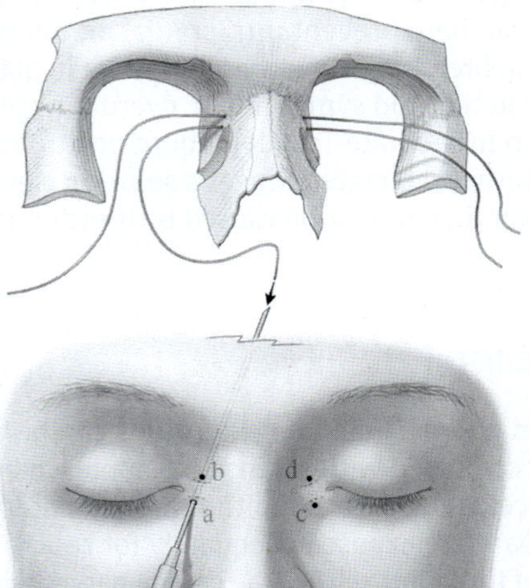

C

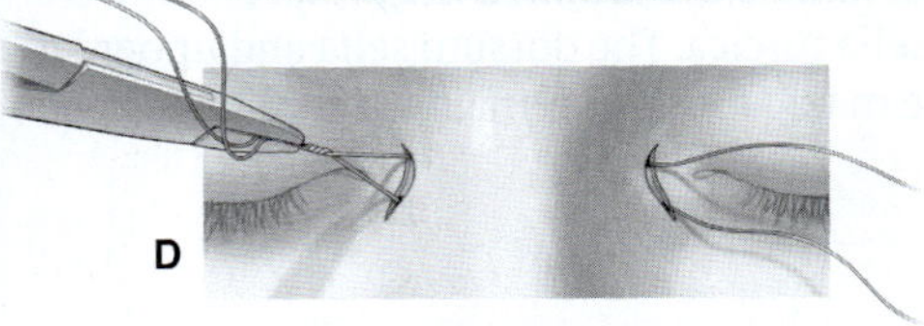

D

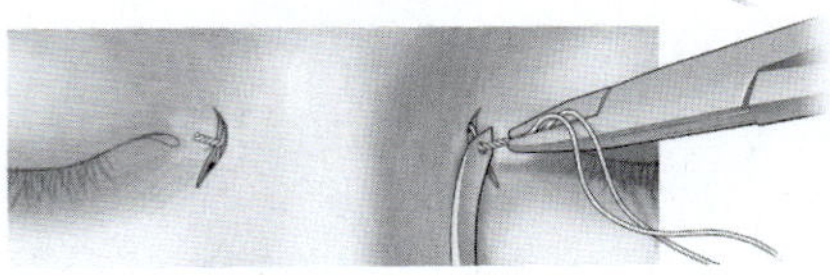

E

Figure 35–5 **(A)** The osteotomy cuts (dashed lines) of the subcranial transbasal approach are outlined. **(B)** Transcranial exposure of the sinonasal cavity is facilitated. **(C)** Two 28-gauge wires are passed through drill holes and turned from the inside-out through the skin of the face. To do so, the skin is perforated with an 18-gauge needle above and below each medial canthus (perforation marks labeled a, b, c, and d). The wires are passed out, and the skin bridge is cut with a no. 15 blade. **(D)** The wires are then twisted clockwise. **(E)** The contralateral wires are pulled tight over a wire passer awl and twisted clockwise. Overhanging wires are buried in subcutaneous tissue. **(F)** The skin incision is closed with 5–0 chromic subcuticular closure. (Figures 35A, B from Lawton MT, Beals SP, Joganic EF, Han PP, Spetzler RF. The transfacial approaches to midline skull base lesions: a classification scheme. Oper Tech Neurosurg 1999;2:1–18, with permission from Elsevier Science Inc. Figures 35C–F from Feiz-Erfan I, Han PP, Spetzler LI. The radical transbasal approach for resection of anterior and midline skull base lesions. J Neurosurg 2005;103:487, with permission from the Journal of Neurosurgery.)

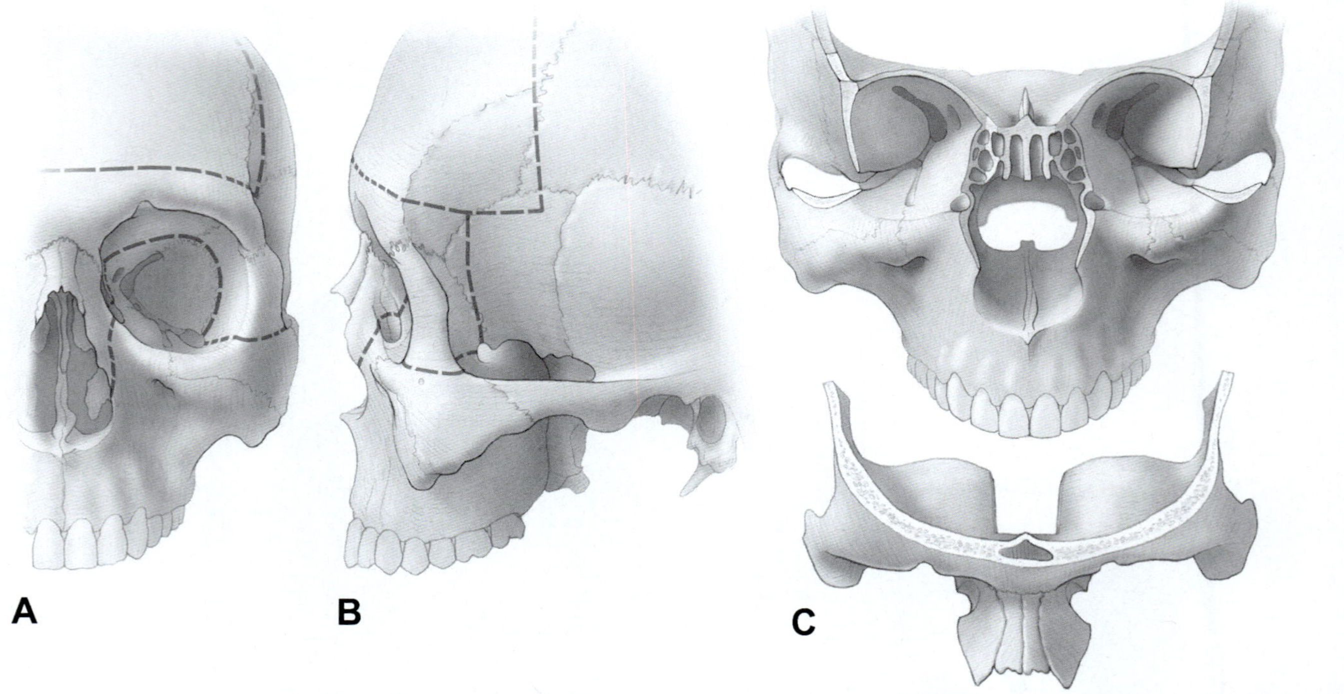

Figure 35–6 **(A)** Osteotomy cuts (dashed lines) for the radical transbasal approach from frontal and **(B)** lateral views. **(C)** Mobilization of the nasofronto-orbital bar achieves extensive exposure of the anterior skull base via this transbasal-type approach. (From Feiz-Erfan I, Han PP, Spetzler LF. The radical transbasal approach for resection of anterior and midline skull base lesions. J Neurosurg 2005;103:486, with permission from the Journal of Neurosurgery.)

Radical Transbasal Approach

The radical transbasal approach is the most extensive version of the transbasal approach. It includes the osteotomies of the orbital bar described for the subcranial transbasal approach but also a complete osteotomy of the lateral orbital wall **(Fig. 35–6)**. Therefore, the initial osteotomy cuts are made with a saw from inside the orbit. The tip of the saw is inserted into the inferior orbital fissure and cut axially from inside the orbit out toward the temporal fossa. For the second cut, the saw is inserted from the temporal fossa into the inferior orbital fissure. The cut proceeds upward, perpendicular toward the anterior fossa. The middle fossa should not be entered. The remainder of the cuts and the closure are performed as for the subcranial transbasal approach.

◆ Postoperative Management

Patients are admitted to the intensive care unit. They can usually be extubated postoperatively. Neurological monitoring is required to rule out pneumocephalus, CSF leakage, infection, or postoperative bleeding. If symptomatic pneumocephalus is diagnosed, bedside decompression can be performed percutaneously. In such instances an elective reintubation can help prevent intracranial air entrapment caused by nasal breathing. If lumbar drains are in place, vigilance is needed to avoid symptomatic overdrainage of CSF. In this case, an immediate Trendelenburg position and injection of intrathecal lactated Ringer's solution can be lifesaving by preventing herniation caused by overdrainage.

◆ Conclusion

The transbasal approach and its extensions can be applied from above or combined with a transfacial approach to obtain craniofacial access. Lesions along the midline anterior and central skull base are exposed adequately for resection. The lateral limits of this approach are the cranial nerves and internal carotid arteries. The posterior limit is the dura over the clivus. The caudal limit is the foramen magnum, and the cranial limit is the sella turcica. The dorsum sella and upper lateral corner of the maxillary sinus remain surgical blind spots.

36

Transmandibular Approaches to the Skull Base

Iman Feiz-Erfan, Salvatore C. Lettieri, Robert F. Spetzler, Randall W. Porter, Stephen P. Beals, Edward F. Joganic, and Franco DeMonte

Skull base surgical approaches that utilize osteotomies of the mandible can be applied to lesions of the clivus, craniocervical junction, and upper anterior cervical spine. They can also be used to reach pathology medial to the carotid artery along the skull base as well as to resect pathology located in the infratemporal fossa. The transmandibular approaches differ according to the location of the mandibular osteotomy, the type of osteotomy, and the soft tissue dissection required. Three variations of the transmandibular approach used to access the central skull base and craniocervical junction are discussed: (1) the median labial-mandibular-glossotomy (LMG), (2) the transmandibular-circumglossal-retropharyngeal (TCR) approach, and (3) the bilateral-sagittal split mandibular osteotomy (BSSMO).

◆ Patient Selection

Typically, patients with primarily extradural tumors in the midline skull base and craniocervical junction or infratemporal fossa and parapharyngeal space are best suited for this procedure.

◆ Preoperative Preparation

Every patient requires PANOREX imaging to rule out the presence of dental hardware or osteomyelitis. Because the oropharyngeal cavity is opened, antibiotic coverage begins preoperatively. Usually gram-positive and - negative coverage and coverage for anaerobic organisms are recommended to treat the surgical field with oropharyngeal flora. A spinal subarachnoid drain can be placed to relieve retraction pressure on the brain. If dural resection and reconstruction are required, lumbar drainage can help to reduce spinal fluid leakage. Pneumatic compression boots are placed at the time of general anesthesia to reduce the risk of deep venous thrombosis. A temporary tracheostomy is usually recommended. It is often placed immediately before the procedure to help maintain and secure the airway intra- and postoperatively. Temporary tarsorrhaphies should be performed to protect the cornea. Because patients will cease for a postoperative period of about two weeks from oral alimentation, an intraoperative feeding tube is frequently placed. Sometimes, a surgically placed feeding tube is necessary if a prolonged period of parenteral nutrition is required.

◆ Operative Procedure

Median Labial-Mandibular-Glossotomy (LMG) Approach

A tracheostomy is performed before the procedure begins. The intraoral cavity and face are prepared and draped in a sterile fashion. A skin incision divides the lower lip in the midline and extends to the chin to the level of the hyoid bone. Different incisions are available to achieve a good cosmetic outcome **(Fig. 36–1A).** The primary difference is the configuration of the incision over the chin.

After the chin is incised, the midline of the mandible is exposed in a subperiosteal fashion between the two mental foramina. A stair-step mandibulotomy is performed between the midline incisors **(Fig. 36–1B).** A right-angle reciprocating saw is used to make the osteotomy.

The miniplates for later fixation of the osteotomies are applied before the osteotomy is performed to insure that the bones are reassembled correctly. Performing a stair-step osteotomy rather than a straight osteotomy enhances the stability of the osteotomy when it is reassembled.

During the osteotomy, the roots of the teeth should not be violated to avoid tooth loss. Although a central incisor may be removed for this osteotomy, it is usually not required.

After the osteotomy is performed, the tongue is grasped with towel clamps or sutures placed on each side of the tip and elevated cranially. The ventral surface of the tongue is exposed. The midline raphe is identified. Using monopolar cautery with a small tip or needle, a midline glossotomy is performed along the raphe. The glossotomy is extended in the midline to the level of the glossal epiglottic fold posteriorly. The incision is also extended anteriorly along the floor of the mouth between the orifices of the sublingual ducts down to the hyoid bone inferiorly **(Fig. 36–1C).**

Next, the oropharynx and most proximal portion of the hypopharynx are exposed. Depending on the location of the lesion, cranial exposure can be obtained by splitting the soft palate and, if necessary, by osteotomizing the hard palate circumferentially. This maneuver exposes the nasopharynx and enhances access to the sphenoid sinus and sella cranially and extends down to the upper cervical spine **(Fig. 36–1D).** This approach provides a midline exposure between the two carotid arteries and hypoglossal nerves. When the LMG approach is completed without osteotomy of the hard palate, the distal clivus and upper cervical spine are exposed **(Fig. 36–1E).**

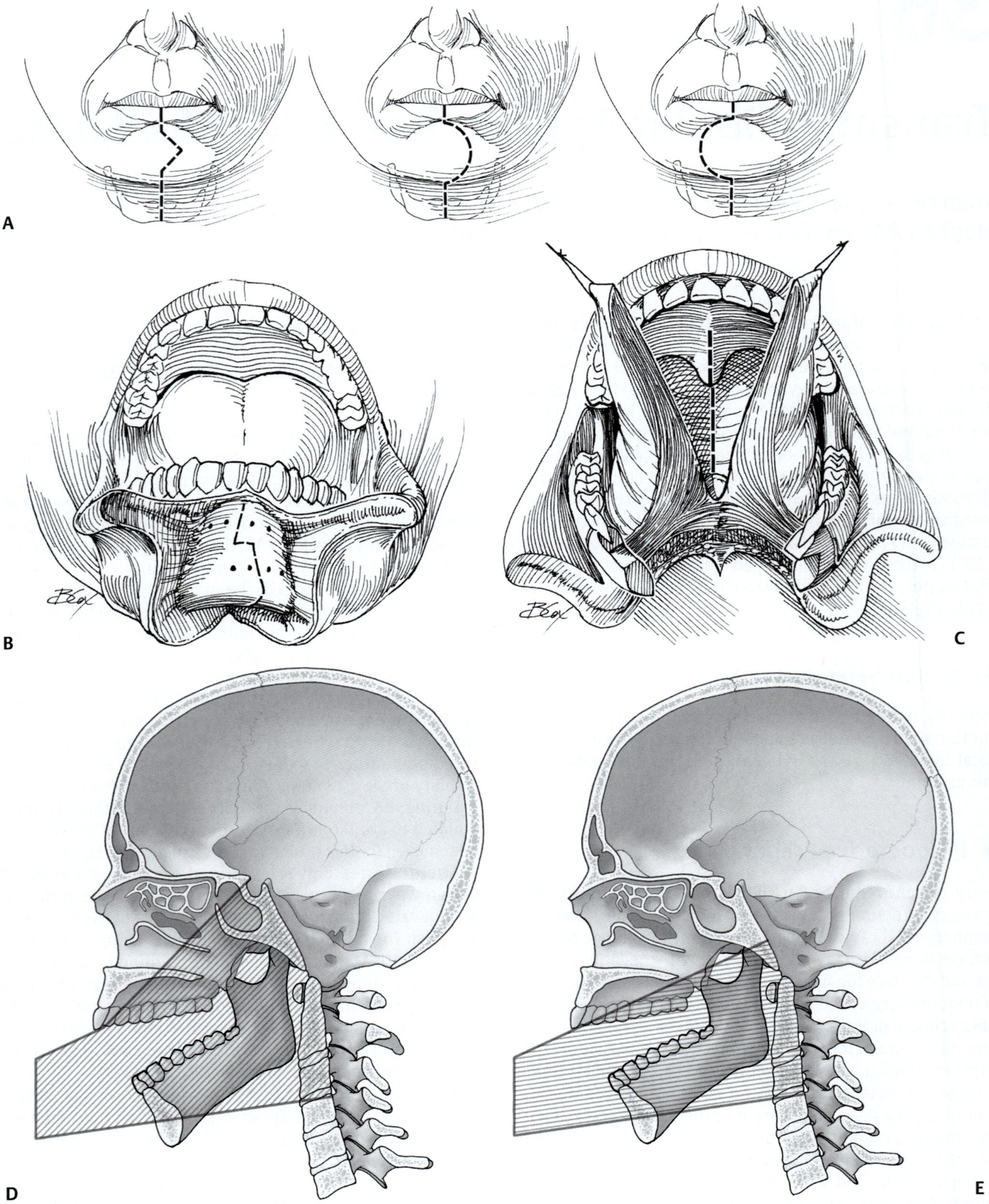

Figure 36–1 **(A)** Three variations of skin incisions (dashed lines) for the labial-mandibular-glossotomy (LMG) approach. **(B)** The lower lip is cut, holes are drilled to preapply miniplates, and the stair-step mandibulotomy is outlined on the exposed mandible. **(C)** The tongue is divided in the midline and elevated to the sides. The uvula can be divided in the midline along the site of the naso-oropharyngeal incision (dashed line). Alternatively, the uvular base can be cut laterally, thereby leaving the structure intact (not shown in figure). **(D)** By osteotomizing the hard palate, the transoral approach to the skull base can be extended to expose the sella, upper clivus, and craniocervical junction (shaded area). **(E)** The LMG approach provides exposure to the lower clivus and upper cervical spine (shaded area).

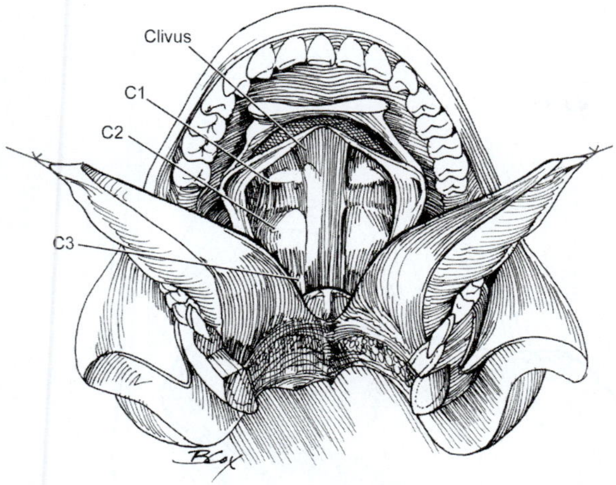

(*Continued*) **Figure 36–1** **(F)** Bony exposure is shown after the LMG approach. (From Barrow Neurological Institute with permission.)

To reach pathology located in the craniocervical junction, clivus, and sphenoid sinus, the pharyngeal mucosa must be incised. Usually, a midline incision is performed with monopolar cautery. After the bony clivus and craniocervical junction are exposed **(Fig. 36–1F),** bone can be removed with drills and rongeurs. After the lesion is removed, the pharyngeal mucosa is sutured together in one layer using absorbable suture material (braided or nonbraided).

If incised, the soft palate is sutured in place using absorbable suture material. If the hard palate was osteotomized temporarily, it can be replaced with miniplates before the soft palate is closed. Placing an obturator may help the palatal mucosa to heal onto the hard palate. The glossotomy is repaired posteriorly to anteriorly and from the dorsal to the ventral surface. Starting posteriorly, the dorsal surface of the tongue is closed with an absorbable suture by inverting the raphe on the surface.

Next the muscle layers are sutured in place. The floor of the mouth is sutured together with absorbable suture. The preapplied miniplates are used to rigidly fix the mandibular osteotomy in an anatomical position. Meticulous reapproximation of the vermilion border is followed by a multilayer closure of the lip. If necessary, drains can be placed and tunneled through a stab incision in the neck. The skin of the neck is closed with nonabsorbable skin stitches. A 5–0 suture is used to close the facial skin.

The Transmandibular-Circumglossal-Retropharyngeal Approach

After the head and neck are draped in a sterile fashion and the intraoral cavity is prepared, a tracheostomy is performed. A skin incision begins just below the tip of the mastoid process and curves beneath the ipsilateral ear. The incision follows a neck crease ~5 cm away from the mandible until the midline is reached. It then proceeds rostrally toward the chin and extends through the lower lip **(Fig. 36–2A).** A skin flap is elevated in a subplatysmal fashion in the upper neck, and the submandibular region is exposed **(Fig. 36–2B).** Care should be taken to avoid injury to the marginal mandibular branch of the facial nerve. The styloid process is palpated and the muscular attachments are separated. The major vessels in the neck, including the common carotid, internal carotid, and external carotid arteries, their branches, and the jugular vein, are exposed and traced superiorly to the skull base. The lingual and hypoglossal nerves are identified and dissected free.

The mandibulotomy is performed as described for the median LMG approach. To avoid the loss of a tooth, a lateral site for a stair-step mandibulotomy can be chosen as an alternative to the midline stair-step mandibulotomy. Performing a stair-step mandibulotomy between the lateral incisor and canine lowers the risk of damaging the roots of the teeth. The roots of the lateral incisor and canines diverge, producing more space to perform an osteotomy between them.

The small needle monopolar cautery is used to incise the ipsilateral side of the floor of the mouth around the base of the tongue. A cuff of tissue is left attached to the mandible for later repair. This incision, which extends circumferentially around the tongue to the anterior tonsillar pillar, allows lateral retraction of the split mandible. During this dissection injury to the lingual nerve should be avoided.

The divided mandible and tongue are retracted. Next, the anterior belly of the gastric muscle and mylohyoid muscle are divided to allow further retraction of the osteotomized mandible. Dividing the external carotid artery distal to the lingual artery allows maximal opening of this corridor, providing access to the parapharyngeal space **(Fig. 36–2C).**

At this point, dissection is tailored to the location of the lesion. If the lesion is primarily located laterally within the infratemporal fossa, the basic approach should be completed. The lesion is usually visualized and can be approached from this territory. If midline access to the clivus and craniocervical junction is needed, the mucosal incision is extended to the hypopharynx, passing lateral to the tonsil and the orifice of the eustachian tube.

The eustachian tube and the levator and tensor veli palatini muscles, which tether the nasopharynx to the skull base, must be divided. Next, the pharynx is dissected off the longus colli muscles and prevertebral fascia to expose the clivus, craniocervical junction, and upper cervical spine. The pharyngeal flap is elevated and rotated medially. If more cranial exposure is needed to reach the sphenoid sinus and pituitary gland, the soft palate must be dissected off the hard palate ~1 cm from the gingival margin. A curved linear incision just crosses the midline anteriorly from the hard palate **(Fig. 36–2D).**

The palatal mucosa is elevated from the hard palate. The greater palatine vessels are cauterized and divided. This palatal flap is retracted contralaterally. Using reciprocating saws, the hard palate can be osteotomized in a circumferential fashion and later replaced with miniplates. Removing the palatal bone exposes the nasal choana.

The lingual nerve is followed cranially to the medial pterygoid muscle on which this nerve lies. Further cranially, the nerve leads to the foramen ovale. The pterygoid plates are removed by dividing the pterygoid muscles, and full exposure of the midline and central skull base to the infratemporal fossa is achieved.

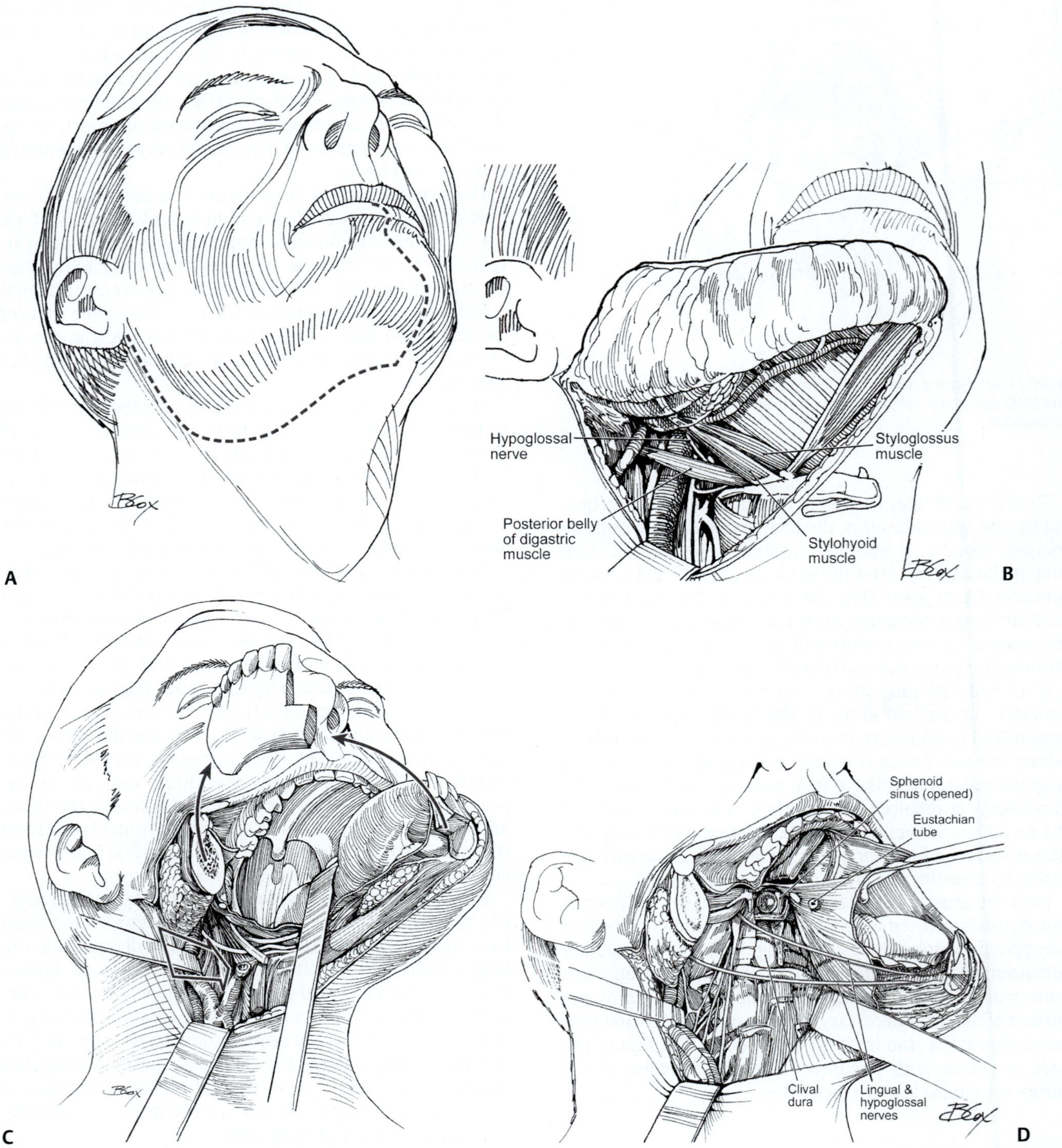

Figure 36–2 **(A)** The skin incision for the transmandibular-circumglossal-retropharyngeal (TCR) approach (dashed line) begins just inferior to the tip of the ipsilateral mastoid process, extends within a neck crease well below the mandible, and reaches the midline of the lower lip. **(B)** The skin flap and platysma are elevated cranially. The submandibular gland is either elevated along the musculocutaneous flap or resected. The styloglossus and stylohyoid muscles, the posterior belly of the digastric muscle, and the hypoglossal nerve are visualized. **(C)** After the stair-step mandibulotomy is completed, dissection proceeds around the base of the tongue ipsilaterally toward the anterior tonsillar pillar. The external carotid artery can be ligated (open arrow) distal to the lingual artery to increase exposure in the surgical corridor. To improve visualization, the ipsilateral mandible (black arrows) is shown completely separated from its proximal origin. **(D)** The palatal mucosa is incised along the ipsilateral gingival margin. The sella, sphenoid sinus, clivus, and upper cervical spine are exposed by retracting the oropharyngeal tube medially to avoid disrupting its mucosal integrity. The posterior nasal cavity can be viewed if its mucosa is opened transorally. (From Barrow Neurological Institute with permission.)

For closure, the pharynx is released from retraction and laid over the prevertebral fascia. The posterolateral mucosal incision is carefully reapproximated. The mucoperiosteal palate incision is reattached to the gingival margin, and the soft palate is reattached with absorbable stitches. A palatal splint that has been fashioned preoperatively is placed to support the palatal mucosa. The floor of the mouth is sutured together with absorbable suture to the tissue cuff, which is medial to the mandible. The mandibulotomy is fixated with the prefitted miniplates and miniscrews. Alternatively, the mandibulotomy can be rigidly fixated first and the oral floor closed thereafter. This strategy eliminates tension on the suture line of the oral floor. The remainder of the skin and lip closure follows that of the LMG approach.

The Bilateral-Sagittal Split Mandibular Osteotomy Approach

The patient's face and oral cavity are prepared and draped in a sterile fashion. This approach is unique because no facial incision is needed. All incisions are within the buccal sulcus. Again, a tracheotomy is placed before surgery to protect the airway. The lower buccal sulcus is infiltrated with local anesthetic and incised with fine-needle monopolar cauterization. The lateral ramus and posterior mandibular body are exposed in a subperiosteal fashion. The lingula of the mandible indicates the medial entry point of the neurovascular bundle that enters on each side of the mandible.

The osteotomy lines are outlined **(Fig. 36–3A–D)**, and miniplates are applied before the osteotomy to ensure correct

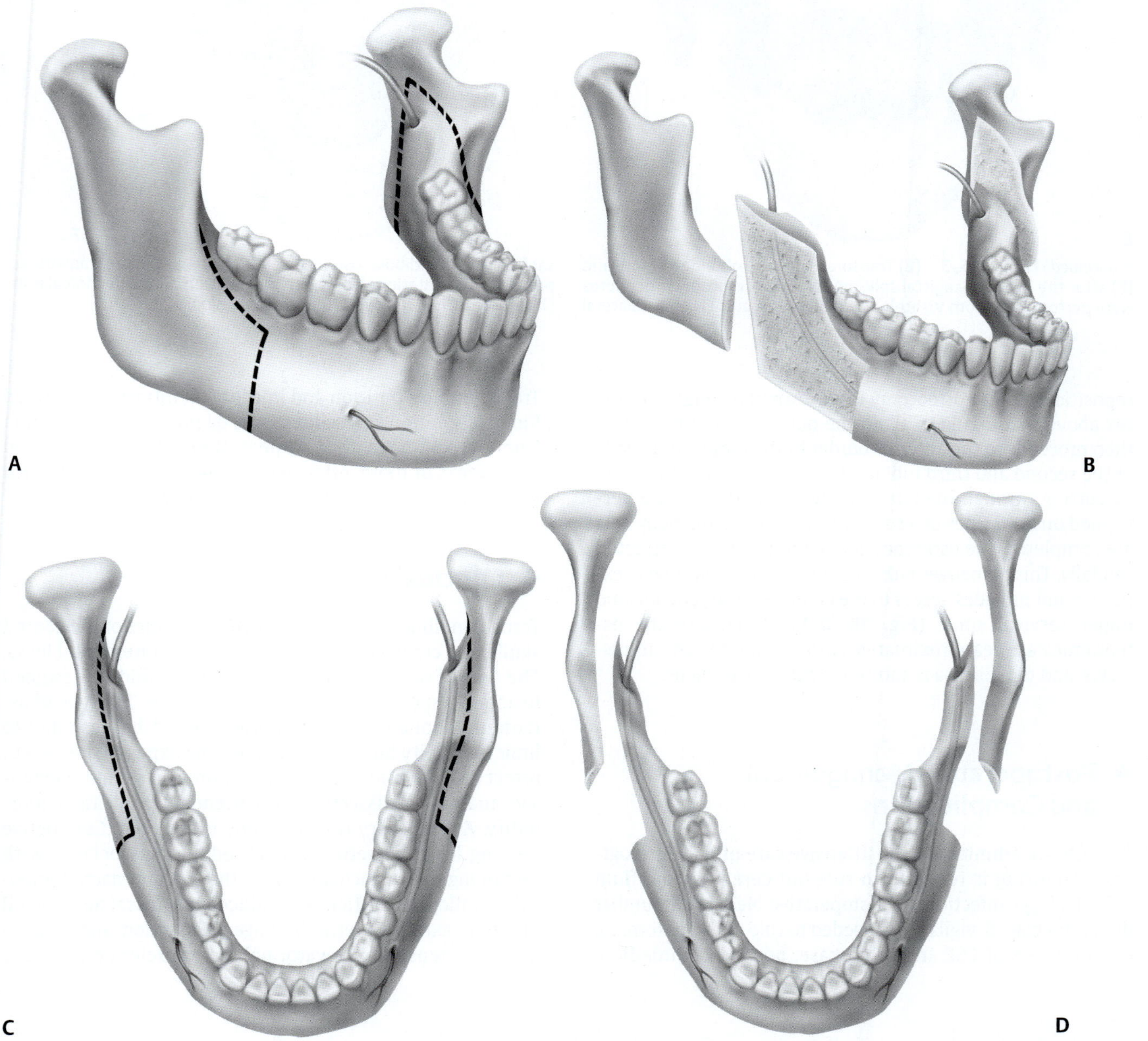

Figure 36–3 Anatomical illustrations of **(A,B)** oblique and **(C,D)** superior views of the mandible **(A,C)** before and **(B,D)** after planned (dashed lines) osteotomies.

(*Continued on page 306*)

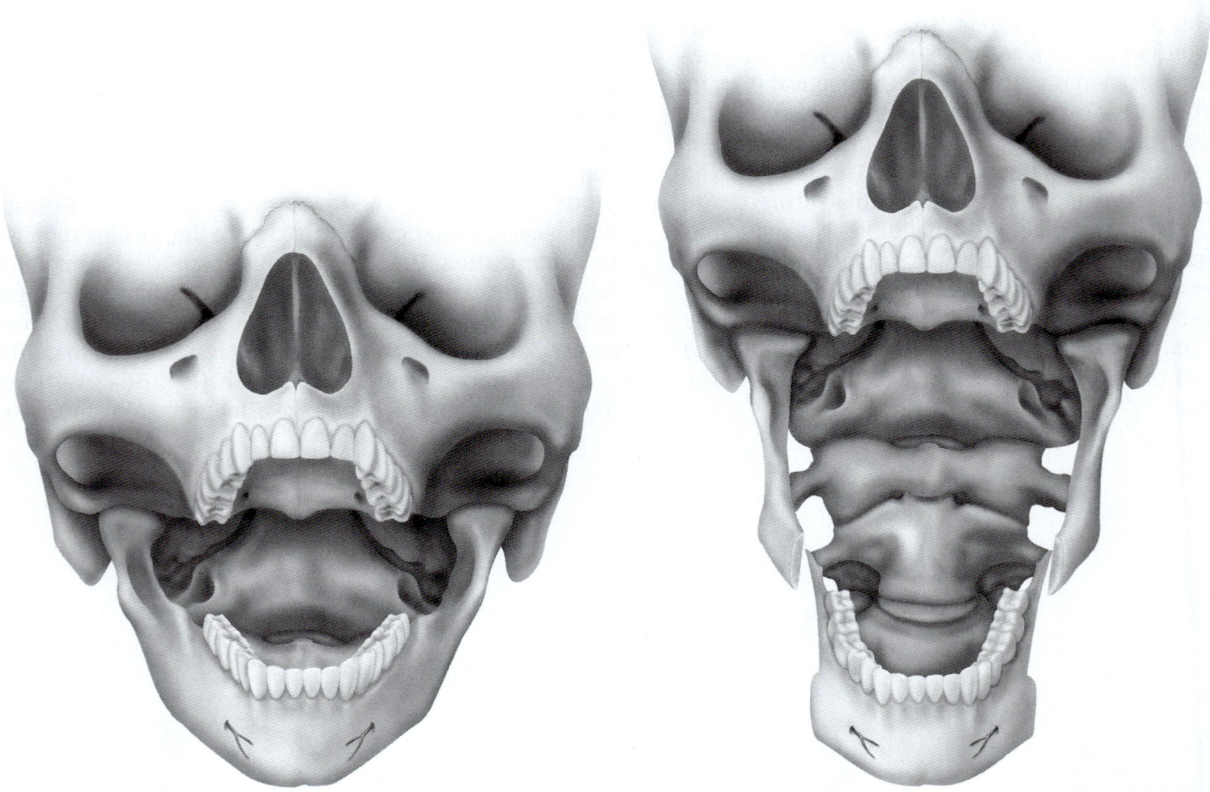

E

F

(*Continued*) **Figure 36–3** **(E)** Transoral exposure obtained before and **(F)** after the bilateral-sagittal split mandibular osteotomy procedures were performed. (From Vishteh AG, Beals SP, Joganic EF, et al. Bilateral sagittal split mandibular osteotomies as an adjunct to the transoral approach to the anterior craniovertebral junction. (From Technical note. J Neurosurg 1999;90:267–270, with permission.)

repositioning. The osteotomy is performed through the cortex above the lingula to avoid the neurovascular bundle. It then proceeds to the anterior border of the ramus to the side of the second and third molars. The osteotomy is completed by cutting through the lateral cortex. Osteotomies are performed on both sides in a similar fashion. After the bony cuts are completed, the osteotomized mandible can be retracted caudally. This maneuver enhances inferior oropharyngeal exposure and provides access to the craniocervical junction and upper cervical spine **(Fig. 36–3E,F).** At closure the osteotomies are reapproximated with miniplates and miniscrews, and the mucosa is sutured in the buccal sulcus.

◆ Postoperative Management and Complications

Patients are admitted to the intensive care unit. Neurological monitoring is required to rule out cerebrospinal fluid (CSF) leakage, infection, or postoperative bleeding. If lumbar drains are placed, vigilance is needed to rule out symptomatic overdrainage of CSF. In such a case, however, immediate Trendelenburg position and injection of intrathecal lactated Ringer's solution can be lifesaving by preventing herniation from overdrainage. Oral alimentation is typically avoided for 2 weeks or more. After swallowing has been determined to be functional, feeding can advance slowly.

◆ Conclusions

Transmandibular approaches enable exposure of the central skull base, craniocervical junction, and infratemporal fossa. The type of transmandibular approach should be designed to access a specific lesion and its extensions. The type of osteotomy applied to the mandible should be designed to limit morbidity but also to enhance the exposure needed to resect a given lesion. All of these approaches require extensive anatomical dissection with attendant predictable morbidity. A temporary tracheostomy is required. Conductive hearing loss and serous otitis media are associated with sectioning the eustachian tube in the TCR approach. Temporary swallowing difficulties induced by glossal and palatal incisions, extensive retropharyngeal dissection, and sectioning of the tensor and levator palatini muscles occasionally necessitate the placement of a gastrostomy tube. Therefore, the advantages of these approaches must be weighed carefully against this potential morbidity.

For extensive lesions involving the midline skull base, especially those with a lateral extension, a wide exposure through a TCR approach is beneficial. Because this approach does not violate the pharynx over the midline, it is particularly useful for lesions with an intradural extension. At closure, the pharynx can resume its anatomical position and buttress the reconstruction of the resection cavity, thus diminishing the risk of CSF leakage when compared with a midline transpharyngeal approach.

When a limited midline exposure of the craniocervical junction is desired and when the opening of the mouth is not wide enough, a BSSMO approach is preferred. No disfiguring facial incisions are required, and intraoral dissection is limited compared with tongue-splitting and retropharyngeal approaches. This approach allows the midline of the mandible to be retracted caudally, thereby enlarging the craniocaudal transoral access to the craniocervical junction. This approach is particularly valuable for patients with rheumatoid arthritis whose mouth opening may be impaired because the temporomandibular joint is involved with the arthritis.

Index

Page numbers followed by *f* or *t* indicate material in figures or tables, respectively.

B

D

E

F

J

N

S

T

U